Schizophrenia

Schizophrenia: from neuroimaging to neuroscience

Edited by

Stephen M. Lawrie
University of Edinburgh Division of Psychiatry,
Royal Edinburgh Hospital, Edinburgh, Scotland, UK

Daniel R. Weinberger
Clinical Brain Disorders Branch, National Institute of Mental Health,
DHHS, Bethesda, Maryland, USA

and

Eve C. Johnstone
University of Edinburgh Division of Psychiatry,
Royal Edinburgh Hospital, Edinburgh, Scotland, UK

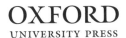

OXFORD
UNIVERSITY PRESS

OXFORD

UNIVERSITY PRESS

Great Clarendon Street, Oxford OX2 6DP

Oxford University Press is a department of the University of Oxford.
It furthers the University's objective of excellence in research, scholarship,
and education by publishing worldwide in

Oxford New York

Auckland Bangkok Buenos Aires Cape Town Chennai
Dar es Salaam Delhi Hong Kong Istanbul Karachi Kolkata
Kuala Lumpur Madrid Melbourne Mexico City Mumbai Nairobi
São Paulo Shanghai Singapore Taipei Tokyo Toronto

Oxford is a registered trade mark of Oxford University Press
in the UK and in certain other countries

Published in the United States
by Oxford University Press Inc., New York

A catalogue record for this title is available from the British Library

Library of Congress Cataloging in Publication Data

Schizophrenia: from neuroimaging to neuroscience/edited by
Stephen M. Lawrie, Daniel R. Weinberger, and Eve C. Johnstone.

Includes bibliographical references and index.
1. Schizophrenia-Imaging. 2. Brain-Imaging. I. Lawrie, Stephen M. II.
Weinberger, Daniel R. (Daniel Roy) III. Johnstone, Eve C.
[DNLM: 1. Schizophrenia-diagnosis. 2. Diagnostic Imaging.
3. Magnetic Resonance Imaging. 4. Schizophrenia-physiopathology.
WM 203 533785 2004]
RC 514.53356 2004 616.89[1] 807548—dc22 2004019166
ISBN 0 19 852596 6 (Hbk: alk paper)

10 9 8 7 6 5 4 3 2 1

Typeset by Newgen Imaging Systems (P) Ltd., Chennai, India
Printed in Great Britain
on acid-free paper by
Biddles Ltd., King's Lynn

Preface

The application of brain imaging techniques to study schizophrenia and other neuropsychiatric disorders, and the complexity of data processing and analysis, is ever increasing. Currently available textbooks on schizophrenia, and those on brain imaging, consider the overlap briefly at most. This book details what structural and functional brain imaging studies have already established about schizophrenia and what developments are likely in the foreseeable future.

The chapters are written by internationally acknowledged experts in the application of a particular research method to schizophrenia and describe the nature of the signal acquired, the main technological problems, the best replicated findings and their specificity, and future possibilities. The book is comprehensively illustrated, and a colour plate section separates the sections on structural and functional imaging approaches. We have endeavored to include sufficient methodological detail to be of value to imaging researchers, while emphasizing a clinical perspective throughout, which should be relevant to clinicians. We hope the readers of this book will appreciate the accessible text (allowing for the occasional mathematical formula) and extensive use of figures and tables.

S.M.L., D.R.W., and E. C. J.

Contents

Contributors

R. Alexander Bantick
The Cyclotron Unit
Clinical Sciences Centre
Imperial College London
The Hammersmith Hospital
London, UK

Mark E. Bastin
Medical and Radiological Sciences
(Medical Physics)
University of Edinburgh
Western General Hospital
Edinburgh, UK

Alessandro Bertolino
Dipartimento di Scienze Neurologiche e
Psichiatriche
Universita' degli Studi di Bari
Bari, Italy
and Department of Radiology
IRCCSS 'Casa Sollievo della Sofferenza'
San Giovanni Rotondo (Foggia)
Italy

Edward T. Bullmore
University of Cambridge
Department of Psychiatry
Brain Mapping Unit
Addenbrooke's Hospital
Cambridge, UK

Tyrone D. Cannon
Department of Psychology
UCLA College of Letters and
  Science
and Departments of Psychiatry and
  Human Genetics
UCLA School of Medicine
Franz Hall
Los Angeles, CA
USA

Nitin Gogtay
Child Psychiatry Branch
National Institute of Mental Health
Bethesda, MD
USA

Paul M. Grasby
The Cyclotron Unit
Clinical Sciences Centre
Imperial College London
The Hammersmith Hospital
London, UK

Andreas Heinz
Department of Psychiatry of the
  Charité
Charité Campus Mitte
Berlin
Germany

Garry D. Honey
University of Cambridge
Department of Psychiatry
Brain Mapping Unit
Addenbrooke's Hospital
Cambridge, UK

Eve C. Johnstone
University of Edinburgh
Division of Psychiatry
Kennedy Tower
Royal Edinburgh Hospital
Morningside Park
Edinburgh, UK

Thomas Koenig
Department of Psychiatric
Neurophysiology
University Hospital of Clinical Psychiatry
Bern
Switzerland

Stephen M. Lawrie
University of Edinburgh
Division of Psychiatry
Kennedy Tower
Royal Edinburgh Hospital
Morningside Park
Edinburgh, UK

Stefano Marenco
Clinical Brain Disorders Branch
National Institute of Mental Health
Intramural Research Program
DHHS
Bethesda, MD
USA

Robert W. McCarley
Boston VA Healthcare System
Clinical Neuroscience Division
Laboratory of Neuroscience
Department of Psychiatry
Harvard Medical School
and McLean Hospital
Brockton, MA
USA

Phillip K. McGuire
Institute of Psychiatry
Division of Psychological Medicine
Section of Neuroimaging
London, UK

Andrew M. McIntosh
University of Edinburgh
Division of Psychiatry
Kennedy Tower
Royal Edinburgh Hospital
Morningside Park
Edinburgh, UK

Andrew J. Montgomery
The Cyclotron Unit
Clinical Sciences Centre
Imperial College London
The Hammersmith Hospital
London, UK

Margaret A. Niznikiewicz
Boston VA Healthcare System
Clinical Neuroscience Division
Laboratory of Neuroscience
Department of Psychiatry
Harvard Medical School
Brockton, MA
USA

David G. C. Owens
University of Edinburgh
Division of Psychiatry
Kennedy Tower
Royal Edinburgh Hospital
Morningside Park
Edinburgh, UK

Judith L. Rapoport
Child Psychiatry Branch
National Institute of
Mental Health
Bethesda, MD
USA

Berenice Romero
Department of Psychiatry of the Charité
Charité Campus Mitte
Berlin
Germany

Timm Rosburg
Department of Epileptology
University of Bonn
Bonn
Germany

Dean F. Salisbury
Boston VA Healthcare System
Clinical Neuroscience Division
Laboratory of Neuroscience
Department of Psychiatry
Harvard Medical School
and Cognitive Neuroscience Laboratory
McLean Hospital
Cambridge, MA
USA

Heinrich Sauer
Department of Psychiatry
Friedrich-Schiller-University Jena
Jena
Germany

Kevin M. Spencer
Boston VA Healthcare System
Clinical Neuroscience Division
Laboratory of Neuroscience
Department of Psychiatry
Harvard Medical School
Brockton, MA
USA

Alexandra Sporn
Child Psychiatry Branch
National Institute of Mental Health
Bethesda, MD
USA

Werner K. Strik
University Hospital of Bern
Clinical Psychiatry
Bern
Switzerland

Paul Thompson
Laboratory of Neuro Imaging
Department of Neurology
Division of Brain Mapping
UCLA School of Medicine
Los Angeles, CA
USA

Arthur W. Toga
Laboratory of Neuro Imaging
Department of Neurology
Division of Brain Mapping
UCLA School of Medicine
Los Angeles, CA
USA

Daniel R. Weinberger
Clinical Brain Disorders Branch
National Institute of Mental Health
Intramural Research Program
DHHS
Bethesda, MD
USA

Abbreviations

ACC	anterior cingulate cortex		DSM	Diagnostic and Statistical Manual of Mental Disorders
AD	Alzheimer's disease			
ADC	apparent diffusion coefficient		DTI	diffusion tensor imaging
ADHD	attention deficit/hyperactivity disorder		DT-MRI	diffusion tensor magnetic resonance imaging
AEF	auditory evoked field		DUP	duration of untreated psychosis
AHC	amygdala–hippocampal complex		DW	diffusion-weighted
AMPT	α-methyl-*para*-tyrosine		DZ	dizygotic
ANIMAL	automatic nonlinear image matching and anatomical labeling		EEG	electroencephalography
			EHRS	Edinburgh High Risk Study
AOS	adult-onset schizophrenia		EPI	echo-planar imaging
BDNF	brain-derived neurotrophic factor		EPS	extrapyramidal side-effects
BFC	bias field corrector		ERP	event related potential
BOLD	blood oxygenation level dependent (signal)		e.s.	effect size
			FA	fractional anisotropy
BP	binding potential		FDG	fluorodeoxyglucose
BPRS	Brief Psychiatric Rating Scale		FEP	first-episode psychosis
cAMP	cyclic adenosine monophosphate		FFTs	Fast Fourier Transforms
CASH	Comprehensive Assessment of Symptoms and History		fMRI	functional magnetic resonance imaging
CAT	computerized axial tomography		FP-CIT	2β-carbomethoxy-3β-(4-iodophenyl)-N-(3-fluoropropyl) nortropane
CBF	cerebral blood flow			
CGAS	Children's Global Assessment Scale			
			FWHM	full-width-at-half-maximum
Cho	choline		GABA	γ-aminobutyric acid
CHRP	Copenhagen High Risk Project		GAF	global assesment of function (scores)
CHRS	Copenhagen High Risk Study		GBR	gamma-band response
β-CIT	2β-carbomethoxy-3β-(4-iodophenyl)tropane		GFS	global field synchronization
			GLM	general linear model
COMT	catechol-*O*-methyl-transferase		GPI	general paralysis of the insane
COS	childhood-onset schizophrenia		HIV	human immunodeficiency virus
CPT	Continuous Performance Task		HMPAO	Hexa-Methyl Propylene Amine Oxime
Cre	creatine			
CSF	cerebrospinal fluid		^{1}H-MRS	proton magnetic resonance spectroscopy
CT	computed tomography			
DA	dopamine		HRF	haemodynamic response function
DAAO	D-amino acid oxidase		HVA	Homovanillic acid
DBM	deformation-based morphometry		IBZM	iodobenzamide
DLPFC	dorsolateral prefrontal cortex		ICBM	International Consortium for Brain Mapping
DRD$_2$	D$_2$ receptor			

ICD	International Classification of Disease	PD	proton density or Parkinson's disease
ICV	intracranial volume	PET	positron emission tomography
IMP	iodoamphetamine	PFC	prefrontal cortex
INSECT	intensity normalized stereotaxic environment for classification of tissue	PGSE	pulsed gradient spin-echo
		PM	post-mortem
		ppm	parts per million
ISI	inter-stimulus interval	PSE	Present State Examination
LFPs	local field potentials	QEEG	quantified electroencephalography
LORETA	low-resolution electromagnetic tomography	QMEG	quantified magnetoencephalography
		QNB	(R,S)-3-quinuclidinyl-4-iodobenzilate
LV	lateral ventricle		
MANCOVA	multivariate analysis of covariance	rCBF	regional cerebral blood flow
		RF	radiofrequency
MDI	multi dimensionally impaired	r.m.s.	root mean squared
MEG	magnetoencephalography	ROI	region of interest
MHPG	3-methoxy-4-hydroxy phenol glycol	SCID	structured clinical interview for DSM-IV
MHRS	Melbourne High Risk Study	SE-EPI	spin-echo echo-planar imaging
MMN	mismatch negativity	SENSE	sensitivity encoding
MMSE	mini-mental state exam	SMA	supplementary motor area
MNI	Montreal Neurological Institute	sMRI	structural magnetic resonance imaging
MPRAGE	magnetization-prepared gradient-echo sequences		
		SNR	signal-to-noise ratio
MR	magnetic resonance	SOAs	stimulus–onset asynchronies
MRI	magnetic resonance imaging	SPD	schizotypal personality disorder
MRS	magnetic resonance spectroscopy	SPECT	single-photon emission computed tomography
MT-MRI	magnetization transfer magnetic resonance imaging		
		SPM	statistical parametric mapping
MZ	monozygotic	SSR	steady state response
N3	non-parametric non-uniform intensity normalization	SSRI	selective serotonin reuptake inhibitors
NAA	N-acetyl-aspartate	STG	superior temporal gyrus
NAAG	N-acetyl-aspartylglutamate	TAC	time activity curve
NAALADase	N-acetylated-α-linked-amino dipeptidase	TBM	transcranial magnetic stimulation
		TE	echo time
NIMH	National Institute of Mental Health	TMS	transcranial magnetic stimulation
NMDA	N-methyl-D-aspartate	TR	repeat time
NMR	nuclear magnetic resonance	UHR	ultra high risk
NOS	not otherwise specified	3V	third ventricle
NRG1	neuroregulin 1	VBM	voxel-based morphometry
NSS	neurological soft signs	VBR	ventricular brain ratio
OC	obstetric complication	VCFS	velo-cardio-facial syndrome
ODD	Oppositional defiant disorder	V_D	volume of distribution
PANSS	positive and negative syndrome scale	WCST	Wisconsin Card Sorting Test
pCPA	p-chlorophenylalanine		

Chapter 1

Early studies of brain anatomy in schizophrenia

Eve C. Johnstone and David G. C. Owens

Introduction

Emil Kraepelin (1856–1927) is generally considered to have defined the disease concept that came to be known as schizophrenia. In defining dementia praecox, he drew together hebephrenia, as described by Hecker (1871), catatonia, as described by Kahlbaum (1874), and his own dementia paranoides, as he regarded them all as manifestations of the same disorder, which typically had its onset in early adult life and had a poor outcome (Kraepelin 1896). Kraepelin was working shortly after the first academic department of psychiatry in Europe had been sent up in Berlin in 1865, the first Chair being held by Wilhelm Griesinger, whose statement 'mental illness is a somatic illness of the brain' (Griesinger 1861) is often quoted. Investigations relating neuropathology to mental disorder were conducted in his department. In the late nineteenth century, there was considerable success in this area (e.g. Wernicke 1881; Alzheimer 1907), although in relation to dementing illnesses rather than schizophrenia. Although Kraepelin defined dementia praecox on the basis of the characteristic course and outcome of a cluster of symptoms and signs, he stated that this was a disorder of which, if 'every detail' were known, a specific anatomical pathology with a specific aetiology would be found. Kraepelin considered that he was defining a clinical syndrome which represented a disease of the brain, the nature of which would be eventually revealed by appropriate investigations. In his book *Dementia praecox and paraphrenia* (Kraepelin 1919), he included a chapter on morbid anatomy and wrote:

> The morbid anatomy of dementia praecox does not show microscopically any striking changes of the cranial contents . . . On the other hand, it has been shown that in the cortex we have to do with severe and widespread disease of the nerve tissue. Alzheimer has described deep spreading changes in the cortical cells, especially in the deep layers; the nuclei are very much swollen, the nuclear membrane greatly wrinkled, the body of the cell considerably shrunk with a tendency to degeneration . . . Nissl invariably saw widespread cellular disease.

Many early investigators of dementia praecox/schizophrenia sought to examine the anatomy of the nervous system and initially neuropathology was the only tool available to them. Pneumoencephalography was introduced in 1919, and in the 1970s both echoencephalography and computed tomography (CT) were used to study the brain.

There have been relatively few echoencephalographic studies as this technique was known to have the possibility of producing unclear results. There was an extensive literature using CT, but since the 1980s this has been superseded by magnetic resonance imaging (MRI). This chapter will cover neuropathological, pneumoencephalographic, echoencephalographic and computed tomography studies up until the early 1980s, when MRI entered general use for visualization of the brain.

Early pathological studies

The first work in this area concerned coarse brain structure, and a number of studies were conducted up until the 1960s. This work has been reviewed by Brown *et al.* (1986) and is summarized in Table 1.1.

There is something of a tendency for the schizophrenic subjects to have lower brain weights, but, clearly, in a number of the studies there are problems concerning the use of control subjects with dementing conditions. Age differences were not always dealt with. Gross appearances were also the subject of studies by Meynert (1884) and Rawlings (1920), both of whom described an appearance of atrophy of the frontal lobes. Histological studies were carried out from the late nineteenth century, and reports of histological abnormalities in the brains of patients with schizophrenia were presented by Alzheimer (Alzheimer 1897, 1913), Wernicke (1900), and Klippel and Lhermitte (1909). They describe changes such as 'lacunae, pyknotic neuronal atrophy, focal demyelination and metachromatic bodies', but there was little consistency among these reports. In 1924, Dunlap conducted a careful comparison of the brains of eight schizophrenic patients who had died at less than 45 years of age and five controls, selected in each case for a cause of death which was not likely to have influenced the structures of the brain. Independent observers conducted cell counts in layers II, III and IV of the frontal cortex. Diverse cellular changes, similar to those described by previous researchers of dementia praecox, were found in both schizophrenic and control brains, and there were no differences between patients and controls. This cast a shadow of scepticism over the histopathological literature on schizophrenia and, although histological work did continue (e.g. Vogt and Vogt 1948), it was generally considered that the positive results reported by early workers reflected the fact that this work was done when histological techniques were in their infancy, and when the need for controlling fixation and staining was not appreciated. Such views may be found in the reviews of David (1957), Dastur (1959), and Corsellis (1976), who stated 'that present histological methods are not adequate to demonstrate any convincing substrate for the subtle and often reversible mental aberrations that go to make up the "functional psychoses"'. Nevertheless, some work did continue, and consideration of the accessible studies between the work of Dunlap in 1924 and the early 1980s does show abnormality, with a degree of consistency in the findings. A number of these studies show gliosis and, in the more recent work, changes in the orientation of cells have been found (see Table 1.2).

Table 1.1 Studies of brain weight in functional psychosis

Study	Patients with schizophrenia [number]	Comparison group [number]	Result	Difference in weight between schizophrenic and control group (g)
Crichton-Browne (1879)	Pre-Kraepelinian diagnoses classified by Brown et al. (1986) as analogous to schizophrenia [63]	Classified by Brown et al. (1986) as analogous to:		
		Affective disorder [58]	Schizophrenic lower	69
		Date onset insanity [32]	Schizophrenic lower	77
		Dementia [234]	Demented lower	16
		Subnormal [9]	Subnormal lower	107
Mittenzweig (1905)	Functional psychotics [185]	Norms of Marchand	Functional psychotic lower	50
Southard (1910)	Dementia praecox [55]	Norms of Vierodt (1906)	Schizophrenic lower	19
Scharpff (1912)	Functional psychotics [101]	Norms of Marchand	Functional psychotic lower	34
Kure and Shimoda (1923)	Dementia praecox [106]	Combined norms of three workers—Taguchi, Hasa, and Kurikawa [referring to >1000 cases]	Schizophrenic lower	63
Lewis (1923)	Dementia praecox [95]	Norms of Vierordt (1906)	Schizophrenic lower	87
	Dementia praecox [95]	*GPI [50]	GPI lower	17
	Dementia praecox [95]	Arteriosclerotic dementia [60]	Schizophrenic lower	16
	Dementia praecox [95]	Senile dementia [75]	Schizophrenic lower	21
Broser (1949)	Schizophrenia with defect state [219]	Norms for Roessle and Roulet (1932)	No difference	1
Tatetsu (1964)	Schizophrenia [41]	Organic brain disease and others [55]	Schizophrenia heavier	58
Wildi et al. (1967)	Drug-free schizophrenia [51]	Various organic diseases [542]	Schizophrenia heavier	64

* GPI = General Paralysis of the Insane - a form of tertiary syphilis

Table 1.2 Accessible controlled histopathological studies in schizophrenic versus control brains until 1982

Study	Numbers of schizophrenics and control brains	Main findings schizophrenics versus controls
Dunlap (1924)	8 schizophrenics versus 5 controls	No differences in cell counts in cerebral cortex
Tatetsu (1964)	41 schizophrenics versus 55 controls	Apical dendritic thickening: cellular and nuclear enlargement in schizophrenics as compare with controls
Nieto and Escobar (1972)	10 schizophrenics versus 3 controls	Diffuse gliosis of reticular formation, hypothalamus, and periventricular grey matter in schizophrenics compared to controls
Fisman (1975)	10 schizophrenics versus 10 controls	Glial knots and perivascular infiltration in region of Vth nerve nucleus in schizophrenics
Dom (1976)	5 schizophrenics versus 8 controls	Diameter of microneurons reduced in striatum in schizophrenics versus controls. Loss of golgi type II neurons in pulvinar in catatonic schizophrenia
Averbach (1981a,b)	12 schizophrenics and 27 controls	Degeneration with lipid–pigment accumulation in cells of ansa pedunculans of substantia innominata of schizophrenics
Hankoff and Peress (1981)	8 schizophrenics versus 19 controls	No glial proliferation in brainstem of schizophrenics
Scheibel and Kovelman (1981)	8 schizophrenics versus 8 controls	Disorientation of hippocampal pyramidal cells and their dendrites in schizophrenics
Stevens (1982)	25 schizophrenics versus 48 controls	Fibrillary gliosis of periventricular structures, including hypothalamus, midbrain tegmentum and substantia innominata in schizophrenics versus controls

The issue of the presence of gliosis has been of considerable recent interest. Although there is gliosis in the brains of schizophrenic patients, there does not appear to be a pathological increase in these brains (Roberts *et al.* 1987; Bruton *et al.*1990). This relative lack of gliosis has been used to support the currently popular view that schizophrenia is a disorder of neurodevelopment.

Pneumoencephalography

The American neurosurgeon Dandy introduced pneumoencephalography in 1919. The technique was applied to the search for disordered anatomy of the brain in schizophrenia a few years later. An example is shown in Fig. 1.1. Jacobi and Winkler (1927) described a high prevalence of cortical and subcortical abnormality in schizophrenic patients. These initial studies stimulated a number of investigations, especially in Germany and Japan, and the more accessible works in this area are summarized in Table 1.3.

In general, most of this literature supports Jacobi and Winkler's view that signs of cerebral atrophy occur in long-standing 'chronic' schizophrenia. However, pneumoencephalography was associated with both methodological and technical problems.

Methodological problems

A number of studies were performed before standardized measures had been described in the evaluation of pneumoencephalography, and reports were based on visual assessments. The work of Storey (1966) has shown that inter-rater reliability is poorer with this method than with linear measures. The problem was confounded by the fact that most assessments were not made blind to the subjects' diagnosis for the purposes of the study. In view of the considerable morbidity and small but definite mortality

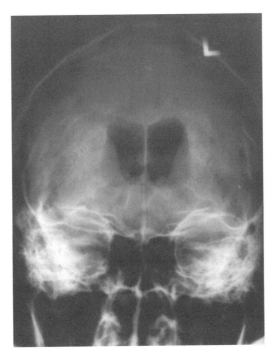

Fig. 1.1 A pneumoencephalogram demonstrating 'dilated' lateral ventricles (kindly provided by Professor Jonathan Best).

Table 1.3 Selected pneumoencephalographic studies in schizophrenia

Study	Number of schizophrenics	Ventricular abnormality	Age	Exchange site	Air inserted (CCs)
Jacobi and Winkler (1927)	19	18 (94.7%)	18–49	Suboccipital	60–145
Moore et al. (1933)	60	25 (41.7%)	17–47	Lumbar	115–235
Lemke (1936)	100	50 (50%)	18–62	Suboccipital	50–60
Donovan et al. (1949)	19	16 (84.2%)	16–60	?	?
Nobile and Brizzi (1953)	43	8 (18.6%)	?	?	50–70
Froshaug and Retterstol (1956)	24	4 (16.7%)	38–55	Lumbar	20–30
Borenstein et al. (1957)	134	118 (88%)	17–60	Lumbar	35–40
Huber (1957)	190	131 (69%)	2nd–6th decade	Lumbar	
Nagy (1959)	226	83 (36.7%)	2nd–7th decade	Suboccipital	50
Bratfos and Sagedal (1960)	40	17 (43%)	?	?	?
Sitnikov (1961)	50	40 (80%)	?	?	?
Haug (1962)	137	66 (49%)	19–59	Lumbar	30
Ansink et al. (1963)	41	10 (24.4%)	21–69	Suboccipital	10
Nagy (1963)	260	152 (58.4%)	Mean 36.1	Suboccipital	50–80
Storey (1966)	18	3 (16.7%)	19–45	Lumbar	40
Asano (1967)	53	34 (64.2%)	Mean 28.9	?	100
Siegel and Heidrich (1970)	350	290 (82.9%)	15–53	Lumbar	60–100
Young and Crampton (1974)	36	24 (66%)	?	?	?
Haug (1982)	38	3 (7.9%)	17–36	Lumbar	30
Total	1838	1092			
Average % abnormality		59.4%			

Frequency of abnormality with lumbar method (n = 951) = 67.3%.
Frequency of abnormality with suboccipital method (n = 646) = 48.5%.

associated with pneumoencephalography (Whittier 1951), the American Roentgen Ray Society decreed in 1929 that it was not appropriate to use normal subjects for control purposes in pneumoencephalography. Many studies in schizophrenia bypassed this difficulty by not including any comparison material at all, while others utilized routine encephalograms performed to exclude potential neurological abnormality but reported as normal, but of course, as Lonnum (1966) has pointed out, 'normal encephalograms are not common in patient populations when strict criteria of normality are applied'. The problem of normal controls was effectively insuperable, but some authors minimized this difficulty by using standardized techniques with blind assessments in samples of different psychiatric diagnoses or in schizophrenics of different clinical types.

Technical problems

Pneumoencephalography is a complex invasive procedure. Most studies did not report their technique, but those that did show substantial variation. Sources of variation include the amount of cerebrospinal fluid (CSF) removed, the amount of air introduced, the site of introduction of the air, the time from introduction of the air to exposure of the film, the position of the head, unequal filling of ventricles, and film focus difference. Volumes of air introduced varied greatly between studies, from Moore and co-workers, who drained the entire cerebrospinal space and introduced an equivalent volume of air (Moore *et al.* 1933, 1935), to Hunter *et al.* (1968), who used a modified technique involving the introduction of only 8 ml of air. While some authors used a volume-for-volume exchange, others introduced a greater quantity of air than CSF withdrawn. The importance of such variation lies in the putative 'ballooning' effect of air on the ventricular system, namely that an introduced gas, especially air at room temperature, inflates the ventricular system, an effect more marked as body temperature expands the gas (Probst 1973). The more gas introduced, or the less room for it to expand, the greater the possible distortion of the ventricles. It has also been suggested that the possibility of this effect is greatest in the third ventricle, especially with the lumbar as opposed to the intracisternal site of exchange. Thus, studies that did not introduce a fixed and smaller amount of air in each subject, at a constant site, present possible sources of variation.

Although it is assumed that most films were taken immediately after the exchange, this may not have been the case. With larger volumes of air, films were sometimes reported at 24 h, especially if ventricular filling was initially unsatisfactory. It has been demonstrated that up to 49% of patients show an absolute increase in ventricular size in 24 h, as opposed to immediate films (Lemay 1967). This is thought to result from resolution of the periventricular oedema-genic effect of an irritant exogenous substance. It is most marked with air (all studies on schizophrenics used air) and less so with oxygen as the exchange gas, and significantly, it is seen most in those with degenerative brain disorders (Lemay 1967). As the worst schizophrenics may be those in whom, by lack of co-operation, satisfactory films are least possible initially and repeats more likely, this could bias findings in favour of apparent dilatation in these subjects. Thus the timing of film exposure may well be important.

These points illustrate the complex dynamic of pneumoencephalography. The fact that most studies were of inadequate design and execution to meet most modern standards is a major bar to acceptance of their findings; it does not, however, justify their being completely disregarded.

The most carefully executed and important studies are probably those of Huber (1957), Haug (1962), Nagy (1963), Storey (1966), and Asano (1967), and these are reviewed briefly. In a series of articles from 1953, culminating in his 1957 monograph, Huber described his pneumoencephalographic work on as total of 195 unselected schizophrenic patients (Huber 1953, 1955, 1957). In addition, he studied 16 atypical schizophrenics and 11 cyclothymics. Most of his subjects were under 50 years of age and he covered all clinical subtypes. He found pathological changes based on standard linear measures in 68.7% of the schizophrenics, especially in the internal liquor spaces, with the third ventricle system most affected. The results could not be attributed to somatic treatment. Huber himself did not conduct a formal statistical evaluation of his data but this was subsequently undertaken by Vogel and Lange (1966). Although Huber's patients were young, statistical analysis revealed an increasing prevalence of abnormality with age, especially in sulcal assessments. However, the abnormalities could not be attributed to age alone. Significant relationships were demonstrated between length of illness and increasing prevalence of severe deficit and, most importantly, between all assessments of ventricular abnormality and increasing severity of deficits, even when the effects of age were removed. Huber subsequently repeated the encephalograms in 27 patients, 19 of whom showed no clinical progression in the degree of their personality deterioration. The radiological appearances of these 19 were unchanged, whereas the eight whose clinical deterioration had progressed all exhibited progression in the pneumoencephalographic abnormalities. However striking his findings, Huber was aware that they appeared qualitatively (at least) non-specific, as he found them in his 'atypical' and 'cyclothymic' groups, although with much lesser frequency.

The work of Haug (1962) is impressive because of his considerable attention to detail and the relative objectivity of his methodology. He assessed the results of pneumoencephalograms in 278 chronic psychiatric in-patients of mixed diagnoses. He accepted that this represented a biased sample, but by using inter-group comparisons his work provided noteworthy findings. Standardized radiological techniques for performing and measuring encephalograms were adhered to, the radiologist being unaware of the psychiatric status. Liberal limits of normality were adopted to minimize inclusion of 'big normal variants' in the pathological groups. Each of the conventional schizophrenic subtypes (except simplex) was represented and a subjective evaluation 'of the presence or absence of dementia' was made. Haug found abnormalities in 84 (61%) of his

137 chronic schizophrenics. These abnormalities predominantly involved the ventricular system, cortical atrophy, when present, being mild and localized. All subtypes were equally affected. There was a highly significant relationship between severe clinical deterioration and definite ventricular dilatation, but no such relationship with cortical changes. The overall prevalence of similar changes in his known organic group was also high, although two-thirds of this category comprised patients diagnosed as having 'reactive psychoses'. None the less, the prevalence of third ventricular and right sella media abnormality was significantly greater in the schizophrenics. In repeat investigations, Haug noted a pathological progression paralleling the clinical one.

The study of Nagy is of interest because of its size. The methodology is less rigorous than that of either Huber or Haug. Nagy (1963) examined pneumoencephalograms from 260 schizophrenic and 133 manic depressive patients, all of whom were female. Of the schizophrenics, 50% had enlarged ventricular indices, while the comparable figure for the manic depressives was 23%. There was a correlation between ventricular enlargement and both impaired social competence and chronicity of course.

Asano (1967) studied 53 young schizophrenics of mean age 28.9 years using a fixed procedure. This included area in addition to linear measures. He found an overall prevalence of abnormality of 64.2% and there was an association with deterioration of function. The ventricular system exhibited abnormalities more frequently than the cortex. Both the third and lateral ventricles showed aberrations with equal frequency.

These authors all show considerable concordance and provide strong evidence that structural brain changes, especially in the form of ventricular dilatation and distortion, may be an integral part of the schizophrenic process. They also suggest that signs of cerebral atrophy may relate to the personality deterioration of the schizophrenic defect. However, Storey (1966), in a small but careful study, could not confirm these findings. He examined the encephalographic data from 18 chronic schizophrenics under 45 years of age. These films were compared with those in age-matched groups selected from the pneumoencephalograms reported as normal in the routine work of the radiology department. Measurements were linear and performed blind by two neuroradiologists. Storey found no difference between patients and controls in the prevalence of abnormality, and no association between pneumoencephalographic variants in age, duration or severity of illness or past somatic treatments. However, this study is marred by the random selection of control pneumoencephalograms, which was not influenced by the provisional diagnosis on which referral for radiological investigations was based. Controls, therefore, had been investigated for conditions such as epilepsy and, as a group, were likely to have had a greater frequency of atrophic change in a normal population.

This literature, although flawed, and concerned with a technique which is now obsolete, remains worthy of attention. Its conclusions are not unanimous but there is a striking degree of consistency in the better studies, and perhaps the most surprising thing about this work, done at a time when there was little to support the implied pathological process underlying schizophrenia apart from articles of faith, was that it gained so little attention. This selective inattention probably has lessons for us still, and surely, as Bliss (1975) has written, 'it may be that these studies are in error, but they cannot be ignored'.

Echoencephalography

Echoencephalography involves transmitting ultrasonic frequencies through the skull and recording echoes, the pattern of which reflects the position of midline structures such as the third ventricle. There have been relatively few studies of schizophrenic patients using echoencephalography, because it is a technique that was rapidly superseded by CT. Ventricular echoes are often unclear and may be affected by factors such as skull thickness. However, the two principal existing studies do provide findings which are reasonably consistent with the results derived using other, less problematic techniques. Holden et al. (1973), examining 79 in-patients with chronic schizophrenia and 79 normal volunteers matched for age and gender, assessed the width of the third ventricle and found that, although there was no overall difference between these groups, within the schizophrenic group, patients with ventricular widening were significantly less likely to respond to antipsychotic medication. In 1976, Daum et al., studying 100 consecutive admissions of various diagnoses to an acute ward, found that third ventricular width was a significant predictor of length of hospital stay, irrespective of diagnosis.

Computer assisted tomography

The method necessary to take imaging in psychiatric disorders forward was provided in 1973 when Godfrey Hounsfield, working for Electrical and Musical Industries (EMI) in London, demonstrated for the first time his technique of computerized axial tomography (CAT). This was the first technique that could safely and non-invasively visualize internal body structures, including soft tissues, without the need for injecting contrast media. Because it was sensitive and had minimal requirements for co-operation by the patient, it was ideal for intra-cranial imaging, especially in psychiatric patients. CAT soon came to mean computer assisted tomography. The procedure involves an X-ray source that rotates in a specified plane around the circumference of a thin cross-section of the head. As the source rotates, voltages are computed for X-ray paths traversing the brain from various angles. The voltage readings are mathematically reconstructed into an image that represents the distribution of densities within that tissue slice. Because the procedure is non-invasive, it allows normal controls to be compared with patients, and the range of appearances in normal subjects to be related to variables such as age (e.g. Barron et al. 1976). The first CT scan in schizophrenia (Johnstone et al. 1976) found the lateral ventricular area to be increased ($P < 0.01$) in a group of chronically institutionalized schizophrenic patients in comparison to an age-matched group of normal controls. A substantial number of studies of CT scans in schizophrenic patients were published in the following years, and accessible early studies are shown in Table 1.4.

Table 1.4 Findings from computed tomography (CT) studies in schizophrenic patients

Study	Sample	Findings
Johnstone et al. (1976)	17 chronic schizophrenics; 8 normal controls	Larger cerebral ventricles in schizophrenics than in controls ($P < 0.01$)
Trimble and Kingsley (1978)	11 schizophrenic patients	7 with early or questionable ventricular enlargement
Campbell et al. (1979)	35 schizophrenic outpatients	6 had 'cortical atrophy'; one patient had ventricular enlargement
Famuyiwa et al. (1979)	45 chronic schizophrenics	31 had abnormal scans
Heath et al. (1979)	85 schizophrenic patients	34 had vermian atrophy
Rieder et al. (1979)	17 schizophrenic outpatients	4 with cortical atrophy
Weinberger et al. (1979a)	58 chronic schizophrenics; 56 normal controls	Ventricles in patients larger than in controls ($P < 0.0001$)
Weinberger et al. (1979b)	60 chronic schizophrenics; 62 normal controls	Wider cortical sulci in patients than in controls (P < 0.05)
Weinberger et al. (1979c)	75 psychiatric patients; 60 chronic schizophrenics	10 schizophrenic patients with atrophy of the anterior cerebellar vermis
Golden et al. (1980a)	42 chronic schizophrenics	60% exceeded normal ventricular size drawn from the literature
Golden et al. (1980b)	24 chronic schizophrenics; 22 'normal' controls	Reduced CAT numbers in several brain regions in the schizophrenics
Owens et al. (1980)	110 in-patients with chronic schizophrenia; 18 non-institutionalized patients with established schizophrenia; 8 patients with first schizophrenic episodes; 10 long-stay in-patients with affective psychoses; 22 non-institutionalized patients with established affective psychoses; 19 outpatients with neurotic disorders	Age significantly correlated with lateral ventricular size, but institutionalized schizophrenics had larger lateral ventricles than neurotics when age was taken into account. Ventricular enlargement was unrelated to past antipsychotics, insulinoma therapy or ECT. Within the institutionalized schizophrenics, ventricular enlargement was significantly associated with impaired social behaviour and the presence of abnormal involuntary movements
Naeser et al. (1981)	17 chronic schizophrenics	Reversed occipital asymmetry three times more frequent than normal
Luchins et al. (1982)	66 right-handed chronic schizophrenics; 100 neurological controls	Patients without atrophy had increased reversals of the usual asymmetry of the frontal and occipital lobes

CAT, computerized axial tomography; ECT, electroconvulsive therapy.

The first demonstration by CT of differences between schizophrenic patients and normal controls, in terms of brain structure (Johnstone *et al.* 1976), met with a mixed and sometimes sceptical response (Jellinek 1976; Marsden 1976), but was soon replicated (Weinberger *et al.* 1979*a*) and the great majority of the studies conducted since that time, as reviewed by Lewis (1990), have confirmed the finding of lateral ventricular enlargement, although there have been some negative studies, for example Jernigan *et al.* (1982*a*, *b*) and Lacano *et al.* (1988). The main assessments used in CT studies were the area measurements of ventricles in relation to the brain-the ventricular brain ratio (VBR). This was the measure that gained the widest acceptance in the psychiatric literature (Weinberger *et al.* 1983). Linear measures were used in some studies, but these correlated relatively poorly with calculated ventricular volumes (Penn *et al.* 1978). The use of attenuation numbers would seem to be a more direct measure than VBR, but their reliability proved to be uncertain (Levi *et al.* 1982). Lateral ventricular size was the measure most commonly studied, but the studies of Weinberger *et al.* (1979*b*) and Tanaka *et al.* (1981) demonstrated 'atrophy' of the cortex, Weinberger *et al.* (1979*c*) also demonstrated cerebral atrophy. In those studies where clinical correlates were sought, it appeared that lateral ventricular enlargement tended to be associated with neuropsychological impairment (Johnstone *et al.* 1978; Donnelly *et al.* 1980), negative rather than positive schizophrenic features (Takahashi *et al.* 1981; Andreasen and Olsen 1982), poor pre-morbid adjustment and relatively poor response to treatment (Weinberger *et al.* 1983), and behavioural deterioration and the presence of spontaneous involuntary movements (Owens *et al.* 1985).

The possibility that the findings could have been due to the effects of treatment was raised early on, but this was discounted by the work of Owens *et al.* (1985), where 112 schizophrenic in-patients were selected from a total sample of 510 individuals conforming to strict diagnostic criteria for schizophrenia. Within this population, it was possible to compare groups of patients who matched in terms of age, sex and measures of severity of illness, who had and had not been heavily treated with specific treatment modalities, e.g. antipsychotic drugs, electroconvulsive therapy (ECT), insulin coma. It was demonstrated in this study that treatment effects could not account for the increased ventricular size shown.

At the time when CT studies of schizophrenia were being conducted, the idea that this condition is a disorder of the brain was not accepted in the way that it is now. The early studies sought to demonstrate that the anatomical differences from controls could be demonstrated reliably and that these were not due to some confounding effect, such as treatment or intercurrent disease. Once these matters had been established, the motivation was generally to establish matters such as the clinical correlates and the timing of changes, with a view to increasing understanding of the nature of the disorder and of its pathological basis. As far as schizophrenia was concerned, CT was a research tool and was not used in clinical practice, either as a diagnostic instrument or as a guide to treatment or prognosis. However, it did have some clinical

utility, as the early studies showed that it could be used to demonstrate unsuspected organic pathology in a small number of people with chronic schizophrenia
(Owens *et al.* 1980).

CT was a great improvement over pneumoencephalography. Initially, pictures were
very imprecise, but resolution improved greatly within a very few years. None the less,
the technique did not allow for a distinction between grey and white matter, so that there
was no possibility of localizing underlying pathology (see, for example, Fig. 1.2). The
procedure also involved exposure to ionizing radiation and there were continuing concerns about the safety of repeated examinations. The technology only permitted an
inference about abnormalities of volume obtained from changes in the area measures of
the lateral ventricular system at its largest. At the time when CT was used in psychiatric
research, the technology did not exist for simultaneous imaging of contiguous slices that
were thin enough (i.e. 1-2 mm) to allow construction of 'near life' volumetric models.

Standardization procedures for repeat scans were imperfect and the issue of whether
or not ventricular enlargement progressed was never satisfactorily resolved with this
technique. The facts that significant ventricular enlargement was shown to be present in
young, first-episode schizophrenic patients (Turner *et al.* 1986) and that a lack of association between duration of illness and ventricular enlargement on CT was repeatedly
shown (Lewis 1990) certainly provide indirect evidence against progression. Most of the
direct evidence that became available from follow-up studies of patients who were
rescanned reported no change in ventricular size (Nasrallah *et al.* 1986; Illowsky *et al.*
1988; Reveley *et al.* 1988), but Kemali *et al.* (1989) found a significant enlargement from
baseline ventricular measures in re-scanned schizophrenic patients versus normal
controls.

In 1984, the first magnetic resonance imaging (MRI) scan study in schizophrenia was
published (Smith *et al.* 1984). MRI was initially referred to as nuclear magnetic

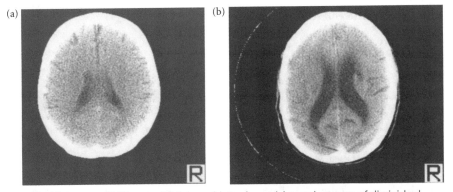

Fig. 1.2 (a) A 'normal' CT scan. (b) Enlarged lateral ventricles and an area of diminished
attenuation on the lateral margin of the right body anteriorly, compatible with infarction, in a
patient with schizophrenia (note also the 'streaking' artefact due to patient motion).

resonance (NMR). This term was used in 1946 by the groups of Bloch and of Purcell to describe the phenomenon whereby the nuclei of certain atoms, when placed in a magnetic field, can be made to absorb or emit radiation. The application of this technique to humans, with the ability to reconstruct the data to create an image, was later developed, with pioneering work being conducted by Mansfield and Maudsley (1977), Lauterbur (1979) and Mallard *et al.* (1979). The images are very much clearer than with CT. Grey and white matter can be differentiated. It is possible to visualize the posterior fossa, which was a considerable problem with early CT, and as the technique does not involve use of ionizing radiation, repeated examinations can be carried out without risk. This technique, therefore, entirely superseded CT for research purposes within a very few years.

However, by the time this happened, the idea that, at least on a group basis, schizophrenia was associated with demonstrable anatomical brain changes as compared with normal controls had achieved general acceptance, and this was largely due to the findings of the CT studies. These were not ignored in the way that the pneumoencephalographic work had been, because, of course, it was possible to have adequate controls in a way that could only be achieved with a non-invasive technique.

In addition to laying the foundations for the detailed studies using MRI which are now being conducted, the CT studies of schizophrenia encouraged a return to neuropathological studies of the disorder, few of which had been undertaken in the middle decades of the twentieth century. The modern work has been admirably reviewed by Harrison (1999). In summary, the findings are that while problems of small sample sizes and differing techniques remain, on macroscopic study strong and consistent support can be found for ventricular enlargement, decreased cortical volume, and disproportionate volume loss from the temporal lobe. Consistent and strong histological findings are of the absence of gliosis as an intrinsic feature, smaller size of cortical and hippocampal neurons, and fewer neurons in dorsal thalamus.

Therefore, in spite of all the problems, it does appear that the identification of the pathological substrate of schizophrenia is in sight.

References

Alzheimer, A. (1897). Beitrage zur pathologischen Anatomie der Hirnrinde und zur anatomischen Grundlage der Psychosen. *Monatsschrift für Psychiatrie und Neurologie*, **2**, 8–120.

Alzheimer, A. (1907). Uber eine eigenartige Erkrankung der Hirnrinde. *Allegemeine Zeitschrift für Psychiatrie und Psychisch-Gerichtlich Medizine*, **64**, 146–8.

Alzheimer, A. (1913). Beiträge zur pathologischen Anatomie der Dementia praecox. *Allgemeine Zeitschrift für Psychiatrie*, **70**, 810–12.

Andreasen, N. C. and Olsen, S. (1982). Negative v positive schizophrenia. Definition and validation. *Archives of General Psychiatry*, **39**, 789–94.

Ansink, B. J. J., Buis, C., Tolsma, F. J. (1963). The pneumoencephalogram in chronic schizophrenics. *Psychiatria, Neurologia, Neurochirurgia* **66**, 120–30.

Asano, N. (1967). In *Pneumoencephalographic study of schizophrenia* (ed. H. Mitsuda), pp. 209-19. Igaku-Shoin, Tokyo.

Averbach, P. (1981*a*). Lesions of the nucleus ansae peduncularis in neuropsychiatric disease. *Archives of Neurology* **38**, 230–5.

Averbach, P. (1981*b*). Structural lesions of the brain in young schizophrenics. *Canadian Journal of Neurological Sciences* **8**, 73–6.

Barron, S. A., Jacobs, L., and Kinkel, W. R. (1976). Changes in size of normal lateral ventricles during aging determined by computerized tomography. *Neurology*, **26**, 1011–13.

Bliss, E. L. (1975). In *Brain damage-evidence from pneumoencephalograms* (ed. S. Wolf and B. B. Berle), pp. 42–5. Plenum Press, New York.

Borenstein, P., Dabbah, M., Metzger, J. (1957). L'encephalographie fractionnee dans les syndromes schizophreniques. *Annals of Medical Psychology* **115**, 385–426.

Bratfos, O., Sagedal, E. (1960). Luftencefalografiske undersokelser hos pasienter innlagt i sinnssykehus. *Nordisk Medicin* **51**, 1606–9.

Broser. (1949). Hirngewicht und Hirnprozess bei Schizophrenie. *Archiv für Psychiatrie und Nervenkrankheiten* **182**, 439–49.

Brown, R., Colter, N., Corsellis, J. A., Crow, T. J., Frith, C. D., Jagoe, R. *et al.* (1986). Post-mortem evidence of structural brain changes in schizophrenia. Differences in brain weight, temporal horn area, and parahippocampal gyrus compared with affective disorder. *Archives of General Psychiatry*, **43**, 36–42.

Bruton, C. J., Crow, T. J., Frith, C. D., Johnstone, E. C., Owens, D. G., and Roberts, G. W. (1990). Schizophrenia and the brain: a prospective clinico-neuropathological study. *Psychological Medicine*, **20**, 285–304.

Campbell, R., Hays, P., Russell, D. B., Zacks, D. J. (1979). CT scan variants and genetic heterogeneity in schizophrenia. *American Journal of Psychiatry* **136**, 722–3.

Corsellis, J. A. N. (1976). In *Psychoses of obscure pathology* (ed. W. B. Blackwood and J. A. N. Corsellis), pp. 903–15. Edward Arnold, London.

Crichton-Browne, J. (1879). On the weight of the brain and its component parts in the insane. *Brain* **2**, 42–67.

Dastur, D. K. (1959). The pathology of schizophrenia. *Archives of Neurology and Psychiatry*, **81**, 601–14.

Daum, C. H., McKinney, W. M., Proctor, R. C., Barnes, R. W., and Potter, P. (1976). Echoencephalographs of 100 consecutive acute psychiatric admissions. *Journal of Clinical Ultrasound*, **4**, 329–33.

David, G. B. (1957). In *The pathological anatomy of the schizophrenias* (ed. D. Richter), pp. 93–130. Pergamon, New York.

Dom, R. (1976). Neostriatal and Thalamic Interneurones: Their role in the pathophysiology of Huntington's Chorea, Parkinson's disease and Catatonic Schizophrenia. *Louvain, Belgium. University of Louvain, PhD Thesis.*

Donnelly, E. F., Weinberger, D. R., Waldman, I. N., and Wyatt, R. J. (1980). Cognitive impairment associated with morphological brain abnormalities on computed tomography in chronic schizophrenic patients. *Journal of Nervous and Mental Disease*, **168**, 305–8.

Donovan, J. F., Galbraith, A. J., Jackson, H. (1949). Some observations on leucotomy and investigations by pneumoencephalography. *Journal of Mental Science* **95**, 655–66.

Dunlap, C. B. (1924). Dementia praecox: some preliminary observations on brains from carefully selected cases and a consideration of certain sources of error. *American Journal of Psychiatry*, **80**, 403–21.

Famuyiwa, O. O., Eccleston, D., Donaldson, A. A., Garside, R. F. (1979). Tardive dyskinesia and dementia. *British Journal of Psychiatry* **135**, 500–4.

Fisman, M. (1975). The brain stem in psychosis. *British Journal of Psychiatry* **126**, 414–22.

Froshaug, H., Retterstol, N. (1956). Clinical and pneumo-encephalographic studies on cerebral atropies of middle age. *Acta Psychiatrica Scandinavica* **106**, 83–102.

Golden, C. J., Moses, J. A., Jr., Zelazowski, R., Graber, B., Zatz, L. M., Horvath, T. B., Berger, P. A. (1980*a*). Cerebral ventricular size and neuropsychological impairment in young chronic schizophrenics. Measurement by the standardized Luria-Nebraska Neuropsychological Battery. *Archives of General Psychiatry* **37**, 619–23.

Golden, C. J., Graber, B., Moses, J. A., Zatz, L. M. (1980*b*). Differentiation of chronic schizophrenics with and without ventricular enlargement by the Luria-Nebraska Neuropsychological Battery. *International Journal of Neuroscience* **11**, 131–8.

Griesinger, W. (1861). *Die Pathologie und Therapie der psychischen Krankheiten*, (1st edn 1845). Krabbe, Stuttgart.

Hankoff, L. D., Peress, N. S. (1981). Neuropathology of the brain stem in psychiatric disorders. *Biological Psychiatry* **16**, 945–52.

Harrison, P. J. (1999). The neuropathology of schizophrenia. A critical review of the data and their interpretation. *Brain*, **122**, 593–624.

Haug, J. O. (1962). Pneumoencephalographic studies in mental disease. *Acta Psychiatrica Scandinavica*, **38**, 1–114.

Haug, J. O. (1982). Pneumoencephalographic evidence of brain atrophy in acute and chronic schizophrenic patients. *Acta Physiologica Scandinavica* **66**, 374–83.

Heath, R. G., Franklyn, D. E., Shraberg, D. (1979). Gross pathology of the cerebellum in patients diagnosed and treated as functional psychiatric disorders. *Journal of Nervous and Mental Disease* **167**, 585–92.

Hecker, E. (1871). Die Hebephrenie Ein Beitrag zur klinischen Psychiatrie. *Archiv für Pathologische, Anatomie und Physiologie und für Klinische Medizin*, **52**, 394–429.

Holden, J. M., Forno, G., Itil, T., and Hsu, W. (1973). Echoencephalographic patterns in chronic schizophrenia (relationship to therapy resistance). *Biological Psychiatry*, **6**, 129–41.

Huber, G. (1953). Zur frage der mit hirnatrophie einhergehenden schizophrenie. *Archiv der Psychiatrie und Zeitschrift fuer Neurologie*, **190**, 429–48.

Huber, G. (1955). Das pneumencephalogramm am beginn schizophrener erkrankungen. *Archiv der Psychiatrie und Zeitschrift fuer Neurologie*, **193**, 406–26.

Huber, G. (1957). *Pneumoencephalographische und Psychopathologische bilder bei Endogenen Psychosen*. Springer-Verlag, Berlin.

Hunter, R., Jones, M., and Cooper, F. (1968). Modified lumbar air encephalography in the investigation of long-stay psychiatric patients. *Journal of Neurological Sciences*, **6**, 593–6.

Illowsky, B. P., Juliano, D. M., Bigelow, L. B., and Weinberger, D. R. (1988). Stability of CT scan findings in schizophrenia: results of an 8 year follow-up study. *Journal of Neurology, Neurosurgery and Psychiatry*, **51**, 209–13.

Jacobi, W. and Winkler, H. (1927). Encephalographische studien an chronisch schizophrenen. *Archiv für Psychiatrie und Nervenkrankheiten*, **81**, 299–332.

Jellinek, E. H. (1976). Cerebral atrophy and cognitive impairment in chronic schizophrenia. *Lancet*, **2**, 1202–3.

Jernigan, T. L., Zatz, L. M., Moses, J. A., Jr, and Berger, P. A. (1982*a*). Computed tomography in schizophrenics and normal volunteers. I. Fluid volume. *Archives of General Psychiatry*, **39**, 765–70.

Jernigan, T. L., Zatz, L. M., Moses, J. A., Jr, and Cardellino, J. P. (1982*b*). Computed tomography in schizophrenics and normal volunteers. II. Cranial asymmetry. *Archives of General Psychiatry*, **39**, 771–3.

Johnstone, E. C., Crow, T. J., Frith, C. D., Husband, J., and Kreel, L. (1976). Cerebral ventricular size and cognitive impairment in chronic schizophrenia. *Lancet*, **2**, 924–6.

Johnstone, E. C., Crow, T. J., Frith, C. D., Stevens, M., Kreel, L., and Husband, J. (1978). The dementia of dementia praecox. *Acta Psychiatrica Scandinavica*, **57**, 305–24.

Kahlbaum, K. L. (1874). *Die Katatonie onder das Spannungirresein. Eine Klinische Form psychischer Krankheit.* Hirschwald, Berlin.

Kemali, D., Maj, M., Galderisi, S., Milici, N., and Salvati, A. (1989). Ventricle-to-brain ratio in schizophrenia: a controlled follow-up study. *Biological Psychiatry*, **26**, 756–9.

Klippel, M. and Lhermitte, J. (1909). Un cas de demence précoce a type catatonique avec autopsie. *Revue Neurologique*, **17**, 157–8.

Kraepelin, E. (1896). *Lehrbuch der Psychiatrie.* Barth, Leipzig.

Kraepelin, E. (1919). *Dementia praecox and paraphrenia*, (trans. R. M. Barclay). Livingstone, Edinburgh.

Kure, S., Shimoda, M. (1923). On the brain of dementia praecox. *Journal of Nervous and Mental Disease* **58**, 338–53.

Lacono, W. G., Smith, G. N., Moreau, M., Beiser, M., Fleming, J. A., Lin, T. Y. *et al.* (1988). Ventricular and sulcal size at the onset of psychosis. *American Journal of Psychiatry*, **145**, 820–4.

Lauterbur, P. C. (1979). Image formation by induced local interactions: examples employing NMR. *Nature*, **242**, 190–1.

Lemay, M. (1967). Changes in ventricular size during and after pneumoencephalography. *Radiology*, **88**, 57–63.

Lemke, R. (1936). Untersuchungen uber die soziale Prognose der Schizophrenie unter besonderer Berucksichtigung des encephalographischen Befundes. *Archiv für Psychiatrie und Nervenkrankheiten* **104**, 89–136.

Levi, C., Gray, J. E., McCullough, E. C., and Hattery, R. R. (1982). The unreliability of CT numbers as absolute values. *American Journal of Radiology*, **139**, 443–7.

Lewis, N. D. C. (1923). *The Constitutional Factors in Dementia Praecox: Particular Attention to the Circulatory System and to Some of Endocrine Glands. Nervous and Mental Disease Monograph Series.* Nervous and Mental Disease Publishing Co., Washington.

Lewis, S. W. (1990). Computerized-tomography in schizophrenia 15 years on. *British Journal of Psychiatry*, **157**, 16–24.

Lonnum, A. (1966). *The clinical significance of ceregbral ventricular enlargement.* Universitetsforlaget, Oslo.

Luchins, D. J., Weinberger, D. R., Wyatt, R. J. (1982). Schizophrenia and cerebral asymmetry detected by computed tomography. *American Journal of Psychiatry* **139**, 753–7.

Mallard, J., Hutchison, J. M., Edelstein, W., Ling, R., and Foster, M. (1979). Imaging by nuclear magnetic resonance and its bio-medical implications. *Journal of Biomedical Engineering*, **1**, 153–60.

Mansfield, P. and Maudsley, A. A. (1977). Medical imaging by NMR. *British Journal of Radiology*, **50**, 188–94.

Marsden, C. D. (1976). Cerebral atrophy and cognitive impairment in chronic schizophrenia. *Lancet*, **2**, 1079.

Meynert, T. (1884). *Psychiatrie.* W. Braumuller, Wien.

Mittenzweig, R. (1905). Hirngewicht und Geisteskrankheit. *Allegemeine Zeitschrift für Psychiatrie und Psychisch-Gerichtlich Medizine* 31–62.

Moore, M., Nathan, D., Elliott, A. R., and Laubach, C. (1933). Encephalographic studies in schizophrenia (dementia praecox): Report of sixty cases. *American Journal of Psychiatry*, **89**, 801–10.

Moore, M. T., Nathan, D., Elliott, A. R., and Laubach, C. (1935). Encephalographic studies in mental disease. *American Journal of Psychiatry*, **92**, 43–67.

Naeser, M. A., Levine, H. L., Benson, D. F., Stuss, D. T., Weir, W. S. (1981). Frontal leukotomy size and hemispheric asymmeteries on computerized tomographic scans of schizophrenics with variable recovery. *Archives of Neurology* **39**, 30–7.

Nagy, K. (1959). Pneumoencephalographische befunde bei akuten und chronischen psychosen. *Archives of Neurology and Psychiatry* **198**, 544–53.

Nagy, K. (1963). Pneumoencephalographische befunde bei endogen psychosen. *Nervenarzt*, **34**, 543–8.

Nasrallah, H. A., Olson, S. C., McCalley-Whitters, M., Chapman, S., and Jacoby, C. G. (1986). Cerebral ventricular enlargement in schizophrenia. A preliminary follow-up study. *Archives of General Psychiatry*, **43**, 157–9.

Nieto, D., Escobar, A. (1972). Major psychoses. In *Pathology of the Nervous System* (ed. J. Minckler), pp. 2654–70, McGraw Hill, New York.

Nobile, S., Brizzi, R. (1953). La pneumoencefalografia negli schizofrenici. *Rivista Sperimentale di Freniatria e Medicina Legale delle Alienazioni Mentali* **7**, 705–13.

Owens, D. G. C., Johnstone, E. C., Bydder, G. M., and Creel, L. (1980). Unsuspected organic disease in chronic schizophrenia demonstrated by computer tomography. *Journal of Neurology, Neurosurgery and Psychiatry*, **43**, 1065–9.

Owens, D. G., Johnstone, E. C., Crow, T. J., Frith, C. D., Jagoe, J. R., and Kreel, L. (1985). Lateral ventricular size in schizophrenia: relationship to the disease process and its clinical manifestations. *Psychological Medicine*, **15**, 27–41.

Penn, R. D., Belanger, M. G., and Yasnoff, W. A. (1978). Ventricular volume in man computed from CAT scans. *Annals of Neurology*, **3**, 216–23.

Probst, F. P. (1973). Gas distension of the lateral ventricles at encephalography. *Acta Radiologica Diagnostica*, **14**, 1–4.

Rawlings, E. (1920). The histopathologic findings in dementia praecox. *American Journal of Insanity*, **76**, 265–84.

Reveley, M. A., Chitkara, B., and Lewis, S. W. (1988). Ventricular and cranial size in schizophrenia: a 4 to 7 year follow-up. *Schizophrenia Research*, **1**, 163.

Rieder, R. O., Donnelly, E. F., Herdt, J. R., Waldman, I. N. (1979). Sulcal prominence in young chronic schizophrenic patients: CT scan findings associated with impairment on neuropsychological tests. *Psychiatry Research* **1**, 1–8.

Roberts, G. W., Colter, N., Lofthouse, R., Johnstone, E. C., and Crow, T. J. (1987). Is there gliosis in schizophrenia? Investigation of the temporal lobe. *Biological Psychiatry*, **22**, 1459–68.

Roessle, R. and Roulet, F. (1932). *Mass und Zahl der Pathologie*. Springer, Berlin.

Scharpff. (1912). Hirngewicht und Psychose. *Archiv für Psychiatrie und Nervenkrankheiten* **49**, 242–52.

Schiebel, A. B., Kovelman, J. A. (1981). Disorientation of the hippocampal pyramidal cell and its process in the schizophrenic patient. *Biological Psychiatry* **16**, 101–2.

Siegel, E., Heidrich, R. (1970). Beziehungen zwischen pneumenzephalographischen und psychopathologischen befunden bei schizophrenie. *Psychiatrie, Neurologie, und Medizinische Psychologie* **22**, 132–7.

Sitnikov, E. M. (1961). Pneumoencephalography in chronis schizophrenic illnesses. *Zhurnal Nevropatologii i Psikhiatrii Imeni S.S. Korsakova* **61**, 1251–4.

Smith, R. C., Calderon, M., Ravichandran, G. K., Largen, J., Vroulis, G., Shvartsburd, A. *et al.* (1984). Nuclear magnetic resonance in schizophrenia: a preliminary study. *Psychiatry Research*, **12**, 137–47.

Southard, E. E. (1910). A study of the dementia praecox group in the light of certain cases showing anomalies or scleroses in particular brain regions. *American Journal of Insanity* **67**, 119–76.

Stevens, J. R. (1982). The neuropathology of schizophrenia. *Psychological Medicine* **12**, 695–700.

Storey, P. B. (1966). Lumbar air encephalography in chronic schizophrenia: a controlled experiment. *British Journal of Psychiatry*, **112**, 135–44.

Takahashi, R., Inanaga, V., Kato, N., Kumashiro, H., Nishimura, T., Okuma, T. *et al.* (1981). In *CT scanning and the investigation of schizophrenia* (ed. C. Perris, G. Struwe, and B. Jansson), pp. 259–68. Elsevier/North Holland, Amsterdam.

Tanaka, Y., Hazama, H., Kawahara, R., and Kobayashi, K. (1981). Computerized tomography of the brain in schizophrenic patients. A controlled study. *Acta Psychiatrica Scandinavica*, 63, 191–7.

Tatetsu, S. (1964). A contribution to the morphological background of shizophrenia. *Acta Neuropathologica* 3, 558–71.

Trimble, M. and Kingsley, D. (1978). Cerebral ventricular size in chronic schizophrenia. *Lancet* i, 278.

Turner, S. W., Toone, B. K., and Breet-Jones, J. R. (1986). CT scan changes in early chronic schizophrenia-their relationship to perinatal trauma, family history and alcohol intake: preliminary findings. *Psychological Medicine*, 14, 219–25.

Vogel, T. and Lange, H.-J. (1966). Pneumencephalographische und psychopathologische bilder bei endogen psychosen. Statistische untersuchungen an dem von G. Huber 1957 veroffentlichten material. *Archiv für Psychiatrie und Nervenkrankheiten*, 208, 371–84.

Vogt, C. and Vogt, O. (1948). Über anatomische substrate bernerkungen zu pathoanatomischen befunden bei schizophrenia. *Artzliche Forschungen*, 3, 1–7.

Weinberger, D. R., Torrey, E. F., Neophytides, A. N., and Wyatt, R. J. (1979*a*). Lateral cerebral ventricular enlargement in chronic schizophrenia. *Archives of General Psychiatry*, 36, 735–9.

Weinberger, D. R., Torrey, E. F., Neophytides, A. N., and Wyatt, R. J. (1979*b*). Structural abnormalities in the cerebral cortex of chronic schizophrenic patients. *Archives of General Psychiatry*, 36, 935–9.

Weinberger, D. R., Torrey, E. F., and Wyatt, R. J. (1979*c*). Cerebellar atrophy in chronic schizophrenia. *Lancet*, 1, 718–19.

Weinberger, D. R., Wagner, R. L., and Wyatt, R. J. (1983). Neuropathological studies of schizophrenia: a selective review. *Schizophrenia Bulletin*, 9, 193–212.

Wernicke, C. (1881). *Lehrbuch der Gehirnkrankheiten für Arzte und Studierende I*. Fischer, Berlin.

Wernicke, C. (1900). *Grundriss der Psychiatrie*. Johannes Barth, Leipzig.

Whittier, J. R. (1951). Deaths related to pneumoencephalography during a six-year period. *Archives of Neurology and Psychiatry*, 65, 463–71.

Wildi, E., Linder, A., Costoulas, G. (1967). Schizophrenie et involution cerebrum sénile. *Psychiatrie et Neurologie* 154, 1–26.

Young, I. J., Crampton, A. R. (1974). Cerebrospinal fluid uric acid levels in cerebral atrophy occurring in psychiatric and neurologic patients. *Biological Psychiatry* 8, 281–92.

Chapter 2

Structural magnetic resonance imaging

Andrew McIntosh and Stephen Lawrie

Introduction

The technique of nuclear magnetic resonance originated before the use of computed tomography. Initially used to image small quantities of biological tissue (Lauterbur 1973), it was much longer before it found a clinical application (Budinger and Lauterbur 1984). The superior spatial resolution of magnetic resonance imaging (MRI) enabled clinicians to visualize demyelinating lesions and was subsequently used to examine the brains of individuals with schizophrenia, in the hope that it might aid diagnosis and further our knowledge of pathophysiology. There were good grounds to think that this would be the case, since the inferior technique of computed tomography (CT) had consistently showed the presence of cortical 'atrophy' and ventricular enlargement.

Almost two decades of structural magnetic resonance imaging (sMRI) research have elapsed and the precise causes of schizophrenia continue to elude researchers. Nevertheless, much more is known about schizophrenia now than was the case 20 years ago. Over 100 studies have compared schizophrenics with healthy controls, and many others have looked at diagnostic, aetiological, and prognostic associations. This chapter will review this body of work, after briefly considering important methodological points.

Structural MRI signal

The brain images created by MRI arise because of the properties of the component tissues, and in particular, the magnetic properties of protons (hydrogen nuclei).

When a tissue is placed in a magnetic field (B_0), a proportion of the hydrogen nuclei will align with the magnetic field and precess around it, at a frequency known as the Lamor frequency, at an angle to the direction of the magnetic field. The hydrogen nuclei will not be in phase with one another (i.e. at the same frequencies, as if 'marching in step with one another'; Suckling and Bullmore 2000) and the tissue itself will generate no coherent signal under these conditions. When a radiofrequency pulse is applied to the tissue, the spinning nuclei tip further from the direction of the field and spin briefly in phase with one another (Fig. 2.1). Over time, the spins of the respective nuclei return to their original state, both by returning to their original angle of spin

Fig. 2.1 The increase in angle of displacement of hydrogen nuclei following the application of a radiofrequency (RF) pulse. After nuclei move from angle α to β they return to the original angle at a rate determined by the T_1 decay constant.

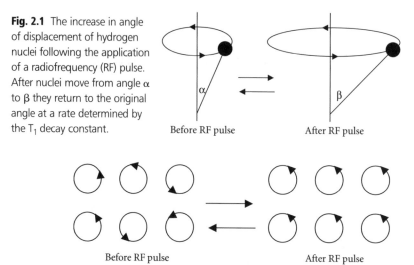

Before RF pulse   After RF pulse

Before RF pulse   After RF pulse

Fig. 2.2 The phasing of hydrogen nuclei after the application of a brief radiofrequency (RF) pulse. The tendency for protons to return (decay) to their original (out of phase) state is summarized using the T_2 constant.

before the field was applied and also by de-phasing with one another. The tendency for nuclei to return from their 'tipped state' to their original angles occurs exponentially and can be summarized using a rate constant called T_1. The tendency for nuclei to de-phase from one another again also occurs exponentially and occurs at a rate that can be expressed using a rate constant known as T_2 (Fig. 2.2).

T_1 is sometimes known as the spin–lattice rate constant, while T_2 is sometimes known as the spin–spin constant. Measuring the decay constants T_1 and T_2, as well as the overall proton density (PD) has many clinical applications, as the values reflect the underlying anatomy and also physiology of the brain. T_1, T_2, and PD signals at each unit of brain volume (voxel) can be presented as a grey-scale image, with the highest signals represented as white voxels and low signals as black. However, a single radio-frequency pulse as described above would produce signals from brain tissue decaying as a function of T_1, T_2, and PD and also from brain tissue on many different slices. For this reason, sequences have been devised which generate signals that are highly dependent upon either the T_1 or T_2 decay constants or on PD, and which are slice selective, acquiring image data from one slice of brain tissue at a time. The most common sequences used are the spin–echo sequence and gradient–echo. Many other sequences exist and the interested reader should refer to Professor Hornak's MRI Tutor website (www.mritutor.com) for further details.

Spin–echo sequence

Spin–echo sequences (Fig. 2.3) involve the application of a radiofrequency pulse at time 0 and, after a time TE/2 later, an inversion pulse of 180° to displace those protons that have

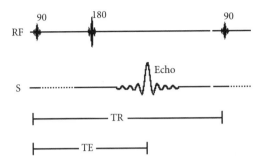

Fig. 2.3 Typical spin–echo scanning sequence. RF, radiofrequency pulse; S, signal; TR, repeat time; TE, echo time. Magnetic field gradients are also applied during the scan in three (*x*, *y*, *z*) dimensions.

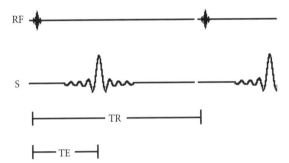

Fig. 2.4 A gradient scanning sequence. RF, radiofrequency pulse; S, signal; TR, repeat time; TE, echo time. Magnetic field gradients are also applied during the scan in three (*x*, *y*, *z*) dimensions.

decayed most from their 'excited' state. Images can be acquired during the period between the first two pulses, or after the 180° pulse and the beginning of the next sequence. By varying the timing of the image acquisition, the echo time (TE), and the repeat times, PD-, T_1-, or T_2-weighted images can be acquired from the same imaging sequence.

Gradient–echo

A typical gradient–echo sequence is shown in Fig. 2.4. The first event in the sequence is the application of a radiofrequency pulse at time 0. This pulse can flip the protons by an angle, usually between 5 and 90 degrees, known as the 'flip angle'. At a given time (TE) after the radiofrequency pulse, the image signal is acquired. After a further interval, the radiofrequency pulse is reapplied and the sequence is repeated. The time between cycles is called the repetition time (TR).

The flip angle, TR, and TE together determine the scan time, image resolution and T_1 or T_2 weighting. Smaller flip angles phase spinning protons but do not displace them very far from their original axes. The images acquired from these sequences tend therefore to be T_2 weighted. Conversely, larger flip angles tend to produce T_1-weighted images. The gradient–echo sequence can also be modified by the application of a 180° pulse before the subsequent cycles. This 'pre' pulse allows the faster acquisition of T_1-weighted images using low flip angles. These sequences are sometimes called magnetization-prepared gradient-echo sequences (MPRAGE).

Measurement of tissue signal

The image itself is created from the measurement of energy 'released' from tissue by several radiofrequency detectors located in a coil placed around the head of the subject. Images are created using Fourier analysis of this information to make a 'back projection' of the properties of the tissue which gave rise to the signal in the first place.

Methodological considerations

Image acquisition

The first MRI study of schizophrenia was conducted by Smith (1984) with only nine schizophrenic subjects and five controls. Although no significant differences in cortical areas were found between the groups, a single, unreliably positioned slice was examined in a small number of subjects. The methods of MRI studies have advanced greatly over the past 20 years, in parallel with advances in the technology of image acquisition and analysis.

The main factors influencing image quality are shown in Box 2.1 (Beck *et al.* 2002; Davidson and Heinrichs 2003). Greater magnetic strength has the effect of increasing signal to noise ratio and provides greater tissue contrast. However, magnetic field strength is usually maximal at the centre or core of the magnet and decays slightly at distances further away from the centre. This 'field inhomogeneity' can lead to differences in tissue contrast and quality, which increases noise and may lead to unreliable results. Conventionally, field inhomogeneity is controlled for by scanning an object of homogeneous density and correcting the images for any inhomogeneity observed in the object. However, the object used is typically a fluid phantom which bears little resemblance to a complex structure such as the brain. Slice thickness is an important consideration in MRI studies of the brain because thinner slices give rise to greater resolution, and brain tissue present at one anatomical level is separated from that at another level more effectively. A signal in one plane of brain tissue from two adjacent regions is sometimes called a 'partial volume'. Early sMRI studies often acquired images from several slices of the brain but left interslice gaps of the brain from which no data were acquired.

Box 2.1 Parameters influencing MRI image quality

- Magnet strength
- Field inhomogeneity
- Time to echo, repeat time, flip angle, etc.
- Slice thickness
- Contiguous versus interleaved versus spaced slices
- Plane of acquisition

This meant that planar or volumetric data on a brain region were often incomplete and potentially inaccurate. Generally, brain 'slicing' is now contiguous. Finally, volumes or areas are commonly acquired as T_1-weighted coronal images and, for most purposes, this is probably adequate. However, some regions (e.g. the hippocampus) are better visualized in an oblique or transverse plane, parallel to the long axis of the structure.

Image analysis

The results from structural magnetic imaging studies are influenced by the method of image analysis as well as the method of image acquisition. Until about 5 years ago, studies almost exclusively used semi-automated methods to extract the brain from the surrounding tissues; followed by manual tracing around regions of interest (ROI) with the aid of a tissue-contrast facility (Fig. 2.5). Tracings were usually made with the aid of an anatomical atlas and using operationalized criteria for delineating brain structures.

Box 2.2 Methods of image analysis

- Region of interest
  - manual
  - semi-automated
  - fully automated
- Voxel based
  - statistical parametric mapping (SPM)
  - other methods (e.g. those based on 'fuzzy logic')

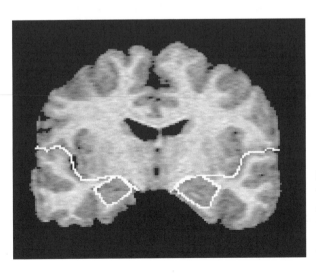

Fig. 2.5 Region of interest tracing of left and right amygdala–hippocampal complexes and temporal lobes, made on a T_1-weighted coronal image.

Volumes were then calculated by multiplying each regional area by the slice thickness, summing all slice volumes over the brain region in question. This technique involves a certain amount of subjectivity and it is essential to first establish adequate inter-rater and intra-rater reliability. Large structures (e.g. whole brain, temporal and frontal lobes) tend to have high measurement reliability, whereas smaller structures (e.g. hippocampus, amygdala, caudate) are generally subject to greater measurement error. In an attempt to measure smaller volumes more reliably, parcellation techniques have been developed. These generally involve tracing in three dimensions simultaneously, but this technique is very time consuming and subjective judgements continue to be necessary (e.g. Caviness *et al.* 2000).

An alternative approach to image analysis has been developed, called 'voxel-based morphometry' (VBM). This involves the transformation of each brain into a common three-dimensional space, and segmentation into grey and white matter and cerebrospinal fluid (CSF). Differences in, for example, grey matter density are then computed by comparing these 'normalized' brains from each group on a voxel by voxel basis (see Chapter 6 for details of this and other automated techniques). VBM avoids subjective judgements about where a region of interest begins and ends, and can be used to investigate very small structures, but the results obtained reflect the statistical probability of differences in tissue density rather than volume, and cannot be interpreted with the same ease as a mean difference in volume. However, studies using both ROI analysis and VBM suggest that the results are generally similar (Wright *et al.* 1999*a*; Lawrie *et al.* 2001; Job *et al.* 2002, 2003).

Patient and control selection

In sMRI studies of patients with schizophrenia, the usual design is to compare a sample of cases with unaffected controls, healthy relatives, or patients with another psychiatric disorder. The primary interest of such a study is to examine whether the volume of a brain region differs between groups. Where a significant difference is shown, the difference is usually attributed to the diagnosis. However, the many differences between controls and established patients with schizophrenia mean that anatomical differences may be attributable to treatment, the effects of an ongoing disease process, or the effect of a risk factor. A more rigorous design is to follow unaffected patients prospectively before and as they become unwell. This is rarely feasible (see later), and for these and other practical reasons the predominant design, as in the rest of medicine, has been the case-control study.

However, case-control studies are susceptible to several sources of bias. First, patients and controls may be dissimilar in many ways, in addition to their diagnostic status. Patients recruited from hospitals are often those with the most severe illnesses, greatest social adversities and complicating factors, e.g. substance misuse. The recruitment of socially comparable well controls is not easy. Non-schizophrenic psychiatric or neurological controls can be used as an alternative control group, being more similar than groups of well volunteers in terms of potential confounders of brain volume, such as social class and educational level, for example. However, healthy controls are almost always required. It is sometimes possible to recruit healthy controls from the non-genetic relatives and social networks of the patients themselves, thereby establishing both a more generally comparable control group and one that may be more committed to the research in question (having first-hand knowledge of the effects of schizophrenia). However, studies using this design run the potential risk that the controls are themselves atypical of unaffected people from the general population. Many studies attempt to match schizophrenic patients to one or more controls for known influences on brain volume (e.g. age, sex, IQ). Matched designs have great value when the potentially confounding variables are well understood and can be measured accurately, but this may well not be the case for schizophrenia. For instance, IQ has been shown to be both a risk factor and a state indicator (Cosway *et al.* 2000), such that matching patients with controls of equal current IQ might effectively select intellectually inferior controls, and vice versa for premorbid IQ matching. There is also the danger of over-matching patients and controls on variables that are important in the pathogenesis of schizophrenia itself (i.e. those on the causal pathway).

An ideal approach might be to select affected subjects and healthy controls randomly from a population. However, this is easier said than done, and still has hazards. Population sampling (e.g. from the electoral register) may select subjects who are relatively affluent and patients who are not representative of patients in general. Ethics committees might be reluctant to agree to the unsolicited approach of potential study participants, and some participants will inevitably refuse to be scanned. This design has obvious theoretical advantages over the hospital-based studies, but the authors are unaware of any examples of using this approach in sMRI studies of schizophrenia.

The influence of methodological and descriptive variables on the results obtained from case-control studies has been examined by very few studies. One study that has assessed the influence of methodological confounds on observed effect sizes is that of Davidson and Heinrichs (2003), using meta-analytic methods. They found that sample size was negatively correlated with effect size overall, suggesting that sampling or publication bias may be an important source of apparent case-control differences in imaging studies of schizophrenia (but see Lawrie and Abukmeil 1998; Wright *et al.* 2000). Davidson and Heinrichs (2003) also reported that the proportion of right-handed males in individual studies was associated with the extent of the differences found (but see Nelson *et al.* 1998). Slice thickness and time to echo were also related to some observed effect sizes, although magnetic strength was not. This study suggests that methodological issues are important sources of potential bias in sMRI research. None the less, these effects are not as large as those of the illness.

Differences between patients with schizophrenia and healthy controls

Very early neuroimaging studies and more modern techniques both agree that the brain in schizophrenia is different from the brain of healthy control subjects. As it has become possible to reliably identify and measure smaller regions of interest within the brain, researchers have identified regions that are more reduced in volume than is the brain as a whole. Several systematic reviews of more than 100 individual controlled studies have summarized our knowledge of the location and extent of these regional differences (Lawrie and Abukmeil 1998; Wright *et al.* 2000; Davidson and Heinrichs 2003). Wright *et al.* (2000) combined MRI studies of the same region of interest using random effects meta-analysis, and is the only one so far to provide statistical summaries of all the regions examined, while the descriptive review by Shenton *et al.* (2001) is the most extensive. We will use these reviews to summarize this extensive literature, highlight studies of particular interest, and mention regions that require further study, rather than exhaustively list all the studies done so far.

Whole brain

Whole brain volume in schizophrenia has been examined in multiple studies and reviewed in several systematic reviews and meta-analyses. Although whole brain volume is reduced compared to controls when studies are combined (Lawrie and Abukmeil 1998; Wright *et al.* 2000), most individual studies fail to find a significant difference between schizophrenics and controls (Shenton *et al.* 2001). The effect size appears to be around –0.31 for grey and –0.19 for white matter. This corresponds to an average volume reduction of 4% in grey matter (95%CI 1–6%) and 2% in white matter (95%CI 0–5%) (Wright *et al.* 2000). Whole brain volume reductions appear to be similarly equivocal in individual first-episode studies, as the majority of studies do not find significant differences (Bilder *et al.* 1994; Lawrie *et al.* 1999; Velakoulis *et al.* 1999), with only the occasional exception (e.g. in adolescents, James *et al.* 1999).

Ventricles and CSF

Most MRI studies measure ventricular size separately for all ventricles and often divide the lateral ventricles into their anterior, inferior and posterior horns, and the ventricular body. In schizophrenia, the lateral and third ventricles are about 20–30% larger than in controls (Lawrie and Abukmeil 1998; Wright *et al.* 2000; Shenton *et al.* 2001). Wright *et al.* (2000) demonstrated that the bodies of the left and right ventricles contributed the largest amount to this effect, being increased in volume by about 48% compared to control subjects, and the frontal horns contributed the least. The fourth ventricle showed a non-significant increase of 7% in schizophrenic compared to control subjects. Studies of first-episode patients and healthy relatives tend to confirm that differences in lateral and third ventricular volumes are present at first presentation (Barr *et al.* 1997; DeLisi *et al.* 1991, 1998).

Prefrontal cortex

Most studies of prefrontal cortex volume in schizophrenia have found lower volumes in schizophrenic patients compared to controls, regardless of whether chronic

(Harvey *et al.* 1993; Andreasen *et al.* 1994*b*) or first-episode patients (Bilder *et al.* 1994; Gur *et al.* 2000*a*) were examined (for a review, see Shenton *et al.* 2001). Overall, the volume reductions appear to be from 2 to 8% (Wright *et al.* 2000). However, since prefrontal cortex accounts for approximately 30% of total cerebral volume, and has diverse regional specialization, the finding of reduced volume is not in itself very revealing. Frontal volume reductions have been further characterized using parcellation or various approaches to computational morphometry. Reductions in anterior cingulate, orbitofrontal, dorsolateral and ventromedial cortices have been found using both parcellation (Crespo-Facorro *et al.* 1999; Goldstein *et al.* 1999; Gur *et al.* 2000*a*) and automated techniques (Chua *et al.* 1997; Gaser *et al.* 1999; Wright *et al.* 1999*a*; Job *et al.*, 2002). However, the studies tend to be small and each individual finding has yet to be broadly replicated.

Temporal lobes

Abnormalities of temporal cortex are well described in schizophrenic patients. Of 51 MRI studies of whole temporal lobe volume in schizophrenia, 61% showed reductions in schizophrenic patients compared to healthy controls (Shenton *et al.* 2001). Wright *et al.* (2000) pooled the results from 25 studies comparing schizophrenic patients with controls, and found a reduction of between 2 and 4% in affected patients. However, temporal lobe reductions are less consistently found in first-episode studies than in chronic patients, but medial temporal lobe volumes remain consistently smaller in comparison to controls (Lieberman *et al.* 1993; Lawrie *et al.* 1999). The reason for this is unclear, but there is some evidence that temporal lobe differences may progress over time (DeLisi *et al.* 1998; Jacobsen *et al.* 1998). Alternatively, the tendency for first-episode studies to be smaller may have led to insufficient statistical power.

Some temporal lobe sub-regions appear to be reduced to a greater extent. Superior temporal gyrus (STG) volume in schizophrenia has been the subject of several studies. The attention this region receives is perhaps because of its close association with language, and because of functional imaging studies which have shown changes in perfusion in schizophrenic subjects with clinical associations. Superior temporal gyrus volume appears to be reduced in schizophrenic subjects compared to controls, with a relatively greater effect on size for the left anterior superior and posterior superior segments (Cohen's d $\approx$ 0.4) (Wright *et al.* 2000). The fusiform gyrus has also been found to be relatively small (Paillere-Martinot *et al.* 2001; Onitsuka *et al.* 2003).

Amygdala

Medial temporal lobe volumes (typically hippocampus and amygdala combined) were significantly reduced in schizophrenic patients compared to controls in 74% of the 49 studies identified by Shenton *et al.* (2001). Of the 44 regions considered by

Wright *et al.* (2000), the left and right amygdalae had two of the largest volume reductions of all (Cohen's $d = -0.72$ and -0.69, for left and right, respectively), being reduced by around 10% in schizophrenic subjects. Wright *et al.* considered ROI studies, where regions were defined using established and operationalized criteria. Further evidence of grey matter loss has come from VBM studies, which have shown reduced amygdala grey matter density in several studies (Wright *et al.* 1999; Job *et al.* 2002) and evidence of abnormal shape (Shenton *et al.* 2002), although there are some contradictory studies (Levitt *et al.* 2001) and some important methodological difficulties associated with its measurement (see David *et al.* 2002).

Hippocampus and parahippocampus

Early studies of the hippocampus in schizophrenia tended to incompletely image the structure, using only a few interleaved slices. The general tendency now to use contiguous slices has greatly improved the accuracy of hippocampal measurement, and there are now more than 30 well-conducted studies which show a reduction of around 6% in both left and right hippocampi compared to healthy controls (Wright *et al.* 2000). The changes also appear to be present at first presentation (e.g. Whitworth *et al.* 1998; Velakoulis *et al.* 1999) although there is some doubt as to whether they may be acquired as patients become unwell (Lawrie *et al.* 2001, 2002) and whether they progress once psychotic symptoms have become established (Gur *et al.* 1998; Jacobsen *et al.* 1998). The pattern of results for left and right parahippocampus is similar (eight studies, >350 subjects, Cohen's d ≈ -0.4 to -0.7), although there is evidence that study results vary by more than one would expect by chance alone, suggesting some unexplained clinical or methodological heterogeneity.

Thalamus

Evidence suggesting a reduced volume of the thalamus in schizophrenia has only become available relatively recently (Andreasen *et al.* 1994*a*; Gur *et al.* 1998; Staal *et al.* 1998; Gilbert *et al.* 2001). However, the thalamus is a collection of several nuclei, and it is difficult both to separate the whole structure from surrounding grey matter and to visualize each individual nucleus with MRI. Voxel-based morphometry studies have not confirmed the results of ROI analyses (Job *et al.* 2002; Kubicki *et al.* 2002), but this may require a specific focus on the thalamus. There is also some evidence that antipsychotic medication may increase thalamic size, further confounding any association with diagnosis (Gur *et al.* 1998).

Basal ganglia and nucleus accumbens

In contrast to other nuclei, there is good evidence that patients with schizophrenia have a larger left and right globus pallidus than healthy subjects of the same age. Several studies (e.g. Kelsoe *et al.* 1988; Jernigan *et al.* 1991) have found increases of around 20% overall (Wright *et al.* 2000), including some data from first-episode studies. However, some studies measure lentiform nucleus rather than globus pallidus and putamen separately, and the evidence for an increased volume of the putamen in chronic patients is somewhat weaker. First-episode studies do not generally find increases in putamen compared to healthy controls, although putamen and globus pallidus volumes are significantly smaller in first-episode compared to chronic patients (Lang *et al.* 2001; Gunduz *et al.* 2002). The possibility that such changes are an effect of antipsychotic treatment has been suggested by several studies which correlate basal ganglia volumes with antipsychotic exposure (e.g. Chakos *et al.* 1994). However, these studies tend to find associations between antipsychotic exposure and caudate volume rather than globus pallidus or putamen volumes as expected. This finding is difficult to explain in the broader context of the MRI literature which does not consistently find increases in caudate volume compared to controls (e.g. Wright *et al.* 2000; 10 studies, 565 patients). There is some evidence that caudate volume is decreased in first-episode patients (Keshavan *et al.* 1998), which might suggest that antipsychotic exposure minimizes these reductions which predate treatment. Overall, the basal ganglia literature is rather inconsistent, potentially due to measurement difficulties or dynamic disease and therapeutic effects. There remains considerable doubt as to whether the basal ganglia are larger, smaller or similar in size before antipsychotic treatment (Lang *et al.* 2001; Gunduz *et al.* 2002; McCreadie *et al.* 2002). No convincing evidence that the nucleus accumbens differs in size between schizophrenia and controls has yet been shown (Gunduz *et al.* 2002).

Insula

The insula is a region of cerebral cortex not usually included within the previously mentioned structures. It lies buried within the depths of the lateral sulcus, concealed by the frontal, temporal and parietal lobes and is situated overlying the site at which the telencephalon and diencephalons fused during embryological development. There is some evidence from both ROI (Kim *et al.* 2003) and VBM (Sigmundsson *et al.* 2001; Kubicki *et al.* 2002; Shapleske *et al.* 2002) that there may be grey matter reductions in the insula in schizophrenic patients compared to controls.

There is therefore what could be called a gross 'neuroanatomy of schizophrenia' (Table 2.1). This now needs to be specified in greater detail and related to the clinical and aetiological features of the disorder. The effects of potential confounders such as gender and co-morbid substance misuse are particularly pertinent in this respect. Gender may have a moderating influence on the neuroanatomy of schizophrenia (Goldstein *et al.* 2002), although the reviews already cited make it clear that this is far from confirmed. Alcohol misuse certainly has neuroanatomical effects, even when drinking does not reach the level of psychological or physical dependence, but the best available evidence is that this exaggerates differences rather than accounting for them (Mathalon *et al.* 2003).

Table 2.1 Summary of sMRI findings in schizophrenia (combines Wright *et al.* 2000; Shenton *et al.* 2001)

Region	Findings
Whole brain volume	50+ studies. Reduced by approximately 2–3%. Grey matter decreased by around 4%. White matter volume may not be different from healthy controls
Frontal lobes	50+ studies. Reductions of approximately 3% compared to controls
Temporal lobes	100+ studies. Whole temporal lobe reduced by approximately 5–6% Reductions also found in planum temporale and anterior/posterior superior temporal gyrus
Hippocampus	10+ studies. Consistent reductions shown in most studies of around 4%
Parahippocampus	10+ studies. Parahippocampus reduced by about 10%
Amygdala	10+ studies. Overall reduced by around 4% compared to controls
Basal ganglia	20+ studies. Increased globus pallidus size by around 20%. Association found between enlargement and antipsychotic exposure, e.g. Chakos *et al.* (1994). Caudate and putamen do not consistently show enlargement
Thalamus	10+ studies. Several negative studies exist but meta-analysis shows significant differences between patients and controls overall
Lateral ventricles	20+ studies. Increased by approximately 20%, although a larger difference is found for the body of the lateral ventricles (47–50%) and the occipital horns (28–31%). Enlargement of lateral ventricles may be greater in men
Third ventricle	30+ studies. Consistently shows enlargement averaging 26% overall

Clinical relationships

Qualitative abnormality and clinical utility

The available evidence, using either CT or MRI, suggests that the rate of unsuspected cerebral abnormality in schizophrenia is higher than in healthy controls (Lawrie *et al.* 1997). The rate at which clinically significant abnormality is detected is somewhat lower, between 0% (Lieberman *et al.* 1992; Harvey *et al.* 1993) and 4–5% (Waddington *et al.* 1990; Lawrie *et al.* 1997) in patients with schizophrenia. In a study of 1000 healthy asymptomatic research volunteers at the National Institutes of Health (Bethesda, USA), only 82% of the MRI results were reported as entirely normal. However, of the 18% showing abnormal findings, 15.1% required no referral; 1.8% required routine referral and 1.1% required urgent referral. None required immediate referral. In subjects grouped for urgent referral, two (possibly three) had primary brain tumours. These results suggest that unsuspected abnormalities are relatively common in patients with schizophrenia and healthy volunteers (Katzman *et al.* 1999), but the rate of clinically significant findings is relatively low and does not justify routine imaging for clinical reasons. There is however, little doubt that benign neurodevelopmental abnormalities are more common in schizophrenic patients than in controls (Lawrie *et al.*, 1997). Although their importance to the neurodevelopmental hypothesis of schizophrenia is acknowledged (Weinberger 1987), their clinical value is somewhat limited and appears to carry no additional treatment implications.

Prospective studies of people at increased risk of schizophrenia have found subtle differences in brain structure which are evident in the premorbid state and which might allow psychosis to be predicted. These studies (which are discussed in detail later in this chapter) have found differences in regions such as the anterior cingulate cortex, amygdala–hippocampus, thalamus, and lateral ventricles, which are greater in the high-risk subjects who eventually become psychotic than those who remain well (e.g. Johnstone *et al.* 2002; Pantelis *et al.*, 2003). The sensitivity and specificity of these measures remains uncertain and will require to be clarified in independent test set samples before the methods can be considered to be clinically useful.

Currently, the role of sMRI in clinical practice appears limited to those patients in whom an underlying lesion is suspected. Even in this situation, the utility of sMRI is somewhat limited. The ability to define and reliably measure smaller and smaller structures means that sMRI may yet be useful clinically to differentiate schizophrenia from other disorders and to predict outcome in those with an established diagnosis. However, even if an MRI measure can be shown to have sufficiently high specificity, the relatively low prevalence of schizophrenia in the general population is likely to restrict its use to people who at are increased risk of schizophrenia for genetic or other reasons.

Diagnostic specificity

Since some symptoms of schizophrenia (e.g. hallucinations, delusions) are also manifest in a number of patients with affective disorder, it is not surprising that these two syndromes show a degree of overlap in their gross neuroanatomy. Several studies have also shown, in families multiply affected by psychosis, that schizophrenia and bipolar disorder do not 'breed true' (Kendler *et al.* 1993; Valles *et al.* 2000). These results suggest that the phenotypes of schizophrenia and bipolar disorder are, at least, imperfectly defined.

Lateral ventricular enlargement has been found in the majority of studies comparing bipolar patients with healthy controls (Jurjus *et al.* 1993; Friedman *et al.* 1999) and has been associated with poor outcome (Johnstone *et al.* 1989*b*) and psychotic symptoms (Kato *et al.* 1994). Although temporal volume reductions are relatively well replicated in schizophrenia, differences between bipolar patients and controls are less consistent (Hauser *et al.* 1989; Harvey *et al.* 1994). Several recent studies have reported no reduction in amygdala volume in affective disorder and three research groups have found an increased volume in bipolar patients (e.g. Altshuler *et al.* 1998). This is a potentially specific neuroanatomical difference between the major psychoses, but requires further replication with direct comparisons between schizophrenic and bipolar patients (see, for example, Kubicki *et al.* 2002). Other cerebral regions have also been examined with respect to diagnostic specificity for schizophrenia as opposed to affective disorder, but the results are in general equivocal (Bearden *et al.* 2001).

MRI findings by symptom and factor

The limitations of a categorical approach to the diagnosis of psychotic illness have long been apparent, even to some of the earliest researchers in the field (e.g. Kraepelin in the twentieth century). Diagnosis frequently fails to predict symptoms, treatment response, or outcome, and many risk factors for schizophrenia are also risk factors for affective disorder. The failings of our current diagnostic systems have led some to speculate that a dimensional approach to diagnosis might be based on safer assumptions (McIntosh et al. 2001; Peralta et al. 2001; Serretti et al. 2001), with some epidemiological support (van Os et al. 1999; Stefanis et al. 2002).

The earliest studies of dimensions of psychopathology and schizophrenia (Liddle 1987, 1992; Liddle and Morris 1991; Liddle et al. 1992; Johnstone and Frith 1996) showed that three syndromes of psychopathology could be identified: reality distortion (delusions and hallucinations), disorganization (thought disorder), and psychomotor poverty (negative symptom) syndromes. Using VBM, Chua (1997) found that there was a significant negative correlation between psychomotor poverty score and the volume of the left prefrontal grey matter, and a significant positive correlation between disorganization and the relative volumes of the hippocampus and the parahippocampal/fusiform gyri. On the other hand, we have related symptom dimensions to volumes in a broad range of psychoses (McIntosh et al. 2001) and have found associations between 'elation' and a larger thalamus and also between 'disorganization' and smaller temporal lobe volumes.

The obvious limitations of diagnoses and the relative complexity of dimensional approaches have led some researchers to look for associations between particular symptoms and brain regions. Studies focusing on hallucinations or delusions have shown a tendency to implicate the temporal lobes, particularly on the left (Barta et al. 1990; Levitan et al. 1999a; Shapleske et al. 2002). Auditory hallucinations have been linked repeatedly to the superior temporal gyrus (STG), and especially the left anterior STG (Levitan et al. 1999b; Rajarethinam et al. 2001). Reductions in left posterior STG grey matter have been found in association with thought disorder (Shenton et al. 1992; Menon et al. 1995; Rajarethinam et al. 2000). Negative symptoms, on the other hand, tend to show an association with smaller prefrontal lobe volumes (Sanfilipo et al. 2000; Gur et al. 2000a). However, there are just as many negative findings for each of these associations. These inconsistencies raise several possibilities. The available studies may have been underpowered and lacking anatomical detail. Symptoms may be better thought of as attributable to disruptions in distributed networks rather than isolated lesions. Alternatively, structural abnormality could be more closely related to psychophysiological abnormality than the clinical features of the current episode.

Neuropsychological associations

It may be that the cerebral disturbance indexed by sMRI is closer to the neuropsychological impairments than the symptoms of schizophrenia; particularly in light of the consistent if non-specific finding of an association between VBR on CT and cognitive deficits. Neuropsychological abnormalities in schizophrenia have been extensively described in many studies. Several studies have also directly related cerebral volumes to neuropsychological performance in schizophrenic subjects. Most have examined executive function or memory (Bornstein *et al.* 1992; Di Michele *et al.* 1992; Nestor *et al.* 1993, 2002; Seidman *et al.* 1994; Bilder *et al.* 1995; Sullivan *et al.* 1996; Torres *et al.* 1997*a*; Baare *et al.* 1999; Levitt *et al.* 1999; Gur *et al.* 2000*b*; Szeszko *et al.* 2000, 2002; Zuffante *et al.* 2001).

Reduced prefrontal lobe volume has been related to both impaired executive function (Szeszko *et al.* 2000) and impaired memory (Seidman *et al.* 1994; Baare *et al.* 1999) although some negative studies do exist—in particular, an attempt to relate working memory to prefrontal cortex (BA 46) (Zuffante *et al.* 2001). Reduced temporal lobe volume has also been associated with impaired memory (Nestor *et al.* 1993; Nestor *et al.* 2002) with similar effects also being found for the hippocampus (Gur *et al.* 2000*b*; O'Driscoll *et al.* 2001) and parahippocampus (Nestor *et al.* 1993). However, again there are several notable negative studies (e.g. Torres *et al.* 1997*b*). Hippocampal volume reduction has also been related to executive function (Bilder *et al.* 1995; Szeszko *et al.* 2000). The latter finding is consistent with the hypothesis of underlying fronto-temporal dysconnectivity in schizophrenia, but could simply reflect the fact that both frontal and temporal structures are necessary for executive and memory function. Interesting suggestions of a relationship between executive function and striatal volume (Stratta *et al.* 1997), and between fusiform gyrus volume and face recognition (Onitsuka *et al.* 2003), have been found, but both await replication.

Duration of illness, progression, and duration of untreated psychosis

Although the vast majority of case-control studies find no association between volume abnormalities and the duration of illness in schizophrenia (Lawrie and Abukmeil, 1998), a number of prospective sMRI studies of schizophrenia have been conducted over the past decade and suggest that there is a progressive element (DeLisi *et al.* 1992, 1995, 1997, 1998; Nair *et al.* 1997; Rapoport *et al.* 1997; Davis *et al.* 1998; Gur *et al.* 1998; Jacobsen *et al.* 1998; Garver *et al.* 2000; Lieberman *et al.* 2001; Mathalon *et al.* 2001; Cahn *et al.* 2002; Ho *et al.*, 2003; Kasai *et al.* 2003). These studies have mainly been conducted on first-episode patients in early adulthood and adolescence, while others have concentrated on older adults with established diagnoses of schizophrenia. There are replicated progressive reductions in the whole brain, frontal and temporal lobes, and of the STG, particularly in the grey matter of first-episode patients. Some studies also show ventricular enlargement, which may be most pronounced in chronic cases. However, these studies do not generally find any compatible clinical progression (Weinberger and McClure 2002). Moreover, it is at least debateable whether such ROI studies have sufficient power to detect differences reliably over relatively short time periods. The question of whether volume reductions over time are specific to schizo-phrenia has been addressed in a single study, which showed no reductions in first-episode affective psychosis over approximately 1.5 years (Kasai *et al.* 2003). These issues are discussed further in Chapter 3.

The finding of progressive volume reductions in schizophrenia has rekindled an interest in neurodegenerative theories, reminiscent of Morel's *démece précoce* (Morel 1860) and Kraepelin's early ideas. Neuropathological studies have consistently failed to find degenerating neurons or gliosis (Harrison 1999), but neurodegeneration is not the only possible explanation for putative progression. Neuronal remodelling, dysregulated apoptosis, excessive synaptic pruning and a loss of dendritic organization could all be part of the explanation. More speculatively, given that neurogenesis is thought to occur in the subventricular zone and dentate gyrus, perhaps the abnormality in schizophrenia is that of reduced formation of new neurons.

The finding of volume reductions in prospective studies of schizophrenic patients and the poor prognostic significance of a long duration between psychotic symptoms and first treatment has led some to speculate that a prolonged duration of untreated psychosis (DUP) may be associated with neurotoxicity. Thus far, only two studies have assessed directly the relationship between DUP and regional brain volumes, and these have found opposing results (Hoff *et al.* 2000; Hietala *et al.* 2003). The evidence for sMRI associations with other aetiological factors is altogether much stronger.

Aetiological associations

Family and twin studies

Structural brain abnormality may be a risk factor for schizophrenia, directly or indir-ectly related to risk factors, an effect of the illness or its treatment, or a combination of these. A family history of schizophrenia has long been established as one of the strongest risk factors for the development of the disorder in unaffected probands (Cannon and Jones 1996). In comparison, other risk factors have generally weaker effects, which are less consistently replicated. The appeal of examining the genetic or at least familial associations of sMRI is therefore obvious. Moreover, the rationale for such studies is relatively strong. First, schizophrenia is associated with cerebral abnormalities and is a highly heritable disorder. Secondly, brain volumes themselves are highly herit-able (Carmelli *et al.* 1998; Baare *et al.* 2001a). Thirdly, they may in themselves be good candidates for both linkage and association analyses (Faraone *et al.* 2003).

Twin studies

Studies of monozygotic (MZ) twins discordant for schizophrenia have the potential to distinguish environmental from genetic effects. In the context of these studies, greater neuroanatomical similarities would be presumed to reflect common genetic effects and differences to reflect environmental effects. However, interpreting such results is limited by the unusual circumstances of twin birth, and differences between twins may be a reflection of different gene expression or gene–environment interaction rather than purely environmental effects. Notwithstanding these limitations, studies of discordant MZ twins have enhanced our understanding of genetic and environmental influences on brain structure in schizophrenia.

In a study of 15 pairs of MZ twins discordant for schizophrenia (Suddath *et al.* 1990), the affected twin had larger ventricles, reduced temporal lobe grey matter and reduced hippocampal volumes. However, no differences were found in either prefrontal lobe volume or white matter. Since prefrontal lobe volume has been shown to be consistently reduced in schizophrenia (Lawrie and Abukmeil 1998; Wright *et al.* 2000) compared to non-related healthy controls, it is possible that a reduced prefrontal lobe volume may be associated with a genetic predisposition to psychosis, while a reduction in temporal lobe grey matter and hippocampal volumes might be associated more closely with the onset of illness itself.

A further study of monozygotic twin pairs discordant for schizophrenia used 15 pairs of discordant monozygotic twins,14 pairs of discordant dizygotic (DZ) twins and 29 healthy twin pairs matched on a number of important confounders of brain volume (Baare *et al.* 2001*b*). Prefrontal brain volumes were smaller in affected versus unaffected monozygotic twins, but this was not apparent for the same sib-wise comparison within the discordant dizygotic twin group. However, irrespective of zygosity, affected twins had smaller whole brain, hippocampal and parahippocampal volumes than their healthy co-twin. Unaffected co-twins had smaller whole brain volumes than twins from unaffected sibships. These findings also suggest that prefrontal brain volumes are associated with the liability to illness and that small whole brain, hippocampal and parahippocampal volumes may also be associated with the development of illness. However, the relationship of these brain regions to genetic vulnerability could not be excluded, due to the relatively small sample sizes, and whole brain volume appeared to be a marker both of illness and genetic vulnerability. A further study specifically examining differences in thalamic and caudate volumes in discordant MZ twins (Bridle *et al.* 2001) found larger caudate nuclei in affected twins but found no differences in thalamic volumes between twin pairs.

In an attempt to further characterize the significance and extent of grey matter deficits in affected and unaffected co-twins, Cannon *et al.* (2002*a*) conducted an automated MRI study of discordant MZ and DZ twins along with a sample of demographically matched control twins. The study used a relatively novel technique of constructing three-dimensional probabilistic maps of the cortex (see Chapter 6). Cortical maps were used to compute three-dimensional vector deformation fields, which allowed researchers to compute a measure to reflect grey matter density at each cortical point. Differences between well twins and their schizophrenic co-twin were found in the region of the dorsolateral prefrontal cortex, superior temporal gyrus, and superior parietal lobule, and were associated with measures of disease severity and cognitive function. No relationship was found with duration of illness or antipsychotic drug treatment. A cortical map of grey matter density associated with genetic proximity to affected patients found deficits in the polar and dorsolateral prefrontal cortex. Medial prefrontal and medial temporal lobe structures could not be assessed in this approach as they cannot be extracted using the surface extraction method employed in the study.

sMRI studies of the 'extended' family

The underlying rationale of examining the first-degree relatives of patients with schizophrenia is that they share approximately 50% of their genome and that common differences versus controls probably reflect genetic factors, while differences between unaffected and affected relatives presumably represent disease-specific effects. A similar degree of abnormality in relatives and patients implies that the volume alterations are not related to the disease itself but are probably related to genetic factors. In some cases, however, studies may be small and of low statistical power, rendering a conclusion of no difference between two groups insecure. It is clear that these studies cannot distinguish genetic and environmental causation, but as schizophrenia is usually found to reflect mainly genetic factors, with a relatively small unique environmental effect, and almost no familial environment involvement (McGuffin *et al.* 1994), the commonalities between patients and their relatives are probably genetic in origin.

Most of these relatives' studies have examined the volumes of the lateral ventricles (LVs) and/or the amygdala–hippocampal complexes (AHCs). Only one study has reported significantly enlarged LVs in relatives as compared to controls (Sharma *et al.* 1998), although most of the studies in siblings (Cannon *et al.* 1998; Seidman *et al.* 1999; Staal *et al.* 2000) or offspring (Schreiber *et al.* 1999; Lawrie *et al.* 2001; Keshavan *et al.* 1997, 2002) give results in that direction. The few comparisons of patients and healthy sibs are, on the other hand, almost universally significant (Cannon *et al.* 1998; Sharma *et al.* 1998; Staal *et al.* 2000; McDonald *et al.* 2002), as are the twin studies, suggesting stronger environmental and phenotypic effects.

However, the evidence from relatives' studies is inconclusive for most other brain regions, in some cases because of insufficient studies and in others due to low power. There are, for example, isolated reports of abnormal cerebral torque (e.g. Sharma *et al.* 1999), but the most consistent abnormalities in patients (Sommer *et al.* 2001) have not been found in relatives (Bartley *et al.* 1993; Frangou *et al.* 1997), and findings of abnormal sylvian fissure (Honer *et al.* 1995) and AHC asymmetry (Schreiber *et al.* 1999) have yet to be replicated (Bartley *et al.* 1993). However, there is a degree of agreement with the twin and automated studies reviewed above for frontal and temporal lobe differences, with the changes greatest in schizophrenic subjects, intermediate in relatives and smallest in controls. The main support for this from ROI studies in relatives is as trends from a large study using sophisticated segmentation algorithms (Cannon *et al.* 1998), and studies contrasting patients with their unaffected relatives (Staal *et al.* 2000, 2002; McDonald *et al.* 2002). Preliminary VBM analyses of the latter study suggest both frontal and temporal reductions, with common genetic and disease effects. Small

(Keshavan *et al.* 1997, 2002; Schreiber *et al.* 1999) and large studies (Lawrie *et al.* 2001) of high-risk offspring have not found such differences, and neither have medium-sized studies which do not control for family membership (Sharma *et al.* 1998). It appears that the relatively small effects require automated approaches and should control for within-family clustering.

The importance of statistical power is illustrated in studies of the third ventricle (3V) and the thalamus (the increase in the former probably reflecting reductions in the latter and other surrounding structures). The only negative studies of the third ventricle in relatives ($n = 15$, Schreiber *et al.*, 1999) and the thalamus ($n = 11$, Keshavan *et al.*, 1997) are the two smallest offspring studies, and Keshavan *et al.* (2002) found thalamus reductions when they increased the sample size to 19. While most of the available literature suggests 3V increases and/or thalamus reductions in relatives more than controls (e.g. Lawrie *et al.* 2001), the only significant patient–relative difference reported is for the thalamus (Staal *et al.* 1998). Thalamus reductions may therefore be genetically mediated risk markers.

However, what the relatives' studies are clear about is that amygdala–hippocampal complex (AHC) reductions are both trait and state related. Relatives have smaller AHCs than controls (Keshavan *et al.* 1997, 2002; Schreiber *et al.* 1999; Seidman *et al.* 1999; Lawrie *et al.* 2001), and schizophrenics have smaller AHCs than relatives (O'Driscoll *et al.* 2001; Lawrie *et al.* 2001; Steel *et al.* 2002), although there are some negative studies (Staal *et al.* 2000). There are suggestions that the reductions may be more marked anteriorly (O'Driscoll *et al.* 2001; Keshavan *et al.* 2002), and on the left side (Lawrie *et al.* 2001; Keshavan *et al.* 2002). However, there is good evidence for hippocampal differences as well (Waldo *et al.* 1994; Harris *et al.* 2002; Narr *et al.* 2002; Seidman *et al.* 2002; van Erp *et al.* 2002a; Schulze *et al.* 2003).

Studies of 'obligate carriers'

Studies of the healthy relatives of schizophrenic subjects have provided a useful design in which to study the effects of genes that raise the liability to schizophrenia. Such studies are generally unconfounded by the effects of medication and are not associated with the expression of the illness itself. However, the proportion of genes shared with the affected relative may be less than 50% and the relative importance of shared genetic factors is likely to be less the more distant the relationship. A potentially stronger design is to consider the unaffected relatives of schizophrenic probands who have both a parent and a child with schizophrenia. Unaffected 'obligate carriers' (Fig. 2.6) can therefore be assumed to have transmitted the genotype from one generation to the next without succumbing to the illness themselves. They also share approximately 50% of their genes with both relatives, and since both are affected, the shared genes are more likely to contain alleles which increase the genetic liability to schizophrenia.

Sharma *et al.* (1998, 1999) were one of the first groups to use the 'obligate carrier' approach to study the effects of genes for schizophrenia. Thirty-one people with

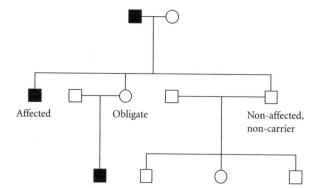

Affected   Obligate   Non-affected,
                                            non-carrier

Fig. 2.6 Idealized family tree demonstrating affected, unaffected, and 'obligate' family members.

schizophrenia were compared to 39 unrelated controls and 57 relatives, of whom 11 were presumed 'obligate carriers'. Obligate carriers had larger left and right lateral ventricles volumes than any other group. A subsequent study by Steel *et al.* (2002) compared six affected sibships of three individuals in which one sibling was an affected subject with schizophrenia, one was a presumed obligate carrier with a child with schizophrenia and one sibling had children who had reached adult life without developing schizophrenia ('non-obligate'). They failed to replicate ventriculomegaly in obligate carriers. In terms of cortical structures, obligates resembled their non-obligate unaffected siblings, both having significantly larger volumes than their affected siblings. However, the amygdala–hippocampal complex was significantly smaller in schizophrenic siblings and their obligate siblings than it was in the non-affected non-obligate sibling. Premorbid IQ, measured by the National Adult Reading Test (NART), was also unexpectedly higher in the sample of obligate carriers.

Studies of familial and sporadic schizophrenia

Studies of the ventricle to brain ratio (VBR) in 'sporadic versus familial' schizophrenia also provide less consensus, as one of the originators of the distinction noted in a review of the early CT studies (Lewis 1990). The rationale is that schizophrenics without an obvious genetic loading are more likely to have had environmental triggers which may increase the VBR, but determining sporadic status is not easy when many healthy relatives are likely to be carrying the gene(s) and, especially in families where there is a poor knowledge of family psychiatric history, an affected subject may be misclassified as 'sporadic' (Johnstone *et al.* 1995). The use of VBR may have further compounded these difficulties by conflating what may be different effects on brain volume and ventricular size in one measure. Indeed, the few sMRI studies to have adopted similar approaches have all reported similar or greater abnormalities in familial cases (Schwarzkopf *et al.* 1991; Roy and Crowe 1994; Falkai *et al.* 2002; Harris *et al.* 2002), with the exception of McDonald *et al.* (2002) and Schulze *et al.* (2003), and some suggest specific genetic effects in frontal and temporal lobes.

Individual gene effects in schizophrenia

Individual gene effects might best be quantified by relating their presence or expression to key clinical features and/or brain imaging findings in both affected subjects and their well relatives. However, to date, very few studies have attempted to relate them to brain structures. Difficulties with this approach are inevitably contingent on the fact that few specific gene effects have been consistently replicated in schizophrenia. Kunugi *et al.* (1999) looked at the relationship between the neurotrophin-3 *A3* allele and regional brain volumes in schizophrenia and bipolar disorder. The results showed *A3* allelic status to be associated with reduced volumes of the hippocampus in schizophrenic but not bipolar subjects. This unconfirmed finding suggests that bipolar subjects may be subject to genetic or environmental factors which ameliorate the effects of this gene. Without further information about the clinical associations of *A3* allelic status it is difficult to draw any firm conclusions from this study. Apolipoprotein E (ApoE) allele status has also been related to hippocampal volume in schizophrenia but the results are inconsistent (Fernandez *et al.* 1999; Hata *et al.* 2002).

Obstetric complications

There is an extensive literature on the clinical effects and imaging abnormalities associated with obstetric complications (OCs). CT has shown associations between OCs and ventriculomegaly in patients and sibs (Reveley *et al.* 1984; DeLisi *et al.* 1986), with a range of adverse neurodevelopmental outcomes. Although many large studies failed to find an association between OCs and increased VBR (Owens *et al.* 1985; Johnstone *et al.* 1989*a*; Jones *et al.* 1994), early data from the Copenhagen High Risk Study (CHRS) strongly suggested a gene–environment interaction, with low birth weight being associated with ventriculomegaly in patients from affected families but not in normal subjects (Silverton *et al.* 1985).

These results have been replicated using sMRI in studies of patients (Alvir *et al.* 1999) and relatives, although there are some negative studies (Sanderson *et al.* 2001). McNeil *et al.* (2000) examined an extended sample of 22 discordant MZ twin pairs and found that those with illness and large (right and total) ventricle volume (but not 3V alone) were more likely to have had labour and neonatal problems, in addition to a prolonged labour. However, adverse events throughout the pregnancy were no more common in patients than in controls. Most recently, Cannon *et al.* (2002*b*) compared 64 patients, 51 of their unaffected sibs and 54 controls for obstetric and perinatal complications. Hypoxic complications interacted with genetic risk to reduce whole brain grey matter volumes (especially in the temporal lobe). Prematurity, small for gestational age status, and prenatal infection had similar effects—they were not associated with adult schizophrenia but rendered the brain more sensitive to the effects of hypoxia.

There is also evidence that OCs are related to small hippocampi in schizophrenia. A small area study of family-history-positive patients found no differences in limbic areas between those with and without birth complications (DeLisi *et al.* 1988), while

Stefanis and colleagues (1999) found a smaller left hippocampus in patients with a history of pregnancy and birth complications, but not in patients from multiply affected families. McNeil *et al.* (2000) reported that intrapair differences in rostral hippocampi volumes between discordant MZ twins were related to prolonged labour. Using original hospital records, and focusing on hypoxic events and 'blue babies', van Erp *et al.* (2002b) found that 72 Finnish patients had smaller hippocampi than 58 siblings, who in turn had smaller volumes than healthy controls, but only patients with documented OCs had smaller hippocampi (sibs with OCs did not). The fact that OC frequency was equal across groups argues against gene–environment co-variation, and the relatively small effect size for hypoxia in the probands (0.24) suggests a sensitivity to the effects of OCs in those destined to become schizophrenic. Further, the intra-class correlations for healthy sibling pairs were higher than for discordant pairs, suggesting that genetic influences on hippocampal volume are larger in health than schizophrenia, and that large genetic variation and/or unique environmental events influence hippocampal volume in patients.

Small and unreplicated studies have reported associations between first-trimester famine (Hulshoff Pol *et al.* 2000) and congenital rubella (Lim *et al.* 1995) with reduced intracranial volume (ICV) in patients with schizophrenia. Sanderson *et al.* (2001) found that patients with a history of early meningitis had reduced AHCs. Season of birth was a widely examined proxy for possible in *utero* infection in CT studies, but most studies find no association between the VBR and time of birth (Silverton *et al.* 1988; DeQuardo *et al.* 1996). However, by far the largest (CT) study did find that patients born between December and April had greater VBRs than those born in other months (Sacchetti *et al.* 1992).

There is therefore fairly strong evidence that OCs, particularly labour complications and documented hypoxia in neonates, interact with genetic risk for schizophrenia to produce larger lateral ventricles and smaller hippocampi. It may be that a genetically small brain and other OCs increase the susceptibility to these effects. The differences may be observable at birth, although there is no direct evidence for this at present.

Prospective study of unaffected individuals at 'high risk' of schizophrenia

High-risk studies follow a cohort of unaffected individuals at increased risk of schizophrenia prospectively through the period of high risk (*c.* age 23 years in males, 26 in women) in the knowledge that some subjects will become affected. This design overcomes several of the difficulties of case-control studies. Imaging findings may be associated with symptoms or neuropsychological performance deficits before and as they arise, and subjects who develop schizophrenia may be scanned before medication has been prescribed.

In spite of the considerable advantages of 'high-risk' studies, they have many practical limitations. Patient attrition, cost and the tendency for both staff and technology to change over time has meant that few centres have exploited this study design successfully. The first high-risk imaging study to be completed was the Copenhagen High Risk Study (CHRS), although the scans (CT) were not repeated over time (Cannon 1989). Two further studies are ongoing, both using sMRI—the Edinburgh High Risk Study (EHRS) and the Melbourne High Risk Study (MHRS).

The Copenhagen High Risk Study

The Copenhagen High Risk Study (Mednick 1966) concerned the children of mothers with schizophrenia. High-risk subjects were compared to healthy controls with no family history of mental illness, matched to high-risk subjects on age, sex, social class, and IQ. The main results suggested that widened fissures and sulci are positively associated to genetic risk but that only schizophrenic subjects have enlarged ventricles (Cannon et al. 1989). A subsequent study of 16 twin pairs discordant for schizophrenia (Zorrilla et al. 1997) found that the sulci to brain ratio and VBR differed between the twin pairs, suggesting an environmental effect or gene–environment interaction.

The Melbourne High Risk Study

Researchers in Melbourne have adopted a different but complementary approach. They have examined groups of people at 'ultra high risk' (UHR) of psychosis, those with first-episode psychosis (FEP, including about 50% with schizophrenia or schizophreniform psychosis), and a large group of healthy controls. The UHR group consisted of referrals to a clinic in Melbourne, of people aged 14–30 with: 'attentuated' partial (positive) psychotic symptoms several times a week for 1 week to 5 years; transient symptoms of less than 1 week's duration in the past year, and/or both trait and state risk factors for psychosis (a family history and a worsening in mental state or general functioning in the past year). Preliminary ROI results suggested non-significant hippocampal reductions in the UHR group and the subgroup of these patients that developed psychosis (Copolov et al. 2000). An early VBM study of nine patients who developed psychosis and 12 who remained well did, however, identify volume reductions in the hippocampus, entorhinal cortex, inferior frontal and fusiform gyri during the transition to psychosis (Pantelis et al. 2002).

Phillips et al. (2002) recently reported on their traced whole brain and hippocampal volumes as possible predictors of psychosis. Between 1995 and 1998, 75% of eligible referrals were scanned, and 5% of scans were lost due to movement artefact, leaving 60 scans. Twenty (33%) of those with usable scans developed an acute psychosis (defined as an increase of one or more points on the Brief Psychiatric Rating Scale (BPRS) or Comprehensive Assessment of Symptoms and History (CASH), several times a week, for more than 1 week) within a year. A Structured Clinical Interview for DSM interview identified diagnoses of schizophrenia spectrum disorder in 11, affective psychosis (3), bipolar disorder (3), and others (3). The UHR groups who did not develop psychosis included four patients with depression and 11 with an anxiety state.

The scans were conducted at two sites and there was a weak tendency for the scanners to deliver different whole brain volumes, and for more of those who developed psychosis (and of one sex) to be scanned at one site (Phillips *et al.* 2002). None the less, controlling for a slightly smaller whole brain, the 60 UHRs has significantly smaller hippocampi (by about 11%, effect size (e.s.) about 0.9) than the controls, but did not differ from the FEPs. However, the UHRs were, on average, 10 years younger and 11 points lower in premorbid IQ than the normals. The 20 who became psychotic were much more closely similar in demographics to the 40 who remained non-psychotic, but, rather counter-intuitively, the (left) hippocampus was *larger* in those who went on to develop a psychosis. These confusing results may be attributable to scanner effects, selection bias, and/or confounding by, for example, other diagnoses or gender.

Pantelis *et al.* (2003) have recently reported on their VBM findings in a slightly extended sample. In 75 people with prodromal symptoms, defined as above, 23 (31%) developed a psychotic disorder (roughly equal numbers of schizophrenia and affective psychoses). Compared to those who did not develop a psychosis, they had less grey matter in right medial temporal, lateral temporal and inferior frontal cortex, and in bilateral cingulate cortex. Twenty-one subjects, 10 of whom had become psychotic (five with schizophrenia), had repeated scans at 1–2 year intervals. They showed reductions over time in left parahippocampal, fusiform, orbitofrontal, and cerebellar grey matter, while those who did not remain psychotic only exhibited cerebellar reductions. These are intriguing results, suggesting grey matter reductions in the run-up to psychosis and immediately after it. However, there are some important issues outstanding—in particular, whether some of those in the UHR group actually had a psychosis before or at study entry, and why the ROI and VBM studies appear to have such different findings.

Edinburgh High Risk Study

The Edinburgh High Risk Study concerns the unaffected young relatives of known patients throughout Scotland, whose consultant knew of a family history of schizophrenia. Healthy family members were included if they had at least two close relatives with a confirmed diagnosis of schizophrenia using the OPCRIT computer program (McGuffin *et al.* 1991). Data were provided by 162 high-risk subjects, and 150 had at least one sMRI scan in the first phase of the study, between 1994 and 1999. Two control groups were also recruited. The first consisted of healthy non-related controls matched as closely as possible for age and sex. The second consisted of patients with first schizophrenic episodes but without a known family history of psychosis. High-risk subjects were further classified, at each of up to 35 interviews so far, into the following categories, according to the Present State Examination (PSE):

0 Symptom free.

1 Any fully rated non-psychotic PSE item (e.g. tension, depression, anxiety).

2 Any partially rated psychotic symptom.

3 Any fully rated psychotic symptom.

4 PSE Catego S+ schizophrenia.

The increased liability to schizophrenia, presumably of genetic origin, was also quantified. Genetic liability to schizophrenia was measured in two ways. The first is an ordinal measure of genetic liability rated, from lowest to highest: two or more second-degree relatives with schizophrenia; one first-degree relative with schizophrenia and one or more second-degree relatives with schizophrenia; and, finally, two or more first-degree relatives with schizophrenia. The other method employs simple matrix algebra to provide a continuous measure of genetic liability, which should, in theory, provide more information about risk (Lawrie *et al.* 2001). High-risk subjects and controls were reassessed every 18 months. Assessments performed included neuropsychological testing and clinical examinations, and a repeat MRI scan of the brain.

Early region-of-interest analysis of the first 100 MRI scans found the amygdala–hippocampal complex to be approximately 4% smaller than that of controls, and about 4% larger than that of subjects with schizophrenia (Lawrie *et al.* 1999). An increase in third ventricular volume was found in high-risk subjects compared to controls, although this was not significant after the correlation in volumes between subjects from the same family had been taken into account (Lawrie *et al.* 2001). VBM confirms these early results and also shows medial prefrontal and temporal lobe reductions in grey matter density with a gradient that is greatest in first episodes, intermediate in high risks and lowest in controls (Job *et al.* 2002, 2003). Within high-risk subjects, higher genetic liability was associated with smaller left and right prefrontal lobes and smaller left and right thalami (Lawrie *et al.* 2001).

Changes in brain size were also measured using repeat scans in the 66 high-risk subjects and 20 healthy controls (Lawrie *et al.* 2002). Changes within the high-risk group were also compared for subgroups according to whether or not they had fully rated psychotic symptoms in the first phase of the study. No differences were found between controls and high-risk subjects as a whole. When high risks with symptoms were compared to those without symptoms, those with psychotic symptoms showed a greater reduction in right temporal lobe volume compared to those without symptoms and similar, though non-significant, differences were also reported in respect of the left temporal lobe and the prefrontal cortex bilaterally. These results have also been replicated using VBM (Job *et al.*, in preparation).

Preliminary analyses of baseline region-of-interest data found that a small thalamus might predict (early) onset of schizophrenia (Johnstone *et al.* 2002). These results have recently been confirmed in the 21 subjects who have developed schizophrenia by the time of writing. The AHC volumes have weaker predictive effects, but they and the thalami appear to reduce further as psychosis develops.

Both sMRI high-risk studies have therefore reported reduced medial temporal lobe structures as a risk marker for schizophrenia and suggest further volume losses around the time of onset.

Conclusions

Although a neuroanatomical profile of schizophrenia is beginning to emerge, the precise nature of the findings requires clarification. In particular, regions with poorly demarcated boundaries are difficult to measure accurately with traditional ROI analysis. Parcellation and VBM are likely to be useful in examining these and small structures with low measurement reliability.

Methodological aspects of sMRI have been shown to exert some influence on the findings of individual studies, but the number and type of patients examined are probably more potent factors. Volume equivalence in a given brain region can only be established by scanning large numbers of representative patients, and few studies could be said to satisfy this criterion. Many twin and family studies assume that equivalence in a regional volume represents a genetic influence, but rarely are the studies sufficiently sized to make this a strong conclusion. Larger studies might also help to clarify the clinical associations of sMRI findings in schizophrenia and whether they extend into other psychoses. On the other hand, given that symptoms and cognitive function are likely to be mediated by networks rather than circumscribed regions of neurons, and potentially affected by pathoplastic effects (e.g. 'personality', life events, and other historical factors), functional imaging is likely to prove more fruitful.

The timing of many findings and the possibility of their progression before and after illness onset is the most controversial issue in sMRI at the present time. Studies of individuals at high risk suggest that some of the changes in schizophrenia predate the disorder and others emerge around onset. Such prospective studies are the best way to establish cause and effect, but are difficult to conduct. Very important information can be more easily obtained from case-control studies that examine the associations between imaging abnormalities and known risk factors for the disorder. At the same time, we need more follow-up studies of people with schizophrenia, with carefully conducted evaluations of both structural volumes and clinical status.

References

Altshuler, L. L., Bartzokis, G., Grieder, T., Curran, J., and Mintz, J. (1998). Amygdala enlargement in bipolar disorder and hippocampal reduction in schizophrenia: an MRI study demonstrating neuroanatomic specificity. *Archives of General Psychiatry*, 55, 663–4.

Alvir, J. M., Woernel, M. G., Gunduz, H., Degreef, G., and Lieberman, J. A. (1999). Obstetric complications predict treatment response in first-episode schizophrenia. *Psychological Medicine*, 29(3), 621–7.

Andreasen, N. C., Arndt, S., Swayze, V., Cizadlo, T., Flaum, M., O'Leary, D. *et al.* (1994a). Thalamic abnormalities in schizophrenia visualized through magnetic resonance image averaging. [comment]. *Science*, 266, 294–8.

Andreasen, N. C., Flashman, L., Flaum, M., Arndt, S., Swayze, V., O'Leary, D. S. *et al.* (1994b). Regional brain abnormalities in schizophrenia measured with magnetic resonance imaging. *Journal of the American Medical Association*, 272, 1763–9.

Baare, W. F., Hulshoff Pol, H. E., Hijman, R., Mali, W. P., Viergever, M. A., and Kahn, R. S. (1999). Volumetric analysis of frontal lobe regions in schizophrenia: relation to cognitive function and symptomatology. *Biological Psychiatry*, **45**, 1597–605.

Baare, W. F., Hulshoff Pol, H. E., Boomsma, D. I., Posthuma, D., de Geus, E. J., Schnack, H. G. *et al.* (2001*a*). Quantitative genetic modeling of variation in human brain morphology. *Cerebral Cortex*, **11**, 816–24.

Baare, W. F., van Oel, C. J., Hulshoff Pol, H. E., Schnack, H. G., Durston, S., Sitskoorn, M. M. *et al.* (2001*b*). Volumes of brain structures in twins discordant for schizophrenia. *Archives of General Psychiatry*, **58**, 33–40.

Barr, W. B., Ashtari, M., Bilder, R. M., Degreef, G., and Lieberman, J. A. (1997). Brain morphometric comparison of first-episode schizophrenia and temporal lobe epilepsy. *British Journal of Psychiatry*, **170**, 515–19.

Barta, P. E., Pearlson, G. D., Powers, R. E., Richards, S. S., and Tune, L. E. (1990). Auditory hallucinations and smaller superior temporal gyral volume in schizophrenia. *American Journal of Psychiatry*, **147**, 1457–62.

Bartley, A. J., Jones, D. W., Torrey, E. F., Zigun, J. R., and Weinberger, D. R. (1993). Sylvian fissure asymmetries in monzygotic twins: a test of laterality in schizophrenia. *Biological Psychiatry*, **34**, 853–63.

Bearden, C. E., Hoffman, K. M., and Cannon, T. D. (2001). The neuropsychology and neuroanatomy of bipolar affective disorder: a critical review. *Bipolar Disorders*, **3**, 106–50.

Beck, B., Plant, D. H., Grant, S. C., Thelwall, P. E., Silver, X., Mareci, T. H. *et al.* (2002). Progress in high field MRI at the University of Florida. *Magma*, **13**, 152–7.

Bilder, R. M., Wu, H., Bogerts, B., Degreef, G., Ashtari, M., Alvir, J. M. *et al.* (1994). Absence of regional hemispheric volume asymmetries in first-episode schizophrenia. *American Journal of Psychiatry*, **151**, 1437–47.

Bilder, R. M., Bogerts, B., Ashtari, M., Wu, H., Alvir, J. M., Jody, D. *et al.* (1995). Anterior hippocampal volume reductions predict frontal lobe dysfunction in first episode schizophrenia. *Schizophrenia Research*, **17**, 47–58.

Bornstein, R. A., Schwarzkopf, S. B., Olson, S. C., and Nasrallah, H. A. (1992). Third-ventricle enlargement and neuropsychological deficit in schizophrenia. *Biological Psychiatry*, **31**, 954–61.

Bridle, N., Pantelis, C., Wood, S. J., Coppola, R., Velakoulis, D., McStephen, M. *et al.* (2001). Thalamic and caudate volumes in monozygotic twins discordant for schizophrenia. *Australian and New Zealand Journal of Psychiatry*, **36**, 347–54.

Budinger, T. F. and Lauterbur, P. C. (1984). Nuclear magnetic resonance technology for medical studies. *Science*, **226**, 95–102.

Cahn, W., Hulshoff Pol, H. E., Lems, E. B. T. E., van Haren, N. E. M., Schnack, H. G., van der Linden, J. A. *et al.* (2002). Brain volume changes in first episode schizophenia. A 1-year follow up study. *Archives of General Psychiatry*, **59**, 1002–10.

Cannon, M. and Jones, P. (1996). Schizophrenia. *Journal of Neurology, Neurosurgery and Psychiatry*, **60**, 604–613.

Cannon, T. D., Mednick, S. A., and Parnas, J. (1989). Genetic and perinatal determinants of structural brain deficits in schizophrenia. *Archives of General Psychiatry*, **46**, 883–9.

Cannon, T. D., van Erp, T. G., Huttunen, M., Lonnqvist, J., Salonen, O., Valanne, L. *et al.* (1998). Regional gray matter, white matter and cerebrospinal fluid distributions in schizophrenic patients, their siblings and controls. *Archives of General Psychiatry*, **59**, 35–41.

Cannon, T. D., Thompson, P. M., van Erp, T. G., Toga, A. W., Poutanen, V. P., Huttunen, M. *et al.* (2002*a*). Cortex mapping reveals regionally specific patterns of genetic and disease-specific gray-matter deficits in twins discordant for schizophrenia. *Proceedings of the National Academy of Sciences USA*, **99**, 3228–33.

Cannon, T. D., van Erp, T. G., Rosso, I. M., Huttunen, M., Lonnqvist, J., Pirkola, T. *et al.* (2002*b*). Fetal hypoxia and structural brain abnormalities in schizophrenic patients, their siblings, and controls. *Archives of General Psychiatry*, **59**, 35–41.

Carmelli, D., DeCarli, C., Swan, G. E., Jack, L. M., Reed, T., Wolf, P. A. *et al.* (1998). Evidence for genetic variance in white matter hyperintensity volume in normal elderly male twins. *Stroke*, **29**, 1177–81.

Caviness, V. S., Makris, N., Lange, N. T., Herbert, M., and Kennedy, D. N. (2000). Advanced applications of MRI in human brain science. *Keio Journal of Medicine*, **49**, 66–73.

Chakos, M. H., Lieberman, J. A., Bilder, R. M., Borenstein, M., Lerner, G., Bogerts, B. *et al.* (1994). Increase in caudate nuclei volumes of first-episode schizophrenic patients taking antipsychotic drugs. *American Journal of Psychiatry* **151**, 1430–6.

Chua, S. E., Wright, I. C., Poline, J. B., Liddle, P. F., Murray, R. M., Frackowiak, R. S. *et al.* (1997). Grey matter correlates of syndromes in schizophrenia. A semi-automated analysis of structural magnetic resonance images[comment]. *British Journal of Psychiatry*, **170**, 406–10.

Copolov, D., Velakoulis, D., McGorry, P., Mallard, C., Yung, A., Rees, S., *et al.* (2000). Neurobiological findings in early phase schizophrenia. *Brain Research Reviews*, **31**, 157–65.

Cosway, R., Byrne, M., Clafferty, R., Hodges, A., Grant, E., Abukmeil, S. S. *et al.* (2000). Neuropsychological change in young people at high risk for schizophrenia: results from the first two neuropsychological assessments of the Edinburgh High Risk Study. *Psychological Medicine*, **30**, 1111–21.

Crespo-Facorro, B., Kim, J. J., Andreasen, N. C., O'Leary, D. S., Wiser, A. K., Bailey, J. M. *et al.* (1999). Human frontal cortex: an MRI-based parcellation method. *Neuroimage*, **10**, 500–19.

David, A. S., Brierley, B., and Shaw, P. (2002). Measuring amygdala volume [comment]. *British Journal of Psychiatry*, **181**, 255–6.

Davidson, L. L. and Heinrichs, R. W. (2003). Quantification of frontal and temporal lobe brain-imaging findings in schizophrenia: a meta-analysis. *Psychiatry Research: Neuroimaging*, **122**, 69–87.

Davis, K. L., Buchsbaum, M. S., Shihabuddin, L., Spiegel-Cohen, J., Metzger, M., Frecska, E. *et al.* (1998). Ventricular enlargement in poor outcome schizophrenia. *Biological Psychiatry*, **43**, 783–93.

DeLisi, L. E., Goldin, L. R., Hamovit, J. R., Maxwell, M. E., Kurtz, D., and Gershon, E. S. (1986). A family study of the association of increased ventricular size with schizophrenia. *Archives of General Psychiatry*, **43**, 148–53.

DeLisi, L. E., Dauphinais, I. D., and Gershon, E. S. (1988). Perinatal complications and reduced size of brain limbic structures in familial schizophrenia. *Schizophrenia Bulletin*, **14**, 185–91.

DeLisi, L. E., Hoff, A. L., Schwartz, J. E., Shields, G. W., Halthore, S. N., Gupta, S. M., *et al.* (1991). Brain morphology in first-episode schizophrenic-like psychotic patients: a quantitative magnetic resonance imaging study. *Biological Psychiatry*, **29**, 159–75 [erratum appears in *Biological Psychiatry*, 1991, **29**(5), 519].

DeLisi, L. E., Hoff, A. L., Kushner, M., Calev, A., and Stritzke, P. (1992). Left ventricular enlargement associated with diagnostic outcome of schizophreniform disorder. *Biological Psychiatry*, **32**, 199–201.

DeLisi, L. E., Tew, W., Xie, S., Hoff, A. L., Sakuma, M., Kushner, M. *et al.* (1995). A prospective follow-up study of brain morphology and cognition in first-episode schizophrenic patients: preliminary findings. *Biological Psychiatry*, **38**, 349–60.

DeLisi, L. E., Sakuma, M., Tew, W., Kushner, M., Hoff, A. L., and Grimson, R. (1997). Schizophrenia as a chronic active brain process: a study of progressive brain structural change subsequent to the onset of schizophrenia. *Psychiatry Research*, **74**, 129–40.

DeLisi, L. E., Sakuma, M., Ge, S., and Kushner, M. (1998). Association of brain structural change with heterogeneous course of schizophrenia from early childhood through five years subsequent to a first hospitalization. *Psychiatry Research*, **84**, 75–88.

DeQuardo, J. R., Goldman, M., and Tendon, R. (1996). VBR in schizophrenia: relationship to family history of psychosis and season of birth. *Schizophrenia Research*, **20**(3), 275–85.

Di Michele, V., Rossi, A., Stratta, P., Schiazza, G., Bolino, F., Giordano, L. *et al.* (1992). Neuropsychological and clinical correlates of temporal lobe anatomy in schizophrenia. *Acta Psychiatrica Scandinavica*, **85**, 484–8.

Falkai, P., Honer, W. G., Alfter, D., Schneider-Axmann, T., Bussfeld, P., Cordes, J., *et al.* (2002). The temporal lobe in schizophrenia from uni- and multiply affected families. *Neuroscience Letters*, **325**, 25–8.

Faraone, S. V., Seidman, L. J., Kremen, W. S., Kennedy, D., Makris, N., Caviness, V. S. *et al.* (2003). Structural brain abnormalities among relatives of patients with schizophrenia: implications for linkage studies. *Schizophrenia Research*, **60**, 125–40.

Fernandez, T., Yan, W. L., Hamburger, S., Rapoport, J. L., Saunders, A. M., Schapiro, M. *et al.* (1999). Apolipoprotein E alleles in childhood-onset schizophrenia. *American Journal of Medical Genetics*, **88**, 211–13.

Frangou, S., Sharma, T., Sigmundson, T., Barta, P., Pearlson, G., and Murray, R. M. (1997). The Maudsley Family Study 4. Normal planum temporale asymmetry in familial schizophrenia. *British Journal of Psychiatry*, **170**, 328–33.

Friedman, L., Findling, R. L., Kenny, J. T., Swales, T. P., Stuve, T. A., Jesberger, J. A. *et al.* (1999). An MRI study of adolescent patients with either schizophrenia or bipolar disorder as compared to healthy control subjects. *Biological Psychiatry*, **46**, 78–88.

Garver, D. L., Nair, T. R., Christensen, J. D., Holcomb, J. A., and Kingsbury, S. J. (2000) Brain and ventricular instability during psychotic episodes of the schizophrenias. *Schizophrenia Research*, **44**, 11–23.

Gaser, C., Volz, H. P., Kiebel, S., Riehemann, S., and Sauer, H. (1999). Detecting structural changes in whole brain based on nonlinear deformations-Application to schizophrenia research. *Neuroimage*, **10**, 107–13.

Gilbert, A. R., Rosenberg, D. R., Harenski, K., Spencer, S., Sweeney, J. A., and Keshavan, M. S. (2001). Thalamic volumes in patients with first-episode schizophrenia. *American Journal of Psychiatry*, **158**, 618–24.

Goldstein, J. M., Goodman, J. M., Seidman, L. J., Kennedy, D. N., Makris, N., Lee, H. *et al.* (1999). Cortical abnormalities in schizophrenia identified by structural magnetic resonance imaging. *Archives of General Psychiatry*, **56**, 537–47.

Goldstein, J. M., Seidman, L. J., O'Brien, L. M., Horton, N. J., Kennedy, D. N., Makris, N. *et al.* (2002). Impact of normal sexual dimorphisms on sex differences in structural brain abnormalities in schizophrenia assessed by magnetic resonance imaging. *Archives of General Psychiatry*, **59**, 154–64.

Gunduz, H., Wu, H., Ashtari, M., Bogerts, B., Crandall, D., Robinson, D. G. *et al.* (2002). Basal ganglia volumes in first-episode schizophrenia and healthy compairson subjects. *Biological Psychiatry*, **51**, 801–8.

Gur, R. E., Cowell, P., Turetsky, B. I., Gallacher, F., Cannon, T., Bilker, W. *et al.* (1998). A follow-up magnetic resonance imaging study of schizophrenia: relationship of neuroanatomical changes to clinical and neurobehavioral measures. *Archives of General Psychiatry*, **55**, 145–52.

Gur, R. E., Cowell, P. E., Latshaw, A., Turetsky, B. I., Grossman, R. I., Arnold, S. E. *et al.* (2000*a*). Reduced dorsal and orbital prefrontal gray matter volumes in schizophrenia. *Archives of*

General Psychiatry, **57**, 761–8 [erratum appears in *Archives of General Psychiatry*, 2000, **57**(9), 858].

Gur, R. E., Turetsky, B. I., Cowell, P. E., Finkelman, C., Maany, V., Grossman, R. I. *et al.* (2000*b*). Temporolimbic volume reductions in schizophrenia. *Archives of General Psychiatry*, **57**, 769–75.

Harris, J. G., Young, D. A., Rojas, D. C., Cajade-Law, A., Scherzinger, A., Nawroz, S. *et al.* (2002). Increased hippocampal volume in schizophrenics' parents with ancestral history of schizophrenia. *Schizophrenia Research*, **55**, 11–17.

Harrison, P. J. (1999). The neuropathology of schizophrenia: a critical review of the data and their interpretation. *Brain*, **122**, 593–624.

Harvey, I., Ron, M. A., Du Boulay, G., Wicks, D., Lewis, S. W., and Murray, R. M. (1993). Reduction of cortical volume in schizophrenia on magnetic resonance imaging. *Psychological Medicine*, **23**, 591–604.

Harvey, I., Persaud, R., Ron, M. A., Baker, G., and Murray, R. M. (1994). Volumetric MRI measurements in bipolars compared with schizophrenics and healthy controls. *Psychological Medicine*, **24**, 689–99.

Hata, T., Kunugi, H., Nanko, S., Fukuda, R., and Kaminaga, T. (2002). Possible effect of the APOE epsilon 4 allele on the hippocampal volume and asymmetry in schizophrenia. *American Journal of Medical Genetics*, **114**, 641–2.

Hauser, P., Altshuler, L. L., Berrettini, W., Dauphinais, I. D., Gelernter, J., and Post, R. M. (1989). Temporal lobe measurement in primary affective disorder by magnetic resonance imaging. *Journal of Neuropsychiatry and Clinical Neurosciences*, **1**, 128–34.

Hietala, J., Canon, T. D., van Erp, T. G., Syva lahti E., Vilkman, H., Laakso, A., *et al.* (2003). Regional brain morphology and duration or illness in never-medicated first-episode patients with schizophrenia. *Schizophrenia Research*, **64**(1), 79–81.

Ho, B. C., Alicata, D., Ward, J., Moser, D. J., O'Leary, D. S., Arndt, S. *et al.* (2003). Untreated initial psychosis: relation to cognitive deficits and brain morphology in first-episode schizophrenia. *American Journal of Psychiatry*, **160**, 142–8.

Hoff, A. L., Sakuma, M., Razi, K., Heydebrand, G., Csernansky, J. G., and DeLisi, L. E. (2000). Lack of association between duration of untreated illness and severity of cognitive and structural brain deficits at the first episode of schizophrenia.[comment]. *American Journal of Psychiatry*, **157**, 1824–8.

Honer, W. G., Bassett, A. S., Squires-Wheeler, E., Falkai, P., Smith, G. N., Lapointe, J. S. *et al.* (1995). The temporal lobes, reversed asymmetry and the genetics of schizophrenia. *NeuroReport*, **7**, 221–4.

Hulshoff Pol, H. E., Hoek, H. W., Susser, E., Brown, A. S., Dingemans, A., Schnack, H. G., *et al.* (2000). Prenatal exposure to famine and brain morphology in schizophrenia. *American Journal of Psychiatry*, **157**, 1170–2.

Jacobsen, L. K., Giedd, J. N., Castellanos, F. X., Vaituzis, A. C., Hamburger, S., Kumra, S. *et al.* (1998). Progressive reduction of temporal lobe structures in childhood-onset schizophrenia. *American Journal of Psychiatry*, **155**, 678–85.

James, A. C., Crow, T. J., Renowden, S., Wardell, A. M., Smith, D. M., and Anslow, P. (1999). Is the course of brain development in schizophrenia delayed? Evidence from onsets in adolescence. *Schizophrenia Research*, **40**, 1–10.

Jernigan, T. L., Zisook, S., Heaton, R. K., Moranville, J. T., Hesselink, J. R., and Braff, D. L. (1991). Magnetic resonance imaging abnormalities in lenticular nuclei and cerebral cortex in schizophrenia. *Archives of General Psychiatry*, **48**, 881–90.

Job, D. E., Whalley, H. C., McConnell, S., Glabus, M., Johnstone, E. C., and Lawrie, S. M. (2002). Structural gray matter differences between first-episode schizophrenics and normal controls using voxel-based morphometry. *Neuroimage*, **17**, 880–9.

Job, D. E., Whalley, H. C., McConnell, S., Glabus, M., Johnstone, E. C., and Lawrie, S. M. (2003). Voxel based morphometry of grey matter densities in subjects at high risk of schizophrenia. *Schizophrenia Research*, **64**(1), 1–13.

Johnstone, E. C. and Frith, C. D. (1996). Validation of three dimensions of schizophrenic symptoms in a large unselected sample of patients. *Psychological Medicine*, **26**, 669–79.

Johnstone, E. C., Owens, D. G., Bydder, G. M., Colter, N., Crow, T. J., and Frith, C. D. (1989*a*). The spectrum of structural brain changes in schizophrenia: age of onset as a predictor of cognitive and clinical impairments and their cerebral correlates. *Psychological Medicine*, **19**, 91–103.

Johnstone, E. C., Owens, D. G., Crow, T. J., Frith, C. D., Alexandropolis, K., Bydder, G. *et al.* (1989*b*). Temporal lobe structure as determined by nuclear magnetic resonance in schizophrenia and bipolar affective disorder. *Journal of Neurology, Neurosurgery and Psychiatry*, **52**, 736–41.

Johnstone, E. C., Lang, F. H., Owens, D. G. C., and Frith, C. D. (1995). Determinants of the extremes of outcome in schizophrenia. *British Journal of Psychiatry*, **167**, 604–9.

Johnstone, E. C., Cosway, R., and Lawrie, S. M. (2002). Distinguishing characteristics of subjects with good and poor early outcome in the Edinburgh High-Risk Study. *British Journal of Psychiatry-Supplementum*, **181**, s26–s29.

Jones, P. B., Harvey, I., Lewis, S. W., Toone, B. K., van Os, J., Williams, M. *et al.* (1994). Cerebral ventricle dimensions as risk factors for schizophrenia and affective psychosis: an epidemiological approach to analysis. *Psychological Medicine*, **24**, 995–1011.

Jurjus, G. J., Nasrallah, H. A., Brogan, M., and Olson, S. C. (1993). Developmental brain anomalies in schizophrenia and bipolar disorder: a controlled MRI study. *Journal of Neuropsychiatry and Clinical Neurosciences*, **5**, 375–8.

Kasai, K., Shenton, M. E., Salisbury, D. F., Hirayasu, Y., Lee, C., Ciszewski, A. A. *et al.* (2003). Progressive decrease of left superior temporal gyrus grey matter volume in patients with first-episode schizophrenia. *American Journal of Psychiatry*, **160**, 156–64.

Kato, T., Shioiri, T., Murashita, J., Hamakawa, H., Inubushi, T., and Takahashi, S. Phosphorus-31 magnetic resonance spectroscopy and ventricular enlargement in bipolar disorder. *Psychiatry Research*, **55**, 41–50.

Katzman, G. L., Dagher, A. P., and Patronas, N. J. Incidental findings on brain magnetic resonance imaging from 1000 asymptomatic volunteers. *Journal of the American Medical Association*, **282**, 36–9.

Kelsoe, J. R. Jr, Cadet, J. L., Pickar, D., and Weinberger, D. R. (1988). Quantitative neuroanatomy in schizophrenia. A controlled magnetic resonance imaging study. *Archives of General Psychiatry*, **45**, 533–41.

Kendler, K. S., McGuire, M., Gruenberg, A. M., O'Hare, A., Spellman, M., and Walsh, D. (1993). The Roscommon Family Study. IV. Affective illness, anxiety disorders, and alcoholism in relatives. *Archives of General Psychiatry*, **50**, 952–60.

Keshavan, M. S., Montrose, D. M., Pierri, J. N., Dick, E. L., Rosenberg, D., Talagala, L. *et al.* (1997). Magnetic resonance imaging and spectroscopy in offspring at risk for schizophrenia: preliminary studies. *Progress in Neuropsychopharmacology and Biological Psychiatry*, **21**, 1285–95.

Keshavan, M. S., Rosenberg, D., Sweeney, J. A., and Pettegrew, J. W. (1998). Decreased caudate volume in neuroleptic-naive psychotic patients. *American Journal of Psychiatry*, **155**, 774–8.

Keshavan, M. S., Dick, E., Mankowski, I., Harenski, K., Montrose, D. M., Diwadkar, V. *et al.* (2002). Decreased left amygdala and hippocampal volumes in young offspring at risk for schizophrenia. *Schizophrenia Research*, **58**, 173–83.

Kim, J. J., Youn, T., Lee, J. M., Kim, I. Y., Kim, S. I., and Kwon, J. S. (2003). Morphometric abnormality of the insula in schizophrenia: a comparison with obsessive-compulsive disorder and normal control using MRI. *Schizophrenia Research*, **60**, 191–8.

Kubicki, M., Shenton, M. E., Salisbury, D. F., Hirayasu, Y., Kasai, K., Kikinis, R. *et al.* (2002). Voxel-based morphometric analysis of gray matter in first episode schizophrenia. *NeuroImage*, 17, 1711–19.

Kunugi, H., Hattori, M., Nanko, S., Fujii, K., Kato, T. and Nanko, S. (1999). Dinucleotide repeat polymorphism in the neurotrophin-3 gene and hippocampal volume in psychoses. *Schizophrenia Research*, 37, 271–3.

Lang, D. J., Kopala, L. C., Vandorpe, R. A., Rui, Q., Smith, G. N., Goghari, V. M. *et al.* (2001). An MRI study of basal ganglia volumes in first-episode schizophrenia patients treated with risperidone. *American Journal of Psychiatry*, 158, 625–31.

Lauterbur, P. C. (1973). Image formation by induced local interactions: examples employing nuclear magnetic resonance. *Nature*, 242, 190–1.

Lawrie, S. M. and Abukmeil, S. S. (1998). Brain abnormality in schizophrenia. A systematic and quantitative review of volumetric magnetic resonance imaging studies. *British Journal of Psychiatry*, 172, 110–20.

Lawrie, S. M., Abukmeil, S. S., Chiswick, A., Egan, V., Santosh, C. G., and Best, J. J. K. (1997). Qualitative cerebral morphology in schizophrenia: a magnetic resonance imaging study and systematic literature review. *Schizophrenia Research*, 25, 155–66.

Lawrie, S. M., Whalley, H. C., Kestelman, J. N., Abukmeil, S. S., Byrne, M., Hodges, A. *et al.* (1999). Magnetic resonance imaging of the brain in people at high risk of developing schizophrenia. *Lancet*, 353, 30–3.

Lawrie, S. M., Whalley, H. C., Abukmeil, S. S., Kestelman, J. N., Miller, P., Best, J. J. K. *et al.* (2001). Brain structure, genetic liability and psychotic symptoms in subjects at high risk of developing schizophrenia. *Biological Psychiatry*, 49, 811–23.

Lawrie, S. M., Whalley, H. C., Abukmeil, S. S., Kestelman, J. N., Miller, P., Best, J. J. *et al.* (2002). Temporal lobe volume changes in people at high risk of schizophrenia with psychotic symptoms. *British Journal of Psychiatry*, 181, 138–43.

Levitan, C., Ward, P. B., and Catts, S. V. (1999). Superior temporal gyral volumes and laterality correlates of auditory hallucinations in schizophrenia. *Biological Psychiatry*, 46, 955–62.

Levitt, J. J., McCarley, R. W., Nestor, P. G., Petrescu, C., Donnino, R., Hirayasu, Y. *et al.* (1999). Quantitative volumetric MRI study of the cerebellum and vermis in schizophrenia: clinical and cognitive correlates. *American Journal of Psychiatry*, 156, 1105–7.

Levitt, J. G., Blanton, R. E., Caplan, R., Asarnow, R., Guthrie, D., Toga, A. W. *et al.* (2001). Medial temporal lobe in childhood-onset schizophrenia. *Psychiatry Research*, 108, 17–27.

Lewis, S. W. (1990). Computerised tomography in schizophrenia 15 years on. *British Journal of Psychiatry*, 157, 16–24.

Liddle, P. F. (1987). Schizophrenic syndromes, cognitive performance and neurological dysfunction. *Psychological Medicine*, 17, 49–57.

Liddle, P. F. (1992). Regional brain abnormalities associated with specific syndromes of persistent schizophrenic symptoms. *Clinical Neuropharmacology*, 15(suppl.), 402A.

Liddle, P. F. and Morris, D. L. (1991). Schizophrenic syndromes and frontal lobe performance. *British Journal of Psychiatry*, 158, 340–5.

Liddle, P. F., Friston, K. J., Frith, C. D., Hirsch, S. R., Jones, T., and Frackowiak, R. S. (1992). Patterns of cerebral blood flow in schizophrenia. *British Journal of Psychiatry*, 160, 179–86.

Lieberman, J., Bogerts, B., Degreef, G., Ashtari, M., Lantos, G., and Alvir, J. (1992). Qualitative assesssment of brain morphology in acute and chronic schizophrenia. *American Journal of Psychiatry*, 149, 784–94.

Lieberman, J. A., Jody, D., Alvir, J. M., Ashtari, M., Levy, D. L., Bogerts, B. *et al.* (1993). Brain morphology, dopamine, and eye-tracking abnormalities in first-episode schizophrenia. Prevalence and clinical correlates. *Archives of General Psychiatry*, 50, 357–68.

Lieberman, J., Chakos, M., Wu, H., Alvir, J., Hoffman, E., Robinson, D. *et al.* (2001). Longitudinal study of brain morphology in first episode schizophrenia. *Biological Psychiatry*, **49**, 487–99.

Lim, K. O., Beal, D. M., Harvey, R. L., Jr, Myers, T., Lane, B., Sullivan, E. V. *et al.* (1995). Brain dysmorphology in adults with congenital rubella plus schizophrenia like symptoms. *Biological Psychiatry*, **37**, 764–76.

Mathalon, D. H., Sullivan, E. V., Lim, K. O., and Pfefferbaum, A. (2001). Progressive brain volume changes and the clinical course of schizophrenia in men: a longitudinal magnetic resonance imaging study. *Archives of General Psychiatry*, **58**, 148–57.

Mathalon, D. H., Pfefferbaum, A., Lim, K. O., Rosenbloom, M. J., and Sullivan, E. V. (2003). Compounded brain volume deficits in schizophrenia-alcoholism comorbidity. *Archives of General Psychiatry*, **60**, 245–52.

McCreadie, R. G., Thara, R., Padmavati, R., Srinivasan, T. N., and Jaipurkar, D. D. (2002). Structural brain differences between never-treated patients with schizophrenia, with and without dyskinesia, and normal control subjects. *Archives of General Psychiatry*, **59**, 332–6.

McDonald, C., Grech, A., Toulopoulou, T., Schulze, K., Chapple, B., Sham, P. *et al.* (2002). Brain volumes in familial and non-familial schizophrenic probands and their unaffected relatives. *American Journal of Medical Genetics* **114**, 616–25.

McGuffin, P., Farmer, A., and Harvey, I. (1991). A polydiagnostic application of operational criteria in studies of psychotic illness. Development and reliability of the OPCRIT system. *Archives of General Psychiatry*, **48**, 764–70.

McGuffin, P., Asherson, P., Owen, M., and Farmer, A. (1994). The strength of the genetic effect. Is there room for an environmental influence in the aetiology of schizophrenia?[comment]. *British Journal of Psychiatry*, **164**, 593–9.

McIntosh, A. M., Forrester, A., Lawrie, S. M., Byrne, M., Harper, A., Kestelman, J. N. *et al.* (2001). A factor model of the functional psychoses and the relationship of factors to clinical variables and brain morphology. *Psychological Medicine*, **31**, 159–71.

McNeil, T. F., Cantor-Graae, E., and Weinberger, D. R. (2000). Relationship of obstetric complications and differences in size of brain structures in monozygotic twin pairs discordant for schizophrenia. *American Journal of Psychiatry*, **157**, 203–12.

Mednick, S. A. (1966). A longitudinal study of children with a high risk for schizophrenia. *Mental Hygiene*, **50**, 522–35.

Menon, R. R., Barta, P. E., Aylward, E. H., Richards, S. S., Vaughn, D. D., Tien, A. Y. *et al.* (1995). Posterior superior temporal gyrus in schizophrenia: grey matter changes and clinical correlates. *Schizophrenia Research*, **16**, 127–35.

Morel, B. A. (1860). *Traité des malades mentales*. Masson, Paris.

Nair, T. R., Christensen, J. D., Kingsbury, S. J., Kumar, N. G., Terry, W. M., and Garver, D. L. (1997). Progression of cerebroventricular enlargement and the subtyping of schizophrenia. *Psychiatry Research*, **74**, 141–50.

Narr, K. L., van Erp, T. G., Cannon, T. D., Woods, R. P., Thompson, P. M., Jang, S. *et al.* (2002). A twin study of genetic contributions to hippocampal morphology in schizophrenia. *Neurobiology of Disease*, **11**, 83–95.

Nelson, M. D., Saykin, A. J., Flashman, L. A., and Riordan, H. J. (1998). Hippocampal volume reduction in schizophrenia as assessed by magnetic resonance imaging: a meta-analytic study [comment]. *Archives of General Psychiatry*, **55**, 433–40.

Nestor, P. G., Shenton, M. E., McCarley, R. W., Haimson, J., Smith, R. S., O'Donnell, B. *et al.* (1993). Neuropsychological correlates of MRI temporal lobe abnormalities in schizophrenia [comment]. *American Journal of Psychiatry*, **150**, 1849–55.

Nestor, P. G., O'Donnell, B. F., McCarley, R. W., Niznikiewicz, M., Barnard, J., Jen, S. Z. *et al.* (2002). A new statistical method for testing hypotheses of neuropsychological/MRI relationships in schizophrenia: partial least squares analysis. *Schizophrenia Research*, **53**, 57–66.

O'Driscoll, G. A., Florencio, P. S., Gagnon, D., Wolff, A. V., Benkelfat, C., Mikula, L. *et al.* (2001). Amygdala-hippocampal volume and verbal memory in first-degree relatives of schizophrenic patients. *Psychiatry Research*, **107**, 75–85.

Onitsuka, T., Shenton, M. E., Kasai, K., Nestor, P. G., Toner, S. K., Kikinis, R. *et al.* (2003). Fusiform gyrus volume reduction and facial recognition in chronic schizophrenia. *Archives of General Psychiatry*, **60**, 349–55.

Owens, D. G., Johnstone, E. C., Crow, T. J., Frith, C. D., Jagoe, J. R., and Kreel, L. (1985). Lateral ventricular size in schizophrenia: relationship to the disease process and its clinical manifestations. *Psychological Medicine*, **15**, 27–41.

Paillere-Martinot, M., Caclin, A., Artiges, E., Poline, J. B., Joliot, M., Mallet, L. *et al.* (2001). Cerebral gray and white matter reductions and clinical correlates in patients with early onset schizophrenia. *Schizophrenia Research*, **50**, 19–26.

Pantelis, C., Velakoulis, D., McGorry, P. D., Wood, S. J., Suckling, J., Phillips, L. J. *et al.* (2002). Left medial temporal volume reduction occurs during the transition from high-risk to first episode psychosis. *Schizophrenia Research*, **41**, 35.

Pantelis, C., Velakoulis, D., McGorry, P. D., Wood, S. J., Suckling, J., Phillips, L. J. *et al.* (2003). Neuroanatomical abnormalities before and after onset of psychosis: a cross-sectional and longitudinal MRI comparison. *Lancet*, **361**, 281–8.

Peralta, V., Cuesta, M. J., Martinez-Larrea, A., and Serrano, J. F. (2001). Patterns of symptoms in neuroleptic-naive patients with schizophrenia and related psychotic disorders before and after treatment. *Psychiatry Research*, **105**, 97–105.

Phillips, L. J., Velakoulis, D., Pantelis, C., Wood, S., Yuen, H. P., Yung, A. R. *et al.* (2002). Non-reduction in hippocampal volume is associated with higher risk of psychosis. *Schizophrenia Research*, **58**, 145–58.

Rajarethinam, R. P., DeQuardo, J. R., Nalepa, R., and Tandon, R. (2000). Superior temporal gyrus in schizophrenia: a volumetric magnetic resonance imaging study. *Schizophrenia Research*, **41**, 303–12.

Rajarethinam, R., DeQuardo, J. R., Miedler, J., Arndt, S., Kirbat, R., Brunberg, J. A. *et al.* (2001). Hippocampus and amygdala in schizophrenia: assessment of the relationship of neuroanatomy to psychopathology. *Psychiatry Research*, **108**, 79–87.

Rapoport, J. L., Giedd, J., Kumra, S., Jacobsen, L., Smith, A., Lee, P. *et al.* (1997). Childhood onset schizophrenia: progressive ventricular change during adolescence. *Archives of General Psychiatry*, **54**, 897–903.

Reveley, A. M., Reveley, M. A., and Murray, R. M. (1984). Cerebral ventricular enlargement in non-genetic schizophrenia: a controlled twin study. *British Journal of Psychiatry*, **144**, 89–93.

Roy, M. A. and Crowe, R. R. (1994). Validity of the familial and sporadic subtypes of schizophrenia. *American Journal of Psychiatry*, **151**, 805–14.

Sacchetti, E., Calzeroni, A., Vita, A., Terzi, A., Pollastro, F., and Cazzullo, C. L. (1992). The brain damage hypothesis of the seasonality of births in schizophrenia and major affective disorders: evidence from computerised tomography. *British Journal of Psychiatry*, **160**, 390–7.

Sanderson, T. L., Doody, G. A., Best, J., Owens, D. G., and Johnstone, E. C. (2001). Correlations between clinical and historical variables, and cerebral structural variables in people with mild intellectual disability and schizophrenia. *Journal of Intellectual Disability Research*, **45**, 2–98.

Sanfilipo, M., Lafargue, T., Rusinek, H., Arena, L., Loneragan, C., Lautin, A. *et al.* (2000). Volumetric measure of the frontal and temporal lobe regions in schizophrenia: relationship to negative symptoms. *Archives of General Psychiatry*, **57**, 471–80.

Schreiber, H., Baur-Seack, K., Kornhuber, H. H., Wallner, B., Freidrich, J. M., De Winter, I. M. *et al.* (1999). Brain morphology in adolescents at genetic risk for schizophrenia assessed by qualitative and quantitative magnetic resonance imaging. *Schizophrenia Research*, **40**, 81–4.

Schulze, K., McDonald, C., Frangou, S., Sham, P., Grech, A., Toulopoulou, T. *et al.* (2003). Hippocampal volume in familial and nonfamilial schizophrenic probands and their unaffected relatives. *Biological Psychiatry*, **53**, 562–70.

Schwarzkopf, S. B., Nasrallah, H. A., Olson, S. C., Bogerts, B., McLaughlin, J. A., and Mitra, T. (1991). Family history and brain morphology in schizophrenia: an MRI study. *Psychiatry Research*, **40**, 49–60.

Seidman, L. J., Yurgelun-Todd, D., Kremen, W. S., Woods, B. T., Goldstein, J. M., Faraone, S. V. *et al.* (1994). Relationship of prefrontal and temporal lobe MRI measures to neuropsychological performance in chronic schizophrenia. *Biological Psychiatry*, **35**, 235–46.

Seidman, L. J., Faraone, S. V., Goldstein, J. M., Kremen, W. S., Horton, N. J., Makris, N. *et al.* (1999). Thalamic and amygdala-hippocampal volume reductions in first degree relatives of patients with schizophrenia: an MRI-based morphometric analysis. *Biological Psychiatry*, **46**, 941–54.

Seidman, L. J., Faraone, S. V., Goldstein, J. M., Kremen, W. S., Horton, N. J., Makris, N. *et al.* (2002). Left hippocampal volume as a vulnerability indicator for schizophrenia. *Archives of General Psychiatry*, **59**, 849.

Serretti, A., Rietschel, M., Lattuada, E., Krauss, H., Schulze, T. G., Muller, D. J. *et al.* (2001). Major psychoses symptomatology: factor analysis of 2241 psychotic subjects. *European Archives of Psychiatry and Clinical Neuroscience*, **251**, 193–8.

Shapleske, J., Rossell, S. L., Chitnis, X. A., Suckling, J., Simmons, A., Bullmore, E. T. *et al.* (2002). A computational morphometric MRI study of schizophrenia: effects of hallucinations. *Cerebral Cortex*, **12**, 1331–41.

Sharma, T., Lancaster, E., Lee, D., Lewis, S., Sigmundson, T., Takei, N. *et al.* (1998). Brain changes in schizophrenia. Volumetric MRI study of families multiply affected by schizophrenia-the Maudsley Family Study 5. *British Journal of Psychiatry*, **173**, 132–8.

Sharma, T., Lancaster, E., Sigmundson, T., Lewis, S., Takei, N., Gurling, H. *et al.* (1999). Lack of normal pattern of cerebral asymmetry in familial schizophrenic patients and their relatives-The Maudsley Family Study. *Schizophrenia Research*, **40**, 111–20.

Shenton, M. E., Kikinis, R., Jolesz, F. A., Pollak, S. D., LeMay, M., Wible, C. G. *et al.* (1992). Abnormalities of the left temporal lobe and thought disorder in schizophrenia. A quantitative magnetic resonance imaging study. *New England Journal of Medicine*, **327**, 604–12.

Shenton, M. E., Dickey, C. C., Frumin, M., and McCarley, R. W. (2001). A review of MRI findings in schizophrenia. *Schizophrenia Research*, **49**, 1–52.

Shenton, M. E., Gerig, G., McCarley, R. W., Szekely, G., and Kikinis, R. (2002). Amygdala-hippocampal shape differences in schizophrenia: the application of 3D shape models to volumetric MR data. *Psychiatry Research*, **115**, 15–35.

Sigmundsson, T., Suckling, J., Maier, M., Williams, S., Bullmore, E., Greenwood, K. *et al.* (2001). Structural abnormalities in frontal, temporal, and limbic regions and interconnecting white matter tracts in schizophrenic patients with prominent negative symptoms. *American Journal of Psychiatry*, **158**, 234–43.

Silverton, L., Finello, K. M., Mednick, S. A., and Schulsinger, F. (1985). Low birth weight and ventricular enlargement in a high-risk sample. *Journal of Abnormal Psychology*, **94**, 405–9.

Silverton, L., Mednick, S. A., and Harrington, M. E. (1988). Birthweight, schizophrenia and ventricular enlargement in a high-risk sample. *Psychiatry*, **51**(3), 272–80.

Smith, R. C., Calderon, M., Ravichandran, G. K., Largen, J., Vroulis, G., Shvartsburd, A. *et al.* (1984). Nuclear magnetic resonance in schizophrenia: a preliminary study. *Psychiatry Research*, **12**, 137–47.

Sommer, I., Ramsey, N., Kahn, R., Aleman, A., and Bouma, A. (2001). Handedness, language lateralisation and anatomical asymmetry in schizophrenia: Meta-analysis. *British Journal of Psychiatry*, **178**, 344–51.

Staal, W. G., Hulshoff Pol, H. E., Schnack, H., van der Schot, A. C. and Kahn, R. S. (1998). Partial volume decrease of the thalamus in relatives of patients with schizophrenia. *American Journal of Psychiatry*, **155**, 1784–6.

Staal, W. G., Hulshoff Pol, H. E., Schnack, H., Hoogendoorn, M. L. C., Jellema, K., and Kahn, R. S. (2000). Structural brain abnormalities in patients with schizophrenia and their healthy siblings. *American Journal of Psychiatry*, **157**, 416–21.

Steel, R., Whalley, H. C., Miller, P., Best, J. J. K., Johnstone, E. C., and Lawrie, S. M. (2002). Structural MRI of the brain in presumed carriers of genes for schizophrenia, their affected and unaffected siblings. *Journal of Neurology, Neurosurgery and Psychiatry*, **72**, 455–8.

Stefanis, N., Frangou, S., Yakeley, J., Sharma, T., O'Connell, P., Morgan, K. *et al.* (1999). Hippocampal volume reduction in schizophrenia: effects of genetic risk and pregnancy and birth complications. *Biological Psychiatry*, **46**, 697–702.

Stefanis, N. C., Hanssen, M., Smirnis, N. K., Avramopoulos, D. A., Evdokimidis, I. K., Stefanis, C. N. *et al.* (2002). Evidence that three dimensions of psychosis have a distribution in the general population. *Psychological Medicine*, **32**, 347–58.

Stratta, P., Mancini, F., Mattei, P., Daneluzzo, E., Casacchia, M., and Rossi, A. (1997). Association between striatal reduction and poor Wisconsin card sorting test performance in patients with schizophrenia. *Biological Psychiatry*, **42**, 816–20.

Suckling, J. and Bullmore, E. T. (2000). Structural magnetic resonance imaging. In *New Oxford Textbook of Psychiatry*, (ed. M. Gelder, J. J. Lopez-Ibor, and N. Andreasen). Oxford University Press, Oxford.

Suddath, R. L., Christison, G. W., Torrey, E. F., Casanova, M. F., and Weinberger, D. R. (1990). Anatomical abnormalities in the brains of monozygotic twins discordant for schizophrenia [comment]. *New England Journal of Medicine*, **322**, 789–794 [erratum appears in *New England Journal of Medicine*, 1990, **322**(22),1616].

Sullivan, E. V., Shear, P. K., Lim, K. O., Zipursky, R. B., and Pfefferbaum, A. (1996). Cognitive and motor impairments are related to gray matter volume deficits in schizophrenia. *Biological Psychiatry*, **39**, 234–40.

Szeszko, P. R., Bilder, R. M., Lencz, T., Ashtari, M., Goldman, R. S., Reiter, G. *et al.* (2000). Reduced anterior cingulate gyrus volume correlates with executive dysfunction in men with first-episode schizophrenia. *Schizophrenia Research*, **43**, 97–108.

Szeszko, P. R., Strous, R. D., Goldman, R. S., Ashtari, M., Knuth, K. H., and Lieberman, J. A. (2002). Neuropsychological correlates of hippocampal volumes in patients experiencing a first episode of schizophrenia. *American Journal of Psychiatry*, **159**, 217–26.

Torres, I. J., Flashman, L. A., O'Leary, D. S., Swayze, V., and Andreasen, N. C. (1997). Lack of an association between delayed memory and hippocampal and temporal lobe size in patients with schizophrenia and healthy controls. *Biological Psychiatry*, **42**, 1087–96.

Valles, V., van Os, J., Guillamat, R., Gutierrez, B., Campillo, M., Gento, P. *et al.* (2000). Increased morbid risk for schizophrenia in families of in-patients with bipolar illness. *Schizophrenia Research*, **42**, 83–90.

van Erp, T. G., Saleh, P. A., Rosso, I. M., Huttunen, M., Lönnqvist, J., Pirkola, T. *et al.* (2002*a*). Contributions of genetic risk and fetal hypoxia to hippocampal volume in patients with schizophrenia or schizoaffective disorder, their unaffected siblings and healthy unrelated volunteers. *American Journal of Psychiatry*, **159**, 1514–20.

van Os, J., Gilvarry, C., Bale, R., Van Horn, E., Tattan, T., White, I., *et al.* (1999). A comparison of the utility of dimensional and categorical representations of psychosis. UK700 Group. *Psychological Medicine*, **29**, 595–606.

Velakoulis, D., Pantelis, C., McGorry, P. D., Dudgeon, P., Brewer, W., Cook, M., *et al.* (1999*a*). Hippocampal volume in first-episode psychoses and chronic schizophrenia: a high-resolution magnetic resonance imaging study [see comments]. *Archives of General Psychiatry*, **56**, 133–41.

Waddington, J. L., O'Callaghan, E., Larkin, C., Redmond, O., Stack, J., and Ennis, J. T. (1990). Magnetic resonance imaging and spectroscopy in schizophrenia. *British Journal of Psychiatry* **57**(suppl 9), s56–s65.

Waldo, M. C., Cawthra, E., Adler, L. E., Dubester, S., Staunton, M., Nagamoto, H. *et al.* (1994). Auditory sensory gating, hippocampal volume and catacholamine metabolism in schizophrenics and their siblings. *Schizophrenia Research*, **12**, 93–105.

Weinberger, D. R. (1987). Implications of normal brain development for the pathogenesis of schizophrenia. *Archives of General Psychiatry*, **44**, 660–9.

Weinberger, D. R. and McClure, R. K. (2002). Neurotoxicity, neuroplasticity, and magnetic resonance imaging morphometry: What is happening in the schizophrenic brain? *Archives of General Psychiatry*, **59**, 553–8.

Whitworth, A. B., Honeder, M., Kremser, C., Kemmler, G., Felber, S., Hausmann, A. *et al.* (1998). Hippocampal volume reduction in male schizophrenic patients. *Schizophrenia Research*, **31**, 73–81.

Wright, I. C., Ellison, Z. R., Sharma, T., Friston, K. J., Murray, R. M., and McGuire, P. K. (1999*a*). Mapping of grey matter changes in schizophrenia. *Schizophrenia Research*, **35**, 1–14.

Wright, I. C., Sharma, T., Ellison, Z. R., McGuire, P. K., Friston, K. J., Brammer, M. *et al.* (1999*b*). Supra-regional brain systems and the neuropathology of schizophrenia. *Cerebral Cortex*, **9**, 366–78.

Wright, I. C., Rabe-Hesketh, S., Woodruff, P. W., David, A. S., Murray, R. M., and Bullmore, E. T. (2000). Meta-analysis of regional brain volumes in schizophrenia. *American Journal of Psychiatry*, **157**, 16–25.

Zorrilla, L. T., Cannon, T. D., Kronenberg, S., Mednick, S. A., Schulsinger, F., Parnas, J. *et al.* (1997). Structural brain abnormalities in schizophrenia: a family study. *Biological Psychiatry*, **42**, 1080–6.

Zuffante, P., Leonard, C. M., Kuldau, J. M., Bauer, R. M., Doty, E. G., and Bilder, R. M. (2001). Working memory deficits in schizophrenia are not necessarily specific or associated with MRI-based estimates of area 46 volumes. *Psychiatry Research*, **108**, 187–209.

Chapter 3

Structural brain MRI studies in childhood-onset schizophrenia and childhood atypical psychosis

Nitin Gogtay, Alexandra Sporn, and
Judith L. Rapoport

Introduction

It had long been thought that serious childhood psychiatric disorders reflect subtle abnormalities of brain development. Newer imaging technologies have been crucial for supporting and extending this view. While the use of ionizing radiation had limited the use of CAT (computerized axial tomography) and PET (positron emission tomography) scanning in children, the advent of magnetic resonance imaging (MRI) and magnetic resonance spectroscopy (MRS) has made brain imaging a key part of child psychiatric research (Gogate *et al.* 2001). These non-invasive and relatively simple techniques allow reliable, automated quantitative measurements of multiple brain regions (Collins *et al.* 1999). Generally regarded as 'minimal risk', it is now possible to gather both normative and disease-specific data in children (Giedd *et al.* 1996, 1999*a*; Thompson *et al.* 2000, 2001).

The study of brain development from childhood to adolescence allows examination during a period of major reorganization. Since 1990 a prospective study of brain development in healthy children aged 4 to 18 has been ongoing at the National Institute of Mental Health (NIMH). This has increased understanding of normal and pathological brain developmental trajectories during childhood and adolescence. These anatomic studies indicate regional heterogeneity in brain cortical development (Berument *et al.* 1999; Giedd *et al.* 1999*a*). Unexpectedly, the corpus callosum matures in a 'back-to-front' manner during this same period (Thompson *et al.* 2000). Ongoing studies of healthy monozygotic and dizygotic twins show that the volume measurements of most brain regions are highly heritable, with the possible and surprising exception of the cerebellar hemispheres (Giedd, unpublished data, July 2004).

As seen in other areas of medicine, early onset populations may have unique and/ or more salient pathophysiology and familial/genetic associations (Childs and Scriver, 1986). Childhood-onset schizophrenia (COS), defined as the onset of psychotic symptoms before the thirteenth birthday, is a rare and severe form of the illness, which is continuous with its adult counterpart (Nicolson and Rapoport, 1999). The availability of funding for studies of pediatric COS subjects and ample age-matched norms has also allowed the study of brain development during early adolescence. Functional studies are rarely feasible with these patients, both because of the severity of illness and the problem of developing equivalent tasks across their age range. Structural brain imaging studies on such cases may, none the less, valuably expand overall understanding of the disease.

This chapter will review structural brain-imaging studies of very early onset schizophrenia. While supportive of a continuity with later onset disorder, these studies also address the possibility of disease-related progressive brain changes.

Childhood-onset schizophrenia

Background

Childhood-onset schizophrenia has been recognized since the early twentieth century (Kraepelin, 1919) and children can be diagnosed with the unmodified Diagnostic and Statistical Manual of Mental Disorders (DSM) criteria for schizophrenia. Such cases are unfamiliar to most child mental health workers, and many patients with affective or other atypical psychoses are often misdiagnosed as COS (Werry, 1992; Gordon *et al.* 1994; McKenna *et al.* 1994). However, these patients provide an important contrast group in their own right. COS subjects resemble poor-outcome adult cases with respect to their insidious onset and poor premorbid functioning. The early developmental abnormalities in social, motor, and language domains in COS are more striking compared to the later-onset cases (Green *et al.* 1992; Alaghband-Rad *et al.* 1995; Hollis, 1995). Additionally, although not observed in the studies of early development of adult-onset schizophrenia (Walker and Lewine, 1990; Done *et al.* 1994; Jones *et al.* 1994), transient autistic symptoms such as hand flapping and echolalia occur in toddler years for a substantial minority of the children (Russell *et al.* 1989; Green *et al.* 1992; Alaghband-Rad *et al.* 1995), probably reflecting more severely compromised early brain development.

NIMH COS cohort

In the ongoing study of childhood-onset schizophrenia at the NIMH, children with early onset psychosis are recruited nationally for diagnostic screening for COS. Diagnosis of COS is confirmed after a 1-month in-patient evaluation, usually followed by a drug-free observation period. To date, 72 patients have participated in the study, including 41 boys and 31 girls, with a mean age of 14.4 ± 2.5 years and mean age of onset of psychosis at 10.3 ± 1.8 years. All subjects receive a structural brain MRI scan, and are prospectively re-scanned at 2-year intervals, thus providing cross-sectional as well as longitudinal structural brain MRI data. Total and regional gray and white matter volume measurements are obtained through an automated system (Giedd *et al.* 1996; Collins *et al.* 1999).

NIMH atypical psychosis cohort

A second common subgroup of patients referred to NIMH as childhood-onset schizo-phrenia, showed only transient psychotic symptoms, but their primary impairment was from disruptive and aggressive behavior. These cases have been studied prospec-tively in parallel with the COS sample. These children reported brief hallucinations and delusions, typically under stress, but had no evidence of formal thought disorder. On presentation, this group could not be categorized into any of the existing DSM syn-dromes and received an umbrella diagnosis of psychosis Not Otherwise Specified (NOS) (Kumra et al. 1998). Due to their impairments in multiple domains, these chil-dren were provisionally called 'multi dimensionally impaired' (MDI) and, along with their families, have been followed longitudinally with childhood-onset schizophrenia patients (Kumra et al. 1998; Nicolson et al. 2001).

These children came with the provisional diagnosis of schizophrenia, and were treated with similar medications (primarily to control behavioral outbursts). This, and their comparable cognitive level, make them an important clinical comparison group for imaging and other studies.

To date, the NIMH 'MDI' cohort consists of 30 children, all with transient psychotic symptoms before age 13. Their mean age at initial contact was 11.6 ± 2.6 years and the large majority were male (26; 86%), a higher proportion than for COS ($x^2 = 5.92$, df = 1, $P = 0.01$). Their psychotic symptoms were brief (i.e. a few minutes) to infrequent (a few times a month). None showed disorganized speech or the negative symptoms common in our children with schizophrenia. While they had few if any friends, this was due to poor social skills rather than a lack of desire for friends. On first contact, none met criteria for major mood disorder or post-traumatic stress disorder, and all but two had co-morbid disruptive behavior disorder [attention deficit/hyperactivity disorder (ADHD) ($n = 20$), oppositional defiant disorder (ODD) ($n = 8$), conduct disorder ($n = 2$)]. Of 25 MDI children followed up to date over a 2–6-year period, over half (16; 64%) were eventually diagnosed with a mood disorder, including schizoaffec-tive disorder manic type (1), bipolar disorder (7), major depressive disorder (7), and dysthymic disorder (1). The remaining 9 (36%) had not developed another disorder at follow-up and they continued to be characterized as 'MDI'.

Brain imaging studies in childhood-onset schizophrenia

Imaging studies of childhood-onset schizophrenia are scarce. One early CT study of 15 adolescents (mean age = 16 ± 1.5) with schizophrenia or schizophreniform disorder demonstrated larger ventricular volume in the schizophrenic group, with a higher ven-tricular brain ratio associated with poor treatment response, as had been described for adult patients (Schulz et al. 1983). A more recent CT study of 19 children with very early onset schizophrenia (mean age = 11.3 ± 2.3) also showed ventricular enlargement (Badura et al. 2001).

Several brain MRI studies of childhood schizophrenia come from the NIMH sample, with more recent contributions from other groups (Sowell *et al.* 2000; Matsumoto *et al.* 2001*a, b*; James *et al.* 2002). All the automated analyses on this population come from the NIMH sample.

Image analysis

We have used a combination of manual, semi-automated user-interactive, and entirely automated approaches. A typical MR image contains millions of volume elements ('voxels'), each of which has a certain intensity value based upon the magnetic characteristics of the tissue within the voxel. One technique we have used, which has not otherwise been applied to schizophrenic brains, combines automated classification of the voxels into gray matter, white matter, or cerebrospinal fluid ('segmentation') with an automated image matching ('normalization') and labeling program to determine which brain structure or region the voxel belongs to. This is illustrated in Fig. 3.1. Most advanced automated image analysis methods use similar techniques (see Chapter 6 for details).

Longitudinal re-scans, together with the fully automated method, enable the study of brain volumetric changes during development in large populations. Although such automated measures carry a distinct advantage of unbiased measurements of brain volume, the 'gold standard' for quantification of many small structures, such as the globus pallidus, hippocampus, amygdala and thalamus, remains hand tracing (Giedd *et al.* 1996).

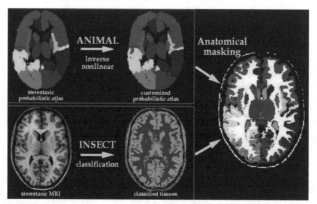

Fig. 3.1 INSECT (intensity normalized stereotaxic environment for classification of tissue) is an automated program for classifying each voxel of a brain MR image into gray matter, white matter, or cerebrospinal fluid, based on the intensity of the voxel. ANIMAL (automatic nonlinear image matching and anatomical labeling) is also an automated approach that labels a voxel's location in space based on prior anatomic knowledge. The MNI (Montreal Neurological Institute) program is unique in that it combines the two techniques. This allows for an automated voxel-intensity and anatomically informed classification of the brain tissue (reproduced from Collins *et al.* 1999, with permission). See Plate 1(a) of the plate section at the centre of this book.

Cross-sectional differences

There is general agreement that children with schizophrenia show increased lateral ventricular volume, decreased total brain volume, decreased gray matter volume, and increased basal ganglia volume (the latter probably secondary to medication) (Frazier *et al.* 1996; Rapoport *et al.* 1997, 1999; Kumra *et al.* 2000; Sowell *et al.* 2000). However, there is less agreement about whether the volume of medial temporal lobe structures is reduced (Jacobsen *et al.* 1996; Matsumoto *et al.* 2001a, b).

An updated comparison of 60 COS (mean age 14.27 ± 2.41 years) with 110 age- (mean age 14.18 ± 2.44) and sex-matched healthy volunteers extends our previous studies. As seen in Table 3.1, the decreased brain volume in COS is due to a robust (10%) decrease in cortical gray matter, while the adjusted white matter volume does not differ significantly between the COS and healthy groups. Of note is the striking reduction in parietal gray matter volume, which may be characteristic of early onset schizophrenia.

A small study of 10 COS subjects (mean age 11 years), using statistical parametric mapping of gray and white matters and cerebrospinal fluid (CSF), found increased ventricular volume and decreased temporal and frontal gray matter volumes (Sowell

Table 3.1 Anatomic brain MRI measures (at initial scan) for COS and age- and sex-matched community controls

Brain region	COS patients, mean ((SD)	Healthy controls, mean ((SD)	ANOVA		ANCOVA	
Automated measures	($n = 60$)	($n = 110$)	*F*	*P*	*F*	*P*
Total cerebral volume	1078.62 (117.96)	1108.05 (116.31)	2.46	0.119	–	–
Total gray matter	687.31 (77.49)	718.05 (76.29)	6.24	0.0135	10.36	0.002
Total white matter	391.31 (50.70)	390.00 (49.50)	0.03	0.870	10.36	0.002[+]
Frontal gray matter	211.91 (25.46)	222.60 (23.03)	7.76	0.006	10.61	0.001
Temporal gray matter	178.08 (20.410)	183.89 (18.83)	3.49	0.064	1.05	0.306
Parietal gray matter	111.92 (13.77)	119.65 (13.52)	12.53	0.0005	17.66	0.00004
Occipital gray matter	61.42 (9.39)	65.55 (10.55)	6.41	0.0123	4.13	0.0436
Lateral ventricles	16.44 (8.42)	11.84 (6.17)	16.54	0.00007[+]	22.97	0.000004[+]

ANOVA and ANCOVA, analysis of variance and covariance (covariate = total cerebral volume).

The mean age for COS (childhood-onset schizophrenia) was 14.27 (SD = 2.41) and for community controls 14.18 (SD = 2.44) (*P* = 0.81).

[+]COS > normal volume.

et al. 2000). While not showing parietal loss, this study did find the ventricular enlargement to be predominantly posterior. As seen below, we believe that the posterior brain regions are selectively affected early in the illness.

Longitudinal (prospective) studies

Prospective longitudinal brain MRI rescan measures for the NIMH COS sample show progressive abnormalities (Fig. 3.2). Increasing ventricular volume, and decreasing total cortical, frontal, temporal, and parietal gray matter volumes were seen 2, 4, and 6 years after their initial scan. Here too, regional gray-white segmentation showed the progressive loss to be for gray matter only (Rapoport *et al.* 1997, 1999; Jacobsen *et al.* 1998; Giedd *et al.* 1999*b*).

More recent studies of adult-onset schizophrenia (AOS), using comparable methodology, have found relatively subtle progressive loss of brain matter (Gur *et al.* 1998; DeLisi 1999*a, b*; Lieberman *et al.* 2001; Mathalon *et al.* 2001). An effect size comparison demonstrates that the progressive changes are more striking during adolescence, at least for very early onset cases (Gogate *et al.* 2001). Figure 3.3 summarizes the effect size comparisons from four of these prospective studies and suggests progressive changes for AOS, and especially COS, in comparison to their respective age-matched healthy controls.

Similarities between the follow-up imaging studies of AOS and COS include progressive ventricular expansion and cortical gray matter loss, mostly in the frontal and temporal regions. In addition to the frontal and temporal gray matter loss, the COS population also showed significant parietal gray matter loss. [The NIMH COS study showed no significant temporal lobe differences on initial scan (Table 3.1).]

The rapid changes seen for COS probably occur only during a limited period, since age of onset is not significantly related to decreased cortical gray matter loss in adult patients (Lim *et al.* 1996; Marsh *et al.* 1997). Moreover, the degree of cortical loss seen in COS would not be sustainable over time without resulting in dementia. Thus, adolescence appears to provide a time-limited window in which progressive brain changes in schizophrenia are most easily observed. The time-limited nature of these

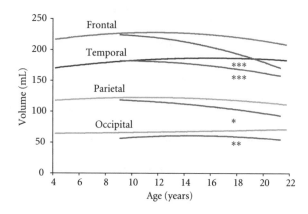

Fig. 3.2 Regional gray matter loss in childhood-onset schizophrenia compared to age- and sex-matched controls; ***, $P = 0.001$; **, $P = 0.02$; *, $P = 0.06$ (from Giedd *et al.* 1999*b*: Rapoport *et al.* 1999).

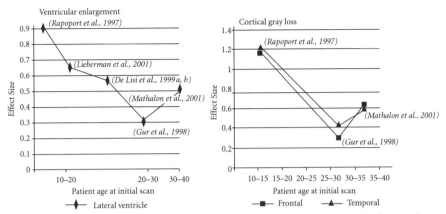

Fig. 3.3 Effect size comparison for MRI studies showing progressive ventricular changes in adult- and childhood-onset schizophrenia at 2-4-year follow-up (from Gogate *et al.* 2001, with permission).

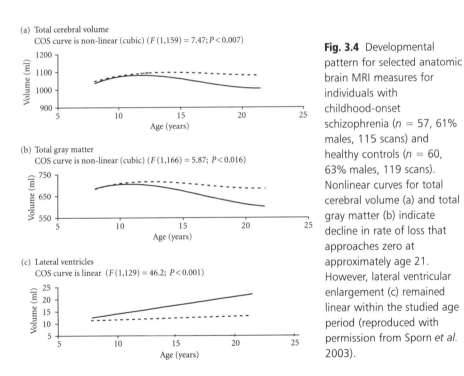

Fig. 3.4 Developmental pattern for selected anatomic brain MRI measures for individuals with childhood-onset schizophrenia (*n* = 57, 61% males, 115 scans) and healthy controls (*n* = 60, 63% males, 119 scans). Nonlinear curves for total cerebral volume (a) and total gray matter (b) indicate decline in rate of loss that approaches zero at approximately age 21. However, lateral ventricular enlargement (c) remained linear within the studied age period (reproduced with permission from Sporn *et al.* 2003).

observations is supported by a very recent longitudinal analysis of our quantitative brain imaging data for a larger group of 36 COS patients with one or more scans, suggesting that the rate of gray matter loss slows as these COS patients reach age 20, as shown in Fig. 3.4 (Sporn *et al.* 2003). We continue to follow these patients and anticipate continued slowing of change with age.

Clinical correlates of gray matter loss

With a larger patient sample, we have been able to examine the clinical correlates of gray matter loss. One regression analysis related demographic, and premorbid characteristics and baseline clinical measures to cortical change; and a second regression analysis related treatment and outcome measures to brain changes. Poor premorbid functioning and baseline clinical severity, as measured by Brief Psychiatric Rating Scale-Child version (BPRS-C) scores, were associated with a faster rate of gray matter reduction (standardized coefficient = 0.34, r^2 = 0.12, $P < 0.05$; and standardized coefficient = 0.31, r^2 = 0.09, $P < 0.05$, respectively) (Sporn et al. submitted). No significant relationships were observed between the rate of cortical gray loss and sex, ethnicity, familial schizotypy, age of onset, duration of illness, full-scale IQ, or information and comprehension subscale raw scores.

Unexpectedly, however, when treatment and outcome measures were examined separately in relation to cortical loss, percentage improvement on the BPRS-C scale was associated with a steeper slope of loss of gray matter, i.e. more improvement was associated with greater gray matter loss (r^2 = 0.22, $P < 0.01$). No other treatment variable, such as medication type, total dose, or dose per weight ratio (in chlorpromazine equivalents), or clinical rating scale scores at follow-up, was associated with the rate of gray matter reduction, nor were there any significant correlations with cognitive test performance. With pooled analyses including baseline, follow-up, and clinical change scores, the clinical improvement measures showed the strongest correlation with the rate of gray matter loss (Sporn et al., submitted). These observations differ from the recent longitudinal analysis of Ho et al. (2003), where recent-onset AOS patients ($n = 73$) and controls ($n = 23$) were followed for 3 years. In this study, poor outcome at follow-up correlated with increased ventricular volume, increased loss of frontal white matter volume, and also with increased frontal CSF volume. However, this study did not show significant gray matter loss in patients.

Disease specificity

A prospective brain MRI study of patients with COS ($n = 23$; mean age = 13.9 ± 2.5 years) and pediatric patients with 'atypical psychosis' (MDI group; $n = 19$; mean age = 13.3 ± 3 years) was carried out using the automatic measures shown in Fig. 3.1, to test the hypothesis that cortical gray matter loss was unique to COS (Gogtay et al. 2004). Both groups of adolescent patients were also compared with age- and sex-matched healthy controls ($n = 38$; mean age = 13.2 ± 3 years). Importantly, the MDI group did not differ from COS with respect to medications, hospitalization, and cognitive functioning. The mean follow-up period was 2.5 ± 0.8 years. The COS group had significantly greater total and regional gray matter loss than did the 'MDI' or healthy control groups (ANOVA post-hoc P values from 0.002 to 0.02), which did not differ significantly from each other (Fig. 3.5). Thus, the progressive cortical loss appears to be specific to schizophrenia. Further evidence of this is provided by the fact that the region-specific gray matter loss in COS during adolescence is in marked contrast with the subtle, global

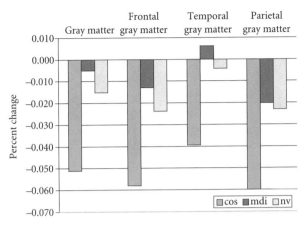

Fig. 3.5 Comparison of change in gray matter volumes over time for age- and sex-matched individuals with childhood-onset schizophrenia (COS, *n* = 23), multi dimensionally impaired (MDI, *n* = 19), and healthy community controls (NV, *n* = 38).

(equal for gray and white matter), and nonprogressive reduction in brain volume seen in adolescent children with ADHD (Castellanos *et al.* 2002; Gogtay *et al.* 2002).

Dynamic mapping of brain development using structural MRI

Most recently, in collaboration with Drs Paul Thompson, Arthur Toga and co-workers at UCLA, longitudinal rescans during adolescence for the NIMH COS sample were analyzed using a cortical pattern matching method (Thompson *et al.* 2001). Three scans per subject obtained at approximately 2-year intervals were examined. In this technique the three-dimensional distribution of gray matter in the brain is first computed and then mathematically compared from one scan to the next. The method utilizes a computational tensor-matching strategy that aligns corresponding landmarks on the cortical surface, over time and across subjects, with greater spatial detail than previously obtainable (Thompson *et al.* 2000). This permits mapping of region-specific brain cortical development across time and between subject groups with high resolution, and thus facilitates the detection of dynamic changes in regional gray matter.

Subtraction maps of the youngest COS and controls show that the parietal gray matter volume loss occurs initially, with frontal and temporal gray matter changes appearing later across the adolescent years. This supports the findings presented earlier, using the more automated quantitative approach, and suggests that the progressive gray matter loss in COS takes place in a regular postero-anterior wave-like fashion (Fig. 3.6).

Understanding of this cortical wave of gray matter loss will rest, in part, on research on the normal pattern of cortical development. It is possible that the back-to-front cortical loss is an exaggeration of a similar pattern in normal cortical development. To examine healthy cortical development utilizing tensor mapping technique, 68 prospective scans from 20 healthy pediatric controls between the ages of 8 and 20 years are currently being processed.

Some support of this back-to-front wave of cortical loss as intrinsic to schizophrenia is provided by our study of full siblings of COS patients. A recent comparison of

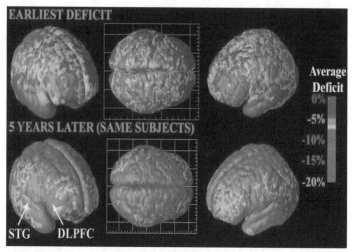

Fig. 3.6 Progressive and region-specific loss of cortical gray matter in childhood-onset schizophrenia compared with age- and sex-matched community controls. STG, superior temporal sulcus; DLPFC, dorsolateral prefontal cortex. Loss of gray matter is shown as deficit per year (reproduced from Thompson *et al.* 2001, with permission). See Plate 1(b) of the plate section at the centre of this book.

15 healthy siblings of COS patients and 32 age- and sex-matched community controls showed that the COS siblings have smaller parietal gray matter volumes (Gogtay *et al.* 2004). This finding was more prominent in younger (age 18 and below) siblings, while the older sibling group showed trends for total and frontal gray matter volume reduction. Although limited by small sample size, these familial findings, if replicated, would suggest that a back-to-front pattern (parieto-frontal) of gray matter loss could be a trait marker in schizophrenia.

Comment and future directions

The data summarized here represent the largest imaging study of early onset schizophrenia, of normal childhood brain development, and the most extensive prospective study of brain changes in schizophrenia at any age. The late progressive loss of gray matter volume is at least consistent with a neuropathology of schizophrenia characterized by reduced neuropil (Harrison 1999; Selemon and Goldman-Rakic 1999; Glantz and Lewis 2000) and with suggestions of widespread disconnectivity between multiple cortical regions (Woods 1998; McGlashan and Hoffman 2000). However, there are alternative interpretations of these findings and a need to link them to the clinical course of schizophrenia.

One version of the neurodevelopmental hypothesis of schizophrenia proposes an early (and fixed) lesion in the pre- or perinatal period, resulting in a disturbed late maturational response (Weinberger 1987). This hypothesis is supported by the animal models of schizophrenia, where developmentally specific early lesions can disrupt the later maturing regions, such as the frontal-limbic circuitry, and that such effects could be the result of the interaction of genetic variability (and vulnerability) and environmental factors (Lipska and Weinberger 1995; Lipska *et al.* 2002). Our data partly support these arguments, as our COS patients also showed more pronounced evidence of early brain impairment, as indicated by their more impaired early development (Alaghband-Rad *et al.* 1995; Nicolson *et al.* 2000). Thus it could be argued that our subjects have a more striking earlier 'lesion' and that this produces more drastic later disturbance of adolescent brain maturation.

An alternate formulation of the neurodevelopmental hypothesis is that of Woods (1998). Based in part on the normal skull size but increased intracranial CSF space in schizophrenia, he proposed that the illness is a progressive neurodevelopmental disorder. It is possible that the neurodevelopmental genes will have multiple roles across different time periods, and that etiological agents causing abnormalities in early development will have related but different effects at later stages, depending upon gene–environment interaction.

It is also possible that the progressive brain changes represent a neuroplastic response to the illness. This might account, in part, for our finding that the decrease in regional and total gray matter showed a significant (albeit inverse) relationship with clinical improvement across this period (Sporn *et al.* submitted). Clearly, a plastic brain response to illness cannot represent the only basis for these changes, as healthy siblings of our probands also show some relative cortical gray matter decrease on initial scans. It may be that early clinical improvement is a by-product of elimination by 'overpruning' of malfunctioning synapses. It is intriguing that the COS slopes seem to diverge from normal around age 10, the mean age of onset of psychosis for this group, but we have no way to address the question of whether the loss 'triggers' the illness.

Further study of these progressive changes is an important future direction for schizophrenia research. Establishing patterns of brain cortical development in normal children will be critical for the interpretation of these findings. The initial relative parietal gray matter loss for COS suggests that clinical and neuroanatomic studies, particularly of 'high-risk' populations should focus more on parietal lobe structure and function. Clinically, tests of visual processing and some attentional functions may be of particular importance during this period (Brody and Pribram 1978; Posner and Dehaene 1994; Creem and Proffitt 2001). Imaging COS probands and their siblings, as well as age- and treatment-matched patient contrast groups, with other modalities such as MRS and Diffusion Tensor Imaging (DTI), may provide complementary data to those presented here.

References

Alaghband-Rad, J., McKenna, K., Gordon, C. T., Albus, K. E., Hamburger, S. D., Rumsey, J. M. *et al.* (1995). Childhood-onset schizophrenia: the severity of premorbid course. *Journal of the American Academy of Child and Adolescent Psychiatry*, **34** (10), 1273–83.

Badura, F., Trott, G. E., Mehler-Wex, C., Scheuerpflug, P., Hofmann, E., Warmuth-Metz, M. *et al.* (2001) A study of cranial computertomograms in very early and early onset schizophrenia. *Journal of Neural Transmission*, **108** (11), 1335–44.

Berument, S. K., Rutter, M., Lord, C., Pickles, A. and Bailey, A. (1999). Autism screening questionnaire: diagnostic validity. *British Journal of Psychiatry*, **175**, 444–51.

Brody, B. A. and Pribram, K. H. (1978). The role of frontal and parietal cortex in cognitive processing: tests of spatial and sequence functions. *Brain*, **101**, 607–33.

Castellanos, F. X., Lee, P. P., Sharp, W., Jeffries, N. O., Greenstein, D. K., Clasen, L. S. *et al.* (2002). Developmental trajectories of brain volume abnormalities in children and adolescents with attention-deficit/hyperactivity disorder. *Journal of the American Medical Association*, **288**, 1740–8.

Childs, B. and Scriver, C. R. (1986). Age at onset and causes of disease. *Perspectives in Biology and Medicine*, **29** (3 Pt 1), 437–60.

Collins, D. L., Zijdenbos, A. P., Baare, W. F. C., and Evans, A. C. (1999). ANIMAL+INSECT: Improved cortical structure segmentation. In: *Proceedings of the Annual Conference on Information Processing in Medical Imaging (IPMI)*, pp. 210–223. Springer, Visegrad, Hungary.

Creem, S. H. and Proffitt, D. R. (2001). Defining the cortical visual systems: 'what', 'where', and 'how'. *Acta Psychologica (Amsterdam)*, **107**, 43–68.

DeLisi, L. E. (1999a). Regional brain volume change over the life-time course of schizophrenia. *Journal of Psychiatric Research*, **33** (6), 535–41.

DeLisi, L. E. (1999b). Defining the course of brain structural change and plasticity in schizophrenia. *Psychiatry Research*, **92** (1), 1–9.

Done, D. J., Crow, T. J., Johnstone, E. C., and Sacker, A. (1994). Childhood antecedents of schizophrenia and affective illness: social adjustment at ages 7 and 11. *British Medical Journal*, **309** (6956), 699–703.

Frazier, J. A., Giedd, J. N., Hamburger, S. D., Albus, K. E., Kaysen, D., Vaituzis, A. C. *et al.* (1996). Brain anatomic magnetic resonance imaging in childhood-onset schizophrenia. *Archives of General Psychiatry*, **53** (7), 617–24.

Giedd, J. N., Snell, J. W., Lange, N., Rajapakse, J. C., Casey, B. J., Kozuch, P. L. *et al.* (1996). Quantitative magnetic resonance imaging of human brain development: ages 4–18. *Cerebral Cortex*, **6** (4), 551–60.

Giedd, J. N., Blumenthal, J., Jeffries, N. O., Castellanos, F. X., Liu, H., Zijdenbos, A. *et al.* (1999a). Brain development during childhood and adolescence: a longitudinal MRI study [letter]. *Nature Neuroscience*, **2**, 861–3.

Giedd, J. N., Jeffries, N. O., Blumenthal, J., Castellanos, F. X., Vaituzis, A. C., Fernandez, T. *et al.* (1999b). Childhood-onset schizophrenia: progressive brain changes during adolescence [see comments]. *Biological Psychiatry*, **46** (7), 892–8.

Glantz, L. A. and Lewis, D. A. (2000). Decreased dendritic spine density on prefrontal cortical pyramidal neurons in schizophrenia [see comments]. *Archives of General Psychiatry*, **57** (1), 65–73.

Gogate, N., Giedd, J., Janson, K., and Rapoport, J. L. (2001). Brain imaging in normal and abnormal brain development: new perspectives for child psychiatry. *Clinical Neuroscience Research*, **1**, 283–90.

Gogtay, N., Giedd, J., and Rapoport, J. L. (2002). Brain development in healthy, hyperactive, and psychotic children. *Archives of Neurology*, **59**, 1244–8.

Gogtay, N., Sporn, A., Clasen, L.S., Nugent, T.F. III, Greenstein, D., Nicholson, R. *et al.* (2004). Comparison of progressive cortical gray matter loss in childhood-onset schizophrenia with that in childhood-onset atypical psychoses. *Archives of General Psychiatry*, **61**, 17–22.

Gordon, C. T., Frazier, J. A., McKenna, K., Giedd, J., Zametkin, A., Zahn, T. *et al.* (1994). Childhood-onset schizophrenia: an NIMH study in progress. *Schizophrenia Bulletin*, **20** (4), 697–712.

Green, W. H., Padron-Gayol, M., Hardesty, A. S., and Bassiri, M. (1992). Schizophrenia with childhood onset: a phenomenological study of 38 cases. *Journal of the American Academy of Child and Adolescent Psychiatry*, **31** (5), 968–76.

Gur, R. E., Cowell, P., Turetsky, B. I., Gallacher, F., Cannon, T., Bilker, W. *et al.* (1998). A follow-up magnetic resonance imaging study of schizophrenia. Relationship of neuroanatomical changes to clinical and neurobehavioral measures. *Archives of General Psychiatry*, **55** (2), 145–52.

Harrison, P. J. (1999). The neuropathology of schizophrenia. A critical review of the data and their interpretation. *Brain*, **122** (Pt 4), 593–624.

Ho, B.-C., Andreasen, N. C., Nopoulos, P., Arndt, S., Magnotta, V., and Flaum, M. (2003). Progressive structural brain abnormalities and their relationship to clinical outcome: a longitudinal magnetic resonance imaging study early in schizophrenia. *Archives of General Psychiatry*, **60** (6), 585–94.

Hollis, C. (1995). Child and adolescent (juvenile onset) schizophrenia. A case control study of premorbid developmental impairments. *British Journal of Psychiatry*, **166** (4), 489–95.

Jacobsen, L. K., Giedd, J. N., Vaituzis, A. C., Hamburger, S. D., Rajapakse, J. C., Frazier, J. A., *et al.* (1996). Temporal lobe morphology in childhood-onset schizophrenia. *American Journal of Psychiatry*, **153** (3), 355–61 [published erratum appears in *American Journal of Psychiatry*, 1996, **153** (6), 851].

Jacobsen, L. K., Giedd, J. N., Castellanos, F. X., Vaituzis, A. C., Hamburger, S. D., Kumra, S. *et al.* (1998). Progressive reduction of temporal lobe structures in childhood-onset schizophrenia. *American Journal of Psychiatry*, **155** (5), 678–85.

James, A. C., Javaloyes, A., James, S., and Smith, D. M. (2002). Evidence for non-progressive changes in adolescent-onset schizophrenia: follow-up magnetic resonance imaging study. *British Journal of Psychiatry*, **180**, 339–44.

Jones, P., Rodgers, B., Murray, R., and Marmot, M. (1994). Child development risk factors for adult schizophrenia in the British 1946 birth cohort. *Lancet*, **344** (8934), 1398–402.

Kraepelin, E. (1919). *Dementia Praecox*. Robert E Krieger, Huntington, NY.

Kumra, S., Jacobsen, L. K., Lenane, M., Zahn, T. P., Wiggs, E., Alaghband–Rad, J. *et al.* (1998). 'Multidimensionally impaired disorder': is it a variant of very early-onset schizophrenia? [see comments]. *Journal of the American Academy of Child and Adolescent Psychiatry*, **37** (1), 91–9.

Kumra, S., Giedd, J. N., Vaituzis, A. C., Jacobsen, L. K., McKenna, K., Bedwell, J. *et al.* (2000). Childhood-onset psychotic disorders: magnetic resonance imaging of volumetric differences in brain structure. *American Journal of Psychiatry*, **157** (9), 1467–74.

Lieberman, J., Chakos, M., Wu, H., Alvir, J., Hoffman, E., Robinson, D. *et al.* (2001). Longitudinal study of brain morphology in first episode schizophrenia. *Biological Psychiatry*, **49**, 487–99.

Lim, K. O., Harris, D., Beal, M., Hoff, A. L., Minn, K., Csernansky, J. G. *et al.* (1996). Gray matter deficits in young onset schizophrenia are independent of age of onset. *Biological Psychiatry*, **40**, 4–13.

Lipska, B. K. and Weinberger, D. R. (1995). Genetic variation in vulnerability to the behavioral effects of neonatal hippocampal damage in rats. *Proceedings of the National Academy of Sciences, USA*, **92** (19), 8906–10.

Lipska, B. K., Halim, N. D., Segal, P. N., and Weinberger, D. R. (2002). Effects of reversible inactivation of the neonatal ventral hippocampus on behavior in the adult rat. *Journal of Neuroscience*, **22**, 2835–42.

Marsh, L., Harris, D., Lim, K. O., Beal, M., Hoff, A. L., Minn, K. *et al.* (1997). Structural magnetic resonance imaging abnormalities in men with severe chronic schizophrenia and an early age at clinical onset. *Archives of General Psychiatry*, **54**, 1104–12.

Mathalon, D. H., Sullivan, E. V., Lim, K. O., and Pfefferbaum, A. (2001). Progressive brain volume changes and the clinical course of schizophrenia in men: a longitudinal magnetic resonance imaging study. *Archives of General Psychiatry*, **58**, 148–57.

Matsumoto, H., Simmons, A., Williams, S., Hadjulis, M., Pipe, R., Murray, R. *et al.* (2001*a*). Superior temporal gyrus abnormalities in early-onset schizophrenia: similarities and differences with adult-onset schizophrenia. *American Journal of Psychiatry*, **158** (8), 1299–304.

Matsumoto, H., Simmons, A., Williams, S., Pipe, R., Murray, R., and Frangou, S. (2001*b*). Structural magnetic imaging of the hippocampus in early onset schizophrenia. *Biological Psychiatry*, **49** (10), 824–31.

McGlashan, T. H. and Hoffman, R. E. (2000). Schizophrenia as a disorder of developmentally reduced synaptic connectivity. *Archives of General Psychiatry*, **57** (7), 637–48.

McKenna, K., Gordon, C. T., Lenane, M., Kaysen, D., Fahey, K., and Rapoport, J. L. (1994). Looking for childhood-onset schizophrenia: the first 71 cases screened [see comments]. *Journal of the American Academy of Child and Adolescent Psychiatry*, **33** (5), 636–44.

Nicolson, R. and Rapoport, J. L. (1999). Childhood-onset schizophrenia: rare but worth studying. *Biological Psychiatry*, **46** (10), 1418–28.

Nicolson, R., Lenane, M., Singaracharlu, S., Malaspina, D., Giedd, J. N., Hamburger, S. D. *et al.* (2000). Premorbid speech and language impairments in childhood-onset schizophrenia: association with risk factors. *American Journal of Psychiatry*, **157** (5), 794–800.

Nicolson, R., Lenane, M., Brookner, F., Gochman, P., Kumra, S., Spechler, L. *et al.* (2001). Children and adolescents with psychotic disorder not otherwise specified: A two to eight year follow up. *Comprehensive Psychiatry*, **42** (4), 319–25.

Posner, M. I. and Dehaene, S. (1994). Attentional networks. *Trends in Neurosciences*, **17**, 75–9.

Rapoport, J. L., Giedd, J., Kumra, S., Jacobsen, L., Smith, A., Lee, P. *et al.* (1997). Childhood-onset schizophrenia. Progressive ventricular change during adolescence [see comments]. *Archives of General Psychiatry*, **54** (10), 897–903.

Rapoport, J. L., Giedd, J. N., Blumenthal, J., Hamburger, S., Jeffries, N., Fernandez, T. *et al.* (1999). Progressive cortical change during adolescence in childhood-onset schizophrenia. A longitudinal magnetic resonance imaging study. *Archives of General Psychiatry*, **56** (7), 649–54.

Russell, A. T., Bott, L., and Sammons, C. (1989). The phenomenology of schizophrenia occurring in childhood. *Journal of the American Academy of Child and Adolescent Psychiatry*, **28** (3), 399–407.

Schulz, S. C., Koller, M. M., Kishore, P. R., Hamer, R. M., Gehl, J. J., and Friedel, R. O. (1983). Ventricular enlargement in teenage patients with schizophrenia spectrum disorder. *American Journal of Psychiatry*, **140** (12), 1592–5.

Selemon, L. D. and Goldman-Rakic, P. S. (1999). The reduced neuropil hypothesis: a circuit based model of schizophrenia [see comments]. *Biological Psychiatry*, **45** (1), 17–25.

Sowell, E. R., Levitt, J., Thompson, P. M., Holmes, C. J., Blanton, R. E., Kornsand, D. S. *et al.* (2000). Brain abnormalities in early-onset schizophrenia spectrum disorder observed with statistical parametric mapping of structural magnetic resonance images. *American Journal of Psychiatry*, **157** (9), 1475–84.

Sporn, A. L., Greenstein, D. K., Gogtay, N., Jeffries, N. O., Lenane, M., Gochman, P., *et al.* (2003). Progressive brain volume loss during adolescence in childhood-onset schizophrenia. *American Journal of Psychiatry*, **160**, 2181–9.

Thompson, P. M., Giedd, J. N., Woods, R. P., MacDonald, D., Evans, A. C., and Toga, A. W. (2000). Growth patterns in the developing brain detected by using continuum mechanical tensor maps. *Nature*, **404**, 190–3.

Thompson, P. M., Vidal, C., Giedd, J. N., Gochman, P., Blumenthal, J., Nicolson, R., *et al.* (2001). From the Cover: Mapping adolescent brain change reveals dynamic wave of accelerated gray matter loss in very early-onset schizophrenia. *Proceedings of the National Academy of Sciences, USA*, **98** (20), 11650–5.

Walker, E. and Lewine, R. J. (1990). Prediction of adult-onset schizophrenia from childhood home movies of the patients. *American Journal of Psychiatry* **147**, 1052–6.

Chapter 4

MR proton spectroscopy

Stefano Marenco, Daniel R. Weinberger,
and Alessandro Bertolino

Basic principles and methodology

Spectroscopy allows determination of the relative concentrations of certain chemicals in the brain through a non-invasive procedure based on a nuclear magnetic resonance (NMR) scan. The technique exploits the properties of magnetic nuclei such as hydrogen (^{1}H) and phosphorus (^{31}P). The magnetic property of these and other nuclei is manifested with their 'spin'. When a nucleus has spin, it creates a small magnetic field, with a specific strength and orientation. Normally, in tissue the magnetic fields of separate nuclei cancel out. In a strong external field (such as provided by a clinical MR scanner) a net magnetization of the tissue occurs due to the magnetic nuclei aligning themselves to the major axis of the field. The nuclei with spin will begin precessing around the axis of net magnetization. One can perturb their precession by applying radiofrequency waves (also called excitation pulses) at a specific frequency (the frequency of precession of the particular spin one wants to image, also called Larmor frequency) and intensity. This will cause the spins to modify their alignment as they absorb energy from the radio waves and then return gradually in sync with the main magnetic field, releasing energy that can be measured by a radio antenna. The release of energy is called relaxation, and it follows exponential decay laws that are described by values such as T_1, T_2, and T_2*. The signal obtained from the antenna can then be decomposed in different frequencies, by a mathematical decomposition process called Fourier Transform. The Fourier Transform yields estimates of power for each frequency measured. Thus, for a given imaging element (or voxel) the power present in a certain frequency band will be roughly proportional to the concentration of the compound that emits that particular frequency when one accounts for factors related to the imaging sequence, for specific characteristics of the tissue and chemical being considered, and of the specific hardware being used.

In Fig. 4.1, a typical proton (^{1}H) spectrum is shown. One can notice several peaks of different amplitudes. The position of the peaks in the spectrum (measured in parts per million, or ppm, relative to a reference frequency, usually that of tetramethylsilane, or TMS, for proton spectra) is caused by the phenomena of chemical shift and spin coupling, and the amplitude of the spectra is modulated by relaxation (mentioned above) and chemical exchange. Chemical shift is caused by clouds of electrons moving around

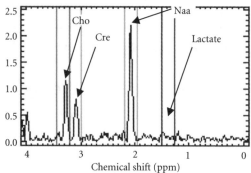

Fig. 4.1 A typical spectrum obtained with a 3T scanner with an echo time (TE) of 280 ms. At this echo time the only metabolites that can clearly be recognized are N-acetyl-aspartate (Naa), choline-containing compounds (Cho), and creatine-containing compounds (Cre), identified by the arrows. Lactate is usually absent in normal brain. The main peaks of interest are identified and the relative limits of the integration peaks are shown as vertical bars surrounding the metabolites.

the nucleus. These electrons produce their own small magnetic field that 'shields' the nucleus, causing it to resonate at a slightly lower frequency (chemical shift). Since each atomic nucleus in each molecule, even if consisting of the same element (e.g. ^{1}H), experiences different shielding, it is possible to recognize different molecules by excitation of only one atomic nucleus. For these molecules to be 'visible' with magnetic resonance spectroscopy (MRS), they have to be naturally abundant and the molecule must be in solution, i.e. freely mobile.

In summary, it is possible to identify different chemical molecules containing ^{1}H as different peaks in a spectrum. Each peak corresponds to one or more molecules and the area under the peak is proportional to the concentration of the molecule.

The metabolites of main interest for ^{1}H studies of schizophrenia are: (1) water at 4.7 ppm, by far the strongest signal in tissue; (2) N-acetyl-aspartate (NAA) at 2 ppm; (3) creatine-containing compounds (Cre) at 3 ppm; and (4) choline-containing compounds (Cho) at 3.2 and 3.9 ppm. Chemical exchange is not critical to the understanding of low-resolution proton spectroscopy of the molecules that are commonly studied in schizophrenia.

Physiology of metabolite peaks that can be observed with proton spectroscopy

N-Acetyl-aspartate

N-Acetyl-aspartate (NAA) is produced primarily in mitochondria of neurons, from aspartate and acetyl-CoA, by the enzyme L-aspartate N-acetyltransferase (Jacobson 1959). It can also derive from the cleavage of N-acetyl-aspartylglutamate (NAAG) by N-acetylated-α-linked-amino dipeptidase (NAALADase) (Slusher *et al.* 1990), although the physiological role of this pathway is uncertain. The synthesis of NAA can be blocked by inhibition of several mitochondrial complexes (Bates *et al.* 1996) or by depletion of glutathione (Heales *et al.* 1995), which indirectly results in mitochondrial dysfunction. Therefore, NAA may index mitochondrial metabolism in addition to neuronal survival (Clark 1998).

NAA can be detected with histochemical techniques, mainly in neurons and mostly pyramidal glutamatergic neurons in the frontal and motor cortices (Moffett *et al.* 1991). However, NAA has also been found in oligodendrocyte cultures (Urenjak *et al.* 1993; Bhakoo and Pearce 2000) and the initial manifestations of Canavan's disease, where excess NAA is present, consist of lesions of white matter rather than gray matter (Matalon *et al.* 1988). Moreover, the main enzyme responsible for the degradation of NAA is found predominantly in oligodendrocytes (Baslow *et al.* 1999). These data point to a role of NAA in white matter.

The precise physiological role of NAA remains undetermined—but see excellent reviews by Tsai and Coyle (1995) and Baslow (2000). Roles in transporting water molecules produced during oxidative metabolism outside of the neuron (Baslow 2002), and as an acetyl donor for the formation of membranes (D'Adamo and Yatsu 1966; Shigematsu *et al.* 1983) have been proposed. Recently, data derived from medial temporal lobe resected from patients with intractable epilepsy (Petroff *et al.* 2002) seem to support a coupling between NAA and glutamate production.

NAA reductions have been reported in disorders where there is neuronal death, such as Alzheimer's disease (AD) (Miller *et al.* 1993; Schuff *et al.* 2002), and metabolic dysfunction, such as human immunodeficiency virus (HIV) infection (Meyerhoff *et al.* 1994). NAA is also reduced in temporal lobe epilepsy (Hugg *et al.* 1993) and its reduction correlates with depression of glucose metabolism, as measured with positron emission tomography (PET) (Lu *et al.* 1997; but see Knowlton *et al.* 2002 for evidence to the contrary). Although neuronal loss is present in these patients, it does not seem to explain the degree of NAA reduction, which may correlate more closely with mitochondrial dysfunction (Petroff *et al.* 2002). The only condition where NAA is unequivocally increased is Canavan's disease, as mentioned above.

NAA reductions have been shown to be at least partially reversible under treatment for multiple sclerosis (De Stefano *et al.* 1995) or HIV (Vion-Dury *et al.* 1995), indicating that NAA reductions should not be interpreted as equivalent to irreversible tissue loss unless there is pathological evidence for this (as in AD).

Choline

The choline (Cho) peak includes several different metabolites, mainly choline, phosphatidylcholine, glycerophosphocholine, phosphocholine, and, to a lesser extent, acetylcholine (Miller 1991). It is still unclear which one of these compounds contributes most to this peak, but glycerophosphocholine (Tan *et al.* 1998) and phosphocholine (Tunggal *et al.* 1990) are the best candidates. Changes of the choline peak are not unequivocally interpretable (for a review, see Boulanger *et al.* 2000). Nevertheless, Cho peak increases have been demonstrated in various disorders where there is excessive membrane breakdown, such as multiple sclerosis (Wolinsky *et al.* 1990; Degaonkar *et al.* 2002) and Huntington's disease (Jenkins *et al.* 1993). The degree to which the choline peak is sensitive to alimentary choline intake is still unclear (Stoll *et al.* 1995; Tan *et al.* 1998).

Creatine

The creatine (Cre) peak includes creatine and creatine phosphate. The latter serves as a reserve for high-energy phosphates and buffers ATP/ADP reservoirs (Miller 1991), while creatine constitutes one of its precursors. Generally, because Cre is thought to be unaffected in several pathological processes, it is used as a reference to normalize other metabolites. In these studies the assumption is that Cre does not change due to the pathological condition examined, but this assumption is rarely tested (for a positive example, see Jenkins *et al.* 2000).

It would be preferable to have absolute measurements of metabolites rather than ratios. Unfortunately, absolute metabolite concentration measurements *in vivo* have important limitations, although several authors currently claim to have achieved this goal.

Other recognizable peaks at short TE

When imaging with short echo times, metabolites such as myoinositol (related to metabolism or possibly to glial integrity) and a peak containing glutamate and γ-aminobutyric acid (GABA) (Glx peak), as well as NAAG (Pouwels and Frahm 1997), can be measured. However, the peaks are not easily differentiated from the background and corrections for unsuppressed water and other macromolecules become critical, creating potential sources of error. Clearly, the techniques that are able to measure GABA, glutamate, and NAAG (all neurotransmitters that have been implicated in the pathogenesis of schizophrenia) are of great potential interest for schizophrenia investigators, but caution is needed when interpreting the results.

Technical aspects of *in vivo* measurements

Many strategies for spectroscopy measurements and data processing are used in the literature. A detailed review is not possible here, but we give a list of some major factors of technical variability, taken from the literature, that can influence the results:

- main field (B_0) strength;
- water suppression, fat suppression;
- acquisition sequence and localization methods (single voxel versus imaging);
- time of echo (TE) and time of repetition (TR);
- filtering, voxel size, and partial volume effects;
- spectral fitting versus integral of the peak;

- modality of spectral exclusion for quality control; and
- ratios of metabolites versus 'absolute' quantification.

For a detailed description of these factors related to MR spectroscopy a useful textbook reference (Salibi and Brown 1998) and a recent review with a methodological focus (Stanley *et al.* 2000) are available.

Proton spectroscopy as a tool to investigate the impact of genetic variation on brain function

Given the important physiological implications of changes in metabolites, proton spectroscopy has been used recently to identify the effects of genetic variations on NAA concentrations. Egan *et al.* (2003) found a reduction in left hippocampal NAA/Cre to be associated with the presence of a variation of the gene encoding brain-derived neurotrophic factor (BDNF). This variation consisted of the substitution of a single amino acid (a methionine for a valine) in the BDNF pro-protein. The authors show that this mutation has important implications in the trafficking of the protein, and probably disrupts its depolarization-induced secretion, which may be critical for the effects of this molecule on long-term potentiation in the medial temporal lobe. Not only was the NAA/Cre ratio reduced in the carriers of the methionine allele, but their performance on an episodic verbal memory task was reduced as compared to the valine allele carriers, and hippocampal blood flow activation measured with functional MRI was also altered. However, it is entirely unclear by which mechanism NAA would be reduced as a consequence of changes in the BDNF genotype.

Other groups have attempted to link NAA to cognitive function and the apolipoprotein E (APOE) gene, since it is known that one form of this gene confers risk for AD and may be associated with reduced memory function. No association has been found between measures of NAA concentrations and this gene in two studies *in vivo* (Bartres-Faz *et al.* 2002; Kantarci *et al.* 2002), including one where left medial temporal lobe measures were performed (Bartres-Faz *et al.* 2002). However, one post-mortem investigation has found that NAA, phosphomonoesthers, and phosphodiesther abnormalities were all accentuated when comparing patients who carried the APOE-4 allele as compared to homozygotes for the APOE-3 allele (Klunk *et al.* 1998).

Findings in schizophrenia

We will focus here on proton studies of schizophrenia. For a review of 31P studies in schizophrenia see Keshavan *et al.* (2000) and Weinberger and Laruelle (2002).

Findings in the medial temporal lobe

Most of the literature on schizophrenia seems to converge on one finding: reduced hippocampal or medial temporal lobe NAA/Cre. This has been shown by Nasrallah *et al.* (1994) in chronic patients treated with neuroleptics, and has been replicated numerous times with single voxel techniques in chronic (Maier *et al.* 1995; Maier and Ron 1996; Yurgelun-Todd *et al.* 1996; Fukuzako *et al.* 1999) and first-episode (Renshaw *et al.* 1995) patients treated with neuroleptics. Cecil *et al.* (1999) studied a region including the superior temporal gyrus and insula, in drug-naïve, first-episode patients, and found significant reductions of NAA/Cre. All studies that have used measures of multiple voxels have found a reduction of NAA/Cre in hippocampus/medial temporal lobe in adults (Bertolino *et al.* 1996, 1998*a*; Deicken *et al.* 1999) and children with schizophrenia (Bertolino *et al.* 1998*b*), in medication-free patients (Bertolino *et al.* 1998*a*), and in the siblings of patients (Callicott *et al.* 1998); the latter suggesting that this is a genetically inherited trait that may predispose to the illness. Most recently, this finding has been replicated yet again, by an imaging study that corrected for cerebrospinal fluid (CSF) contributions to the imaging voxels and estimated absolute concentrations of NAA (Weber-Fahr *et al.* 2002). No differences were found for Cho and Cre in this study, and this may help interpret the prior studies where only ratios could be assessed. However, the authors do not separate out gray and white matter, and analyze results only from two voxels inside the hippocampal formation. There is a need for further studies of this kind and improved quantitative assessment of individual metabolites.

The literature also includes some negative results. For example Bartha *et al.* (1999) could not demonstrate a reduction of absolute NAA concentrations in the left mesial temporal lobe, using a method that fits the metabolites based on *a priori* knowledge and modeling of the various components of the spectrum. They studied first-episode and never-treated patients. Similarly, Buckley *et al.*(1994), Heimberg *et al.*(1998), and Kegeles *et al.* (2000) could not find medial temporal lobe differences from controls in patients with schizophrenia.

There may be several reasons for these discrepancies. For example, several of these studies did not match patients and normal controls for age (Maier and Ron 1996; Yurgelun-Todd *et al.* 1996; Cecil *et al.* 1999). The lack of a correlation of their NAA measures with age may be due to small sample sizes over a limited age span. Another aspect of this literature is that although the majority of studies use a ratio of NAA to Cre, several studies used different ratios that are not necessarily related. For example, Nasrallah *et al.* (1994) used a ratio of NAA to the spectrum between 9 and 12 ppm (this is the only study using this ratio). Maier *et al.* (1995) used a ratio to unsuppressed water, but it is unclear how they accounted for the contribution of CSF to the volume of interest. Similarly, Bartha *et al.* (1999) used a ratio to water, but apparently assumed that the relative contributions of gray matter, white matter, and CSF are constant across subjects. Deicken *et al.* (1999) used an institutional measure of absolute NAA corrected for coil loading and amplifier settings.

Another important factor to consider is the time of echo of the signal acquisitions. In a recent meeting abstract (Ke *et al.* 2002), a significant shortening in NAA T_2 was reported between patients with schizophrenia and normal controls. If this were the case, one would expect larger differences between patients and controls in studies performed with longer TE, when T_2 signal loss is more prominent. Indeed, all studies performed with a TE above 100 ms found reduced absolute NAA or NAA/Cre values, while studies with short to moderate TE (20–70 ms) are evenly divided between studies that find a reduction and those that do not. If confirmed, differences in T_2 relaxation time of NAA in schizophrenia could be of great interest. T_2 is related to the molecular environment of the measured protons and finding what alters NAA signal might be an important clue to the pathophysiology of schizophrenia. However, this also raises the possibility that T_2 differences could artifactually reduce NAA signals in patients. Finally, there are significant differences in the composition of patient cohorts: degree of chronicity, male/female assortment, schizophrenia subtypes, medications, and use of benzodiazepines prior to the scan vary widely.

Despite the inconsistencies in methodology, the literature appears fairly concordant in supporting a reduction of NAA or NAA/Cre in the medial temporal lobe in schizophrenia. Although some have interpreted this reduction as related to neuron death, this appears to be unlikely in the light of neuropathological findings, even very recent ones (Walker *et al.* 2002) that do not find neuronal loss in the hippocampus. The MRI and neuropathological literature support a relative functional deficiency of hippocampal circuits associated with reduced neuropil in schizophrenia (Weinberger 1999).

Findings in prefrontal areas

Prefrontal areas of the brain have been investigated as a site of particular neuronal pathology in schizophrenia (Weinberger *et al.* 2001). Investigation of prefrontal areas with MRS has followed. Finding an abnormality of NAA in dorsolateral prefrontal cortex (PFC) would be expected to reflect reduced neuronal function and to be a possible hallmark of the illness (Weinberger *et al.* 2001). Some of the strongest evidence supporting the central role of the prefrontal cortex in mediating negative symptoms and in regulating dopamine release in the basal ganglia has been achieved with MRS.

The first obstacle to the interpretation of this literature is that the positioning of voxels for analysis has been very heterogeneous. We will try to categorize the studies, based on which section of the frontal lobes they cover, assuming that there is some functional specificity (and therefore neurochemical diversity) between different prefrontal areas.

Prefrontal areas: dorsolateral prefrontal cortex

The work by Bertolino and colleagues at the NIMH has addressed the pathophysiology of prefrontal abnormalities in NAA/Cre in detail, generating important new knowledge in the field. Besides finding reduced NAA/Cre in the PFC in patients on and off medications (Bertolino *et al.* 1996, 1998*a*) and in children with schizophrenia (Bertolino *et al.* 1998*b*), correlations have emerged between reductions in NAA/Cre in the PFC and increased negative symptoms (Callicott *et al.* 2000*a*), and reduced regional cerebral blood flow activation or altered blood oxygenation level dependent (BOLD) signal during the execution of tasks that engage the frontal lobe (Bertolino *et al.* 2000*b*;

Callicott *et al.* 2000*b*), stressing the functional significance of NAA abnormalities in this area. The paper by Bertolino *et al.* (2000*b*) examined two cohorts of patients with schizophrenia and matched normal controls performing two different tasks that engage the prefrontal cortex by activating a working memory network: the Wisconsin Card Sorting Test (WCST) and the N-Back. These subjects received a spectroscopy study at rest and a PET cerebral blood flow (CBF) study during the execution of either task. In patients with schizophrenia, NAA/Cre values specifically in the PFC predicted the degree of blood flow activation in an extended working memory network. Callicott *et al.* (2000*b*) analyzed the relationship of NAA/Cre values in the PFC and changes in BOLD response during the execution of the N-Back with fMRI. They found an inverse correlation between NAA/Cre in the PFC and BOLD activation in patients with schizophrenia: the greater the neuronal pathology (low NAA/Cre) the larger the change in BOLD signal during the N-Back task. The patients also had increased BOLD responses compared to the controls, which was interpreted as lower efficiency in processing the demands of the working memory task. Both schizophrenia cohorts had reduced NAA/Cre in the PFC as compared to normal values; however, no correlation between reduced NAA/Cre and fMRI signal were present in the hippocampus, which also showed altered fMRI signal (Callicott *et al.*2000*b*). Therefore, although the direction of the abnormality in BOLD signal measured with fMRI, and CBF measured with PET, is opposite, in both cases the NAA/Cre level *specifically* in the dorsal PFC predicted the degree of abnormality in activation of the working memory network in patients with schizophrenia.

Negative findings have been reported in dorsolateral PFC. A lack of statistically significant reductions of NAA/Cre has been shown (Stanley *et al.* 1996; Block *et al.* 2000) (although these authors do find NAA/Cho reductions), even with methodology entirely consistent with prior positive studies (Callicott *et al.* 1998). This is possibly because of variations in patient cohorts.

Despite these isolated negative findings, the pathophysiological implications of reduced NAA/Cre for schizophrenia have been shown to be extensive. For example, reduced blood flow activation in the PFC during a working memory task (Berman *et al.* 1986; Weinberger *et al.* 1986) has been linked to increased dopamine metabolism in the basal ganglia (Meyer-Lindenberg *et al.* 2002) and to cognitive dysfunction in patients with schizophrenia. The increased release of dopamine in the basal ganglia of patients with schizophrenia has, in turn, been linked to positive symptoms, since dopamine blockers are effective in reducing them. It has also been observed that especially patients with acute illness exacerbation show increased dopamine release in the basal ganglia (Laruelle *et al.* 1996, 1999; Breier *et al.* 1997). Bertolino *et al.* (2000*a*) linked these observations to reductions in NAA/Cre in the PFC of patients with schizophrenia. They showed a negative correlation between NAA/Cre in the PFC and the degree of dopamine release in the basal ganglia, as measured by the displacement of [^{11}C]raclopride by amphetamine. Moreover, Bertolino *et al.* (1999) showed that

NAA/Cre in the PFC correlated negatively with D_2 receptor availability in the basal ganglia, as measured by binding potential for IBZM (a iodinated D_2 ligand). This correlation was not found in any other region explored and was interpreted to mean that a dysfunction of PFC (resulting in low NAA/Cre) was related to lower baseline dopamine levels in the basal ganglia (resulting in higher binding potential of IBZM, a ligand that can be displaced by endogenous dopamine). Current evidence indicates that NAA reduction in the PFC is likely not of a genetic origin, since it is not found in siblings of patients with schizophrenia (as opposed to medial temporal lobe NAA reduction: Callicott et al. 1998). A recent study (Kinney et al. 2000) has shown that prefrontal NAA/Cre is negatively correlated, although weakly, to the severity of obstetric complications. The only available investigation of subjects at risk for schizophrenia studied with spectroscopy in the anterior cingulate region (Keshavan et al. 1997) found a trend towards a reduction of NAA/Cho. Therefore, it is likely that environmental causation interacts with a genetic predisposition to dysfunctional medial temporal lobe circuits, to cause failure of prefrontal circuits in early adulthood (Weinberger 1986).

Prefrontal areas: frontal-pole white matter and superior frontal gyrus

The majority of spectroscopy studies focusing on the frontal lobe have been performed with single voxels placed in the white matter of the frontal pole, sometimes including the cortex of the superior frontal gyrus. The first investigation to be conducted in this area was by Buckley et al. (1994). They found a weak reduction of NAA/(NAA + Cre + Cho) and an increase in Cho. More substantial reductions of NAA/Cre were found by Choe et al. (1994) in 23 drug-naïve chronic patients with schizophrenia, then replicated in a larger study of 34 patients and 20 normal controls (Choe et al. 1996), as well as by Cecil et al. (1999), who studied patients in their first episode of illness with minimal neuroleptic exposure, Deicken et al. (1997a) and Steel et al. (2001). Lim et al. (1998) found selective reductions of NAA in white matter of prefrontal and parietal white matter. Although extremely useful in accounting for partial volume effects of gray and white matter, their sophisticated technique did not allow for more detailed regional analysis. This is important especially for gray matter, since one of the assumptions of their work is that NAA concentration is stable across functionally distinct cortical areas (e.g. dorsolateral and medial prefrontal cortices).

Fukuzako et al. (1995) and Heimberg et al. (1998) found no difference between fairly large samples of patients and normal controls in a predominantly white matter region of the prefrontal lobe. In conclusion, most studies appear to find reductions of NAA/Cre or NAA in the white matter of the prefrontal lobe, independent of the type of methodology used. There are inconsistencies, but these are most likely due to the types of patients included. Regarding differences in T_2, the above mentioned abstract by Ke et al. (2002) shows more pronounced shortening of the T_2 of NAA in prefrontal white matter. This may explain the higher degree of consistency of long and short TE studies in this area.

Prefrontal areas: medial prefrontal cortex and cingulate gyrus

Several authors have focused on medial prefrontal cortex and the anterior cingulate gyrus. Bartha *et al.* (1997) found increased glutamine in the medial prefrontal cortex, in patients who had no prior history of treatment with antipsychotics, which may be compatible with reduced glutamate transmission. It has to be stressed that the variability of the measurement of glutamine was very high (50% of the mean), therefore raising the concern that one cannot obtain reliable estimates of metabolites with low signal, the peaks of which are sometimes difficult to differentiate from surrounding ones. Theberge *et al.* (2002) have recently replicated the finding of an increased amount of glutamine in a separate set of 21 drug-naïve patients, with a 4T magnet that allows quantification of metabolites in smaller voxels. No significant difference in NAA between patients and controls was found in either study. This was also the case in Bertolino *et al.* (1996) and Delamillieure *et al.* (2002).

Reductions of NAA/Cre or absolute NAA measures were found by Deicken *et al.* (1997*b*), Do *et al.* (2000), and in selected populations, e.g. in a few patients with the deficit syndrome (Delamillieure *et al.* 2000), in children with schizophrenia (Thomas *et al.* 1998), and in patients taking typical neuroleptics (Ende *et al.* 2000). Yamasue *et al.* (2002) found reduced NAA/Cho and increased Cho/Cre in the anterior cingulate of patients with schizophrenia treated with typical neuroleptics versus controls, reminiscent of the results by Buckley *et al.* (1994).

None of the above-mentioned studies that use 'absolute' measures of NAA, except for Theberge *et al.* (2002), takes into account the content of CSF in the measured region, a potentially important confound for cortical measurements. Bartha *et al.* (1997) and Theberge *et al.* (2002) use a reference to water corrected for various factors, which may be prone to errors. As frequently the case in the spectroscopy literature, the exact location of the voxels analyzed in these studies differed, and therefore it is unclear whether these studies are fully comparable.

In conclusion, the evidence for a medial prefrontal reduction in NAA is not consistent and further studies are needed to confirm and characterize it.

Findings in the cerebellum

Deicken *et al.* (2001) have found reduced NAA and Cre concentrations in the cerebellar vermis, which were independent of gray matter composition of the voxels. Other studies conducted with fairly large voxels have been negative (Eluri *et al.* 1998; Tibbo *et al.* 2000), as was as a post-mortem study (Omori *et al.* 1997). However, Eluri *et al.* (1998) did find reduced NAA/Cre in the pons of patients with schizophrenia. The results of all of these studies may be questionable given the enhanced pulsatility of these regions under the effect of the cardiac cycle.

Findings in the thalamus

Heimberg *et al.* (1998), Deicken *et al.* (2000), Omori *et al.* (2000), Auer *et al.* (2001), and Ende *et al.* (2001) found reductions in of NAA the thalamus, but Bertolino *et al.*

(1996, 1998a), Delamillieure *et al.* (2002), Hagino *et al.* (2002), and Theberge *et al.* (2002) did not find changes in NAA/Cre or NAA/Cho in this brain region. The mediodorsal nucleus of the thalamus is possibly the only brain region where careful and replicated studies have found a reduction in neuronal counts in patients with schizophrenia compared with normal controls post-mortem (Pakkenberg 1992; Popken *et al.* 2000; Young *et al.* 2000). Therefore a reduction in NAA, but possibly also in Cre, may be expected. On the other hand, an increase in Cho would not be expected, given the lack of gliosis in schizophrenia. Ende *et al.* (2001) found a reduction in Cho, possibly indicating a reduction in synapse formation; however, none of the other investigations mentioned here showed positive findings for Cho. Most papers published on the thalamus are lacking corrections for partial voluming of gray and white matter, and voxel sizes (4–6 mm) are typically larger than the mediodorsal nucleus itself, therefore it is not clear whether the observed reductions of NAA are compatible with the neuropathological findings. In Deicken *et al.* (2000), special care was dedicated to placing a single voxel 1.5 mm in volume within the boundaries of the thalamus. Theberge *et al.* (2002) found an increase in left thalamic glutamine similar to their finding in the anterior cingulate region.

Findings in the basal ganglia

Other spectroscopy studies in schizophrenia have focused on the basal ganglia. Bertolino *et al.* (1996, 1998a), Heimberg *et al.* (1998), and Ohara *et al.* (2000) found no difference between patients with schizophrenia and controls in metabolite ratios in the putamen, but older studies found small reductions in NAA/Cho bilaterally (Fujimoto *et al.* 1996) or in the left caudate (Shioiri *et al.* 1996) of patients with schizophrenia. More recently, Bustillo *et al.* (2002b) found elevations of choline in the left caudate nucleus of 11 antipsychotic naïve patients with schizophrenia, compared with age-matched controls. The weight of the evidence is therefore for elevated choline, at least in the caudate, while results in the putamen are negative. This choline elevation has been interpreted by Bustillo *et al.* (2002b) as possibly reflecting decreased glucose metabolism, or possibly a dysfunction in phospholipid membrane formation.

The effects of neuroleptics

Neuroleptics have been found to increase NAA/Cre values in the dorsolateral prefrontal cortex in patients with schizophrenia (Bertolino *et al.*, 2001). This study included 23 patients, 14 of which were treated with atypical antipsychotics. The atypical antipsychotics appeared to have a somewhat greater effect in elevating NAA/Cre in the dorsolateral prefrontal cortex than typical neuroleptics.

Somewhat similar results were found by Braus *et al.* (2001) in the anterior cingulate. NAA, after correction for age, correlated significantly and positively with time of exposure to atypical neuroleptics in 12 patients, while there was a tendency to decrease over time in the group of 11 patients who had been treated exclusively with typicals. Also the findings by Heimberg *et al.* (1998) seem to indicate higher values of NAA/Cre in the frontal lobe of patients treated with atypical versus typical antipsychotics, although the number of subjects in the two groups was very small (two and four, respectively).

Bustillo *et al.* (2001) reported that patients treated with haloperidol had lower NAA than patients treated with clozapine, and that only those treated with haloperidol had significantly lower values than normal. In a longitudinal study, the same group found that frontal white matter NAA decreased in all but one patient after treatment with quietiapine or haloperidol (Bustillo *et al.* 2002*a*). These results were interpreted as an indication of a possibly toxic effect of neuroleptics on prefrontal NAA. All the studies cited above remain somewhat inconclusive though, since they generally compare two different cohorts of patients, or it is difficult to separate the effects due to illness duration and neuroleptic exposure. Evidence available to this point, on the overall effect of neuroleptics on frontal lobe NAA, remains controversial.

There is one report that looked at the peak representing glutamate, glutamine, and GABA (Glx peak) before and after treatment with olanzapine (Goff *et al.* 2002). They found that although this peak did not change overall, it did increase in those patients who had improvement in negative symptoms. A prior study that followed 34 neuroleptic-naïve patients and chronic patients during 4–6 months of treatment with mostly typical neuroleptics found a reduction of the Glx peak (Choe *et al.* 1996). This study had also observed increases in the Glx peak at baseline (prior to neuroleptic treatment), therefore indicating a normalization of this parameter during the initial treatment phases. Two notes of caution are necessary in assessing these conflicting results: (1) the peak is difficult to detect and therefore the measurement is prone to errors; (2) attribution of changes in this peak to glutamate, and particularly to synaptically released glutamate, is questionable.

Glutathione measures as a proxy for oxidative metabolism

Although not commonly used, proton spectroscopy may be able to provide a measure of cerebral oxidative metabolism by measuring the levels of glutathione *in vivo*. This is achieved by observing the cysteine peak at 2.95 ppm. Work by Do *et al.* (2000) indicates that this measurement is feasible and to some extent quantifiable. This group found a 50% reduction in glutathione in the medial prefrontal cortex of 14 patients with schizophrenia (nine of which were naïve or off medications for at least 6 months), the largest difference ever reported for any metabolite. This agreed with smaller reductions (27%) in the gluthatione found in the CSF. NAA was also reduced in a subsample of these patients. This is interesting because a study in rats had previously demonstrated that glutathione depletion is associated with mitochondrial dysfunction and reductions of NAA concentrations (Heales *et al.* 1995). Therefore, it is plausible that NAA and glutathione reduction and mitochondrial dysfunction may all be observed at the same time. Although of interest, this work on glutathione lacks replication and a demonstration of relationship to symptoms or other key aspects of the illness.

New techniques

New techniques for the measurement of GABA (Rothman *et al.* 1993; Shen *et al.* 2002) are becoming available, but have not yet been employed in the study of schizophrenia. More recently, spectroscopic techniques able to measure neuronal metabolism have emerged (Rothman *et al.* 1992; Shen and Rothman 2002). These techniques study the metabolic cycle of glutamate and glutamine by administering ^{13}C-labeled glucose that gets incorporated into glutamate and rapidly exchanged with glutamine proportionally to excitatory metabolism. An analogous technique has been developed to study GABA metabolism, therefore assessing inhibitory metabolism. Although still in their infancy and still using quite large voxels, these techniques represent an interesting development of spectroscopy techniques.

Conclusion

MR spectroscopy has made important contributions to understanding the pathophysiology of schizophrenia. Further advances will likely derive by replicating and extending associations of NAA measures with genetic variants that may influence the schizophrenia phenotype, such as brain-derived neurotrophic factor (Egan *et al.* 2003). As our understanding of the function of NAA increases, so will our ability to interpret findings in the literature. Moreover, improvements in the image acquisition techniques and in absolute quantification of metabolites *in vivo* will advance our understanding further, especially when complemented by the study of new metabolites. In short, MR spectroscopy is an important tool in the study of the complex abnormalities of brain function associated with schizophrenia.

References

Auer, D. P., Wilke, M., Grabner, A., Heidenreich, J. O., Bronisch, T., and Wetter, T. C. (2001). Reduced NAA in the thalamus and altered membrane and glial metabolism in schizophrenic patients detected by 1H-MRS and tissue segmentation *Schizophrenia Research*, **52**, 87–99.

Bartha, R., Williamson, P. C., Drost, D. J., Malla, A., Carr, T. J., Cortese, L. *et al.* (1997). Measurement of glutamate and glutamine in the medial prefrontal cortex of never-treated schizophrenic patients and healthy controls by proton magnetic resonance spectroscopy *Archives of General Psychiatry*, **54**, 959–65.

Bartha, R., al-Semaan, Y. M., Williamson, P. C., Drost, D. J., Malla, A. K., Carr, T. J. *et al.* (1999). A short echo proton magnetic resonance spectroscopy study of the left mesial-temporal lobe in first-onset schizophrenic patients *Biological Psychiatry*, **45**, 1403–11.

Bartres-Faz, D., Junque, C., Clemente, I. C., Lopez-Alomar, A., Bargallo, N., Mercader, J. M. *et al.* (2002). Relationship among (1)H-magnetic resonance spectroscopy, brain volumetry and genetic polymorphisms in humans with memory impairment *Neuroscience Letters*, **327**, 177–80.

Baslow, M. H. (2000). Functions of N-acetyl-L-aspartate and N-acetyl-L-aspartylglutamate in the vertebrate brain: role in glial cell-specific signaling. *Journal of Neurochemistry*, **75**, 453–9.

Baslow, M. H. (2002). Evidence supporting a role for N-acetyl-L-aspartate as a molecular water pump in myelinated neurons in the central nervous system. An analytical review. *Neurochemistry International*, **40**, 295–300.

Baslow, M. H., Suckow, R. F., Sapirstein, V., and Hungund, B. L. (1999). Expression of aspartoacylase activity in cultured rat macroglial cells is limited to oligodendrocytes. *Journal of Molecular Neuroscience*, **13**, 47–53.

Bates, T. E., Strangward, M., Keelan, J., Davey, G. P., Munro, P. M., and Clark, J. B. (1996). Inhibition of N-acetylaspartate production: implications for 1H MRS studies in vivo. *Neuroreport*, **7**, 1397–400.

Berman, K. F., Zec, R. F., and Weinberger, D. R. (1986). Physiologic dysfunction of dorsolateral prefrontal cortex in schizophrenia. II. Role of neuroleptic treatment, attention, and mental effort. *Archives of General Psychiatry*, **43**, 126–35.

Bertolino, A., Nawroz, S., Mattay, V. S., Barnett, A. S., Duyn, J. H., Mooren, C. T. *et al.* (1996). Regionally specific pattern of neurochemical pathology in schizophrenia as assessed by multislice proton magnetic resonance spectroscopic imaging. *American Journal of Psychiatry*, **153**, 1554–63.

Bertolino, A., Callicott, J. H., Elman, I., Adler, C., Mattay, V. S., Shapiro, M. *et al.* (1998a). Regionally specific neuronal pathology in untreated patients with schizophrenia: a proton magnetic resonance spectroscopic imaging study. *Biological Psychiatry*, **43**, 641–8.

Bertolino, A., Kumra, S., Callicott, J. H., Mattay, V. S., Lestz, R. M., Jacobsen, L. *et al.* (1998b). Common pattern of cortical pathology in childhood-onset and adult-onset schizophrenia as identified by proton magnetic resonance spectroscopic imaging. *American Journal of Psychiatry*, **155**, 1376–83.

Bertolino, A., Knable, M. B., Saunders, R. C., Callicott, J. H., Kolachana, B., Mattay, V. S. *et al.* (1999). The relationship between dorsolateral prefrontal N-acetylaspartate measures and striatal dopamine activity in schizophrenia *Biological Psychiatry*, **45**, 660–7.

Bertolino, A., Breier, A., Callicott, J. H., Adler, C., Mattay, V. S., Shapiro, M. *et al.* (2000a). The relationship between dorsolateral prefrontal neuronal N-acetylaspartate and evoked release of striatal dopamine in schizophrenia *Neuropsychopharmacology*, **22**, 125–32.

Bertolino, A., Esposito, G., Callicott, J. H., Mattay, V. S., Van Horn, J. D., Frank, J. A. *et al.* (2000b). Specific relationship between prefrontal neuronal N-acetylaspartate and activation of the working memory cortical network in schizophrenia. *American Journal of Psychiatry*, **157**, 26–33.

Bertolino, A., Callicott, J. H., Mattay, V. S., Weidenhammer, K. M., Rakow, R., Egan, M. *et al.* (2001). The effect of treatment with antipsychotic drugs on brain N-acetylaspartate measures in patients with schizophrenia. *Biological Psychiatry*, **49**, 39–46.

Bhakoo, K. K. and Pearce, D. (2000). In vitro expression of N-acetyl aspartate by oligodendrocytes: implications for proton magnetic resonance spectroscopy signal in vivo. *Journal of Neurochemistry*, **74**, 254–62.

Block, W., Bayer, T. A., Tepest, R., Traber, F., Rietschel, M., Muller, D. J. *et al.* (2000). Decreased frontal lobe ratio of N-acetyl aspartate to choline in familial schizophrenia: a proton magnetic resonance spectroscopy study. *Neuroscience Letters*, **289**, 147–51.

Boulanger, Y., Labelle, M., and Khiat, A. (2000). Role of phospholipase A(2) on the variations of the choline signal intensity observed by 1H magnetic resonance spectroscopy in brain diseases. *Brain Research Brain Research Reviews*, **33**, 380–9.

Braus, D. F., Ende, G., Weber-Fahr, W., Demirakca, T., and Henn, F. A. (2001). Favorable effect on neuronal viability in the anterior cingulate gyrus due to long-term treatment with atypical antipsychotics: an MRSI study. *Pharmacopsychiatry*, **34**, 251–3.

Breier, A., Su, T. P., Saunders, R., Carson, R. E., Kolachana, B. S., de Bartolomeis, A. *et al.* (1997). Schizophrenia is associated with elevated amphetamine-induced synaptic dopamine concentrations: evidence from a novel positron emission tomography method. *Proceedings of the National Academy of Sciences, USA*, **94**, 2569–74.

Buckley, P. F., Moore, C., Long, H., Larkin, C., Thompson, P., Mulvany, F. *et al.* (1994). 1H-magnetic resonance spectroscopy of the left temporal and frontal lobes in schizophrenia: clinical, neurodevelopmental, and cognitive correlates. *Biological Psychiatry*, **36**, 792–800.

Bustillo, J. R., Lauriello, J., Rowland, L. M., Jung, R. E., Petropoulo, H., Hart, B. L. *et al.* (2001). Effects of chronic haloperidol and clozapine treatments on frontal and caudate neurochemistry in schizophrenia. *Psychiatry Research*, **107**, 135–49.

Bustillo, J. R., Lauriello, J., Rowland, L. M., Thomson, L. M., Petropoulos, H., Hammond, R. *et al.* (2002a). Longitudinal follow-up of neurochemical changes during the first year of antipsychotic treatment in schizophrenia patients with minimal previous medication exposure. *Schizophrenia Research*, **58**, 313–21.

Bustillo, J. R., Rowland, L. M., Lauriello, J., Petropoulos, H., Hammond, R., Hart, B. *et al.* (2002b). High choline concentrations in the caudate nucleus in antipsychotic-naive patients with schizophrenia. *American Journal of Psychiatry*, **159**, 130–3.

Callicott, J. H., Egan, M. F., Bertolino, A., Mattay, V. S., Langheim, F. J., and Fraňk J. A. *et al.* (1998). Hippocampal N-acetyl aspartate in unaffected siblings of patients with schizophrenia: a possible intermediate neurobiological phenotype. *Biological Psychiatry*, **44**, 941–50.

Callicott, J. H., Bertolino, A., Egan, M. F., Mattay, V. S., Langheim, F. J., and Weinberger, D. R. (2000a). Selective relationship between prefrontal N-acetylaspartate measures and negative symptoms in schizophrenia. *American Journal of Psychiatry*, **157**, 1646–51.

Callicott, J. H., Bertolino, A., Mattay, V. S., Langheim, F. J., Duyn, J., Coppola, R. *et al.* (2000b). Physiological dysfunction of the dorsolateral prefrontal cortex in schizophrenia revisited. *Cerebral Cortex*, **10,** 1078–92.

Cecil, K. M., Lenkinski, R. E., Gur, R. E., and Gur, R. C. (1999). Proton magnetic resonance spectroscopy in the frontal and temporal lobes of neuroleptic naive patients with schizophrenia. *Neuropsychopharmacology*, **20**, 131–40.

Choe, B. Y., Kim, K. T., Suh, T. S., Lee, C., Paik, I. H., Bahk, Y. W. *et al.* (1994). 1H magnetic resonance spectroscopy characterization of neuronal dysfunction in drug-naive, chronic schizophrenia. *Academic Radiology*, **1**, 211–16.

Choe, B. Y., Suh, T. S., Shinn, K. S., Lee, C. W., Lee, C., and Paik, I. H. (1996). Observation of metabolic changes in chronic schizophrenia after neuroleptic treatment by in vivo hydrogen magnetic resonance spectroscopy. *Investigative Radiology*, **31**, 345–52.

Clark, J. B. (1998). N-acetyl aspartate: a marker for neuronal loss or mitochondrial dysfunction. *Developmental Neuroscience*, **20**, 271–6.

D'Adamo, A. F., Jr and Yatsu, F. M. (1966). Acetate metabolism in the nervous system. N-acetyl-L-aspartic acid and the biosynthesis of brain lipids *Journal of Neurochemistry*, **13**, 961–5.

Degaonkar, M. N., Khubchandhani, M., Dhawan, J. K., Jayasundar, R., and Jagannathan, N. R. (2002). Sequential proton MRS study of brain metabolite changes monitored during a complete pathological cycle of demyelination and remyelination in a lysophosphatidyl choline (LPC)-induced experimental demyelinating lesion model. *NMR in Biomedicine*, **15**, 293–300.

Deicken, R. F., Zhou, L., Corwin, F., Vinogradov, S., and Weiner, M. W. (1997a). Decreased left frontal lobe N-acetylaspartate in schizophrenia. *American Journal of Psychiatry*, **154**, 688–90.

Deicken, R. F., Zhou, L., Schuff, N., and Weiner, M. W. (1997b). Proton magnetic resonance spectroscopy of the anterior cingulate region in schizophrenia. *Schizophrenia Research*, **27**, 65–71.

Deicken, R. F., Pegues, M., and Amend, D. (1999). Reduced hippocampal N-acetylaspartate without volume loss in schizophrenia *Schizophrenia Research*, **37**, 217–23.

Deicken, R. F., Johnson, C., Eliaz, Y., and Schuff, N. (2000). Reduced concentrations of thalamic N-acetylaspartate in male patients with schizophrenia. *American Journal of Psychiatry*, **157**,644–7.

Deicken, R. F., Feiwell, R., Schuff, N., and Soher, B. (2001). Evidence for altered cerebellar vermis neuronal integrity in schizophrenia. *Psychiatry Research*, **107**, 125–34.

Delamillieure, P., Fernandez, J., Constans, J. M., Brazo, P., Benali, K., Abadie, P. *et al.* (2000). Proton magnetic resonance spectroscopy of the medial prefrontal cortex in patients with deficit schizophrenia: preliminary report. *American Journal of Psychiatry*, **157**, 641–3.

Delamillieure, P., Constans, J. M., Fernandez, J., Brazo, P., Benali, K., Courtheoux, P. *et al.* (2002). Proton magnetic resonance spectroscopy (H-1 MRS) in schizophrenia: Investigation of the right and left hippocampus, thalamus, and prefrontal cortex. *Schizophrenia Bulletin*, **28**, 329–39.

De Stefano, N., Matthews, P. M., and Arnold, D. L. (1995). Reversible decreases in N-acetylaspartate after acute brain injury. *Magnetic Resonance in Medicine*, **34**, 721–7.

Do, K. Q., Trabesinger, A. H., Kirsten-Kruger, M., Lauer, C. J., Dydak, U., Hell, D. *et al.* (2000). Schizophrenia: glutathione deficit in cerebrospinal fluid and prefrontal cortex in vivo. *European Journal of Neuroscience*, **12**, 3721–8.

Egan, M. F., Kojima, M., Callicott, J. H., Goldberg, T. E., Kolachana, B. S., Bertolino, A. *et al.* (2003). The BDNF val66met polymorphism affects activity-dependent secretion of BDNF and human memory and hippocampal function. *Cell*, **112**, 257–69.

Eluri, R., Paul, C., Roemer, R., and Boyko, O. (1998). Single-voxel proton magnetic resonance spectroscopy of the pons and cerebellum in patients with schizophrenia: a preliminary study. *Psychiatry Research*, **84**, 17–26.

Ende, G., Braus, D. F., Walter, S., Weber-Fahr, W., Soher, B., Maudsley, A. A. *et al.* (2000). Effects of age, medication, and illness duration on the N-acetyl aspartate signal of the anterior cingulate region in schizophrenia. *Schizophrenia Research*, **41**, 389–95.

Ende, G., Braus, D. F., Walter, S., and Henn, F. A. (2001). Lower concentration of thalamic n-acetylaspartate in patients with schizophrenia: a replication study. *American Journal of Psychiatry*, **158**, 1314–16.

Fujimoto, T., Nakano, T., Takano, T., Tokeuchi, K., Yamada, K., Fukuzako, T. *et al.* (1996). Proton magnetic resonance spectroscopy of basal ganglia in chronic schizophrenia. *Biological Psychiatry*, **40**, 14–18.

Fukuzako, H., Takeuchi, K., Hokazono, Y., Fukuzako, T., Yamada, H., Hashiguchi, T. *et al.* (1995). Proton magnetic resonance spectroscopy of the left medial temporal and frontal lobes in chronic schizophrenia: preliminary report. *Psychiatry Research*, **61**, 193–200.

Fukuzako, H., Kodama, S., Fukuzako, T., Yamada, K., Doi, W., Sato, D. *et al.* (1999). Subtype-associated metabolite differences in the temporal lobe in schizophrenia detected by proton magnetic resonance spectroscopy. *Psychiatry Research*, **92**, 45–56.

Goff, D. C., Hennen, J., Lyoo, I. K., Tsai, G., Wald, L. L., Evins, A. E. *et al.* (2002). Modulation of brain and serum glutamatergic concentrations following a switch from conventional neuroleptics to olanzapine. *Biological Psychiatry*, **51**, 493–7.

Hagino, H., Suzuki, M., Mori, K., Nohara, S., Yamashita, I., Takahashi, T. *et al.* (2002). Proton magnetic resonance spectroscopy of the inferior frontal gyrus and thalamus and its relationship to verbal learning task performance in patients with schizophrenia: a preliminary report. *Psychiatry and Clinical Neurosciences*, **56**, 499–507.

Heales, S. J., Davies, S. E., Bates, T. E., and Clark, J. B. (1995). Depletion of brain glutathione is accompanied by impaired mitochondrial function and decreased N-acetyl aspartate concentration. *Neurochemistry Research*, **20**, 31–8.

Heimberg, C., Komoroski, R. A., Lawson, W. B., Cardwell, D., and Karson, C. N. (1998). Regional proton magnetic resonance spectroscopy in schizophrenia and exploration of drug effect. *Psychiatry Research*, **83**, 105–15.

Hugg, J. W., Laxer, K. D., Matson, G. B., Maudsley, A. A., and Weiner, M. W. (1993). Neuron loss localizes human temporal lobe epilepsy by in vivo proton magnetic resonance spectroscopic imaging. *Annals of Neurology*, **34**, 788–94.

Jacobson, K. B. (1959). Studies on the roles of N-acetylaspartic acid in mammalian brain. *Journal of General Physiology*, **43**, 323–33.

Jenkins, B. G., Koroshetz, W. J., Beal, M. F., and Rosen, B. R. (1993). Evidence for impairment of energy metabolism in vivo in Huntington's disease using localized 1H NMR spectroscopy. *Neurology*, **43**, 2689–95.

Jenkins, B. G., Klivenyi, P., Kustermann, E., Andreasson, O. A., Ferrante, R. J., Rosen, B. *et al.* (2000). Nonlinear decrease over time in N-acetyl aspartate levels in the absence of neuronal loss and increases in glutamine and glucose in transgenic Huntington's disease mice. *Journal of Neurochemistry*, **74**, 2108–19.

Kantarci, K., Smith, G. E., Ivnik, R. J., Petersen, R. C., Boeve, B. F., Knopman, D. S. *et al.* (2002). 1H magnetic resonance spectroscopy, cognitive function, and apolipoprotein E genotype in normal aging, mild cognitive impairment and Alzheimer's disease. *Journal of International Neuropsychological Society*, **8**, 934–42.

Ke, Y., Coyle, J. T., Simpson, N. S., Gruber, S. A., Renshaw, P. F., and Yurgelun-Todd, D. A. (2002). Brain NAA T2 values are significantly lower in schizophrenia. *Tenth Meeting of the International Society for Magnetic Resonance Imaging*, p. 976

Kegeles, L. S., Shungu, D. C., Anjilvel, S., Chan, S., Ellis, S. P., Xanthopoulos, E. *et al.* (2000). Hippocampal pathology in schizophrenia: magnetic resonance imaging and spectroscopy studies. *Psychiatry Research*, **98**, 163–75.

Keshavan, M. S., Montrose, D. M., Pierri, J. N., Dick, E. L., Rosenberg, D., Talagala, L. *et al.* (1997). Magnetic resonance imaging and spectroscopy in offspring at risk for schizophrenia: preliminary studies. *Progress in Neuropsychopharmacology and Biological Psychiatry*, **21**, 1285–95.

Keshavan, M. S., Stanley, J. A., and Pettegrew, J. W. (2000). Magnetic resonance spectroscopy in schizophrenia: Methodological issues and findings—Part II. *Biological Psychiatry*, **48**, 369–80.

Kinney, D. K., Steingard, R. J., Renshaw, P. F., and Yurgelun-Todd, D. A. (2000). Perinatal complications and abnormal proton metabolite concentrations in frontal cortex of adolescents seen on magnetic resonance spectroscopy. *Neuropsychiatry Neuropsychology and Behavioral Neurology*, **13**, 8–12.

Klunk, W. E., Panchalingam, K., McClure, R. J., Stanley, J. A., and Pettegrew, J. W. (1998). Metabolic alterations in postmortem Alzheimer's disease brain are exaggerated by Apo-E4. *Neurobiology of Aging*, **19**, 511–15.

Knowlton, R. C., Abou-Khalil, B., Sawrie, S. M., Martin, R. C., Faught, R. E., and Kuzniecky, R. I. (2002). In vivo hippocampal metabolic dysfunction in human temporal lobe epilepsy. *Archives of Neurology*, **59**, 1882–6.

Laruelle, M., Abi-Dargham, A., van Dyck, C. H., Gil, R., D'Souza, C. D., Erdos, J. *et al.* (1996). Single photon emission computerized tomography imaging of amphetamine-induced dopamine release in drug-free schizophrenic subjects. *Proceedings of the National Academy of Sciences, USA*, **93**, 9235–40.

Laruelle, M., Abi-Dargham, A., Gil, R., Kegeles, L., and Innis, R. (1999). Increased dopamine transmission in schizophrenia: relationship to illness phases. *Biological Psychiatry*, **46**, 56–72.

Lim, K. O., Adalsteinsson, E., Spielman, D., Sullivan, E. V., Rosenbloom, M. J., and Pfefferbaum, A. (1998). Proton magnetic resonance spectroscopic imaging of cortical gray and white matter in schizophrenia. *Archives of General Psychiatry*, **55**, 346–52.

Lu, D., Margouleff, C., Rubin, E., Labar, D., Schaul, N., Ishikawa, T. *et al.* (1997). Temporal lobe epilepsy: correlation of proton magnetic resonance spectroscopy and 18F-fluorodeoxyglucose positron emission tomography. *Magnetic Resonance in Medicine*, **37**, 18–23.

Maier, M. and Ron, M. A. (1996). Hippocampal age-related changes in schizophrenia: a proton magnetic resonance spectroscopy study. *Schizophrenia Research*, **22**, 5–17.

Maier, M., Ron, M. A., Barker, G. J., and Tofts, P. S. (1995). Proton magnetic resonance spectroscopy: an in vivo method of estimating hippocampal neuronal depletion in schizophrenia. *Psychological Medicine*, **25**, 1201–9.

Matalon, R., Michals, K., Sebesta, D., Deanching, M., Gashkoff, P., and Casanova, J. (1988). Aspartoacylase deficiency and N-acetylaspartic aciduria in patients with Canavan disease. *American Journal of Medical Genetics*, **29**, 463–71.

Meyerhoff, D. J., MacKay, S., Poole, N., Dillon, W. P., Weiner, M. W., and Fein, G. (1994). N-acetylaspartate reductions measured by 1H MRSI in cognitively impaired HIV-seropositive individuals. *Magnetic Resonance Imaging*, **12**, 653–9.

Meyer-Lindenberg, A., Miletich, R. S., Kohn, P. D., Esposito, G., Carson, R. E., Quarantelli, M. *et al.* (2002). Reduced prefrontal activity predicts exaggerated striatal dopaminergic function in schizophrenia. *Nature Neuroscience*, **5**, 267–71.

Miller, B. L. (1991). A review of chemical issues in 1H NMR spectroscopy: N-acetyl-L-aspartate, creatine and choline *NMR in Biomedicine*, **4**, 47–52.

Miller, B. L., Moats, R. A., Shonk, T., Ernst, T., Woolley, S., and Ross, B. D. (1993). Alzheimer disease: depiction of increased cerebral myo-inositol with proton MR spectroscopy. *Radiology*, **187**, 433–7.

Moffett, J. R., Namboodiri, M. A., Cangro, C. B., and Neale, J. H. (1991). Immunohistochemical localization of N-acetylaspartate in rat brain. *Neuroreport*, **2**, 131–4.

Nasrallah, H. A., Skinner, T. E., Schmalbrock, P., and Robitaille, P. M. (1994). Proton magnetic resonance spectroscopy (1H MRS) of the hippocampal formation in schizophrenia: a pilot study. *British Journal of Psychiatry*, **165**, 481–5.

Ohara, K., Isoda, H., Suzuki, Y., Takehara, Y., Ochiai, M., Takeda, H. *et al.* (2000). Proton magnetic resonance spectroscopy of lenticular nuclei in simple schizophrenia. *Progress in Neuropsychopharmacology and Biological Psychiatry*, **24**, 507–19.

Omori, M., Pearce, J., Komoroski, R. A., Griffin, W. S., Mrak, R. E., Husain, M. M. *et al.* (1997). In vitro 1H-magnetic resonance spectroscopy of postmortem brains with schizophrenia. *Biological Psychiatry*, **42**, 359–66.

Omori, M., Murata, T., Kimura, H., Koshimoto, Y., Kado, H., Ishimori, Y. *et al.* (2000). Thalamic abnormalities in patients with schizophrenia revealed by proton magnetic resonance spectroscopy. *Psychiatry Research*, **98**, 155–62.

Pakkenberg, B. (1992). The volume of the mediodorsal thalamic nucleus in treated and untreated schizophrenics. *Schizophrenia Research*, **7**, 95–100.

Petroff, O. A., Errante, L. D., Rothman, D. L., Kim, J. H., and Spencer, D. D. (2002). Neuronal and glial metabolite content of the epileptogenic human hippocampus. *Annals of Neurology*, **52**, 635–42.

Popken, G. J., Bunney, W. E., Potkin, S. G., and Jones, E. G. (2000). Subnucleus-specific loss of neurons in medial thalamus of schizophrenics. *Proceedings of the National Academy of Sciences, USA*, **97**, 9276–80.

Pouwels, P. J. and Frahm, J. (1997). Differential distribution of NAA and NAAG in human brain as determined by quantitative localized proton MRS. *NMR in Biomedicine*, **10**, 73–8.

Renshaw, P. F., Yurgelun-Todd, D. A., Tohen, M., Gruber, S., and Cohen, B. M. (1995). Temporal lobe proton magnetic resonance spectroscopy of patients with first-episode psychosis. *American Journal of Psychiatry*, **152**, 444–6.

Rothman, D. L., Novotny, E. J., Shulman, G. I., Howseman, A. M., Petroff, O. A., Mason, G. *et al.* (1992). 1H-[13C] NMR measurements of [4–13C]glutamate turnover in human brain. *Proceedings of the National Academy of Sciences, USA*, **89**, 9603–6.

Rothman, D. L., Petroff, O. A., Behar, K. L., and Mattson, R. H. (1993). Localized 1H NMR measurements of gamma-aminobutyric acid in human brain in vivo. *Proceedings of the National Academy of Sciences, USA*, **90**, 5662–6.

Salibi, N. and Brown, M. A. (1998). *Clinical MR spectroscopy. First principles.* Wiley Liss, New York.

Schuff, N., Capizzano, A. A., Du, A. T., Amend, D. L., O'Neill, J., Norman, D. *et al.* (2002). Selective reduction of N-acetylaspartate in medial temporal and parietal lobes in AD. *Neurology*, **58**, 928–35.

Shen, J. and Rothman, D. L. (2002). Magnetic resonance spectroscopic approaches to studying neuronal: glial interactions. *Biological Psychiatry*, **52**, 694–700.

Shen, J., Rothman, D. L., and Brown, P. (2002). In vivo GABA editing using a novel doubly selective multiple quantum filter. *Magnetic Resonance in Medicine*, **47**, 447–54.

Shigematsu, H., Okamura, N., Shimeno, H., Kishimoto, Y., Kan, L., and Fenselau, C. (1983). Purification and characterization of the heat-stable factors essential for the conversion of lignoceric acid to cerebronic acid and glutamic acid: identification of N-acetyl-L-aspartic acid. *Journal of Neurochemistry*, **40**, 814–20.

Shioiri, T., Hamakawa, H., Kato, T., Murashita, J., Fujii, K., Inubushi, T. *et al.* (1996). Proton magnetic resonance spectroscopy of the basal ganglia in patients with schizophrenia: a preliminary report. *Schizophrenia Research*, **22**, 19–26.

Slusher, B. S., Robinson, M. B., Tsai, G., Simmons, M. L., Richards, S. S., and Coyle, J. T. (1990). Rat brain N-acetylated alpha-linked acidic dipeptidase activity. Purification and immunologic characterization. *Journal of Biological Chemistry*, **265**, 21297–301.

Stanley, J. A., Williamson, P. C., Drost, D. J., Rylett, R. J., Carr, T. J., Malla, A. *et al.* (1996). An in vivo proton magnetic resonance spectroscopy study of schizophrenia patients. *Schizophrenia Bulletin*, **22**, 597–609.

Stanley, J. A., Pettegrew, J. W., and Keshavan, M. S. (2000). Magnetic resonance spectroscopy in schizophrenia: methodological issues and findings—part I. *Biological Psychiatry*, **48**, 357–68.

Steel, R. M., Bastin, M. E., McConnell, S., Marshall, I., Cunningham-Owens, D. G., Laurie, S. M. *et al.* (2001). Diffusion tensor imaging (DTI) and proton magnetic resonance spectroscopy (1H MRS) in schizophrenic subjects and normal controls. *Psychiatry Research*, **106**, 161–70.

Stoll, A. L., Renshaw, P. F., De Micheli, E., Wurtman, R., Pillay, S. S., and Cohen, B. M. (1995). Choline ingestion increases the resonance of choline-containing compounds in human brain: an in vivo proton magnetic resonance study. *Biological Psychiatry*, **37**, 170–4.

Tan, J., Bluml, S., Hoang, T., Dubowitz, D., Mevenkamp, G., and Ross, B. (1998). Lack of effect of oral choline supplement on the concentrations of choline metabolites in human brain. *Magnetic Resonance in Medicine*, **39**, 1005–10.

Theberge, J., Bartha, R., Drost, D. J., Menon, R. S., Malla, A., Takhar, J. *et al.* (2002). Glutamate and glutamine measured with 4.0 T proton MRS in never-treated patients with schizophrenia and healthy volunteers. *American Journal of Psychiatry*, **159**, 1944–6.

Thomas, M. A., Ke, Y., Levitt, J., Caplan, R., Curran, J., Asarnow, R. *et al.* (1998). Preliminary study of frontal lobe 1H MR spectroscopy in childhood-onset schizophrenia. *Journal of Magnetic Resonance Imaging*, **8**, 841–6.

Tibbo, P., Hanstock, C. C., Asghar, S., Silverstone, P., and Allen, P. S. (2000). Proton magnetic resonance spectroscopy (1H-MRS) of the cerebellum in men with schizophrenia. *Journal of Psychiatry and Neuroscience*, **25**, 509–12.

Tsai, G. and Coyle, J. T. (1995). N-acetylaspartate in neuropsychiatric disorders. *Progress in Neurobiology*, **46**, 531–40.

Tunggal, B., Hofmann, K., and Stoffel, W. (1990). In vivo 13C nuclear magnetic resonance investigations of choline metabolism in rabbit brain. *Magnetic Resonance in Medicine*, **13**, 90–102.

Urenjak, J., Williams, S. R., Gadian, D. G., and Noble, M. (1993). Proton nuclear magnetic resonance spectroscopy unambiguously identifies different neural cell types. *Journal of Neuroscience*, **13**, 981–9.

Vion-Dury, J., Nicoli, F., Salvan, A. M., Confort-Gouny, S., Dhiver, C., and Cozzone, P. J. (1995). Reversal of brain metabolic alterations with zidovudine detected by proton localised magnetic resonance spectroscopy. *Lancet* **345** 60–1.

Walker, M. A., Highley, J. R., Esiri, M. M., McDonald, B., Roberts, K.C., Evans, S. P. *et al.* (2002). Estimated neuronal populations and volumes of the hippocampus and its subfields in schizophrenia. *American Journal of Psychiatry*, **159**, 821–8.

Weber-Fahr, W., Ende, G., Braus, D. F., Bachert, P., Soher, B. J., Henn, F. A. *et al.* (2002). A fully automated method for tissue segmentation and CSF-correction of proton MRSI metabolites corroborates abnormal hippocampal NAA in schizophrenia. *Neuroimage*, **16**, 49–60.

Weinberger, D. R. (1986). The pathogenesis of schizophrenia: a neurodevelopmental theory. In *The neurology of schizophrenia* (ed. H. A. W. Nasrallah, D. R.), pp. 397–406. Elsevier, Amsterdam.

Weinberger, D. R. (1999). Cell biology of the hippocampal formation in schizophrenia. *Biological Psychiatry*, **45**, 395–402.

Weinberger, D. R. and Laruelle, M. (2002). Neurochemical and neuropharmacologic imaging in schizophrenia. In *Neuropsychopharmacology: The fifth generation of progress* (ed. K. L. Davis, D. Charney, J. T. Coyle, and C. Nemeroff), pp. 833–55. Lippincott Williams & Wilkins, Philadelphia, PA.

Weinberger, D. R., Egan, M. F., Bertolino, A., Callicott, J. K., Mattay, V. S., Lipska, B. K. *et al.* (2001). Prefrontal neurons and the genetics of schizophrenia. *Biological Psychiatry*, **50**, 825–44.

Wolinsky, J. S., Narayana, P. A., and Fenstermacher, M. J. (1990). Proton magnetic resonance spectroscopy in multiple sclerosis. *Neurology*, **40**, 1764–9.

Yamasue, H., Fukui, T., Fukuda, R., Yamada, H., Yamasaki, S., Kuroki, N. *et al.* (2002). 1H-MR spectroscopy and gray matter volume of the anterior cingulate cortex in schizophrenia. *Neuroreport*, **13**, 2133–7.

Young, K. A., Manaye, K. F., Liang, C. L., Hicks, P. B., and German, D. C. (2000). Reduced number of mediodorsal and anterior thalamic neurons in schizophrenia. *Biological Psychiatry*, **47**, 944–53.

Yurgelun-Todd, D. A., Renshaw, P. F., Gruber, S. A., Ed, M., Waternaux, C., and Cohen, B. M. (1996). Proton magnetic resonance spectroscopy of the temporal lobes in schizophrenics and normal controls. *Schizophrenia Research*, **19**, 55–9.

Chapter 5

Diffusion tensor magnetic resonance imaging

Mark E. Bastin and Stephen M. Lawrie

Introduction

A large body of evidence from *in vivo* imaging and post-mortem studies suggests that the brains of patients with schizophrenia are both structurally and functionally compromised. The most replicated gross morphometric findings from magnetic resonance (MR) imaging studies are enlarged lateral ventricles and reduced cerebral volume, specifically temporal lobe and amygdala/hippocampal complex, compared with age- and gender-matched controls (Lawrie and Abukmeil 1998). Segmentation studies suggest that these volume deficits occur more often in cortical grey matter than white (Zipursky *et al.* 1992; Schlaepfer *et al.* 1994). However, while abnormalities of white matter volume are not as widely reported (Wright *et al.* 2000), there are compelling data from other types of imaging to suggest that white matter function may also be substantially affected in schizophrenia. For example, magnetization transfer MR imaging (MT-MRI), which provides a quantitative measure of macromolecular structural integrity, has demonstrated differences in fronto-temporal regions and interhemispheric connections between schizophrenic and control brains (Foong *et al.* 2000*a*, 2001; Bagary *et al.* 2003). These differences are most likely related to myelin and axonal abnormalities. Proton MR spectroscopy (^{1}H-MRS), which provides a localized insight into brain biochemistry *in vivo*, has further shown significantly reduced *N*-acetyl-aspartate (NAA) signal in the white matter of schizophrenic patients with abnormally small grey, but not white, matter volumes (Lim *et al.* 1998). Since NAA is thought to be a putative marker for healthy neurons, a reduced NAA signal may indicate compromised neuronal connectivity. Support for the hypothesis that a cortical disconnection syndrome plays a core role in schizophrenia comes from functional imaging studies which have found abnormal fronto-temporal activation in verbal fluency and related tasks (Friston and Frith 1995; Frith *et al.* 1995; Fletcher *et al.* 1999; Lawrie *et al.* 2002). Frontal–parietal connections may also be affected as they are also known to modulate selective attention, a cognitive feature commonly impaired in schizophrenia (Kastner and Ungerleider 2000).

Unfortunately, while both MT-MRI and ^{1}H-MRS can detect subtle brain pathology, neither modality allows the direct mapping of white matter connectivity. However, this situation has recently been remedied with the introduction of diffusion tensor MR imaging (DT-MRI). This technique measures the three-dimensional mobility of water molecules *in vivo* from sets of diffusion-weighted MR images. Since water molecules diffuse preferentially along axons rather than across them, the measurement of diffusion anisotropy from the diffusion tensor can provide detailed information on fibre-tract orientation and other architectural features of brain tissue. Such information may prove to be invaluable in the study and characterization of a wide range of neurological disorders, including schizophrenia. Therefore, in order to provide the reader with a detailed understanding of this new and potentially very important imaging modality, a description of the background and methodology of diffusion MR imaging and its extension to DT-MRI are presented in detail below. We then discuss the results obtained from the small number of DT-MRI studies of adult-onset schizophrenia undertaken so far, and how these data add to our current understanding of this condition. Finally, ways are suggested in which future studies could be improved in terms of both methodology and experimental design.

In vivo diffusion magnetic resonance imaging

Diffusion in fluid systems where the concentration of molecular species is uniform and stable is usually described using statistical methods that determine the probability of a particle moving a certain distance over a measurement of time. In this stochastic model of diffusion, the microscopic random motions of each molecule, caused by repeated collisions with other molecules, are driven by the ambient thermal energy of the fluid. These molecular motions are termed random walks, since the magnitude and direction of each trajectory are unrelated to those of the previous path. In an isotropic medium, such as pure water, all directions are equivalent, so that after a sufficiently large number of collisions there will be no net bulk displacement of a molecule from its starting position. There will, however, be a spherical region around this starting location in which the molecule can be expected to be found at any given time point. Specifically, it can be shown that the probability of finding a labelled molecule initially at location z_1 at a new location z_2 after a certain diffusion time (τ_D) has a Gaussian distribution with zero mean. The mean-square displacement in three dimensions ($<z_2>$) that occurred during τ_D can then be related to the self-diffusion coefficient (D) using the Einstein equation

$$<z^2> = 6D\tau_D \qquad [5.1]$$

This equation indicates that the mean-squared displacement of a molecule from its initial location is directly proportional to the diffusion time, while D characterizes the mobility of molecules in a given fluid at a specific temperature.

In biological tissue, the presence of multiple cellular compartments with semipermeable barriers causes the diffusion of water protons to depart significantly from that seen in unrestricted isotropic diffusion in an infinite medium. Membranes and organelles that may be partially permeable now restrict water molecules. Thus, they cannot travel unhindered between two points, but must travel tortuous paths to cover any given distance. In this situation, the mean-square displacement remains proportional to τ_D, although D now has a smaller value than that measured for free diffusion. For example, typical measured values for the diffusion coefficient of water in brain parenchyma range from 700 to 1000 $\times$ 10^{-6} mm^2 s^{-1}, while D of pure water is 3080 $\times$ 10^{-6} mm^2 s^{-1} at 37.4°C. To reflect the fact that water diffusion is now governed both by temperature and interactions with the cellular microstructure, the diffusion coefficient of water measured by MR imaging is termed the apparent diffusion coefficient (ADC).

Methods

The measurement of brain water diffusion *in vivo* is typically achieved using a fast pulsed gradient spin-echo (PGSE) sequence designed to generate two-dimensional diffusion-weighted (DW) MR images in the axial, coronal, or sagittal plane (Stejskal and Tanner 1965; Turner and Le Bihan 1990). In this method, diffusion sensitivity is achieved by inserting two strong magnetic field gradient pulses symmetrically around the 180° refocusing pulse in the frequency-encoding (g_x), phase-encoding (g_y), or slice-selection (g_z) channels, or combinations thereof, in a spin-echo sequence (see Fig. 5.1a). Measurements of water diffusion are then obtained along the direction in which the diffusion sensitizing gradient is applied. The duration and separation of these gradient pulses are classically represented as δ and Δ, respectively. The purpose of these gradient pulses is to label magnetically protons attached to diffusing molecules, which then act like endogenous tracers, the motion of which can be monitored. This encoding of diffusion effects can be understood as follows. During the first gradient pulse, protons experience different magnetic field strengths depending on their location in the magnet bore, with the result that they accumulate different phase shifts. For stationary protons these induced phase shifts are exactly reversed by the second gradient pulse played out after the 180° refocusing pulse. However, diffusing protons will not experience the same net gradient field during the two pulses, due to their random motions. This will result in imperfect refocusing of the spin-echo, leading to signal attenuation. Ideally, to define precisely the diffusion time of this experiment, Δ should be much larger than δ, and the gradients should be infinitely short pulses of large amplitude. However, the finite rise times and maximum gradient strengths available on current whole-body clinical scanners mean that this condition is rarely met in practice. The presence of such finite duration pulses, means that the diffusion time is more difficult to define exactly, although $\tau_D = \Delta - \delta/3$ is often used rather than $\tau_D = \Delta$ (Stejskal and Tanner 1965). Furthermore, the extended duration of these diffusion sensitizing pulses means that long echo times (TE) are needed in order to achieved an adequate diffusion-related signal attenuation. Thus, DW images are inherently also T$_2$-weighted.

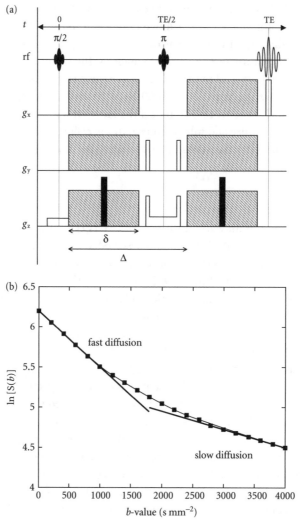

Fig. 5.1 (a) Schematic diagram of a PGSE sequence designed to measure diffusion effects simultaneously in the frequency-encoding (g_x), phase-encoding (g_y), and slice-selection (g_z) directions. Ideally, the diffusion gradients should be infinitely short pulses of large amplitude (black gradients), although the finite rise times and maximum gradient strengths available on current whole-body clinical scanners mean that this condition is rarely met in practice (shaded gradients). (b) Plot of the natural log of signal intensity ($\ln[S(b)]$) versus b-value for white matter in the human brain, assuming slow exchange between fast- and slow-diffusion components (Clark and Le Bihan 2000).

The signal intensity in a generic DW spin-echo experiment is given by

$$S(b) = S_0 e^{-\gamma^2 \delta^2 G^2 \left(\Delta - \frac{\delta}{3} \right) \text{ADC}} = S_0 e^{-b\text{ADC}}$$ [5.2]

where S_0 is the T_2-weighted signal intensity, γ is the gyromagnetic ratio, G is the diffusion gradient strength, and b is the gradient factor, or b-value, that determines the degree of diffusion weighting employed in the sequence. A two-dimensional map of the spatial distribution of ADC values of brain water can then be determined by measuring the slope of a plot of $\ln[(S(b)]$ versus b on a voxel-by-voxel basis. In the simplest type of DW imaging experiment, the measured signal intensity is assumed to be a monotonic function of b. Estimates of S_0 and the ADC can then be determined by fitting a straight line to values of $\ln[S(b)]$ obtained at two different b-values, namely b_{max} and b_{min}. The most common implementation of these so-called two-point sampling schemes involves acquiring a baseline T_2-weighted image ($b_{min} \sim 0$ s mm^{-2}) and one or more DW images at b_{max}. The choice of b_{max} for this experiment is, however, complicated by the fact that $S(b)$ has been found not to be a mono-exponential function of b at large values of diffusion weighting. Measurements of the ADC in both human and rat brain have shown that this curve is, in reality, bi-exponential (Niendorf *et al.* 1996; Clark and Le Bihan 2000), with two regions in which $\ln[S(b)]$ is proportional to b. The first of these regions, characterized by what has been called the fast diffusion component (ADC$_{fast}$), is in the range $b \sim 0$–1500 s mm^{-2}, while the second, corresponding to the slow diffusion component (ADC$_{slow}$), is in the range $b \sim 2500$–4000 s mm^{-2} (see Fig. 5.1b). The exact origin of these fast and slow water diffusion components has yet to be determined, but it may be that the fast diffusion component originates from extracellular water and the slow component from intracellular water (Nicholson and Sykova 1998). Unfortunately, this interpretation is complicated by the discrepancy between the estimated volume fraction of ADC$_{fast}$ ($f_{fast} \sim 0.65$) and the known volume fraction of the extracellular space ($f_{extra} \sim 0.2$). Therefore, to avoid underestimating the fast diffusion component by including data from the slow diffusion component, the majority of studies use sampling schemes with b_{max} in the range 1000–1500 s mm^{-2}.

Fast imaging

The addition of large diffusion-encoding gradients into a spin-echo sequence makes it highly sensitive to involuntary patient motion. This is because even sub-millimetre displacements during the experiment will induce significant phase errors within and between consecutive phase-encoding steps. Such bulk motion will then totally obscure the signal from the small (10–20 μm) random molecular motions that are to be measured. This problem can be addressed in several ways, namely by: (1) collecting all the imaging data as rapidly as possible in a single-shot acquisition or parallel imaging technique such as sensitivity encoding (SENSE); (2) correcting the motion-induced phase errors in a multi-shot acquisition using a reference phase provided by a navigator echo; and (3) employing sequences that are largely insensitive to bulk motion.

By far the most common single-shot DW acquisition is that based on spin-echo echo-planar imaging (EPI). This is because not only can individual DW images be collected as rapidly as every 150 ms or so, but also because EPI provides images that have a relatively high spatial resolution, with good signal-to-noise characteristics and low radiofrequency (RF) power deposition (Turner and Le Bihan 1990). Unfortunately, the low image bandwidth in the phase-encoding direction means that EPI also suffers from artefacts caused by susceptibility changes at tissue boundaries, and from geometric image distortions created by the significant eddy currents arising from the diffusion sensitizing gradients. Several solutions to these problems have been suggested in the literature (Jezzard and Balaban 1995; Haselgrove and Moore 1996; Alexander *et al.* 1997; Jezzard *et al.* 1998; Bastin 1999, 2001; Papadakis *et al.* 2000*a*; Schmithorst and Dardzinski 2002). An alternative approach to single-shot DW-EPI is provided by SENSE (Pruessmann *et al.* 1999). In this method, phase encoding is achieved using an array of coils with different spatial sensitivities. This enables the number of phase-encoding steps to be reduced by a factor R, typically 2–8, where R is the ratio between the number of phase-encoding steps required for a standard single-coil acquisition and that required for SENSE. Although reducing the number of phase-encoding steps lowers the signal-to-noise ratio (SNR) of the DW images, the decrease in effective acquisition time has been shown to reduce blurring, chemical shift, and susceptibility artefacts (Bammer *et al.* 2002).

These EPI artefacts can also be significantly reduced in a multi-shot acquisition with navigator echo. In such sequences, two 180° refocusing pulses follow the initial 90° pulse, resulting in the formation of two spin-echo signals. One of these signals is phase encoded as normal, while the other is the non-phase-encoded navigator echo. The data from the navigator echo signal are then used to correct both intraview and view-to-view phase errors resulting from rigid body motions (Anderson and Gore 1994; Ordidge *et al.* 1994). Another highly effective multi-shot method of collecting DW images is provided by line scan diffusion MR imaging (Gudbjartsson*et al.* 1996; Buchsbaum *et al.* 1998). In this scheme, a two-dimensional DW image is formed from the sequential collection of many spin-echo column excitations. This acquisition method makes the sequence largely insensitive to bulk patient motion, chemical shift, and susceptibility artefacts. However, it takes longer to generate two-dimensional DW images than EPI, and this is not commonly available on clinical scanners.

One further point to note is that although these techniques do significantly reduce the effects of gross patient motion, pulsatile brain motion arising from the cardiac cycle can still introduce artefacts into the final DW images. For example, pulsatile brain motion has been shown to affect posterior regions in and inferior to the corpus callosum in EPI-based acquisitions (Skare and Andersson 2001). Such artefacts are most easily removed by gating the acquisition to the cardiac cycle using a peripheral-gating device attached to the subject's finger. The repetition time of the acquisition, typically between 10 and 20 RR periods, depending on the heart rate, is then chosen to allow sufficient time for the DW images to be collected, reconstructed, and stored by the scanner hardware.

Diffusion anisotropy

Figure 5.2 shows single-shot T_2-weighted and DW-EP images acquired from a healthy female volunteer. In the three DW-EP images, diffusion gradients have been applied sequentially along the superior/inferior (b), left/right (c) and anterior/posterior (d) gradient directions, respectively. In the three DW images, the contrast clearly depends on the direction of the applied diffusion gradient, with white matter structures running perpendicular to the diffusion gradient direction being brighter that those running parallel. This directional dependence arises because water molecules diffuse preferentially along the long axes of axons rather than across them. As discussed below, this diffusion anisotropy can be measured quantitatively from the diffusion tensor. However, this figure also shows why it is important to remove these diffusion anisotropy effects when calculating the ADC. This is usually achieved by determining the ADC in three orthogonal directions from Equation 5.2 and then calculating a mean rotationally invariant ADC (<ADC>) from these data (Ulug *et al.* 1997).

The origin of anisotropic water diffusion in white matter could arise from any longitudinally orientated neuronal structures that provide barriers to water molecules in directions perpendicular to the principal axonal axis. Three such structures are the myelin sheath around the axons, the axonal membrane, and the three-dimensional axonal cytoskeleton consisting of microtubes, neurofilaments, and inter-connecting microfilaments. Diffusion parallel to the length of the axon could also be aided by fast

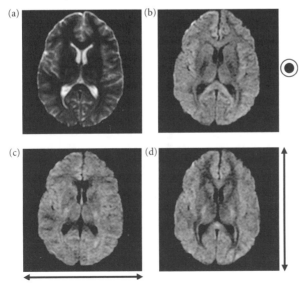

Fig. 5.2 Single-shot T_2-weighted (a) and DW-EP (b–d) images acquired at the level of the third ventricle from a 33-year-old female volunteer. In the three DW-EP images, diffusion gradients have been applied sequentially along (b) the superior/inferior $(g_x\, g_y\, g_z) = (0\ 0\ 1)$, (c) the left/right $(1\ 0\ 0)$, and (d) the anterior/posterior $(0\ 1\ 0)$ gradient directions, respectively. Note how the contrast varies with diffusion gradient direction in the three DW-EP images.

axonal transport. However, extensive *in vivo* and *in vitro* experiments on various non-myelinated neuronal fibres (Beaulieu and Allen 1994 *a*; Huppi *et al.* 1998; Gulani *et al.* 2001), axons with large axoplasmic spaces (Beaulieu and Allen 1994*b*), and neurons in which fast axonal transport has been inhibited (Beaulieu and Allen 1994*a*), indicate that the primary determinant of anisotropic water diffusion is the dense packing of axonal membranes hindering water mobility, with myelin playing an important, but secondary role. Therefore, at the low values of diffusion-weighting used in most human studies ($b < 1500$ s mm^{-2}), diffusion anisotropy probably arises directly from the anisotropic tortuosity of the extracellular space. For example, in a bundle of tightly packed axonal fibres, water molecules would actually have to travel a distance of $\pi d/2$ to appear to diffuse over a distance of the fibre diameter, d. Thus, the ADC measured perpendicular to the fibres would then be, on average, only 40% of that measured parallel to them, a value which fits reasonably well with literature data (Le Bihan *et al.* 1993).

Diffusion tensor magnetic resonance imaging

The tendency of axonal membranes to bias the random motion of water molecules along the principal axes of white matter fibre bundles means that diffusion can only be fully characterized if both its magnitude and directionality can be determined. Since white matter fibres are orientated in a three-dimensional space, diffusion *in vivo* can be represented mathematically by a second-order symmetric tensor (Basser *et al.* 1994). The apparent diffusion tensor of water (**D**) has the form

$$\mathbf{D} = \begin{pmatrix} D_{xx} & D_{xy} & D_{xz} \\ D_{xy} & D_{yy} & D_{yz} \\ D_{xz} & D_{yz} & D_{zz} \end{pmatrix} \qquad [5.3]$$

where D_{xx}, D_{yy}, and D_{zz} represent diffusion fluxes along the x, y, and z directions, and D_{xy}, D_{xz}, and D_{yz} represent correlations between diffusion fluxes in orthogonal directions. This tensor is symmetric; that is, it has only three unique off-diagonal elements (e.g. $D_{xy} = D_{yx}$), because it represents the diffusion of an uncharged moiety, namely water. For charged molecules, $D_{xy} \neq D_{yx}$, so **D** would have six unique off-diagonal elements.

In the tensor model of water diffusion, the signal intensity obtained in a generic DW spin-echo experiment is

$$S(\mathbf{b}) = S_0 e^{-\sum_{i}^{3} \sum_{j}^{3} b_{ij} D_{ij}} \qquad [5.4]$$

where S_0 is the T_2-weighted signal intensity and b_{ij} is a matrix of gradient factors which determines the degree of diffusion weighting in all directions represented in **D**. Values for the **b**-matrix are calculated numerically from the precise gradient waveforms used in the imaging sequence (Mattiello *et al.* 1997). Using multivariate linear regression, the six independent elements of **D** ($[D_{xx} \, D_{yy} \, D_{zz} \, D_{xy} \, D_{xz} \, D_{yz}]$) and

$\ln(S_0)$ are estimated statistically by minimizing the sum of the squares of the differences between the measured DW spin-echo signal intensities and those theoretically predicted by Equation [5.4] (Basser *et al.* 1994; Pierpaoli *et al.* 1996). This is achieved by applying diffusion gradients along n non-collinear directions at m gradient strengths (b-values) and measuring the signal intensity as a function of the **b**-matrix. Thus, once the **b**-matrix corresponding to each DW image has been calculated, estimates of **D** and the T_2-weighted signal intensity can be determined on a voxel-by-voxel basis.

In the simplest possible DT-MRI experiment, a T_2-weighted EP image ($b_{min} \sim$ 0 s mm^{-2}) and six DW-EP images ($b_{max} \sim$ 1000–1500 s mm^{-2}) are collected for each slice location (Basser and Pierpaoli 1998; Shrager and Basser 1998). Although this experiment provides values of **D** in the quickest manner, the calculation of **D** becomes deterministic rather than statistical. Thus, no error estimates of **D** or regression coefficients indicating the goodness of fit can be obtained. Furthermore as already discussed above, since a mono-exponential decay in $\ln[S(b)]$ versus b is assumed, only **D** for the fast diffusion component can be measured (Clark *et al.* 2002). If the variance of **D** is required, then additional measurements of the DW signal intensity can be obtained either by acquiring DW images at two or more non-zero b-values (Xing *et al.* 1997; Armitage and Bastin 2001), or by collecting DW images in which diffusion gradients are applied in more than six non-collinear directions.

Diffusion gradient orientation

Since the diffusion gradient-encoding scheme may influence the estimation of **D**, various methods have been suggested by which optimum sets of diffusion gradient direction vectors can be chosen. These schemes fall broadly into three main categories: (1) heuristic methods based on the 13 non-collinear gradient directions corresponding to the face centres

$$\mathbf{G}_1 = [(1\ 0\ 0), (0\ 1\ 0), (0\ 0\ 1)] \qquad [5.5]$$

edge bisectors

$$\mathbf{G}_2 = \frac{1}{\sqrt{2}}[(1\ 0\ 1), (0\ 1\ 1), (1\ 1\ 0)] \qquad [5.6]$$

and

$$\mathbf{G}_3 = \frac{1}{\sqrt{2}}[(-1\ 0\ 1), (0\ 1\ -1), (-1\ 1\ 0)] \qquad [5.7]$$

and body diagonals of a unit cube,

$$\mathbf{G}_4 = \frac{1}{\sqrt{3}}[(1\ 1\ 1), (1\ 1\ -1), (-1\ 1\ 1)(1\ -1\ 1)]; \qquad [5.8]$$

(2) methods that chose directions based on landmarks of geometric polyhedra, and (3) numerically optimized methods that seek to maximize or minimize a specific criterion. Examples of heuristic encoding schemes include orthogonal gradient encoding ($\mathbf{G}_1 + \mathbf{G}_2$), double oblique gradient encoding ($\mathbf{G}_2 + \mathbf{G}_3$), orthogonal/tetrahedral hybrid encoding ($\mathbf{G}_1 + \mathbf{G}_4$), decahedral gradient encoding ($\mathbf{G}_2 + \mathbf{G}_3 + \mathbf{G}_4$) and complete heuristic gradient encoding ($\mathbf{G}_1 + \mathbf{G}_2 + \mathbf{G}_3 + \mathbf{G}_4$). Geometric polyhedra that can be used for diffusion gradient encoding include the dodecahedron, BuckyBall, and the family of regular icosahedral polyhedra (Hasan *et al.* 2001). Perhaps the most commonly used numerically optimized method is that suggested by Jones *et al.* (1999*a*). In this scheme, which is based on an analogy with electrostatic repulsion, *n* non-collinear gradient directions are chosen using a criterion that maximized the separation between *n* electrical charges placed randomly on a sphere. Schematic diagrams for four examples of these diffusion gradient-encoding schemes are shown in Fig. 5.3.

There is still some debate about which of these methods provides the optimum sampling scheme. For example, Hasan *et al.* (2001) found that there is no significant advantage in using more than six directions if icosahedron sampling is employed.

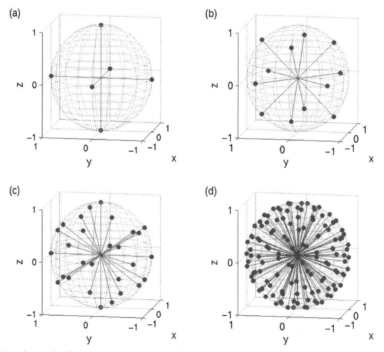

Fig. 5.3 Schematic diagrams showing n gradient vectors (and their reflections through the origin) for four different diffusion gradient encoding schemes: (a) *n* = 3 orthogonal gradient encoding, i.e. **G**₁ (see Fig. 5.2); (b) *n* = 6 double oblique gradient encoding, i.e. **G**₂ + **G**₃; (c) *n* = 15 regular icosahedral polyhedra encoding (Hasan et al. 2001); and (d) *n* = 64 numerically optimized encoding (Jones et al. 2002*b*).

Conversely, Skare *et al.* (2000*a*) and Papadaksi*et al.* (2000*b*) have shown that the precision of the estimation of **D** is improved if there are a greater number of diffusion gradient direction vectors orientated uniformly in space. High angular sampling schemes certainly reduce the potential dependence of the measured **D** on diffusion gradient direction, and are required if non-Gaussian (non-tensorial) diffusion behaviour is to be observed (Frank 2001).

Quantitative diffusion parameters

The three-dimensional information on the diffusion of water molecules *in vivo* contained in **D** is best understood in terms of the diffusion ellipsoid. In this graphical description of **D**, the surface of the ellipsoid represents the mean-squared displacement of a water molecule from the origin in the measurement time τ_D, while its orientation indicates the orthotropic axes of the medium. The shape of the diffusion ellipsoid is fully characterized by six parameters, namely the magnitude of the three scalar diffusivities along the three orthogonal axes that describe the orientation of the ellipsoid relative to the magnet coordinate system. By diagonalizing **D**, that is rotating the magnet coordinate system on to the principal coordinate system of the diffusion ellipsoid, it is possible to determine the eigenvalues ($\lambda_i = 1,2,3$) and eigenvectors ($\varepsilon_i = 1,2,3$) of **D**, which are the effective principal diffusivities of water molecules along the orthotropic axes of the medium (Basser 1995). The largest principal diffusivity and its corresponding axis are called λ_1 and ε_1, while the smallest principal diffusivity and its axis are termed λ_3 and ε_3. In an isotropic medium, where there is no preferred direction for random water motions, the diffusion ellipsoid is spherical, with all three principal diffusivities being approximately equal (see Fig. 5.4a). In a highly anisotropic medium, where one direction is preferred over the others, λ_1 will be much larger than λ_2 and λ_3, and the diffusion ellipsoid will be elongated in the direction of λ_1 (see Fig. 5.4b). This prolate diffusion can be seen in large white matter fibre tracts, where water diffuses predominantly along the direction of the fibres and only to a lesser extent across them. Finally, λ_1 and λ_2 can be approximately equal, but much greater than λ_3. In this situation, the diffusion ellipsoid has a 'pancake' shape (see Fig. 5.4c).

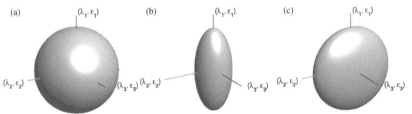

Fig. 5.4 Schematic diagram showing the diffusion ellipsoid shape for (a) isotropic diffusion, $\lambda_1 \sim \lambda_2 \sim \lambda_3$; (b) prolate diffusion, $\lambda_1 \gg \lambda_2 \sim \lambda_3$; and (c) oblate diffusion, $\lambda_1 \sim \lambda_2 \gg \lambda_3$. Isotropic diffusion is seen in CSF and grey matter regions, prolate diffusion is seen in coherently organized white matter structures, and oblate diffusion is seen in white matter regions when two or more white matter fibre tracts intersect.

The physiological origin of this oblate diffusion is difficult to explain, but may result from random measurement noise, partial volume effects, or the crossing of two or more fibre bundles.

Although the diffusion ellipsoid presents a clear visual representation of **D**, it does not provide quantitative scalar measures of diffusion that can be used to compare different patient populations. To address this problem, a number of diffusion indices, which condense the diffusion tensor information into simple scalar parameters, have been suggested. These diffusion parameters can then be thought of as quantitative histological or physiological stains that may be used to evaluate brain structure and function. The simplest of such quantitative diffusion indices is the mean diffusivity ($<D>$)

$$<D> = \frac{(\lambda_1 + \lambda_2 + \lambda_3)}{3}$$ [5.9]

which measures the size of the diffusion ellipsoid. This parameter is the tensor equivalent of $<ADC>$ obtained from the three orthogonal gradient encoding experiment. However, $<D>$ provides no indication of the shape of the diffusion ellipsoid. Such information can be obtained from diffusion anisotropy indices, which provide an indication of the eccentricity of the diffusion ellipsoid. However, the calculation of diffusion anisotropy is complicated by the effect that random measurement noise present in the component DW images has on the calculation of the eigenvalues of **D**. It has been shown that experimental noise causes the largest and smallest eigenvalues, λ_1 and λ_3, to diverge from their true infinite SNR values (Pierpaoli and Basser 1996; Bastin *et al.* 1998). This effect can artefactually increase the measured diffusion anisotropy in indices that require the eigenvalues to be sorted by their magnitude, e.g. λ_1/λ_3. To reduce this noise sensitivity, fully quantitative diffusion anisotropy indices are constructed from either all three eigenvalues of **D** or from scalar invariants which characterize the geometric properties of the diffusion ellipsoid (Ulug and van Zijl 1999). Perhaps the most often quoted rotationally invariant diffusion anisotropy index is the fractional anisotropy (FA)

$$FA = \sqrt{\frac{3}{2}} \sqrt{\frac{(\lambda_1 - <D>)^2 + (\lambda_2 - <D>)^2 + (\lambda_3 - <D>)^2}{\lambda_1^2 + \lambda_2^2 + \lambda_3^2}}$$ [5.10]

which measures the fraction of the total magnitude of **D** that is anisotropic, and takes a value of 0 for isotropic diffusion ($\lambda_1 = \lambda_2 = \lambda_3$) and 1 for completely anisotropic diffusion ($\lambda_1 > 0; \lambda_2 = \lambda_3 = 0$). This index is popular because it provides a higher SNR and better depiction of diffusion anisotropy effects than other rotationally invariant indices, such as the relative anisotropy or volume ratio (Papadakis *et al.* 1999).

Examples of two-dimensional maps of the T_2-weighted signal intensity, $<D>$ and FA obtained from a healthy female volunteer are shown in Fig. 5.5. In these maps,

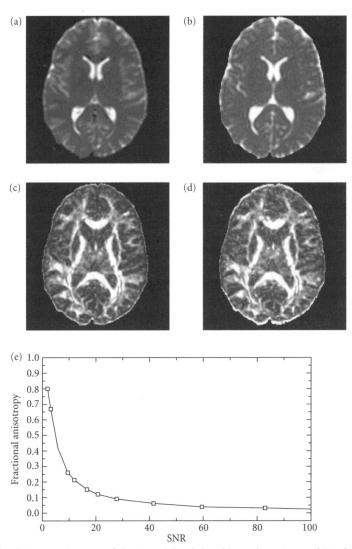

Fig. 5.5 (a–d) Parametric maps of the T_2-weighted signal intensity, $<D>$ and FA obtained from a 33-year-old female volunteer. Maps (a–c) have been calculated from DW-EP images corrected for the effects of eddy current distortions (Bastin 1999), while (d) was calculated from uncorrected DW-EP images. The blurring at grey/white matter tissue interfaces and rim artefacts in this map compared to (c) is clearly evident. (e) Plot of FA versus SNR for an isotropic medium obtained from numerical simulations. Note the significant overestimation of FA when SNR falls below approximately 20.

cerebrospinal fluid (CSF) is clearly visible as regions with high D and low diffusion anisotropy, while the major white matter fibre tracks are highlighted in the FA map due to their high diffusion anisotropy. Average values for $<D>$ and FA for CSF, white and grey matter obtained from five healthy volunteers are shown in Table 5.1. These

Table 5.1 Values of the mean diffusivity (<D>) and fractional anisotropy (FA) for various different brain regions obtained from five volunteers (Ulug and van Zijl 1999)

Brain region	<D> ($\times 10^{-6}$ mm^2 s^{-1})	FA
CSF	3250 ± 120	0.45 ± 0.03
Grey		
Cortical grey	930 ± 20	0.31 ± 0.02
Thalamus	730 ± 50	0.43 ± 0.07
Caudate nucleus	680 ± 70	0.41 ± 0.08
Lentiform nucleus	720 ± 90	0.42 ± 0.09
Average grey	760 ± 11	0.39 ± 0.06
White		
Corpus callosum (genu)	750 ± 100	0.78 ± 0.03
Corpus callosum (splenium)	880 ± 100	0.81 ± 0.03
Internal capsule (post. limb)	690 ± 30	0.74 ± 0.04
Internal capsule (ant. limb)	700 ± 10	0.71 ± 0.06
External capsule/extremum	730 ± 40	0.58 ± 0.03
Optic radiation	710 ± 30	0.64 ± 0.04
Frontal/parietal white matter	770 ± 30	0.64 ± 0.04
Average white	750 ± 0.07	0.70 ± 0.04

data show that CSF has high <D> and low FA values. Grey and white matter have similar values of <D>, but, as expected, the diffusion anisotropy of white matter is significantly greater than that of grey matter.

Unfortunately, while rotationally invariant diffusion anisotropy indices are less susceptible to experimental noise than indices that require magnitude sorting of the eigenvalues, diffusion anisotropy is still overestimated, especially in isotropic structures (see Fig. 5.5e), if the SNR value of the DW images is less than approximately 20–25 (Pierpaoli and Basser 1996; Bastin *et al.* 1998). Since the SNR value for a DW image collected at 1.5 Tesla with standard acquisition parameters (e.g. TE of 100 ms, a slice thickness of 5 mm and a b-value of 1000 s mm^{-2}) is typically 10–12, ameliorating the effects of noise is critical to the accurate quantification of diffusion anisotropy. The easiest solution to this problem is just to collect multiple acquisitions and magnitude average the DW images to provide a suitable SNR. However, this approach extends the length of the examination and may be problematic when imaging sick patients. Other methods which use both the eigenvalues and eigenvectors of **D** to reduce the noise sensitivity of diffusion anisotropy measurements have therefore been suggested (Pierpaoli and Basser 1996; Basser and Pajevic 2000; Skare *et al.* 2000*b*). Such schemes are generally based on the assumption that there is some temporal or spatial correlation between the eigenvectors of voxels in coherently organized white matter.

For example, Sun *et al.* (2001) have shown that assessing eigenvector orientational coherence in the same voxel from repeated experiments can reduce the number of acquisitions required to measure accurate diffusion anisotropy values compared with standard eigenvalue-only based indices. Alternatively, non-linear smoothing can be applied to the diffusion data prior to the calculation of **D** to reduce random noise in the raw DW images, and hence improve the SNR and accuracy of diffusion anisotropy measurements (Parker *et al.* 2000).

Finally, the accurate calculation of diffusion anisotropy requires DW images that are free from artefacts. Typically, the most significant distortions that need to be removed from DW-EP imaging data are those arising from eddy currents induced by the diffusion sensitizing gradients. These image distortions take the form of translation, shearing, and scaling of the image (Haselgrove and Moore 1996), and lead to the misregistration of individual DW-EP images in a data set, even in the absence of patient motion. This causes errors in the measured diffusion anisotropy, blurring at grey/white matter tissue interfaces, and rim artefacts (see Fig. 5.5d). Such distortions can be reduced significantly using optimized gradient waveforms (Alexander *et al.* 1997), collection of some form of calibration scan to correct the imaging data (Jezzard *et al.* 1998; Bastin 1999; Papadakis *et al.* 2000a), or by direct warping of distorted DW images on to undistorted baseline images (Ghanei *et al.* 2000; Bastin 2001). The removal of eddy current distortions can also be combined with image registration to remove bulk scan-to-scan patient motion. However, care must be taken that the original orientational information contained within the individual DW images is not lost when these various image warps are applied (Alexander *et al.* 2001).

Tractography

DT-MRI data not only provide scalar measures of diffusion anisotropy, but also have the potential to map white matter fibre tract trajectories *in vivo* (see Fig. 5.6). The three-dimensional tracking of white matter fibres, or tractography, can be achieved using the information contained within the eigenvectors of **D**. Tractography is based on the assumption that the eigenvector associated with the largest diffusivity (eigenvalue) lies parallel to the local fibre direction in large white matter fibre bundles. However, tracking fibres in three dimensions is a complex problem, requiring the component DW images to have good spatial resolution, be relatively free from artefacts and have a high SNR, so that algorithms can track the direction of principal eigenvectors through many contiguous slices (Tournier *et al.* 2002). Furthermore, the image voxels should be near-isotropic (e.g. $2.5 \times 2.5 \times 2.5$ mm) to remove any bias in the diffusion anisotropy measurements that could arise from the orientation of the imaging plane (Jones *et al.* 2002b).

A number of different approaches have been suggested which allow white matter fibres to be followed *in vivo* (Pajevic and Pierpaoli 1999; Jones *et al.* 1999b; Basser *et al.* 2000; Poupon *et al.* 2001; Sato *et al.* 2001; Mori *et al.* 2002). In the simplest terms,

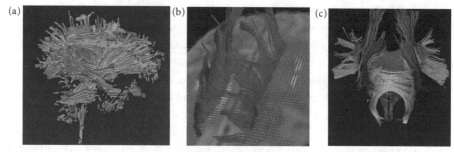

Fig. 5.6 Examples of *in vivo* tracking of white matter fibre bundles from DT-MRI data. (a) The three-dimensional information contained within **D** can be visualized by identifying regions of linear (white matter tracts) and planar (crossing fibres) diffusion and representing them as red streamtubes and green streamsurfaces, respectively. This figure shows geometric models representing the diffusion metric data obtained from a 33-year-old female volunteer. Such methods provide a powerful way of tracking fibres throughout the entire brain. The number of linear, planar, and spherical diffusion voxels in a region can also be determined (Zhang *et al.* 2004). A more standard approach is to depict the direction of fastest diffusion ε_1 using streamlines. Such an analysis is shown for the same volunteer at the level of the centrum semiovale (b) and for the whole brain (c). See Plate 2(a) of the plate section at the centre of this book.

tractography algorithms work by propagating a continuous streamline from an initial seed-point in the direction of the principal eigenvector of a set of voxels whose diffusion anisotropy is above a certain empirically determined threshold. If, over a certain specified distance, the track breaks, or its curvature becomes too great, then it is terminated. These methods allow the topology of major white matter fibre tracts, such as the corpus callosum, internal and external capsule, and pyramidal tract, to be determined, information that is lost when scalar indices derived from **D** are used to compare differences in local brain structure. More advanced algorithms determine the connectivity between brain regions using probabilistic methods (Koch *et al.* 2002; Behrens *et al.* 2003). Such approaches use probability density functions defined at each point in the brain to define the underlying fibre structure, thereby identifying regions of crossing fibres, which are not well described by the single tensor model.

While comparisons of scalar diffusion tensor data can be achieved using manual placement of regions-of-interest (ROIs) on parametric maps obtained from individual subjects, or from voxel-by-voxel and ROI analysis of group-averaged data sets (Buchsbaum *et al.* 1998; Virta *et al.* 1999), there is, as yet, no consensus on how to group-average tensor or tractography data. Jones *et al.* (2002*a*) have recently described an elegant method for generating a generic map of brain connectivity, or 'connectogram', from a group of subjects, i.e. performing tractography on population-averaged diffusion tensor data. Their method involves the generation of a diffusion tensor template in standard space, the co-registration of each individual data set to the template while preserving the principal eigenvector direction, and then creating metrics of the central tendency of the distribution of tensors for each voxel within the standard space. While this approach is very promising, doubts remain about the effect of smoothing on the integrity of the original data, and how differing degrees of brain atrophy may complicate the registration used for spatial normalization.

Application to schizophrenia

There are now more than 10 published studies which have used DT-MRI to investigate whether the brains of schizophrenic patients exhibit abnormal white matter structure compared with healthy age- and sex-matched controls (see Table 5.2). These studies are predicated on the assumption that diffusion parameters derived from $\mathbf{D}$ are sensitive indices of axonal integrity. Thus, reduced FA suggests structural damage and disrupted organization of white matter fibre tracts, while increased $<D>$ suggests oedema, demyelination, and/or axonal loss. Comparison of the data obtained from patient and control groups is then achieved using either a region-of-interest (ROI) or voxel-based (e.g. SPM) approach.

In the first of these studies, Buchsbaum *et al.* (1998) acquired both line-scan DT-MRI and fluoro-2-deoxy-D-glucose positron-emission tomography (PET) data from five patients (three men, two women) and six controls. They found that, compared with controls, schizophrenics had significantly reduced diffusion anisotropy in prefrontal cortical white matter and significantly lower glucose metabolic rates both in this region and in the striatum. The correlations between frontal and striatal metabolism were also lower in the patients. This, they argue, provides structural and functional evidence for diminished fronto-striatal connectivity in schizophrenia. Lim *et al.* (1999) also found reduced white matter diffusion anisotropy in 10 male patients who had no white matter volume deficits. These white matter diffusion abnormalities were widespread, affecting both hemispheres and extending from frontal to occipital regions. By defining small ROIs in the genu and splenium, Foong *et al.* (2000*b*) investigated whether there were any structural abnormalities in the corpus callosum of 20 (15 men, 5 women) schizophrenics. They found that $<D>$ was significantly increased while the FA was significantly reduced in the splenium, but not the genu, in the schizophrenic group compared with the controls. They suggest that this difference may indicate a focal disruption of commissural connectivity in schizophrenia. Agartz *et al.* (2001) replicated this finding of reduced diffusion anisotropy in the splenium of the corpus callosum in 20 schizophrenic patients (11 men, nine women) and 24 controls. Minami *et al.* (2003) found a significant bilateral reduction in FA throughout all white matter regions in 12 patients compared with 11 healthy controls. They also found that higher FA of left frontal white matter correlated significantly with higher dosage of antipsychotic medication. These results, they argue, suggest that schizophrenia is associated with a widespread disruption in white matter myelination, a distortion that is affected by antipsychotics.

Table 5.2 Controlled DT-MRI studies in schizophrenia

Study	Subjects (patients: controls)	Methods	$(b_{min}:b_{max})$ s mm^{-2}	Results
Buchsbaum et al. (1998)	(5:6)	1.5T GE Signa; line scan DWI; voxel based analysis	(5:1005)	↓ FA in right PFC and putamen. No relation to duration or memory
Lim et al. (1999)	(10:10) all male	DW-EPI; ROI analysis	(0:860)	↓ FA throughout WM but especially in PFC; despite no differences in WM volume
Foong et al. (2000b)	(20:25)	1.5T GE Signa; DW-EPI; ROI analysis	(0:700)	↑ <D> and ↓FA in splenium but not genu of corpus callosum
Agartz et al. (2001)	(20:24)	1.5T GE Signa; DW-EPI; voxel-based analysis	(0:1000)	↑ <D> throughout GM and WM. ↓FA in splenium, but not attributable to WM loss
Steel et al. (2001)	(10:10)	2T Elscint; DW-EPI; ROI analysis	(0:687)	No differences in FA. No correlation with duration or NAA concentrations
Foong et al. (2002)	(14:19)	As Foong et al. (2000b), but voxel-based analysis and registration failed in 12 subjects	(0:700)	No differences in <D> or FA of WM
Kubicki et al. (2002)	(15:18) all male	1.5T GE Signa; line-scan DWI; ROI analysis	(5:1000)	Uncinate fasciculus FA group by side interaction; FA correlated with cognitive dysfunction
Begré et al. (2003)	(7:7) first episodes	1.5T Siemens; DW-EPI; ROI analysis	Not stated	No differences in FA; correlation between more anterior α EEG activity and lower FA of both hippocampi in schizophrenics
Burns et al. (2003)	(30:30)	1.5T GE Signa; DW-EPI; voxel-based analysis with automated ROI placement	(0:1000)	↓ FA in arcuate and uncinate fasciculi, not attributable to WM loss

Table 5.2 (continued)

Study	Subjects (patients: controls)	Methods	$(b_{min}:b_{max})$ s mm^{-2}	Results
Minami *et al.* (2003)	(12:11)	1.5T GE Signa; DW-EPI; ROI analysis	(0:2000)	↓ FA throughout WM
Kubicki *et al.* (2003*b*)	(16:18)	As 2002 with: segmentation of cingulum bundle	(5:1000)	↓ FA bilaterally and correlated with cognitive deficits of left side
Wang *et al.* (2003)	(29:20)	1.5T GE; DW-EPI; ROI analysis	(0:1000)	No <*D*> or FA differences in cerebellar peduncles

<*D*>, mean diffusivity; DW-EPI, diffusion-weighted echo-planar imaging; FA, fractional anisotropy; GM, grey matter; NAA, *N*-acetyl-aspartate; PFC, prefrontal cortex; ROI, regions of interest; SE-EPI, spin-echo echo-planar imaging; WM, white matter.

Conversely, Steel *et al.* (2001) and Foong *et al.* (2002) failed to find significant differences in diffusion parameters between schizophrenics and controls in studies involving 10 (5 men, 5 women) and 14 (11 men, 3 women) patients, respectively. However, both studies had significant methodological and experimental design problems that would have reduced their ability to detect potential population differences. Specifically, in both studies the number of patients examined was relatively small, while the quality of the DT-MRI data was not optimal. For example, the <*D*> and FA maps presented by Steel and co-workers are poor, while no eddy current correction was performed on the DW images acquired by Foong *et al.* Notwithstanding these problems, the study by Foong *et al.* (2002) is especially interesting, given that they were unable to replicate the findings of their earlier study (Foong *et al.* 2000*b*) when a subset of the data was re-analysed using SPM. They argue that using voxel-based methods to analyse DT-MRI data is problematic since SPM assumes that the data have a Gaussian distribution (Ashburner and Friston 2000), which is not the case for diffusion anisotropy data. In addition, the operations of spatial normalization and Gaussian smoothing performed by SPM will alter the orientational information contained within the original diffusion anisotropy maps. This will reduce the probability of being able to detect subtle changes in patient groups, especially if the number of subjects studied is small. They therefore suggest that the ROI approach is probably a more reliable method of detecting changes in white matter fibre tracts, especially if these are large enough for the ROI to be reliably placed. Two further studies report negative results: a small study of first-episode patients (Begré *et al.* 2003) and a study that performed an ROI analysis of the cerebellar peduncles (Wang *et al.* 2003).

There is an observable trend in the literature towards testing more specific anatomical hypotheses. Recently, results from several such hypothesis-driven studies have been

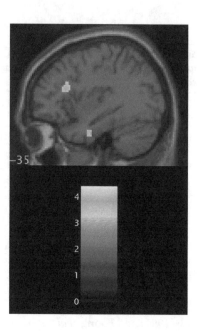

Fig. 5.7 Statistical parametric map overlaid on a T_1-weighted image, showing FA reduction in the left uncinate fasciculus and left arcuate fasciculus for 30 schizophrenic patients compared with 30 matched controls (Burns *et al.* 2003). The threshold for the analysis was set at $P = 0.001$ (uncorrected). The colour bar shows Z values corresponding to colours in the figure. See Plate 2(b) of the plate section at the centre of this book.

reported. In these studies, Kubicki *et al.* (2002, 2003*a*, *b*) and Burns *et al.* (2003) have tested the specific hypothesis that schizophrenia is a disorder of cortical connectivity affecting the white matter tracts linking temporal and frontal lobes. In 15 male patients, Kubicki *et al.* (2002) found a lack of the normal left-greater-than-right asymmetry in the diffusion anisotropy of the uncinate fasciculus in control subjects. A much less ambiguous result is provided by the study of Burns *et al.* (2003), which found significantly reduced diffusion anisotropy in the left uncinate fasciculus and left arcuate fasciculus in 30 (15 men, 15 women) patients (see Fig. 5.7), without any corresponding reduction in white matter density. Kubicki *et al.* (2003*b*) have recently found reduced FA in the cingulum bundle, caudal to the genu of the corpus callosum. Burns *et al.* did not find this, but differences in ROI placement might be responsible. Finally, in an intriguing combined DT/MT-MRI study, reported in a conference abstract, Kubicki *et al.* (2003*a*) found evidence for joint abnormalities in frontal regions, but DT-MRI differences only in the arcuate fasciculus and corpus callosum. The MT-MRI reductions are similar to those previously reported by another group (Bagary *et al.* 2003).

Conclusions

It is clear that DT-MRI provides a very valuable tool for investigating possible white matter structural abnormalities in schizophrenia. Although the first few published studies were essentially 'look and see' experiments, the recent studies by Kubicki *et al.* (2002, 2003*a*, *b*) and Burns *et al.* (2003) have attempted to test more specific hypotheses of cortical disconnectivity. Such anatomically precise hypothesis-driven studies, with sufficient size to detect subtle white matter changes in different patient populations, point the way to future studies, which should aim to determine the exact relationship between the anatomical findings of disconnectivity and the clinical features of schizophrenia. However, to unlock the full potential of this exciting new imaging modality, researchers must employ the best available data acquisition and image processing methodologies. As discussed above, the accurate estimation of diffusion tensor parameters *in vivo* requires the collection of sets of high SNR DW images of the best possible spatial resolution, free from bulk patient motion artefacts (and ideally pulsatile brain motions) and eddy current induced distortions. High angular resolution diffusion gradient sampling in an isotropic voxel acquisition scheme probably provides the optimum form of diffusion data from which to measure diffusion anisotropy and to track fibre bundles in three dimensions. However, significant investment in complex image-processing techniques is also required to extract all the information that is potentially available in DT-MRI data. With such refinements, DT-MRI has the potential to provide unique data about brain connectivity and how it is altered in neuropsychiatric disorders such as schizophrenia.

References

Agartz, I., Andersson, J. L., and Skare, S. (2001). Abnormal brain white matter in schizophrenia: a diffusion tensor imaging study. *Neuroreport*, **12**, 2251–4.

Alexander, A. L., Tsuruda, J. S., and Parker, D. L. (1997). Elimination of eddy current artifacts in diffusion-weighted echo-planar images: the use of bipolar gradients. *Magnetic Resonance in Medicine*, **38**, 1016–21.

Alexander, D. C., Pierpaoli, C., Basser, P. J., and Gee, J. C. (2001). Spatial transformations of diffusion tensor magnetic resonance images. *IEEE Transactions in Medical Imaging*, **20**, 1131–9.

Anderson, A. W. and Gore, J. C. (1994). Analysis and correction of motion artifacts in diffusion weighted imaging. *Magnetic Resonance in Medicine*, **32**, 379–87.

Armitage, P. A. and Bastin, M. E. (2001). Utilizing the diffusion-to-noise ratio to optimize magnetic resonance diffusion tensor acquisition strategies for improving measurements of diffusion anisotropy. *Magnetic Resonance in Medicine*, **45**, 1056–65.

Ashburner, J. and Friston, K. J. (2000). Voxel-based morphometry—the methods. *Neuroimage*, 11, 805–21.

Bagary, M. S., Symms, M. R., Barker, G. J., Mutsatsa, S. H., Joyce, E. M. and Ron, M. A. (2003). Gray and white matter brain abnormalities in first-episode schizophrenia inferred from magnetization transfer imaging. *Archives of General Psychiatry*, **60**, 779–88.

Bammer, R., Auer, M., Keeling, S.L., Augustin, M., Stables, L. A., Prokesch, R. W. *et al.* (2002). Diffusion tensor imaging using single-shot SENSE-EPI. *Magnetic Resonance in Medicine*, **48**, 128–36.

Basser, P. J. (1995). Inferring microstructural features and the physiological state of tissues from diffusion-weighted images. *NMR in Biomedicine*, **8**, 333–44.

Basser, P. J. and Pajevic, S. (2000). Statistical artifacts in diffusion tensor MRI (DT-MRI) caused by background noise. *Magnetic Resonance in Medicine*, **44**, 41–50.

Basser, P. J. and Pierpaoli, C. (1998). A simplified method to measure the diffusion tensor from seven MR images. *Magnetic Resonance in Medicine*, **39**, 928–34.

Basser, P. J., Mattiello, J., and LeBihan, D. (1994). Estimation of the effective self-diffusion tensor from the NMR spin echo. *Journal of Magnetic Resonance*, **103**, 247–54.

Basser, P. J., Pajevic, S., Pierpaoli, C., Duda, J., and Aldroubi, A. (2000). *In vivo* fiber tractography using DT-MRI data. *Magnetic Resonance in Medicine*, **44**, 625–32.

Bastin, M. E. (1999). Correction of eddy current-induced artefacts in diffusion tensor imaging using iterative cross-correlation. *Magnetic Resonance Imaging*, **17**, 1011–24.

Bastin, M. E. (2001). On the use of the FLAIR technique to improve the correction of eddy current induced artefacts in MR diffusion tensor imaging. *Magnetic Resonance Imaging*, **19**, 937–50.

Bastin, M. E., Armitage, P. A., and Marshall, I. (1998). A theoretical study of the effect of experimental noise on the measurement of anisotropy in diffusion imaging. *Magnetic Resonance Imaging*, **16**, 773–85.

Beaulieu, C. and Allen, P. S. (1994*a*). Determinants of anisotropic water diffusion in nerves. *Magnetic Resonance in Medicine*, **31**, 394–400.

Beaulieu, C. and Allen, P. S. (1994*b*). Water diffusion in the giant axon of the squid: implications for diffusion-weighted MRI of the nervous system. *Magnetic Resonance in Medicine*, **32**, 579–83.

Begré, S., Federspiel, A., Kiefer, C., Schroth, G., Dierks, T., and Strik, W. K. (2003). Reduced hippocampal anisotropy related to anteriorization of alpha EEG in schizophrenia. *Neuroreport*, **14**, 739–42.

Behrens, T. E., Johansen-Berg, H., Woolrich, M. W., Smith, S. M., Wheeler-Kingshott, C. A., Boulby, P. A., et al. (2003). Non-invasive mapping of connections between human thalamus and cortex using diffusion imaging. *Nature Neuroscience*, **6**, 750–7.

Buchsbaum, M. S., Tang, C. Y., Peled, S., Gudbjartsson, H., Lu, D., Hazlett, E. A. et al. (1998). MRI white matter diffusion anisotropy and PET metabolic rate in schizophrenia. *Neuroreport*, **9**, 425–30.

Burns, J., Job, D., Bastin, M. E., Whalley, H., Macgillivray, T., Johnstone, E. C. et al. (2003). Structural disconnectivity in schizophrenia: a diffusion tensor magnetic resonance imaging study. *British Journal of Psychiatry*, **182**, 439–43.

Clark, C. A. and Le Bihan, D. (2000). Water diffusion compartmentation and anisotropy at high b values in the human brain. *Magnetic Resonance in Medicine*, **44**, 852–9.

Clark, C. A., Hedehus, M., and Moseley, M. E. (2002). *In vivo* mapping of the fast and slow diffusion tensors in human brain. *Magnetic Resonance in Medicine*, **47**, 623–8.

Fletcher, P., McKenna, P. J., Friston, K. J., Frith, C. D., and Dolan, R. J. (1999). Abnormal cingulate modulation of fronto-temporal connectivity in schizophrenia. *Neuroimage*, **9**, 337–42.

Foong, J., Maier, M., Barker, G. J., Brocklehurst, S., Miller, D. H., and Ron, M. A. (2000*a*). In vivo investigation of white matter pathology in schizophrenia with magnetisation transfer imaging. *Journal of Neurology, Neurosurgery and Psychiatry*, **68**, 70–4.

Foong, J., Maier, M., Clark, C. A., Barker, G. J., Miller, D. H., and Ron, M. A. (2000*b*). Neuropathological abnormalities of the corpus callosum in schizophrenia: a diffusion tensor imaging study. *Journal of Neurology, Neurosurgery and Psychiatry*, **68**, 242–4.

Foong, J., Symms, M. R., Barker, G. J., Maier, M., Woermann, F. G., Miller, D. H. et al. (2001). Neuropathological abnormalities in schizophrenia: evidence from magnetization transfer imaging. *Brain*, **124**, 882–92.

Foong, J., Symms, M. R., Barker, G. J., Maier, M., Miller, D. H., and Ron, M. A. (2002). Investigating regional white matter in schizophrenia using diffusion tensor imaging. *Neuroreport*, **13**, 333–6.

Frank, L. R. (2001). Anisotropy in high angular resolution diffusion-weighted MRI. *Magnetic Resonance in Medicine*, **45**, 935–9.

Friston, K. J. and Frith, C. D. (1995). Schizophrenia: a disconnection syndrome? *Clinical Neuroscience*, **3**, 89–97.

Frith, C. D., Friston, K. J., Herold, S., Silbersweig, D., Fletcher, P., Cahill, C. *et al.* (1995). Regional brain activity in chronic schizophrenic patients during the performance of a verbal fluency task. *British Journal of Psychiatry*, **167**, 343–9.

Ghanei, A., Soltanian-Zadeh, H., Jacobs, M. A., and Patel, S. (2000). Boundary-based warping of brain MR images. *Journal of Magnetic Resonance Imaging*, **12**, 417–29.

Gudbjartsson, H., Maier, S. E., Mulkern, R. V., Morocz, I. A,, Patz, S., and Jolesz, F. A. (1996). Line scan diffusion imaging. *Magnetic Resonance in Medicine*, **36**, 509–19.

Gulani, V., Webb, A. G., Duncan, I. D., and Lauterbur, P. C. (2001). Apparent diffusion tensor measurements in myelin-deficient rat spinal cords. *Magnetic Resonance in Medicine*, **45**, 191–5.

Hasan, K. M., Parker, D. L., and Alexander, A. L. (2001). Comparison of gradient encoding schemes for diffusion-tensor MRI. *Journal of Magnetic Resonance Imaging*, **13**, 769–80.

Haselgrove, J. C. and Moore, J. R. (1996). Correction for distortion of echo-planar images used to calculate the apparent diffusion coefficient. *Magnetic Resonance in Medicine*, **36**, 960–4.

Huppi, P. S., Maier, S. E., Peled, S., Zientara, G. P., Barnes, P. D., Jolesz, F. A. *et al.* (1998). Microstructural development of human newborn cerebral white matter assessed *in vivo* by diffusion tensor magnetic resonance imaging. *Pediatric Research*, **44**, 584–90.

Jezzard, P. and Balaban, R. S. (1995). Correction for geometric distortion in echo planar images from B0 field variations. *Magnetic Resonance in Medicine*, **34**, 65–73.

Jezzard, P., Barnett, A. S., and Pierpaoli, C. (1998). Characterization of and correction for eddy current artifacts in echo planar diffusion imaging. *Magnetic Resonance in Medicine*, **39**, 801–12.

Jones, D. K., Horsfield, M. A., and Simmons, A. (1999*a*). Optimal strategies for measuring diffusion in anisotropic systems by magnetic resonance imaging. *Magnetic Resonance in Medicine*, **42**, 515–25.

Jones, D. K., Simmons, A., Williams, S. C., and Horsfield, M. A. (1999*b*). Non-invasive assessment of axonal fiber connectivity in the human brain via diffusion tensor MRI. *Magnetic Resonance in Medicine*, **42**, 37–41.

Jones, D. K., Griffin, L. D., Alexander, D. C., Catani, M., Horsfield, M. A., Howard, R. *et al.* (2002*a*). Spatial normalization and averaging of diffusion tensor MRI data sets. *Neuroimage*, **17**, 592–617.

Jones, D. K., Williams, S. C., Gasston, D., Horsfield, M. A., Simmons, A., and Howard, R. (2002*b*). Isotropic resolution diffusion tensor imaging with whole brain acquisition in a clinically acceptable time. *Human Brain Mapping*, **15**, 216–30.

Kastner, S. and Ungerleider, L. G. (2000). Mechanisms of visual attention in the human cortex. *Annual Review of Neuroscience*, **23**, 315–41.

Koch, M. A., Norris, D. G., and Hund-Georgiadis, M. (2002). An investigation of functional and anatomical connectivity using magnetic resonance imaging. *Neuroimage*, **16**, 241–50.

Kubicki, M., Westin, C. F., Maier, S. E., Frumin, M., Nestor, P. G., Salisbury, D. F. *et al.* (2002). Uncinate fasciculus findings in schizophrenia: a magnetic resonance diffusion tensor imaging study. *American Journal of Psychiatry*, **159**, 813–20.

Kubicki, M., Westin, C. F., Frumin, M., Ersner-Hershfield, H., Jolesz, F. A., McCarley, R. W. *et al.* (2003*a*). DTI and MTR abnormalities in schizophrenia—voxel wise analysis of white matter integrity. *Schizophrenia Research*, **60**, 199.

Kubicki, M., Westin, C. F., Nestor, P. G., Wible, C. G., Frumin, M., Maier, S. E. *et al.* (2003*b*). Cingulate fasciculus integrity disruption in schizophrenia: A magnetic resonance diffusion tensor imaging study. *Biological Psychiatry*, **54**, 1171–80.

Lawrie, S. M. and Abukmeil, S. S. (1998). Brain abnormality in schizophrenia. A systematic and quantitative review of volumetric magnetic resonance imaging studies. *British Journal of Psychiatry*, **172**, 110–20.

Lawrie, S. M., Buechel, C., Whalley, H. C., Frith, C. D., Friston, K. J., and Johnstone, E. C. (2002). Reduced frontotemporal functional connectivity in schizophrenia associated with auditory hallucinations. *Biological Psychiatry*, **51**, 1008–11.

Le Bihan, D., Turner, R., and Douek, P. (1993). Is water diffusion restricted in human brain white matter? An echo-planar NMR imaging study. *Neuroreport*, **4**, 887–90.

Lim, K. O., Adalsteinsson, E., Spielman, D., Sullivan, E. V., Rosenbloom, M. J., and Pfefferbaum, A. (1998). Proton magnetic resonance spectroscopic imaging of cortical gray and white matter in schizophrenia. *Archives of General Psychiatry*, **55**, 346–52.

Lim, K. O., Hedehus, M., Moseley, M., de Crespigny, A., Sullivan, E. V., and Pfefferbaum, A. (1999). Compromised white matter tract integrity in schizophrenia inferred from diffusion tensor imaging. *Archives of General Psychiatry*, **56**, 367–74.

Mattiello, J., Basser, P. J., and Le Bihan, D. (1997). The b matrix in diffusion tensor echo-planar imaging. *Magnetic Resonance in Medicine*, **37**, 292–300.

Minami, T., Nobuhara, K., Okugawa, G., Takase, K., Yoshida, T., Sawada, S., *et al.* (2003). Diffusion tensor magnetic resonance imaging of disruption of regional white matter in schizophrenia. *Neuropsychobiology*, **47**, 141–5.

Mori, S., Kaufmann, W. E., Davatzikos, C., Stieltjes, B., Amodei, L., Fredericksen, K., *et al.* (2002). Imaging cortical association tracts in the human brain using diffusion-tensor-based axonal tracking. *Magnetic Resonance in Medicine*, **47**, 215–23.

Nicholson, C. and Sykova, E. (1998). Extracellular space structure revealed by diffusion analysis. *Trends in Neuroscience*, **21**, 207–15.

Niendorf, T., Dijkhuizen, R. M., Norris, D. G., van Lookeren Campagne, M., and Nicolay, K. (1996). Biexponential diffusion attenuation in various states of brain tissue: implications for diffusion-weighted imaging. *Magnetic Resonance in Medicine*, **36**, 847–57.

Ordidge, R. J., Helpern, J. A., Qing, Z. X., Knight, R. A., and Nagesh, V. (1994). Correction of motional artifacts in diffusion-weighted MR images using navigator echoes. *Magnetic Resonance Imaging*, **12**, 455–60.

Pajevic, S. and Pierpaoli, C. (1999). Color schemes to represent the orientation of anisotropic tissues from diffusion tensor data: application to white matter fiber tract mapping in the human brain. *Magnetic Resonance in Medicine*, **42**, 526–40.

Papadakis, N. G., Xing, D., Houston, G. C., Smith, J. M., Smith, M. I., James, M. F. *et al.* (1999). A study of rotationally invariant and symmetric indices of diffusion anisotropy. *Magnetic Resonance Imaging*, **17**, 881–92.

Papadakis, N. G., Martin, K. M., Pickard, J. D., Hall, L. D., Carpenter, T. A., and Huang, C. L. (2000*a*). Gradient preemphasis calibration in diffusion-weighted echo-planar imaging. *Magnetic Resonance in Medicine*, **44**, 616–24.

Papadakis, N. G., Murrills, C. D., Hall, L. D., Huang, C. L., and Carpenter, T. A. (2000*b*). Minimal gradient encoding for robust estimation of diffusion anisotropy. *Magnetic Resonance Imaging*, **18**, 671–9.

Parker, G. J., Schnabel, J. A., Symms, M. R., Werring, D. J., and Barker, G. J. (2000). Nonlinear smoothing for reduction of systematic and random errors in diffusion tensor imaging. *Journal of Magnetic Resonance Imaging*, **11**, 702–10.

Pierpaoli, C. and Basser, P. J. (1996). Toward a quantitative assessment of diffusion anisotropy. *Magnetic Resonance in Medicine*, **36**, 893–906.

Pierpaoli, C., Jezzard, P., Basser, P. J., Barnett, A., and Di Chiro, G. (1996). Diffusion tensor MR imaging of the human brain. *Radiology*, **201**, 637–48.

Poupon, C., Mangin, J., Clark, C. A., Frouin, V., Regis, J., Le Bihan, D. *et al.* (2001). Towards inference of human brain connectivity from MR diffusion tensor data. *Medical Image Analysis*, **5**, 1–15.

Pruessmann, K. P., Weiger, M., Scheidegger, M. B., and Boesiger, P. (1999). SENSE: sensitivity encoding for fast MRI. *Magnetic Resonance in Medicine*, **42**, 952–62.

Sato, T., Hasan, K., Alexander, A. L., and Minato, K. (2001). Structural connectivity in white matter using the projected diffusion-tensor distance. *Medinfo*, **10**, 929–32.

Schlaepfer, T. E., Harris, G. J., Tien, A. Y., Peng, L. W., Lee, S., Federman, E. B. *et al.* (1994). Decreased regional cortical gray matter volume in schizophrenia. *American Journal of Psychiatry*, **151**, 842–8.

Schmithorst, V. J. and Dardzinski, B. J. (2002). Automatic gradient preemphasis adjustment: a 15-minute journey to improved diffusion-weighted echo-planar imaging. *Magnetic Resonance in Medicine*, **47**, 208–12.

Shrager, R. I. and Basser, P. J. (1998). Anisotropically weighted MRI. *Magnetic Resonance in Medicine*, **40**, 160–5.

Skare, S. and Andersson, J. L. (2001). On the effects of gating in diffusion imaging of the brain using single shot EPI. *Magnetic Resonance Imaging*, **19**, 1125–8.

Skare, S., Hedehus, M., Moseley, M. E., and Li, T. Q. (2000*a*). Condition number as a measure of noise performance of diffusion tensor data acquisition schemes with MRI. *Journal of Magnetic Resonance*, **147**, 340–52.

Skare, S., Li, T., Nordell, B., and Ingvar, M. (2000*b*). Noise considerations in the determination of diffusion tensor anisotropy. *Magnetic Resonance Imaging*, **18**, 659–69.

Steel, R. M., Bastin, M. E., McConnell, S., Marshall, I., Cunningham-Owens, D. G., Lawrie, S. M., Johnstone, E. C. *et al.* (2001). Diffusion tensor imaging (DTI) and proton magnetic resonance spectroscopy (1H MRS) in schizophrenic subjects and normal controls. *Psychiatry Research*, **106**, 161–70.

Stejskal, E. O. and Tanner, J. E. (1965). Spin diffusion measurements: spin echoes in the presence of a time-dependent field gradient. *Journal of Physical Chemistry*, **42**, 288–92.

Sun, S. W., Song, S. K., Hong, C. Y., Chu, W. C., and Chang, C. (2001). Improving relative anisotropy measurement using directional correlation of diffusion tensors. *Magnetic Resonance in Medicine*, **46**, 1088–92.

Tournier, J. D., Calamante, F., King, M. D., Gadian, D. G., and Connelly, A. (2002). Limitations and requirements of diffusion tensor fiber tracking: an assessment using simulations. *Magnetic Resonance in Medicine*, **47**, 701–8.

Turner, R. and Le Bihan, D. (1990). Single-shot diffusion imaging at 2.0 tesla. *Journal of Magnetic Resonance*, **86**, 445–52.

Ulug, A. M. and van Zijl, P. C. (1999). Orientation-independent diffusion imaging without tensor diagonalization: anisotropy definitions based on physical attributes of the diffusion ellipsoid. *Journal of Magnetic Resonance Imaging*, **9**, 804–13.

Ulug, A. M., Beauchamp, N. Jr, Bryan, R. N., and van Zijl, P. C. (1997). Absolute quantitation of diffusion constants in human stroke. *Stroke*, **28**, 483–90.

Virta, A., Barnett, A., and Pierpaoli, C. (1999). Visualizing and characterizing white matter fiber structure and architecture in the human pyramidal tract using diffusion tensor MRI. *Magnetic Resonance Imaging*, **17**, 1121–33.

Wang, F., Sun, Z., Du, X., Wang, X., Cong, Z., Zhang, H. *et al.* (2003). A diffusion tensor imaging study of middle and superior cerebellar peduncle in male patients with schizophrenia. *Neuroscience Letters*, **348**, 135–8.

Wright, I. C., Rabe-Hesketh, S., Woodruff, P. W., David, A. S., Murray, R. M., and Bullmore, E. T. (2000). Meta-analysis of regional brain volumes in schizophrenia. *American Journal of Psychiatry*, **157**, 16–25.

Xing, D., Papadakis, N. G., Huang, C. L., Lee, V. M., Carpenter, T. A., and Hall, L. D. (1997). Optimised diffusion-weighting for measurement of apparent diffusion coefficient (ADC) in human brain. *Magnetic Resonance Imaging*, **15**, 771–84.

Zang, S., Bastin, M. E., Laidlaw, D. H., Sinha, S., Armitage, P. A., and Deisboeck, T. S. (2004). Visualization and analysis of white matter structural asymmetry in diffusion tensor MR imaging data. *Magnetic Resonance in Medicine*, **51**, 140–7.

Zipursky, R. B., Lim, K. O., Sullivan, E. V., Brown, B. W., and Pfefferbaum, A. (1992). Widespread cerebral gray matter volume deficits in schizophrenia. *Archives of General Psychiatry*, **49**, 195–205.

Chapter 6

Automated analysis of structural MRI data

Paul M. Thompson, Judith L. Rapoport,
Tyrone D. Cannon, and Arthur W. Toga

Introduction

Recent advances in medical imaging have revolutionized our ability to investigate disease. Current brain mapping initiatives are charting brain structure and function in thousands of subjects [e.g. Rapoport *et al.* (1999): $N = 1000+$ children and adolescents; Mazziotta *et al.* (2001): $N = 7000$, including 5800 genotyped subjects and 342 mono- and dizygotic twins]. An urgent goal of these projects is to analyze patterns of altered brain structure and function in disorders such as schizophrenia, Alzheimer's disease, and abnormal childhood development.

   The near-exponential pace of data collection (Fox 1997) has stimulated the development of image analysis algorithms that compare, pool, and average brain data across whole populations. Even so, brain structure is complex and varies dramatically across normal subjects, so systematic patterns of altered structure are hard to detect. This statistical challenge has ignited the rapidly growing field of computational anatomy (Fischl and Dale 2000; Thompson *et al.* 2000*b*; Miller *et al.* 2002; Ashburner *et al.* 2003). This field combines new approaches in computer vision, anatomical surface modeling (Fischl and Dale 2000; Thompson *et al.* 2000; Gerig *et al.*, 2001), differential geometry (Miller *et al.*, 2002), and statistical field theory (Friston *et al.* 1995; Worsley *et al.* 1999; Taylor and Adler 2003) to capture anatomic variation, encode it and detect group-specific patterns. Many computational anatomy techniques are highly automated, making studies of brain structure feasible on a scale not previously imaginable, with extraordinary power to explore disease effects.

Increased automation

As brain mapping analyses begin to draw upon hundreds or even thousands of images (Evans *et al.* 1994, $N = 305$; Good *et al.* 2001*b*, $N = 465$; Mazziotta *et al.* 2001; $N = 851$), computational approaches must distil information from these images in a highly automated way. Extracting scientifically useful data requires a sequence of image processing steps, and these are becoming increasingly easy to apply. Automated scalp editing, image registration, warping, and tissue classification methods are making it faster to pre-process brain images (Toga 1998; Woods *et al.* 1998; Ashburner and Friston 1999; Shattuck and Leahy 2001; Smith *et al.* 2002). Brain parcellation and labeling algorithms are also approaching human accuracy in delineating anatomy (Collins *et al.* 1995; Fischl *et al.* 2000; Pitiot *et al.* 2002). Last, but not least, signal detection methods are being rapidly optimized, drawing on groundbreaking research in image statistics (Gaussian field theory, statistical flattening, and nonparametric methods), as well as novel data transformations (tensor maps, scale space, adaptive filters, etc.). These mathematical developments benefit large-scale clinical and basic science studies, as well as smaller ones where sample sizes or detection power are limited (Thompson *et al.* 2000*a*, 2001*b*).

Statistical atlases

Statistics that describe how brain structure and function vary in a population can also empower the automated analysis of new images (Ashburner *et al.* 1998; Gee and Bajcsy 1998; Dinov *et al.* 2000). Computational brain atlases, for example, warehouse this statistical information in standard three-dimensional coordinate systems (Mazziotta *et al.* 2001; Thompson *et al.*, 2002). Computational algorithms can then use normative criteria to find structures in new images, and also to map patterns of abnormalities in disease. They can also uncover surprising relationships between genotype and phenotype (Styner and Gerig 2001; Thompson *et al.* 2001*a*; Cannon *et al.* 2002), and dynamic brain changes in response to therapy (Haney *et al.* 2001; Toga and Thompson 2003*b*). Due to hardware and network advances, large image analyses can now be run on remote, or distributed, servers. Supercomputing resources can then be harnessed to mine brain data for population trends (Toga *et al.* 2001; cf. Collins *et al.* 2002; Warfield *et al.* 1998).

Organization of this chapter

In this chapter, we review computational methods to detect structural differences in the brain. We describe the mathematical concepts underlying several common approaches, including voxel-based morphometry, deformation morphometry, and tensor-based morphometry, as well as shape modeling and traditional volumetrics (see Fig. 6.1; Table 6.1 summarizes these concepts). We also cover hybrid approaches (e.g. cortical pattern matching) that analyze shape and tissue distribution in the same analysis. Each technique is optimized to detect specific features, and has its own strengths and limitations. We highlight illustrative clinical findings from studies of development, dementia, and schizophrenia. We also describe newer techniques that map patterns of brain change over time (e.g. to study disease progression or medication effects). Finally we describe how imaging statistics can be expanded to assess genetic effects on brain structure, in family, twin, or allele-based designs.

Table 6.1 Classes of morphometric methods. While not an exhaustive list, this table describes some key methods for analyzing MRI data. Each of these methods can be used to identify group differences in brain structure

Method	Principle	Methods papers
VBM	Maps group differences in gray matter, white matter, CSF at each voxel in stereotaxic space	Ashburner and Friston (2000), Davatzikos *et al.* (2001), Good *et al.* (2001*a,b*)
DBM	Analyzes brain shape differences based on deformations that map each brain to a common anatomic template	Ashburner *et al.* (1998), Gaser *et al.* (1999), Thompson *et al.* (2000*a*), Miller *et al.* (2002)
TBM	Analyzes local compression or dilation required to warp a baseline image on to an atlas or onto a later one from the same subject	Davatzikos *et al.* (1996), Fox *et al.* (1998), Thompson *et al.* (2000*a*)
Cortical mapping	Sulcal matching is performed on extracted cortical surface models prior to comparing gray matter measures, shape differences, asymmetries	MacDonald (1998), Fischl and Dale (2000), Thompson *et al.* (2001*b,c,d*)
Shape modeling	Three-dimensional geometric models of anatomical curves or surfaces are averaged and compared	Thompson *et al.* (1996*a,b*), Joshi *et al.* (1997), Csernansky *et al.* (2000), Gerig *et al.* (2001)
Parcellation	Regions of interest are manually traced or automatically labeled on images, and volumes are compared across groups	Collins *et al.* (1995), Kennedy *et al.* (1998), Fischl *et al.* (1999)

VBM, voxel-based morphometry; DBM, deformation-based morphometry; TBM, tensor-based morphometry; CSF, cerebrospinal fluid.

Goals

Morphometric methods are powerful in a variety of settings. Identifying structures with altered volume or shape can help us to understand the biological basis of a disease, pin-pointing when and where deficits occur. Gross structural changes may indicate cellular processes such as neuronal loss or atrophy, delayed myelination, or aberrant migration and connectivity (Bogerts 1999; Falkai *et al.* 1999; Goldman-Rakic and Selemon 1998; Weinberger *et al.* 2001; Weinberger and McClure 2002). Structural changes can also be correlated with functional, metabolic, spectroscopic, or architectonic data (McCarley *et al.* 1999; Buchsbaum *et al.* 2002). If structural measures link with behavioral or cognitive measures, or with clinical outcomes, they may provide a biological marker, or 'endophenotype', for a disease. MRI studies reveal early brain changes in subjects at genetic risk for Alzheimer's disease (ApoE4 carriers; Laakso *et al.*, 2000), and can expedite early diagnosis and treatment. They can uncover drug effects in clinical trials (Fox *et al.* 1999, 2000, 2001). Dynamic brain maps, in particular, capture how the brain changes over time. They reveal growth spurts in childhood

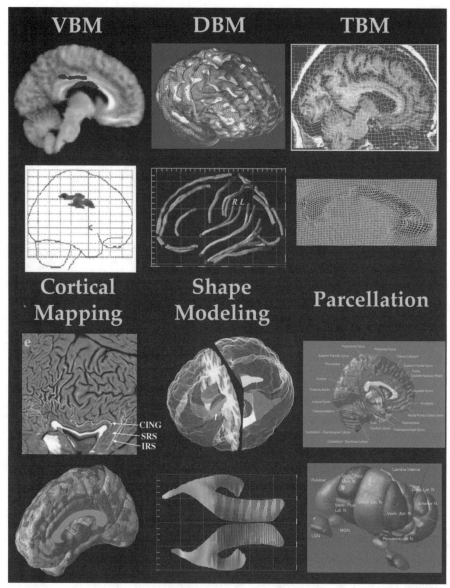

Fig. 6.1 Taxonomy of methods for analyzing MRI data. This schematic illustrates six major types of analysis of structural images, showing some of the data used in each case (see Table 6.1 for the key concepts underlying each method). Voxel-based morphometry (VBM; top left panels) compares anatomy voxel by voxel to find voxels (shown here in blue) where the tissue classification (gray, white matter, CSF) depends on diagnosis or other factors. Results are typically plotted in stereotaxic space (lower panel), and their significance assessed using random field or permutation methods (see text for details). Deformation-based morphometry (DBM) can be used to analyze shape differences in the cortex, or brain asymmetries (colored sulci: red colors show regions of greatest asymmetry). Tensor-based morphometry (TBM) uses

(Thompson *et al.* 2000*a*), gray matter loss in adolescence (Giedd *et al.* 1999*a,b*; Sowell *et al.*, 1999*a,b*), and dynamic waves of brain changes in dementia and schizophrenia (Thompson *et al.* 2001, 2002). These maps can also clarify how disease processes spread dynamically in the brain (Thompson *et al.* 2001*b,d*, 2002). Statistics of these brain changes can also be stored in digital brain atlases. These can be used in medication studies to map where therapy is slowing down a disease process (Haney *et al.* 2001). Deficits can also be compared across cohorts, including chronic, first-episode and early-onset patients, or subgroups with different symptom profiles (Giedd *et al.* 1999*a,b*; Job *et al.* 2002; Narr *et al.* 2002). Screening relatives is also vital for early diagnosis and understanding disease transmission. Structural image analyses can now produce *genetic brain maps* (Thompson *et al.* 2001*a*, 2002). These pinpoint deficit regions in genetically at-risk relatives (Baare *et al.* 2001; Cannon *et al.* 2002; Narr *et al.* 2002). Genetic designs reveal regions where brain structure is under strongest genetic control, linking structural variation with heritable differences in cognitive function (Thompson *et al.* 2001*a*; Posthuma *et al.* 2002). The computational format of these large-scale brain atlases makes it easy to stratify them to search for differences in subpopulations with known environmental risk, or with allelic variations at candidate loci, to identify possible pathogenic factors and explore their effects.

Automated and manual approaches

Brain image analysis is considerably faster when some or all of the image-processing steps are automated. Traditionally, manually intensive approaches (such as tracing three-dimensional regions of interest on brain images) have been the mainstay of structural image analysis. They reveal a consistent pattern of deficits in the dementias (Mega *et al.*, 2000) and schizophrenia (Lawrie and Abukmeil 1998), and provide fundamental data on brain growth in childhood and adolescence (Jernigan *et al.* 2001; Kennedy *et al.* 1998). Manually derived measures also continue to provide extremely

---

three-dimensional warping fields with millions of degrees of freedom (top) to recover and study local shape differences in anatomy across subjects or over time (red colors indicate growth rates in the corpus callosum of a young child). Other methods focus on structures such as the cerebral cortex, which can be flattened to assist the analysis (bottom left), or the lateral ventricles ('shape modeling'). If anatomic structures are represented as parametric surface meshes (Thompson *et al.* 2000*d*), their shapes can be compared, their variability can be visualized, or they can be used to show where gray matter is lost (e.g. in Alzheimer's disease: bottom left panel, red colors denote greatest gray matter loss in the limbic and entorhinal areas). Fine-scale anatomical parcellation (lower right) can be used compare structure volumes across groups, or to create hand-labeled templates that can be automatically warped onto new MRI brain datasets, creating regions of interest where analyses are performed. [VBM data courtesy of Elizabeth Sowell, Ph.D. (adapted from Sowell *et al.* 2000) and parcellation data courtesy of Jacopo Annese, Ph.D., UCLA Laboratory of Neuro Imaging]. See Plate 3 of the plate section at the centre of this book.

valuable information (Lawrie *et al.* 2002), and serve as a gold standard to validate newer, more automated techniques (Job *et al.* 2002; Tisserand *et al.* 2002).

In this chapter, we focus on more automated techniques for analyzing MRI data. We compare these with standard volumetric measures in terms of the results they have found, their statistical power and biases, and the range of features they assess. Despite the overarching goal of automating image analyses, often significant information is gained by combining manual approaches with more automated ones. For example, sulci may be traced manually on a cortical model extracted automatically, to increase the power of a gray matter analysis (see Fig. 6.2; Davatzikos *et al.* 2001; Thompson *et al.* 2001*a,b,c,d*). Automated labelings of the brain may also be corrected manually for greater accuracy (Collins *et al.* 2002; see Fig. 3.1).

Image pre-processing

Magnetic resonance imaging (MRI) is now the modality of choice for clinical and basic science studies of brain structure (Toga and Mazziotta 2002). Three-dimensional MR images provide high-resolution maps of anatomy (even permitting the measurement of cortical thickness; MacDonald 1998; Fischl and Dale 2000). They also provide excellent tissue contrast to differentiate tissue types, such as gray matter, white matter, and CSF. They are sensitive to disease-specific changes in anatomy, including progressive gray matter loss and ventricular enlargement in dementia and schizophrenia, as well as white matter and vascular lesions. A variety of tools have been developed to analyze these images, linking patterns of altered brain structure with diagnosis, symptoms, or demographic factors (Fig. 6.2). We describe some of these key processing steps next.

The first step in most structural image analyses involves placing MRI data from different subjects into a common three-dimensional coordinate system, or stereotaxic space (Collins *et al.* 2002). The success of brain mapping has been promoted by the international adoption of a coordinate-based three-dimensional reference system for brain data. This helps to pool data across subjects and studies. Images and brain maps are aligned with a standard brain template, typically one based on the Talairach stereotaxic atlas (Talairach and Tournoux 1988). Anatomical maps and locations can then be referenced in standard coordinates; mathematical techniques can average images across subjects, detect disease-specific patterns, hemispheric asymmetries, and subtle group differences in cortical function, in whole populations.

Stereotaxic coordinates

The first brain atlas used widely in brain mapping was that defined by the neurosurgeon Jean Talairach (Talairach and Tournoux 1988). Using a stereotaxic device anchored to a patient's skull, neurosurgeons can accurately position surgical apparatus within a patient's brain to target biopsy locations, epileptic foci, and vascular lesions identified in three-dimensional reference coordinates. The Talairach atlas was developed before intraoperative imaging, to make it easier to identify deep nuclei in

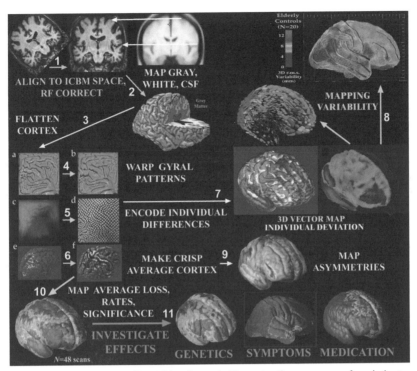

Fig. 6.2 An image analysis pipeline. This schematic illustrates the sequence of analysis steps in an MRI study (Thompson *et al.* 2001*b*). By using several of these processing modules, an investigator can create maps that reveal how brain structure varies in large populations, differs in disease, and is modulated by genetic or therapeutic factors. This approach aligns new three-dimensional MRI scans from patients and controls (1) with an average brain template based on a population (here the ICBM template is used, developed by the International Consortium for Brain Mapping). Tissue classification algorithms then generate maps of gray matter, white matter, and CSF (2). To help compare cortical features from subjects whose anatomy differs, individual gyral patterns are flattened (3) and aligned with a group average gyral pattern (4). If a color code indexing three-dimensional cortical locations is flowed along with the same deformation field (5), a crisp group average model of the cortex can be made (6), relative to which individual gyral pattern differences (7), group variability (8) and cortical asymmetry (9) can be computed. Once individual gyral patterns are aligned to the mean template, differences in gray matter distribution or thickness (10) can be mapped, pooling data from homologous regions of cortex. Correlations can be mapped between disease-related deficits and genetic risk factors (11). Maps may also be generated visualizing linkages between deficits and clinical symptoms, cognitive scores, and medication effects. The only steps here that are currently not automated are the tracing of sulci on the cortex (3a). Some manual editing may also assist algorithms that delete dura and scalp from images, especially if there is very little CSF in the diploic space (e.g. in normal children). See Plate 4 of the plate section at the centre of this book.

stereotaxic coordinates. At the time, these structures were imaged with very limited resolution using pneumoencephalography.

Talairach space

In addition to a series of labeled anatomical plates, reconstructed from histologic material, Talairach defined a mechanism to transfer new images on to the atlas. In the Talairach stereotaxic system, piecewise affine transformations are applied to 12 rectangular regions of brain, defined by vectors from the anterior and posterior commissures to the extrema of the cortex. These transformations reposition the anterior commissure of the subject's scan at the origin of the three-dimensional coordinate space, vertically align the interhemispheric plane, and horizontally orient the line connecting the two commissures. Each point in the incoming brain image, after it is 'warped' into the atlas space, is labeled by an (x,y,z) address referable to the atlas brain. Originally developed for surgery, the Talairach stereotaxic system rapidly became an international standard for reporting functional activation sites in PET studies, allowing researchers to compare and contrast results from different laboratories (Fox *et al.* 1985, 1988; Friston *et al.* 1989, 1991).

MRI brain templates

The Talairach templates were based on post-mortem sections of the brain of a single 60-year-old female subject, and the atlas plates had a variable slice separation (3–4 mm), and inconsistent data from orthogonal planes. To address these limitations, a composite T_1-weighted MRI dataset was constructed from 305 young normal subjects (239 males, 66 females; age: 23.4 ± 4.1 years) whose scans were individually mapped into the Talairach system by a nine-parameter linear transformation, intensity normalized, and averaged on a voxel-by-voxel basis (Evans *et al.*, 1994). The resulting average brain made it easier to develop automated image alignment methods to map new MRI and PET data into a common space (Fig. 6.2, top left). The International Consortium for Brain Mapping (ICBM; Mazziotta *et al.* 1995, 2001) subsequently applied the same image-averaging procedure to a subset of 152 brains. This produced a template that is widely used as part of the Statistical Parametric Mapping image analysis package (SPM99/SPM2; Friston *et al.* 1995 and see http://www.fil.ion.ucl.ac.uk/spm).

Automatically aligning new data to an atlas

New MR data are typically aligned with an atlas template by defining a measure of intensity similarity between the overlapping dataset and atlas. This measure of fit is optimized by tuning the parameters of the alignment transformation until the similarity is maximized (Woods *et al.* 1998; Ashburner 2001). Intensity-based registration measures include three-dimensional cross-correlation (Collins *et al.* 1994a,b, 1995), ratio image uniformity (Woods *et al.* 1992, 1993), or mutual information (Viola and Wells, 1995; Wells *et al.* 1997), or the summed squared differences in intensity between the scans (Christensen *et al.* 1993, 1996; Ashburner *et al.* 1998; Woods *et al.* 1998). Both linear (global) transforms, and nonlinear transforms may be used (nonlinear techniques are reviewed in detail in Toga 1998; Thompson *et al.* 2000*b*). Registration algorithms therefore make it feasible to automatically map new subjects' MRI data to an atlas coordinate space based directly on the Talairach reference system.

Analysis of brain data in a stereotaxic space makes it easier to:

1 compare data across groups, experiments, and data modalities, or over time;

2 define spatial masks to restrict the analysis to a particular anatomical region;

3 employ powerful statistical methods based on random-field theory;

4 gather spatial statistics (sometimes called 'priors') to guide the behavior of an image analysis algorithm (e.g. a tissue classifier); and

5 rapidly re-analyze data using different processing streams (Collins *et al.*, 2002).

In addition to the ICBM template described previously, some groups have aligned data to special templates that reflect the anatomy of Alzheimer's patients (Thompson *et al.* 2000), or children (Wilke *et al.* 2002). Holmes *et al.* (1998) averaged together 27 scans of a single subject, to create a high-resolution MRI atlas template. Kochunov *et al.* (2001) adjusted the shape of this template to the population mean. High-dimensional warping algorithms (Thompson *et al.*, 2000*a,d*) may also be employed to create customized anatomic templates, with the mean shape and intensity for the specific group being studied, with well-resolved cortical features in their mean locations. All these templates can be used in the image analyses described next.

Voxel-based morphometry

Voxel-based morphometry (VBM; Wright *et al.* 1995; Ashburner and Friston 2000) is perhaps the simplest and fastest approach to detecting group differences in brain structure. VBM has been used to study aging and gender effects in normal subjects (Sowell *et al.* 1999*a,b*; Maguire *et al.* 2000; Good *et al.* 2001*a,b*) as well as Alzheimer's disease (Mummery *et al.* 2000; Baron *et al.* 2001), frontotemporal and Lewy body dementia (O'Brien *et al.* 2001; Rosen *et al.* 2002; cf. Studholme *et al.* 2001), Parkinson's disease, and even herpes simplex encephalitis (Gitelman *et al.* 2001). One of its earliest applications was to map gray matter deficits in chronic schizophrenia (Wright *et al.* 1995), and subsequently these deficits were replicated in first-episode (Job *et al.* 2002) and childhood-onset patients (Thompson *et al.* 2001*d*). Typically, the following steps are used.

Tissue classification

MR images are first segmented using a tissue classifier, producing images showing the spatial distribution of gray matter, white matter, and CSF (Fig. 6.1). Tissue classifiers may be supervised (where a user selects some points representing each tissue class to guide classification) or unsupervised (no user intervention). Bayesian segmentation methods (Warfield *et al.* 1998; Ashburner and Friston 2000; Shattuck and Leahy 2001) assign each image voxel to a specific class based on its intensity value as well as prior information on the likely spatial distribution of each tissue in the image. The classification step may be preceded by digital filtering to reduce intensity inhomogeneities due to fluctuations and susceptibility artifacts in the scanner magnetic field. This step is often called RF (radiofrequency) correction or bias correction. Well-validated RF-correction methods include N3 (nonparametric nonuniform intensity normalization), which is based on histogram entropy maximization (Sled *et al.* 1998), and BFC (bias field corrector; Shattuck and Leahy 2001). Arnold *et al.* (2001) compares these and other approaches. In so-called 'expectation-maximization' techniques, RF-correction and tissue-classification steps are combined, using one to help estimate the other in an iterative sequence (Warfield *et al.* 1998).

Jacobian modulation

In VBM, segmented gray matter images are warped to the standard ICBM brain template, or to an average gray matter image representative of the group being studied. Linear (uniform scale and shears) or full nonlinear (warping) transforms may be applied. Since this warping transformation changes the shape of the brain being measured, the intensity in the gray matter image (usually ones, as the image is binary) is divided by the local volumetric expansion factor to preserve the total amount of tissue in the original images (Davatzikos 1998; Goldszal *et al.* 1998; Good *et al.* 2001*a,b*). This step is known as the 'Jacobian modulation' or 'volume preservation' step, and it sensitizes the analysis to true volumetric differences between groups, rather than just differences in the proportion of gray matter after spatial normalization. Regions compressed by the warping transform have their gray matter measure (known as gray matter 'density' or 'concentration') increased. The local expansion factor, or Jacobian, is computed from the deformation gradient, or Jacobian matrix, of the three-dimensional warping field. After spatial normalization, the same voxel location in each image corresponds roughly to the same brain structure (see later for caveats). Normalized gray matter images are then smoothed with a filter (typically a Gaussian or box filter with 8–15 mm full width at half maximum (FWHM); see Salmond *et al.* 2002, for different choices). By the 'matched filter theorem', larger filters optimize detection of diffuse or widespread effects, at the expense of blurring observations from different anatomic regions. This smoothing: (1) partly accounts for registration errors and reduces inter-individual variance, increasing detection sensitivity; and (2) makes the data better approximations to a Gaussian random field. There is some inherent data averaging when applying a filter, and the Central Limit Theorem states that the average of many observations drawn from non-normal distributions still tends to be normally distributed. This normality of the residuals is a requirement if parametric statistics are used in later processing.

Statistical parametric maps

Statistical analysis in VBM typically proceeds by fitting the general linear model (GLM) to the data (gray matter density) from all subjects at each voxel. This identifies voxels where tissue density relates to diagnosis, cognitive scores, etc., after discounting confounding effects (e.g. age, IQ, etc.). As in volumetric studies, a measure of total gray matter or whole-brain volume may also be used as a covariate of interest, and to detrend brain size effects from the data.[1]

Including the overall amount of gray matter as a covariate in the model enables the detection of regionally specific differences in gray matter density, over and above any global differences. Multiple regression and ANOVA, used widely in volumetric analysis, are special cases of the GLM, and are widely used. A statistical parametric map (SPM; Friston *et al.* 1995) is generated in which each voxel contains a statistic quantifying the group difference at that stereotaxic position. At each voxel, the actual statistic is compared with a reference (or *null*) distribution for the statistic (e.g. the values it takes when groups are sampled from the same population, and no effect is present). This gives a *P* value for how likely it is that such a difference could occur by accident, if only that voxel were assessed. Although VBM is designed to evaluate group differences, it is also possible to compare a single subject with a group, so long as the data are first smoothed with a filter of at least 12 mm FWHM. This smoothing is necessary to guard against non-normality of the residuals, which occurs when one of the groups examined consists of only a single subject (Salmond *et al.* 2002).

Caveats

Some caveats are required in interpreting the findings of VBM, because it can infer local anatomical differences: (1) from systematic registration errors in one group relative to the other; and (2) from systematic shifts in unaffected regions that result from differences in truly affected structures (Bookstein 2001). VBM findings can, however, be confirmed using shape-based or volumetric methods (see below for an effect characterized with both techniques).

Example in childhood-onset schizophrenia

Figure 6.3(a) shows an example from a VBM study of childhood-onset schizophrenia (COS; Sowell *et al.* 2000). In COS, as in adult-onset schizophrenia, the third and lateral

---

[1] Brain size confounds. Note that if the groups being compared have differences in average brain size, it may be surprisingly difficult to detrend brain size effects from local measures. Artifactual regional effects may then appear that are, in fact, attributable to variations in overall brain size [this is not just an issue with VBM but with all stereotaxic comparison methods; see Thompson *et al.* (2003) for a review of its impact on reports of sex differences in the corpus callosum]. Because brain substructures do not scale linearly with brain volume (Jäncke *et al.* 1997), the mean location of a given structure linearly mapped into stereotaxic space may differ in small and large brains. To avoid these effects masquerading as local differences, the dependency of warping fields on brain scale can be modeled using multiple regression (Stuart *et al.* 2001), and used to adjust the voxel level effects.

(a)

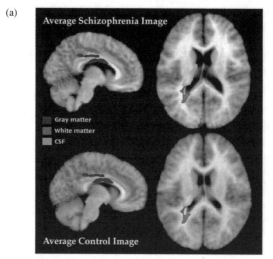

Comparison of gray matter distribution
between child and adolescent groups (*N*= 18)

(b)

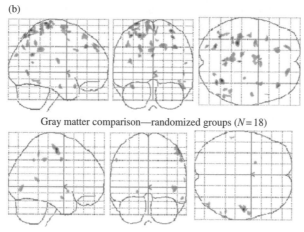

Fig. 6.3 Voxel-based morphometry (figure courtesy of Elizabeth Sowell, data from Sowell *et al.* 1999a). Changes in stereotaxic tissue distribution can be assessed by comparison of binary maps of each tissue class (gray matter, white matter, CSF), after alignment of individual data into stereotaxic space. In (a), voxels with significant differences were assessed between patients with childhood-onset schizophrenia (*N* = 9) and matched controls (*N* = 10; Sowell *et al.* 1999a). Voxels with significant differences in each tissue class were mapped on to orthogonal slices from the averaged patient image (top row), and the same slices of the average control image. In (b), regions of profound gray matter reduction are observed between childhood and adolescence (top panels; *P* < 0.05, permutation test; data from Sowell *et al.* 1999a). Differences in local gray matter content are assessed by fitting a linear statistical model at each voxel, to assess the significance of gray matter reductions with increasing age. The significance of the effect is then assessed by creating a voxel-by-voxel map

ventricles are enlarged. In Fig. 6.3, voxel-level differences between groups are detected in the vicinity of the occipital horns. These voxels contain white matter in controls and CSF in patients. In the average patient image, an arching of the corpus callosum, in the midsagittal plane, places CSF into voxels that are classified as gray matter in controls. These voxels appear in the map of gray matter differences. In this study, volumetric analyses of the lateral ventricles in native image data space confirmed significantly higher volume in posterior, but not anterior, regions (Sowell *et al.* 2000), suggesting that VBM may be a rapid way to identify these volumetric differences.

Several other groups have applied VBM in cohort studies of schizophrenia, finding stereotaxic differences in tissue distribution (Wright *et al.* 1995; Ananth *et al.* 2002; Suzuki *et al.* 2002). In a recent longitudinal study of childhood-onset schizophrenia, we used a variant of VBM (called cortical pattern matching; see below) to detect a wave of progressive cortical gray matter loss, spreading from parietal to frontal and temporal brain regions. This wave of loss spread and intensified over a 5-year period and correlated with global assessments of function (Children's Global Assessment Scale scores; Thompson *et al.* 2001*d*). Wilke *et al.* (2002) noted a similar link between gray matter loss and global assessment of function (GAF) scores in 48 adult-onset schizophrenia patients and 48 controls analyzed with VBM. The more severely ill patients had greater gray matter deficits in the left inferior frontal and inferior parietal lobes. A similar VBM study of first-episode patients (Job *et al.* 2002) identified significant gray matter deficits in the right anterior cingulate, right medial frontal lobe, left middle temporal gyrus, and left limbic and postcentral regions of the left hemisphere. In a recent, very large study (159 patients and 158 controls), Hulshoff Pol *et al.* (2002*b*) detected decreased gray matter density in the left hippocampus and amygdala, consistent with the reduced hippocampal volumes found consistently in volumetric studies of schizophrenia (Lawrie and Abukmeil 1998).

Multiple comparisons correction

In VBM or any statistical mapping approach, a vast number of voxels are assessed (typically millions). *P* values must therefore be corrected for multiple comparisons before the significance of the overall map is assessed, unless there was an *a priori* hypothesis of

---

of these statistics, and examining the null distribution of features that occur in these maps under the null hypothesis of no difference between groups (see Bullmore *et al.* 1999; Thompson *et al.* 2000*b*). To control for false positives, distributions for peak values in the maps, or extents of clusters above a given threshold, can be derived from the theory of stationary Gaussian fields. If the stationarity assumption is violated, some small regions may appear to be significantly different (null map; bottom panels), even if the groups are randomized and there are no true differences. To avoid this, the empirical distribution of different statistical features can be assessed directly from the data by randomly assigning subjects to groups and tabulating a reference distribution, relative to which experimental differences can be assessed.

an effect at a specific stereotaxic voxel. Bonferroni corrections, which adjust P values based on the total number of independent tests, are not used because data at neighboring voxels are highly correlated. Approaches to obtain corrected P values include the theory of stationary Gaussian random fields (Friston *et al.* 1995; Frackowiak *et al.* 1997), and nonparametric methods such as permutation (Bullmore *et al.* 1999; Thompson *et al.* 2000*b*; Nichols and Holmes 2002). Gaussian field theory models the distributions of features in statistical maps that would be found by accident, if the null hypothesis of no significant difference between groups were true. Experimental effects are compared with these null distributions, to check if they could have occurred by accident, or whether there is enough evidence to reject the null hypothesis of no differences between groups. Distributions of the following features were modeled: (1) the maximum value (or peak height, Z_{max}) of the statistic found in the map, and (2) the size of the largest connected cluster of voxels above a given threshold. Null distributions for more complex features can also be derived mathematically, such as the number of clusters exceeding a given height and spatial extent, or the total spatial extent of these clusters. These features are thought of as measurements of 'rising swells or waves in a choppy (noisy) sea' (Lange 1996), where the roughness of the sea is estimated from the data. To estimate the probability that the maximum value of the map (Z_{max}) is greater than a given threshold t under the null hypothesis (i.e. when no difference is present), Worsley *et al.* (1994*a,b*) used the expected Euler characteristic $E[\chi(A(t))]$ of a binarized map thresholded at t, so that for high t,

$$\Pr(Z_{max} > t) \cong E[\chi(A(t))] = \lambda(V)|\Lambda|^{1/2} (2\pi)^{-(D+1)/2} \cdot He_D(t) \exp(-t^2/2). \qquad (6.1)$$

Here $\lambda(V)$ and D are the volume and dimension of the search region, and $He_D(t)$ is the Dth-order Hermite polynomial. The roughness tensor, Λ (or its inverse, the smoothness tensor, Λ^{-1}), is crucial for estimating P values. It is defined as the covariance matrix of the partial derivatives of the residuals along each of the D coordinate axes, with variances $Var[\partial X/\partial x_i]$ on the diagonal and off-diagonal elements $Cov[\partial X/\partial x_i, \partial X/\partial x_j]$. Once these parameters are estimated, a significance level can be assigned to the overall map, so long as the theoretical assumptions are not violated.

Statistical flattening

An underlying assumption of the above parametric approach is that the process is a stationary Gaussian field, i.e. its statistical characteristics, including its roughness parameter $|\Lambda|$ (or its inverse, the smoothness $|\Lambda|^{-1}$), are constant across all voxels in the image. This assumption is reasonable for functional imaging data, but is violated for structural imaging data. Binary structure masks, for example, are constant across large regions, and even after smoothing the signal changes more rapidly at the edges of structures (Worsley *et al.* 1999). The distribution of cluster sizes that occur by accident is therefore skewed towards larger cluster sizes in smooth image regions, resulting in more false positives (and false negatives in rough regions) than predicted by formulae for stationary fields. To address this, Worsley *et al.* (1999) suggested a statistical flattening approach in which the data are warped into a new space, which may have higher dimension than the data, so that in the new space the smoothness of the normalized residuals of the statistical model is stationary. The P value for cluster sizes above a threshold can then be applied using size measurements in the new space, or by estimating the effective resolution of the field directly from the normalized residuals (Worsley *et al.* 1999). Thompson *et al.* (2000*b*) proposed an alternative statistical flattening approach, where a partial differential equation:

$$g^{ij} (\partial^2 \mathbf{u}/\partial r^i \partial r^j) + \partial/\partial \mathbf{u}^j (S^{ij})\mathbf{u}_r i = 0 \qquad (6.2)$$

is run in the image, to generate a deformed grid $\mathbf{u}(\mathbf{r})$ whose deformation gradient tensor approximates the smoothness S^{ij} of the normalized residuals (here g^{ij} is the contravariant metric tensor of the grid). Relative to this new computational grid, the residuals are stationary and isotropic, and P values for the gray matter reductions can be evaluated with standard formulae.

Nonparametric methods: permutation

A final approach to estimate P values for significant features in statistical maps is to estimate their distribution under the null hypothesis by permutation (Bullmore *et al.*, 1999; Sowell *et al.*, 1999*a,b*; Thompson *et al.* 2000*b*, 2001*a,b*, 2002). This nonparametric approach avoids assumptions about the spatial autocorrelation of the process, and has been successful in functional imaging as well (Nichols and Holmes, 2002). Subjects are randomly assigned to groups and the distribution of accidental clusters is tabulated empirically. The overall 'corrected' P value for the effect in the true grouping is given by the proportion of random maps that have an effect at least as strong as the real map (usually this is very small). In a recent study of gray matter changes in adolescence (Sowell *et al.* 1999*a*), we found specific reductions in gray matter in dorsal frontal and parietal cortices (Fig. 6.3b; $P < 0.05$, permutation test). Random permutations revealed that false-positive clusters occurred (on average 5.8 per simulation), but the number of suprathreshold clusters (57) was significantly higher in the real experiment than predicted by the null distribution (Fig. 6.3b). In these experiments, a region of interest may also be specified in advance to constrain the search for significant results, leading to increases in statistical power (Thompson *et al.* 2002).

Anatomical surface modeling

Anatomical surface modeling (Thompson *et al.* 1996*a,b*, 2002; Gerig *et al.* 2001) provides an alternative approach to map group differences in brain structure. Three-dimensional surface models are built to represent anatomical structures in each scan. By imposing a regular mesh structure on structures in different subjects, average models can be created to represent a particular group. Asymmetries, profiles of group variability, and individual or group differences are visualized locally. Rather than contrasting image intensities at each image voxel across subjects (as in VBM), differences in the shapes of structures are measured and mapped. Shape measures can be sensitive to disease-specific changes, even when volumetric measures are not (Narr *et al.* 2000). Narr *et al.* (2000) observed that callosal area did not discriminate schizophrenic groups from healthy controls, while shape measures provided a distinct group separation. Wang *et al.* (2001) found that hippocampal shape descriptors had greater power to distinguish patients from controls than volumetry, while others have argued that each approach provides complementary information (Gerig *et al.* 2001; Golland *et al.* 2001; Thompson *et al.* 2001*b*).

Surface averaging techniques have mapped local profiles of ventricular expansion and cortical asymmetries in dementia, autism, and schizophrenia (Fig. 6.3; Blanton *et al.* 2000; Thompson *et al.* 2000*c*; Narr *et al.* 2002), as well as subtle or pre-clinical hippocampal changes (Csernansky *et al.* 1998; Narr *et al.* 2001*a*). Thinning effects have also been localized at the callosal isthmus in Alzheimer's disease (Thompson *et al.* 1998), as have growth profiles in childhood (Thompson *et al.* 2000*a*). Parametric mesh models have also visualized patterns of callosal arching in chronic and first-episode schizophrenia patients, as well as high-risk relatives (Narr *et al.* 2000, 2002). They have also found gender × disease interactions in schizophrenia (Narr *et al.* 2000) and callosal alterations in fetal alcohol syndrome (Sowell *et al.* 2001; see also Bookstein *et al.* 2001).

Generating surfaces

Some surface models are easy to extract automatically. Examples include the cortex (MacDonald *et al.* 2000; Fischl and Dale 2000; Shattuck and Leahy 2001; Ratnanather *et al.* 2001), cerebellar surface, corpus callosum (Pitiot *et al.* 2002), and hippocampus (Haller *et al.* 1997; Joshi *et al.* 1997). Structures that are more difficult to extract automatically can be traced manually in serial sections, or in three dimensions, using a formal anatomical protocol with quantified reliability (e.g. Sowell *et al.* 2001; Hayashi *et al.* 2002). Manual traces are subsequently converted to uniform mesh format using a regridding algorithm, which makes the sampled points spatially uniform (Thompson *et al.* 1996*a,b*). In many morphometric studies, manual and automated methods are combined, for greatest accuracy. For example, the cortex may be extracted automatically, but gyral landmarks may be traced on it manually by trained raters.

Anatomical averaging

An average anatomical surface is generated for a group of subjects by averaging the vector locations of corresponding surface points across the subject group. This process is repeated for each point on the surface. If $r_i(u,v)$ is the three-dimensional position in stereotaxic space of the point with parametric coordinates (u,v) on the ith subject's mesh, a group average surface model is given by another mesh of the form:

$$r_\mu(u,v) = \left(\frac{1}{N}\right)\sum_{i=1}^{n} r_i(u,v), \quad \text{for all } (u,v). \tag{6.3}$$

Information on anatomic variability may be shown as a variability map (Thompson *et al.* 1996, 1998). To map variability, individual deviations from the average surface are measured by computing three-dimensional displacement maps (Fig. 6.4). These are patterns of three-dimensional displacement vectors that would be required to reshape the average surface into that of a specific individual. If surface locations $\mathbf{r}_i(u,v)$ in subject i, are indexed by parametric coordinates (u,v), then deviations of these locations in individual i from the mean anatomical surface are given by the set of displacement vectors:

$$\mathbf{d}_i(u,v) = \mathbf{r}_i(u,v) - \mathbf{r}_\mu(u,v), \tag{6.4}$$

for all pairs of corresponding grid points $\mathbf{r}_i(u,v)$ and $\mathbf{r}_\mu(u,v)$. For each (u,v), the associated displacement maps $\mathbf{d}_i(u,v)$ represent a sample of (vector) observations from a zero-mean, spatially anisotropic probability distribution (Thompson *et al.* 1996).

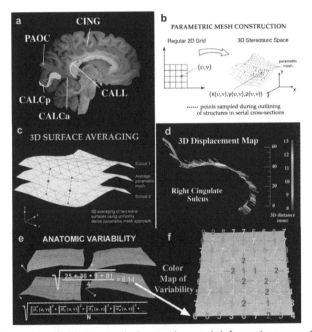

Fig. 6.4 Surface mesh models, anatomical averaging, and deformation maps. Parametric surface modeling is a morphometric approach that makes it easier to compare anatomical models from multiple subjects, as well as make average models for disease and control groups. An algorithm converts a set of digitized points on an anatomical structure boundary [e.g. deep sulci (a)] into a parametric grid of uniformly spaced points in a regular rectangular mesh stretched over the surface [(b); Thompson *et al.* 1996a,b]. By averaging nodes with the same grid coordinates across subjects (c), an average surface is produced for the group. Information on each subject's individual differences is retained as a vector-valued displacement map (d, e). This map indicates how that the subject deviates locally from the average anatomy. The root mean square magnitude (e) of these deviations provides a variability measure, the values of which can be visualized using a color code (f). These maps can illustrate variability in different anatomic systems (f) and detect typical (i.e. average) patterns of brain structure in different anatomic systems.

The variability of the surface points can be encoded using the covariance matrix, or tensor, of the deformation maps:

$$\Psi(u,v) = \left[\frac{1}{(N-1)}\right]\sum_{i=1}^{N} \mathbf{d}_i(u,v)\,\mathbf{d}_i(u,v)^{\mathrm{T}}. \tag{6.5}$$

This matrix stores the shape, or preferred directions, of anatomic variability in the brain (Thompson *et al.* 1996a,b; Cao and Worsley 1999). The simplest measure of anatomic variability is the root mean square magnitude of the three-dimensional displacement vectors, assigned to each point, in the surface maps from individual to average. This variability pattern can be visualized as a color-coded map. This map picks out highly variable regions, such as the occipital horns of the ventricles (Fig. 6.5), and the gyral patterns of the perisylvian cortices.

Application to Alzheimer's disease

An illustrative application of surface modeling is the analysis of ventricular anatomy in Alzheimer's disease. Two features emerge in the average anatomical maps (Fig. 6.5) that may be difficult to localize with conventional volumetry. First, the ventricles are larger in Alzheimer's disease than in healthy controls; secondly, a marked ventricular asymmetry (left larger than right) appears in the occipital horns. Considerable anatomic variation (*red colors in Plate 3*), in occipital horn regions, obscures these average patterns in individual datasets. Once identified, these features can be assessed statistically in new datasets, or an individual anatomy can be compared with the average maps in the atlas.

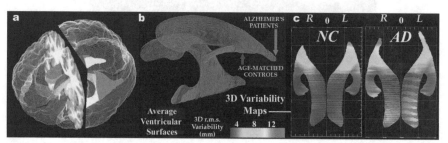

Fig. 6.5 Anatomical averaging, applied in a study of aging and Alzheimer's disease. In a group of elderly Alzheimer's disease patients and matched healthy controls, three-dimensional parametric surface meshes (Thompson *et al.* 1996a,b) were used to model 14 ventricular elements (a). Surface meshes were averaged by hemisphere in each group. (b) An average model for Alzheimer's patients (AD) is superimposed on an average model for matched normal controls (NC). Occipital horns are enlarged in the AD patients, and there is high stereotaxic variability (c) in both groups. Extreme variability at the occipital horn tips also contrasts sharply with the stability of septal and temporal ventricular regions. A top view of these averaged surface meshes reveals localized asymmetry, variability, and displacement within and between groups. These subcortical asymmetries emerge only after averaging anatomical maps in groups of subjects. (See Shape Modeling in Plate 3 of the plate section at the centre of this book.)

Corpus callosum shape in schizophrenia

The averaging of parametric mesh models can also be used to help us to understand how shape modeling relates to voxel-based morphometry. Narr *et al.* (2000) created average models of the *corpus callosum* in 25 chronic schizophrenia patients and 28 matched normal controls (in this case anatomical curves were averaged rather than surfaces, but the principle is the same). An increased curvature, or arching, of the corpus callosum was observed in patients, with stronger effects in males than in females (see Fig. 6.6). These findings complement the periventricular changes mapped in the childhood-onset cohort using VBM (Fig. 6.3; Sowell *et al.* 2000*a*,*b*). Both techniques suggest that the bowing effect may be secondary to third ventricle enlargement. While VBM surveys the whole

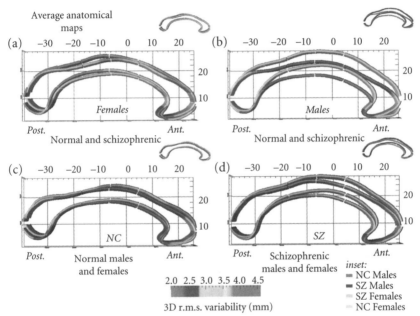

Fig. 6.6 Averaging corpus callosum models in schizophrenia [data from Narr *et al.* (2000), courtesy of Katherine Narr]. Midsagittal corpus callosum boundaries were averaged from 25 patients with chronic schizophrenia (DSM-III-R criteria; 15 males, 10 females; age: 31.1 ± 5.6 years) and from 28 control subjects matched for age (30.5 ± 8.7 years), gender (15 males, 13 females) and handedness (one left-handed subject per group). Profiles of anatomic variability around the group averages are shown as a root mean square (r.m.s.) deviation from the mean. Anatomical averaging reveals a significant bowing effect in the schizophrenic patients relative to controls. Male patients show a significant increase in curvature for superior and inferior callosal boundaries ($P < 0.001$), with a highly significant sex by diagnosis interaction ($P < 0.004$). Separate group averages show that the disease induces less bowing in females (a) than in males (b). Gender differences are not apparent in controls (c), but a clear gender difference is seen in the schizophrenic patients (d). Abnormalities localized in a disease- specific atlas can therefore be analyzed to reveal interactions between disease and demographic parameters.

brain at once, and does not require a priori assumptions about the location or extent of the regions of interest, shape averaging produces a crisp average anatomical boundary that reveals a clearly localized shape difference in patients. In the next section we see how analysis of shape (through deformations) may be combined with a simultaneous analysis of voxel-level differences in gray matter, so that the two effects can be studied in tandem.

Cortical mapping

Individual variations in gyral patterns are so extreme that it is difficult to identify group patterns of cortical organization or pinpoint disease effects. The cortex also changes over time, as in aging, Alzheimer's disease (Mega *et al.* 2000), or development (Sowell *et al.* 1999*a,b*; Blanton *et al.* 2000; Thompson *et al.* 2000*a*, 2001*d*). Cortical pattern matching methods, which encode both gyral pattern and gray matter variation, can substantially improve the statistical power and ability to localize these changes. In schizophrenia, cortical mapping reveals a progressive spread of cortical gray matter deficits in childhood-onset cases (Thompson *et al.* 2001*d*), and deficits can be related to genetics (Cannon *et al.* 2002), symptoms (Vidal *et al.* 2001), and underlying functional activations (Rasser *et al.* 2003). These cortical analyses tease apart the effects of gyral shape variation from gray matter change, as well as cortical asymmetries. As such, these techniques are hybrids between voxel-based methods (such as VBM) that assess tissue distribution, and deformation-based methods that map shape differences using high-dimensional warping transforms. To illustrate these techniques, we describe how to compare and average sulcal patterns and gray matter maps across subjects, groups, and over time, and map their variations and asymmetries.

Cortical parameterization

Many automated algorithms have been developed to extract cortical surface models from three-dimensional MRI data (MacDonald 1998; Shattuck and Leahy 1999; Fischl *et al.* 2000). Some of these impose a tiled, parametric grid structure on the anatomy, which supplies a coordinate framework for subsequent computations. In several approaches (Fischl *et al.* 1999; Haker *et al.* 1999; Shattuck and Leahy 2001), a white matter segmentation is generated first. Its topology is then corrected using graph theoretic methods that remove holes, or artifactual bridges between white matter regions that are not truly connected (Han *et al.* 2001; Shattuck and Leahy 2001). The surface is tiled using triangulation methods such the Marching Cubes algorithm (Lorensen and Cline 1987; analogous methods can be used to recover the gray matter-CSF interface). The gridded surface is then inflated, using iterative smoothing, to a spherical shape. By inverting this inflation mapping, a spherical coordinate system can be projected back on to the three-dimensional model, or the three-dimensional surface may be flattened to a two-dimensional plane prior to computing group differences (Fig. 6.7; Thompson *et al.* 1997, 2001; Angenent *et al.* 1999; Drury *et al.* 2000).

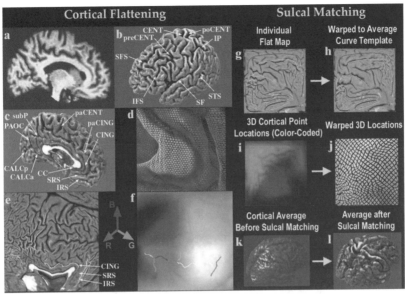

Fig. 6.7 Cortical mapping techniques used to measure differences across subjects and across time. Using cortical flattening (a–f), and sulcal matching (g–l), an average model of the cortex (l) can be built for a group of subjects. Sulcal landmarks are defined on individual cortices, and this enables data to be averaged from corresponding regions of cortex across subjects, reinforcing systematic features. See text for details of this procedure. [Sulci shown in (b), (c) include the superior and inferior frontal (SFS, IFS), pre- and postcentral (preCENT, poCENT), central (CENT), intraparietal (IP), superior temporal (STS), Sylvian fissures (SF), paracentral (paCENT), cingulate (CING) and paracingulate (paCING), subparietal (subP), callosal (CC), superior and inferior rostral (SRS, IRS), parieto-occipital (PAOC), anterior and posterior calcarine (CALCa/p) sulci.]. See Plate 5 of the plate section at the centre of this book.

Matching cortical patterns

Cortical anatomy can be compared, between any pair of subjects, by computing the warped mapping that elastically transforms one cortex into the shape of the other. Due to variations in gyral patterning, cortical differences among subjects will be severely underestimated unless elements of the gyral pattern are matched from one subject to another. This matching is also required for cortical averaging; otherwise, corresponding gyral features will not be averaged together.

To find good matches among cortical regions, we perform the matching process in the cortical surface's parametric space, which permits more tractable mathematics (Fig. 6.7). This vector flow field in the parametric space indirectly specifies a correspondence field in three dimensions, which drives one cortical surface into the shape of another. This mapping can also be constructed so it exactly matches a network of consistently occurring landmark curves (Thompson *et al.* 2000*d*) with their

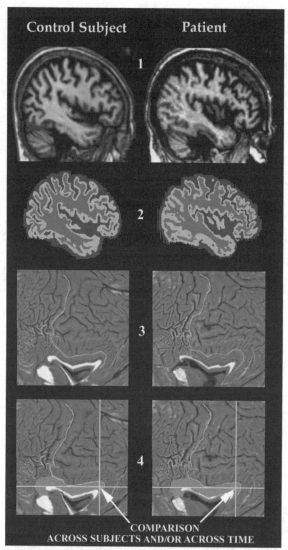

Fig. 6.8 Image-processing steps applied in a cortical pattern-matching study. This flow chart illustrates the key steps used to process the MRI brain scans in a study of cortical gray matter differences between patients and controls. This study uses cortical pattern matching (Thompson *et al.* 2001*b*) to control, as far as possible, for individual sulcal pattern differences. Example brain MRI datasets are shown from a healthy control subject (left column) and from a patient (in this case, a patient with Alzheimer's disease; right column). First, the MRI images (stage 1) have extracerebral tissues deleted from the scans and the individual pixels are classi-fied as gray matter, white matter or CSF (stage 2). After flattening a three-dimensional geometric model of the cortex (stage 3), features such as the central sulcus, and cingulate sulcus may be reidentified. An elastic warp is applied (stage 4), moving these features and entire gyral regions into the same reference position in flat space. After aligning sulcal

counterparts in the target brain, producing a transform that stores detailed information on morphometric differences.

Sulcal alignment

Figure 6.7e shows three-dimensional sulcal landmarks in an individual subject that have been flattened into a two-dimensional square. With the shape-averaging techniques introduced earlier (to average models of the corpus callosum), an average set of flattened sulci can be created for the group of subjects under study (Fig. 6.7). An elastic warp is then applied to each individual's flat map that drives individual landmarks on to this average set of curves (see Thompson *et al.* 2002 for the mathematics). This warping adjusts for cortical patterning differences. Cortical data, such as gray matter density mapped in each individual (Fig. 6.8), or even functional imaging data (Rex *et al.* 2000; Zeineh *et al.* 2001; Rasser *et al.* 2003), can then be carefully aligned across subjects before averaging and comparison. Figure 6.8 shows how this technique aligns maps of gray matter density from homologous cortical regions across subjects. The resulting maps of gray matter density can be analyzed for group differences using VBM-style techniques (examples in dementia and schizophrenia are described below). Cortical pattern matching can also increase detection sensitivity for group effects (Davatzikos *et al.* 2001; Thompson *et al.* 2001*b*), while retaining quantitative measures of gyral pattern differences.

Cortical averaging

In the processing sequence shown in Fig. 6.7, a well-resolved average three-dimensional cortical model can also be created for a group of subjects. A color code, storing three-dimensional cortical locations in each individual, is plotted in flat space, and this color image is convected along with the warp that aligns that individual flattened data to the average. The resulting warped color images can be averaged across subjects and decoded to produce a crisp cortical model, with well-defined sulcal features in their mean geometric locations (Thompson *et al.* 2000*d*).

Deformation-based morphometry

Deformations that align individual anatomies with an average template or an atlas standard can be analyzed to detect group differences in anatomy (a technique called 'deformation-based morphometry'; Thompson *et al.* 1997; Gaser *et al.* 1999;

---

patterns from all individual subjects, group comparisons can be made at each two-dimensional pixel (cross-hairs) that effectively compare gray matter measures across corresponding cortical regions. In this study, the cortical measure that is compared, across groups, and over time, is the amount of gray matter (stage 2) lying within 15 mm of each cortical point. The results of these statistical tests can then be plotted back on to an average three-dimensional cortical model made for the group (Fig. 6.7), and the findings can be visualized as a color-coded map.

Ashburner 2001; Good *et al.* 2001*a*,*b*). Deformation fields are a rich source of morphometric data and their statistics can be stored in an atlas, providing criteria for abnormal anatomy (see Fig. 6.9). Depending on the approach, warping fields may be computed by matching cortical surfaces (as is the case in Fig. 6.9), or by algorithms that warp the entire three-dimensional image on to a neuroanatomic template (e.g. Ashburner *et al.* 1998; see also Toga 1998 for a review). Depending on whether these fields are stored as three-dimensional deformation vectors (Thompson *et al.* 1997; Cao and Worsley 1999), or as a set of basis function coefficients that parameterize the nonlinear warp (Csernansky *et al.* 1998; Ashburner 2001), the analysis of structural differences proceeds a little differently. Deformation fields represented as basis function coefficients can be analyzed using a spectral methods (Joshi *et al.* 1997; Csernansky *et al.* 1999; Miller *et al.* 2002), Riemannian shape manifolds (Bookstein 1997), or with multivariate methods such as canonical variates analysis (Ashburner *et al.* 1998). Most approaches perform statistical analysis on the coefficients of functions that warping algorithms use to represent the deformation fields, such as discrete cosines (Ashburner *et al.* 1998), polynomials (Woods *et al.* 1998), spherical harmonics (Thompson *et al.* 1996*a*,*b*; Gerig *et al.* 2001), or eigenfunctions of self-adjoint differential operators (Miller *et al.* 2002). We describe two such approaches next (others are reviewed in Thompson *et al.* 2000*b*).

Multivariate analysis of deformation fields

Ashburner *et al.* (1998) developed a multivariate statistical approach, based on deformations that match individual anatomies to an atlas, to compare the gross morphometry of male and female brains. They also studied the effects of handedness on brain asymmetry and brain structure. The set of deformation mappings was compacted using principal components analysis, producing a set of vectors with new coefficients (20 parameters accounting for 96% of the variance of the estimated mappings). By performing MANCOVA (multivariate analysis of covariance) on these new vectors, effects of confounding factors that might affect brain structure (e.g. age), and even interactions between variables, were quantified or discounted. If the data vectors, covariates of interest, and confounds are represented by matrices $\mathbf{A}$ ($m \times n$), $\mathbf{C}$ ($m \times c$) and $\mathbf{G}$ ($m \times g$), then variance due to the confounds $\mathbf{G}$ is eliminated with $\mathbf{A_a} = \mathbf{A} - \mathbf{G}(\mathbf{G^T G})^{-1}\mathbf{G^T A}$, and the design matrix is orthogonalized with respect to $\mathbf{G}$ with $\mathbf{C_a} = \mathbf{C} - \mathbf{G}(\mathbf{G^T G})^{-1}\mathbf{G^T C}$. The decrease in predictability of the deformations, once the effects of interest are discounted, is measured using the Wilk's Lambda statistic (Krzanowski, 1988):

$$\Lambda = \frac{\det(\mathbf{W})}{\det(\mathbf{B+W})} \tag{6.6}$$

where $\mathbf{B} = \mathbf{T^T T}$, $\mathbf{W} = (\mathbf{A_a} - \mathbf{T})^T(\mathbf{A_a} - \mathbf{T})$, $\mathbf{T} = \mathbf{C_a}((\mathbf{C_a^T C_a})^{-1}\mathbf{C_a^T A_a})$.

Here Λ has an approximate null distribution of $\exp[\chi^2_{nc}/((n - c - 1)/2 - (m - c - g))]$, where χ^2_{nc} is a χ^2 statistic with nc degrees of freedom. The results of such analyses are a significance value (P value) for the effect (e.g. of disease or handedness, on anatomy), and one or more canonical vectors (or deformations that are eigenvectors of the fitted effects, **B**) which caricature the effect (Ashburner *et al.* 1998).

Random vector fields

A second approach for analyzing deformation fields compiles statistics on the deformation vectors required to align each individual anatomy with an atlas standard. In a random vector field approach (Thompson *et al.* 1997; Cao and Worsley 1999), affine components of the deformation fields are first factored out. After this, the deformation vector required to match the structure at position **x** in the average cortex with its counterpart in subject i can be modeled as:

$$\mathbf{W}_i(\mathbf{x}) = \mu(\mathbf{x}) + \Sigma(\mathbf{x})^{1/2}\varepsilon_i(\mathbf{x}). \tag{6.7}$$

Here $\mu(\mathbf{x})$ is the mean deformation vector for the population (which approaches the zero vector for large N), $\Sigma(\mathbf{x})$ is a nonstationary, anisotropic covariance tensor field estimated from the mappings, $\Sigma(\mathbf{x})^{1/2}$ is the upper triangular Cholesky factor tensor field, and $\varepsilon_i(\mathbf{x})$ is a trivariate random vector field, the components of which are independent zero-mean, unit variance, stationary random fields. This three-dimensional probability distribution makes it possible to visualize the principal directions (eigenvectors) as well as the magnitude of gyral pattern variability, as a 'tensor map' (see Fig. 6.9). The significance of a difference in brain structure between two subject groups (e.g. patients and controls) of N_1 and N_2 subjects is assessed by calculating the sample mean and variance of the deformation fields ($j=1,2$):

$$\mathbf{W}_j^\mu(\mathbf{x}) = \sum_{i=1}^{N_j} \frac{\mathbf{W}_{ij}(\mathbf{x})}{N_j}$$

$$\Psi(\mathbf{x}) = \left(\frac{1}{N_1 + N_2 - 2}\right) \left\{ \sum_{j=1}^{2} \sum_{i=1}^{N_j} [\mathbf{W}_{ij}(\mathbf{x}) - \mathbf{W}_j^\mu(\mathbf{x})][\mathbf{W}_{ij}(\mathbf{x}) - \mathbf{W}_j^\mu(\mathbf{x})]^{\mathrm{T}} \right\} \tag{6.8}$$

and computing the following statistical map (Thompson *et al.* 1997; Cao and Worsley 2001):

$$T^2(\mathbf{x}) = \left\{ \frac{N_1 N_2}{(N_1 + N_2)(N_1 + N_2 - 2)} \right\} [\mathbf{W}_2^\mu(\mathbf{x}) - \mathbf{W}_1^\mu(\mathbf{x})]^{\mathrm{T}} [\Psi(\mathbf{x})]^{-1} [\mathbf{W}_2^\mu(\mathbf{x}) - \mathbf{W}_1^\mu(\mathbf{x})]. \tag{6.9}$$

Under the null hypothesis, $(N_1 + N_2 - 2)T^2(\mathbf{x})$ is a stationary Hotelling's T^2-distributed random field. At each point, if we let $\nu = (N_1 + N_2 - 2)$ and we let the dimension of the search space be $d = 3$, then:

$$F(\mathbf{x}) = \left(\frac{\nu - d + 1}{d}\right) T^2(\mathbf{x}) \sim F_{d,(\nu-d+1)}. \tag{6.10}$$

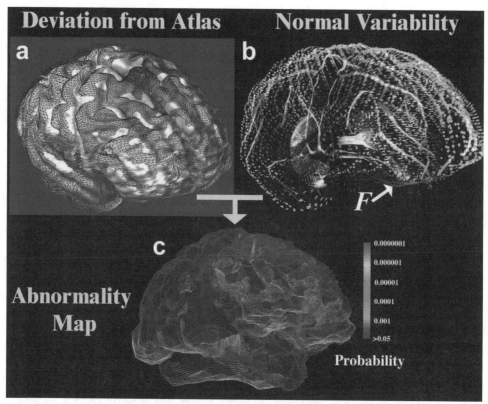

Fig. 6.9 Mapping abnormal cortical shape with deformation-based morphometry. Due to individual anatomical differences, an individual subject's brain will deviate from an anatomic atlas or from an average cortical model prepared for a group (a; white mesh). However, elastic warping algorithms can apply local dilations and contractions to the average brain model, deforming its shape to match the individual anatomy so that key surfaces and landmarks correspond. These deformations also store detailed information on how specific individuals [e.g. brown mesh (a)] deviate from the atlas. Mean anatomical shapes and confidence limits on normal variation (b) can be computed. If individual deviations (a) are calibrated against the probability distributions that capture normal variation, abnormality maps (c) may be generated. These indicate the probability of finding the anatomy in its observed configuration in a normal population. Here, in a patient with mild Alzheimer's disease, atrophic changes are easiest to detect in orbitofrontal regions where normal variation is least (labeled F in (b); red colors in (c); data from Thompson *et al.* 1997, 1998). See Plate 6(a) of the plate section at the centre of this book.

In other words, the field can be transformed point-wise to a Fisher–Snedecor *F* distribution (Thompson *et al.* 1997), and these statistics of abnormality can be plotted in color across the cortex. Figure 6.9 shows the approach applied to detect atrophy in Alzheimer's disease (Thompson *et al.* 1997). Note the broad region of abnormality detected in orbitofrontal cortex (Fig. 6.9). Validation studies on normal elderly subjects revealed that these atrophic changes were specific to patients, and were not detected in controls.

Mapping brain asymmetry

Brain asymmetry may also be studied by analysis of variance in three-dimensional deformation fields. Structural brain asymmetry is linked with functional lateralization (Toga and Thompson 2003a), handedness (Witelson 1989), and language function (Davidson and Hugdahl 1994), and may be diminished in some brain disorders, including schizophrenia (cf. Kikinis *et al.* 1994; Narr *et al.* 2001b; Crow 2002). To visualize the average magnitude of brain asymmetries in a group of subjects, three-dimensional deformation fields can be recovered for each subject, matching each brain hemisphere with a reflected version of the opposite hemisphere (cf. Thompson *et al.* 1998; Wang *et al.* 2001). The pattern of mean brain asymmetry for a group of 20 subjects is shown in Fig. 6.10. The resulting asymmetry fields $\mathbf{a}_i(\mathbf{r})$ (at parameter space location $\mathbf{r}$ in subject i) can be treated as observations from a spatially parameterized random vector field, with mean $\mu_\mathbf{a}(\mathbf{r})$ and a nonstationary covariance tensor $\Sigma_\mathbf{a}(\mathbf{r})$. The significance α of deviations from symmetry can be assessed using a T^2 or F statistic, and ultimately a P value, that indicates evidence of significant asymmetry in cortical patterns between hemispheres (Fig. 6.10).

Using this mapping technique, we showed that brain asymmetry increases during childhood and adolescence (Sowell *et al.* 2001). There are also significant asymmetries in distribution of gray matter in the brain (Watkins *et al.* 2001; Thompson *et al.* 2002), and in the degree to which genes affect brain structure (Thompson *et al.* 2001a). Encoded knowledge on the statistics of brain asymmetry can also help detect departures from normal asymmetry and even the emergence of lesions (sometimes termed 'dissymmetry': see Thirion *et al.* 2000; Joshi *et al.* 2001).

Applications of deformation-based morphometry

Gaser *et al.* (1999, 2001) have used deformation-based morphometry to study differences in brain shape and ventricular expansion in schizophrenia. In a validation study, Gaser *et al.* (2001) used the image deformation algorithm of Ashburner *et al.* (1998) to warp MRI datasets on to a standard brain template. They compared ventricle to brain ratios derived from manual tracings with those derived by integrating the Jacobian determinant (i.e. the 'expansion factor') of the deformation fields, computed automatically, over the ventricular region. The high intraclass correlation between manual and automated measures of ventricular volume ($r = 0.96$) supported the validity of using DBM to examine local and global brain morphology.

Applications in dementia and schizophrenia

Dynamically spreading tissue loss in dementia

Figure 6.11 shows the cortical pattern-matching method applied to a longitudinal study of brain change. A dynamically spreading wave of gray matter loss is visualized in the brains of patients with Alzheimer's disease (AD) as it spreads over time from

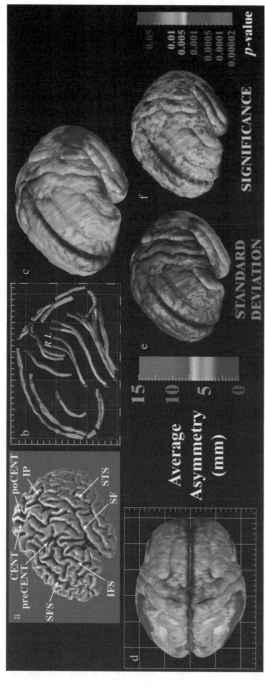

Fig. 6.10 Multi-subject maps of brain asymmetry. Image analysis techniques make it possible to distinguish systematic asymmetries in a population, or a specific group of subjects, from random fluctuations in anatomy (Thompson et al. 2001a). After aligning and scaling individual MRI scans into a standard three-dimensional space, three-dimensional curves representing the primary sulcal pattern are digitized (a). [Sulci include central (CENT), precentral (preCENT), postcentral (poCENT), intraparietal (IP), superior frontal (SFS), inferior frontal (IFS), superior temporal (STS) and Sylvian fissures (SF).] Averaging these curves across 20 normal subjects (b), the magnitude of asymmetry in the average anatomy is shown in color (red colors denote greater asymmetry; note this is a slightly different concept from the averaged 'individual asymmetry', which would also incorporate a measure of random variability; see next panels). Extension of these methods to surfaces (c, d) reveals prominent asymmetries in Broca's anterior speech area and in language regions surrounding the Sylvan fissure. By comparing the average magnitude of the individual asymmetries to their standard error, regions of significant asymmetry are identified (f). See Plate 6(b) of the plate section at the centre of this book.

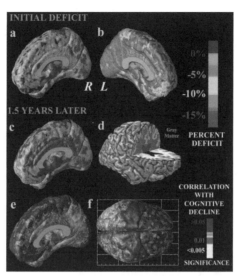

Fig. 6.11 Mapping disease progression and linking structural change with cognitive decline in dementia. Gray matter deficits occurring during the development of Alzheimer's disease are detected by comparing average profiles of gray matter between patients and controls at a baseline scan [mean mini-mental state exam (MMSE) score = 18; panels (a) and (b)] and at their follow-up scan 1.5 years later [mean MMSE =13; (c)]. The average percent loss in patients is shown, for a gray matter density measure derived automatically from each scan (d). Profound loss engulfs the left medial wall [>15%; (b)]. On the right, however, the deficits in temporo-parietal and entorhinal territory (a) spread forwards into the cingulate 1.5 years later (c), after a 5-point drop in average MMSE. Note the division between limbic and frontal zones, with different degrees of impairment (c). The corpus callosum is indicated in white; maps of gray matter change are not defined here, as it is a white matter commissure. Maps (d) and (e) show the significance of the linkage between gray matter reductions and cognition, as measured by MMSE score. Variations in temporal, parietal, and ultimately frontal (f) tissue are linked with cognitive status. Less gray matter is strongly correlated with worse cognitive performance, in all regions with prominent deficits. Linkages are most strongly detected in the left hemisphere medial temporo-parietal zones. As expected, no linkages are found with sensorimotor gray matter variation [*blue strip* in (f)], which is not significantly in deficit in late AD. See Plate 7 of the plate section at the centre of this book.

temporal and limbic cortices into frontal and occipital brain regions, sparing sensorimotor cortices. The maps are based on 52 high-resolution MRI scans of 12 AD patients (age: 68.4 ± 1.9 years) and 14 elderly matched controls (age: 71.4 ± 0.9 years), scanned longitudinally (two scans; interscan interval: 2.1 ± 0.4 years). Three key features are apparent: overall, gray matter loss rates were faster in AD (5.3 ± 2.3%/year) than in healthy controls (0.9 ± 0.9%/year in controls). Secondly, these shifting deficits are asymmetrical (left hemisphere > right), and correlate with progressively declining cognitive status [see map of voxelwise correlations with mini-mental state exam (MMSE) scores]. Finally, cortical tissue is lost in a well-defined sequence as the disease progresses, approximately mirroring the sequence of metabolic decline in PET studies and neurofibrillary tangle accumulation seen cross-sectionally at autopsy. These processes can be observed in video format on the Internet (Thompson *et al.* 2003; see URL). The goal of these dynamic maps is to uncover the path of degeneration for different brain systems, and define possible MRI-based markers for drug trials.

Childhood-onset schizophrenia

Figure 6.12 shows a similar application of cortical pattern matching to detect a spreading wave of gray matter loss in childhood-onset schizophrenia (Thompson *et al.* 2001*d*, 2002). Twelve very early onset schizophrenic patients were scanned three times over a period of 5 years, as were 12 healthy controls matched for age, gender, and demographics. At each scan, a measure of the local quantity of gray matter density was made at each point on the cerebral cortex. The average pattern of changes was mapped in both patients and controls, using cortical pattern matching to help compare data across time, and average data from corresponding regions of cortex. At their first scan (an average of 1.5 years after initial diagnosis, at age 13), patients showed a 10% gray matter deficit in a small region of the parietal cortex. Over the five succeeding years, this brain tissue loss swept forward into dorsolateral prefrontal and temporal cortices, where deficits were not found initially. Male and female patients showed similar patterns of spreading deficits, reaching a 20–25% average loss in some regions. Group

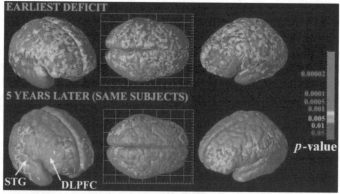

Fig. 6.12 Dynamic brain maps: mapping brain changes in schizophrenia. Derived from high-resolution magnetic resonance images (MRI scans), the images were created after repeatedly scanning 12 subjects with childhood-onset schizophrenia over 5 years, and comparing them with 12 matched, healthy controls, scanned at the same ages and intervals. Severe loss of gray matter is indicated (red and pink colors), while stable regions are in blue. STG denotes the superior temporal gyrus, and DLPFC denotes the dorsolateral prefrontal cortex. Video sequences showing these dynamic changes can be viewed on the Internet at http://www.loni.ucla.edu/~thompson/MOVIES/SZ/sz.html (Reprinted with permission from Thompson *et al.* (2001*d*) *Proceedings of the National Academy of Sciences of the USA*, **98** (20), 11650–5.)

differences were highly significant ($P < 0.01$, permutation test), relative to both healthy controls and non-schizophrenic controls matched for medication and IQ. The mapping technique also agreed with more conventional methods, in which the lobar gray matter volumes were compared over time. Rapoport *et al.* (1999) found that the healthy controls lost cortical gray matter in the frontal (2.6%) and parietal lobes (4.1%); patients had faster losses in frontal (10.9%) and parietal (8.5%) regions, and they also suffered a decrease in temporal gray volume (7%), which remained stable in the controls.

Genetic brain maps

Cortical mapping can also identify deficit patterns associated with genetic risk for schizophrenia. Genetic brain maps (Fig. 6.13) use twin data to fit genetic models to imaging data at each voxel (Thompson *et al.* 2001*a*, 2002). This can show which aspects of brain structure are under strongest genetic control. In disease studies (Cannon *et al.* 2002), they can also reveal brain regions at genetic risk for deficits. To see how this approach works, consider the maps in Fig. 6.13a, b. These are computed from MRI scans of normal twins. Figure 6.13a shows the correlation in gray matter density between identical (monozygotic) twins, who have exactly the same genes. Red colors denote regions where twins are extremely similar in their quantity of gray matter. Figure 6.13b shows the gray matter correlations for fraternal (dizygotic) twins, who share on average half their genes. These correlations are substantially less. If only the environment were important in determining these differences (rather than genetic factors), it would not matter whether the twins were identical or fraternal. However, the heritability map (Fig. 6.13c) shows that gray matter density in certain parts of the brain is statistically more closely matched in the identical twins than in twins who were less similar genetically. Frontal gray matter volumes were found to be under strong genetic control, and correlated with individual differences in intellectual function (IQ; Plomin and Kosslyn 2001; Posthuma *et al.* 2002).

Discordance maps and allelic variation

In a discordant twin study (Cannon *et al.* 2002), we also measured differences in cortical gray matter distribution between monozygotic (MZ) twins discordant for schizophrenia, averaging the results across discordant pairs. In the identical twins we examined, the schizophrenic member of each pair showed statistically significant deficits (between 5 and 8%) in superior parietal and dorsolateral prefrontal cortices, and in the left superior temporal gyrus (Fig. 6.13d). No significant differences were found between discordant co-twins in primary somatosensory or primary motor areas. In the frontal and temporal regions, deficits were found to be highly heritable. The liability map shows regions where deficits were found in healthy relatives of patients. These deficits were statistically linked with the degree of genetic affinity to a patient (i.e. worse deficits in MZ than DZ relatives). This shows that these particular

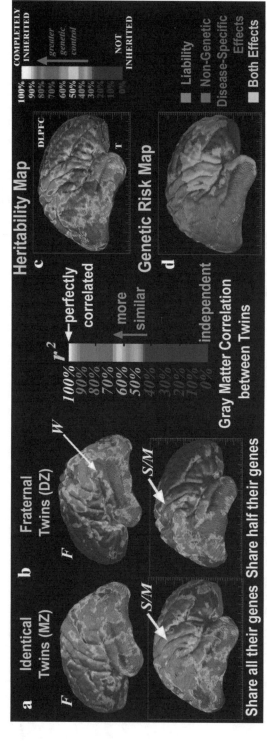

Fig. 6.13 Genetic influences on brain structure: mapping heritability and liability. Color-coded maps (a, b) show local gray matter correlations between monozygotic (MZ) and dizygotic (DZ) twins. (c): A map of heritability statistics (h^2, computed from Falconer's heritability formula) estimates the proportion of anatomic variation attributable to genetic factors. An anatomical band encompassing frontal, sensorimotor, and parietal cortices (red colors) is under strong genetic control. In (d), the liability map (green colors) reveals frontal brain regions where gray matter deficits are found in healthy MZ and DZ twins of schizophrenia patients. Greater deficits are found in relatives who are genetically closer to a patient. Red colors show regions with deficits in schizophrenic twins relative to their genetically identical healthy MZ co-twins. Disease-specific differences must be due, in part, to non-genetic factors. [(a)–(c) Adapted with permission from Thompson et al. (2001a) Nature Neuroscience, **4** (12), 1253–8; (d) adapted from Cannon et al. (2002) Proceedings of the National Academy of Sciences of the USA, **99** (5), 3228–33]. See Plate 8 of the plate section at the centre of this book.

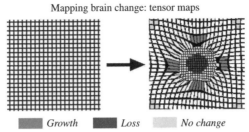

Mapping brain change: tensor maps

| ▨ *Growth* | ■ *Loss* | ▤ *No change* |

Fig. 6.14 Tensor-based morphometry. Patterns of local volumetric growth and loss can be estimated from a deformation map that captures brain changes over time, or even shape differences between an individual or a brain atlas. The determinant of the deformation gradient, i.e. the Jacobian or local expansion factor, is typically shown in color. Tensor maps distinguish local volume changes from volume-preserving shifts in anatomy.

deficits are mediated in part by genetic differences. Similarly, genetic liability was shown to result in increased bowing of the corpus callosum, using shape-averaging methods (Narr *et al.* 2002; cf. Hulshoff Pol *et al.* 2002*a*,*b*).

Tensor maps of brain change

Strategies to map brain changes are of immense value in basic and clinical neuro-science. For longitudinal studies, specialized algorithms have been developed to map patterns of brain change over time, in individuals scanned at multiple time points. These techniques can capture the dynamics of brain growth and loss in development and aging. If they are sufficiently sensitive, they can also assess drugs that aim to decelerate or arrest these changes, pinpointing where tumor growth, gray matter loss, or other atrophic processes are speeding up or slowing down.

Tensor maps

Maps of brain change over time may also be based on a tensor mapping concept. In this approach, a high-dimensional elastic deformation, or warping field, is calculated, typically with millions of degrees of freedom, which drives an image of a subject's anatomy at a baseline timepoint to match its shape in a later scan (see Fig. 6.14). The tensor that is mapped, in this context, is the gradient of the deformation field: mathematically it is equivalent to a 3×3 matrix attached to each point in the anatomy, which describes the principal directions of deformation at that point. The determinant of this matrix, called the Jacobian, is often used to summarize the transformation: this single number represents the local expansion factor (plotted in Fig. 6.14), and can be converted into a growth rate based on the time interval between scans. A notable feature of tensors, relative to displacement vectors, is that they distinguish intrinsic volumetric changes from bulk shifts in anatomy: unlike displacement vectors, tensors are invariant to translational shifts of a structure in stereotaxic space, but they are still sensitive to intrinsic volumetric changes. This distinction can help in studying disease effects, as

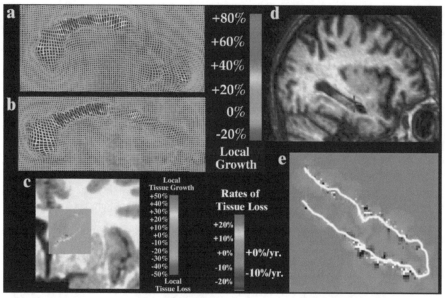

Fig. 6.15 Visualizing growth and atrophy. If follow-up (longitudinal) images are available, the dynamics of brain change can be measured with tensor mapping approaches (Thompson *et al.* 2000a). These maps show local rates of tissue growth or loss. Fastest growth is detected in the isthmus of the corpus callosum in two young girls identically scanned at ages 6 and 7 (a), and at ages 9 and 13 (b). Maps of loss rates in tissue can be generated for the developing caudate [(c), here in a 7- to 11-year-old child], and for the degenerating hippocampus [(d), (e)]. In (e), a female patient with mild Alzheimer's disease was imaged with high-resolution MRI at the beginning and end of a 19-month interval. The patient, aged 74.5 years at first scan, exhibits faster tissue loss rates in the hippocampal head (10% per year, during this interval) than in the fornix. These maps can elucidate the dynamics of therapeutic response in an individual or a population (Haney *et al.* 2001), and may be useful in mapping acute changes in the basal ganglia secondary to antipsychotic medication (Chakos *et al.* 1995).

intrinsic changes in some structures may cause other structures to shift translationally. These two types of changes will usually not be distinguished by voxel-based methods, unless structures are perfectly aligned using high dimensional registration (Bookstein, 2001).

Figure 6.15 shows typical results of a tensor mapping approach we developed to map brain growth in young children. An anterior-to-posterior wave of growth was found in the brains of children scanned repeatedly between the ages of 3 and 15 (Thompson *et al.* 2000a). Parametric surface meshes were built to represent anatomical structures in a series of scans over time, and these were matched using a fully volumetric deformation. Dilation and contraction rates, and even the principal directions of growth, can be derived by examining the eigenvectors of the deformation gradient tensor, or the local Jacobian matrix of the transform that maps the earlier anatomy on to the later

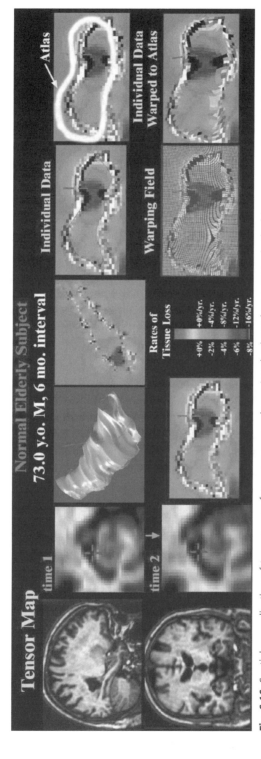

Fig. 6.16 Spatial normalization of tensor maps for group comparisons. Local volume loss patterns in the hippocampus of an elderly subject (here, over a 6-month interval) are hard to appreciate from raw MRI data (left). They can be localized by using three-dimensional surface models to drive a three-dimensional continuum-mechanical partial differential equation (PDE) from which dynamic statistics of loss are derived. Comparison and averaging of this loss rate data across subjects requires a second PDE to convect the attribute data on to an average neuroanatomic atlas (final four panels).

one (Fig. 6.14). By analyzing the deformation fields, tensor maps can be created to reflect the magnitude and principal directions of tissue dilation or contraction. This mapping process is illustrated in Fig. 6.15. The validity of the approach can also be assessed by visualizing 'null maps' of brain change over short intervals. Of particular interest is the pattern of rapid volumetric loss, adjacent to a region of rapid volumetric gain, in the caudate nucleus of a child scanned at ages 7 and 11. The increased spatial detail afforded by these mapping approaches makes them of particular interest for assessing fine-scale caudate changes in response to antipsychotic medications. These drug effects have been reported volumetrically but are currently poorly understood (Chakos *et al.* 1995).

Voxel compression mapping

Tensor maps may also be used to map tissue loss rates over time in patients with dementia (Fig. 6.16) (Janke *et al.* 2001; Thompson *et al.* 2001*b,c*) and multiple sclerosis (Janke *et al.* 2001). Freeborough and Fox (1998) implemented a fluid-matching algorithm to visualize how brain structure locally contracts and expands in a longitudinal study of Alzheimer's disease. Calling the technique 'voxel compression mapping', they also used the Jacobian of the deformation field to compute local atrophy and expansion (see also Thompson *et al.* 2000*a*; Crum *et al.* 2001). These changes were displayed as a color-coded map overlaid on the original scan, which indicates where tissue is lost. In clinical studies using this method, Fox *et al.* (2001) found characteristic patterns of atrophy in the different dementias. Alzheimer's disease patients showed diffuse atrophy, but more regionally selective atrophy was found in individuals with frontotemporal dementia. Janssen *et al.* (2002) suggested that voxel compression maps may even identify regional brain atrophy prior to clinical diagnosis in both Alzheimer's disease and frontotemporal dementia, underscoring the clinical potential of these methods. Strategies for pooling these maps across subjects, in dynamic brain atlases, are reviewed in Toga and Thompson (2003). Once registered across subjects, the resulting Jacobian determinant images may be analyzed using voxel-based methods, an approach known as tensor-based morphometry (TBM; Davatzikos *et al.* 1996; Chung *et al.* 2001; Ashburner *et al.* 2003).

Conclusion

In this chapter, we reviewed some of the major types of morphometric methods for mapping disease-related alterations in brain structure. As image analysis methods become increasingly automated, and as the scope and power of brain imaging studies expands to larger and more complex studies, substantial benefits will accrue. For schizophrenia research in particular, key information is likely to come from the large-scale integration of neuroimaging data across patient cohorts. These include chronic, first-episode, and early-onset patients, as well as data from at-risk relatives and those in the prodromal phase of the disorder. Automated tools can then further stratify these cohorts by symptom profiles, therapeutic response, and currently identified risk factors, to better understand the links between neuroimaging markers and the clinical course of the illness.

In addition, genetic brain maps combine mathematical methods from neuroimaging and genetics. They fit genetic models to voxel-based measures, and assess the results with techniques from imaging statistics and random field theory (Thompson *et al.* 2002). They are also beginning to provide biological markers for brain regions at risk in schizophrenia. In future, similar statistical maps may be useful in large cohort studies to assess how brain structure depends on allelic variation at candidate susceptibility loci (Thompson *et al.* 2002). Continued hybridization of methods from genetics and brain imaging is likely to accelerate our understanding of genetic risks and the time-course of schizophrenia, including its development and progression.

Acknowledgments

This work was supported by National Institute of Mental Health Intramural funding (to J.L.R.), by an NIMH research grant (to T.D.C.), and by research grants (to P.T. and A.W.T.) from the National Center for Research Resources (P41 RR13642 and RR00865), the National Library of Medicine (LM/MH05639), National Institute of Neurological Disorders and Stroke and the NIMH (NINDS/NIMH NS38753 and MH65166), and by the *Human Brain Project* (P20 MH/DA52176). Special thanks go to our colleagues Elizabeth Sowell, Katherine Narr, Christine Vidal, Kiralee Hayashi, Jacopo Annese, Jay Giedd, Greig de Zubicaray, Andrew Janke, Jaakko Kaprio, David MacDonald, Alan Evans, Roger Woods, Colin Holmes, John Bacheller, and John Mazziotta, and many others whose support has been invaluable in these investigations.

References

Ananth, H., Popescu, I., Critchleym H. D., Good, C. D., Frackowiak, R. S., and Dolan, R. J. (2002). Cortical and subcortical gray matter abnormalities in schizophrenia determined through structural magnetic resonance imaging with optimized volumetric voxel-based morphometry. *American Journal of Psychiatry,* **159** (9), 1497–505.

Angenent, S., Haker, S., Tannenbaum, A., and Kikinis, R. (1999). Conformal geometry and brain flattening. *Proceedings of MICCAI 1999*, pp. 271–8.

Arnold, J. B., Liow, J. S., Schaper, K. A., Stern, J. J., Sled, J. G., Shattuck, D. W. *et al.* (2001). Qualitative and quantitative evaluation of six algorithms for correcting intensity nonuniformity effects. *Neuroimage*, **13** (5), 931–43.

Ashburner, J. (2001). *Computational neuroanatomy*. PhD Thesis, University of London, England.

Ashburner, J. and Friston, K. J. (1999). Nonlinear spatial normalization using basis functions. *Human Brain Mapping*, **7** (4), 254–66.

Ashburner, J. and Friston, K. J. (2000). Voxel-based morphometry—the methods. *Neuroimage*, **11** (6), 805–21.

Ashburner, J. and Friston, K. J. (2001). Why voxel-based morphometry should be used. *Neuroimage*, **14**, 1238–43.

Ashburner, J., Neelin, P., Collins, D. L., Evans, A. C., and Friston, K. J. (1997). Incorporating prior knowledge into image registration. *Neuroimage*, **6** (4), 344–52.

Ashburner, J., Hutton, C., Frackowiak, R., Johnsrude, I., Price, C., and Friston, K. (1998). Identifying global anatomical differences: Deformation-based morphometry. *Human Brain Mapping*, **6** (5–6), 348–57.

Ashburner, J., Csernansky, J., Davatzikos, C., Fox, N. C., Frisoni, G., and Thompson, P. M. (2003). Computational neuroanatomy: Towards a computer-assisted diagnosis of degenerative brain diseases based on magnetic resonance imaging. *Lancet Neurology* **2** (2), 79–88.

Baare, W. F., Hulshoff Pol, H. E., Boomsma, D. I., Posthuma, D., de Geus, E. J., Schnack, H. G. *et al.* (2001). Quantitative genetic modeling of variation in human brain morphology. *Cerebral Cortex*, **11** (9), 816–24.

Baron, J. C., Chetelat, G., Desgranges, B., Perchey, G., Landeau, B., de la Sayette, V. *et al.* (2001). In vivo mapping of gray matter loss with voxel-based morphometry in mild Alzheimer's disease. *Neuroimage*, **14** (2), 298–309.

Blanton, R. E., Levitt, J. L., Thompson, P. M., Capetillo-Cunliffe, L. F., Sadoun, T., Williams, T. *et al.* (2000). Mapping cortical variability and complexity patterns in the developing human brain. *Psychiatry Research*, **107**, 29–43.

Bogerts, B. (1999). The neuropathology of schizophrenic diseases: Historical aspects and present knowledge. *European Archives of Psychiatry and Clinical Neuroscience*, **249** (Suppl. 4), 2–13.

Bookstein, F. L. (1997). Landmark methods for forms without landmarks: Morphometrics of group differences in outline shape. *Medical Image Analysis*, **1** (3), 225–43.

Bookstein, F. (2001). Voxel-based morphometry should not be used with imperfectly registered images. *Neuroimage*, **14** (6), 1454–62.

Bookstein, F. L., Sampson, P. D., Connor, P. D., and Streissguth, A. P. (2002). Midline corpus callosum is a neuroanatomical focus of fetal alcohol damage. *Anatomical Record*, **269** (3), 162–74.

Buchsbaum, M. S., Shihabuddin, L., Hazlett, E. A., Schroder, J., Haznedar, M. M., Powchik, P. *et al.* (2002). Kraepelinian and non-Kraepelinian schizophrenia subgroup differences in cerebral metabolic rate. *Schizophrenia Research*, **55** (1–2), 25–40.

Bullmore, E. T., Suckling, J., Overmeyer, S., Rabe-Hesketh, S., Taylor, E., and Brammer, M. J. (1999). Global, voxel, and cluster tests, by theory and permutation, for a difference between two groups of structural MR images of the brain. *IEEE Transactions on Medical Imaging*, **18**, 32–42.

Cannon, T. D., Thompson, P. M., van Erp, T., Toga, A. W., Poutanen, V.-P., Huttunen, M. *et al.* (2002). Cortex mapping reveals regionally specific patterns of genetic and disease-specific gray-matter deficits in twins discordant for schizophrenia. *Proceedings of the National Academy of Sciences USA*, **99**, 3228–33.

Cao, J. and Worsley, K. J. (1999). The geometry of the Hotelling's T-squared random field with applications to the detection of shape changes. *Annals of Statistics*, **27**, 925–42.

Chakos, M. H., Lieberman, J. A., Alvir, J., Bilder, R., and Ashtari, M. (1995). Caudate nuclei volumes in schizophrenic patients treated with typical antipsychotics or clozapine. *Lancet*, **18**, 345 (8947), 456–7.

Christensen, G. E., Rabbitt, R. D., and Miller, M. I. (1993). A deformable neuroanatomy textbook based on viscous fluid mechanics. *27th Annual Conference on Information Sciences and Systems*, pp. 211–16.

Christensen, G. E., Rabbitt, R. D., and Miller, M. I. (1996). Deformable templates using large deformation kinematics. *IEEE Transactions on Image Processing*, **5** (10), 1435–47.

Chung, M. K., Worsley, K. J., Paus, T., Cherif, C., Collins, D. L., Giedd, J. N. *et al.* (2001). A unified statistical approach to deformation-based morphometry. *Neuroimage*, **14** (3), 596–606.

Collins, D. L., Neelin, P., Peters, T. M., and Evans, A. C. (1994*a*). Automatic 3D intersubject registration of MR volumetric data into standardized Talairach Space. *Journal of Computer Assisted Tomography*, **18** (2), 192–205.

Collins, D. L., Peters, T. M., and Evans, A. C. (1994*b*). An automated 3D non-linear image deformation procedure for determination of gross morphometric variability in the human brain. *Proceedings Visualization in Biomedical Computing (SPIE)*, **3**, 180–90.

Collins, D. L., Holmes, C. J., Peters, T. M., and Evans, A. C. (1995). Automatic 3D model-based neuroanatomical segmentation. *Human Brain Mapping*, **3**, 190–208.

Collins, D. L., Montagnat, J., Zijdenbos, A. P., Evans, A. C., and Arnold, D. L. (2001). Automated estimation of brain volume in multiple sclerosis with BICCR. In *Proceedings of the Annual Symposium on Information Processing in Medical Imaging* (ed. M. F. Insana and R.M. Leahy), vol. 2082 of LNCS, pp. 141–7. Springer, Berlin.

Collins, D. L., Zijdenbos, A. P., Paus, T., and Evans, A. C. (2002). Use of registration for cohort studies, In *Medical Image Registration*, (eds. J. Hajinal, D. Hawker, and D. Hill), CRC Press, Boca Raton, Fl.

Crow, T. J. (2002). Handedness, language lateralisation and anatomical asymmetry: Relevance of protocadherin XY to hominid speciation and the aetiology of psychosis: Point of view. *British Journal of Psychiatry*, **181**, 295–7.

Crum, W. R., Scahill, R. I., and Fox, N. C. (2001). Automated hippocampal segmentation by regional fluid registration of serial MRI: Validation and application in Alzheimer's disease. *Neuroimage*, **13**, 847–55.

Csernansky, J. G., Joshi, S., Wang, L., Haller, J. W., Gado, M., Miller, J. P. *et al.* (1998). Hippocampal morphometry in schizophrenia by high dimensional brain mapping. *Proceedings of the National Academy of Sciences USA*, **95** (19), 11406–11.

Csernansky, J. G., Wang, L., Joshi, S., Miller, J. P., Gado, M., Kido, D. *et al.* (2000). Early DAT is distinguished from aging by high-dimensional mapping of the hippocampus. Dementia of the Alzheimer type. *Neurology*, **55** (11), 1636–43.

Davatzikos, C. (1998). Mapping image data to stereotaxic spaces: Applications to brain mapping. *Human Brain Mapping*, **6** (5–6), 334–8.

Davatzikos, C., Vaillant, M., Resnick, S. M., Prince, J. L., Letovsky, S., and Bryan, R. N. (1996). A computerized approach for morphological analysis of the corpus callosum. *Journal of Computer Assisted Tomography*, **20** (1), 88–97.

Davatzikos, C., Genc, A., Xu, D., and Resnick, S. M. (2001). Voxel-based morphometry using the RAVENS maps: Methods and validation using simulated longitudinal atrophy. *Neuroimage*, **14** (6), 1361–9.

Davidson, R. J. and Hugdahl, K. (1994). *Brain asymmetry*. MIT Press, Cambridge, MA.

Dinov, I. D., Mega, M. S., Thompson, P. M., Lee, L., Woods, R. P., Holmes, C. J., *et al.* (2000). *Analyzing functional brain images in a probabilistic atlas: A validation of sub-volume thresholding*. *Journal of Computer Assisted Tomography*, **24** (1),128–38.

Drury, H. A., Van Essen, D. C., Corbetta, M., and Snyder, A. Z. (2000). Surface-based analyses of the human cerebral cortex. In *Brain warping*, (ed. A. W. Toga), Chapter 19. Academic Press, San Diego.

Evans, A. C., Collins, D. L., Neelin, P., MacDonald, D., Kamber, M., and Marrett, T. S. (1994). Three-dimensional correlative imaging: Applications in human brain mapping. In *Functional neuroimaging: Technical foundations*, (ed. R. W. Thatcher, M. Hallett, T. Zeffiro, E. R. John, and M. Huerta), pp. 145–62. Academic Press, San Diego, CA.

Falkai, P., Honer, W. G., David, S., Bogerts, B., Majtenyi, C., and Bayer, T. A. (1999). No evidence for astrogliosis in brains of schizophrenic patients. A post-mortem study. *Neuropathology and Applied Neurobiology*, **25** (1), 48–53.

Fischl, B. and Dale, A. M. (2000). Measuring the thickness of the human cerebral cortex from magnetic resonance images. *Proceedings of the National Academy of Sciences USA*, **97** (20), 11050–5.

Fischl, B., Sereno, M. I., Tootell, R. B. H., and Dale, A. M. (1999). High-resolution inter-subject averaging and a coordinate system for the cortical surface. *Human Brain Mapping*, **8** (4), 272–84.

Fischl, B., Salat, D. H., Busa, E., Albert, M., Dieterich, M., Haselgrove, C. *et al.* (2002). Whole brain segmentation: Automated labeling of neuroanatomical structures in the human brain. *Neuron*, **33** (3), 341–55.

Fox, N. C. and Freeborough, P. A. (1997). Brain atrophy progression measured from registered serial MRI: Validation and application to Alzheimer's disease. *Journal of Magnetic Resonance Imaging*, **7**, 1069–75.

Fox, N. C., Scahill, R. I., Crum, W. R., and Rossor, M. N. (1999). Correlation between rates of brain atrophy and cognitive decline in AD. *Neurology*, **52**, 1687–9.

Fox, N. C., Cousens, S., Scahill, R., Harvey, R. J., and Rossor, M. N. (2000). Using serial registered brain magnetic resonance imaging to measure disease progression in Alzheimer disease: Power calculations and estimates of sample size to detect treatment effects. *Archives of Neurology*, **57**, 339–44.

Fox, N. C., Crum, W. R., Scahill, R. I., Stevens, J. M., Janssen, J. C., and Rossor, M. N. (2001). Imaging of onset and progression of Alzheimer's disease with voxel-compression mapping of serial magnetic resonance images. *Lancet*, **358**, 201–5.

Fox, P. T. (1997). The growth of human brain mapping. *Human Brain Mapping*, **5** (1), 1–2.

Fox, P. T., Perlmutter, J. S., and Raichle, M. (1985). A stereotactic method of localization for positron emission tomography. *Journal of Computer Assisted Tomography*, **9** (1), 141–53.

Fox, P. T., Mintun, M. A., Reiman, E. M., and Raichle, M. E. (1988). Enhanced detection of focal brain responses using inter-subject averaging and change distribution analysis of subtracted PET images. *Journal of Cerebral Blood Flow and Metabolism*, 8, 642–53.

Frackowiak, R. S. J., Friston, K. J., Frith, C. D., Dolan, R. J., and Mazziotta, J. C. (1997). *Human brain function*. Academic Press, San Diego, CA.

Freeborough, P. A. and Fox, N. C. (1998). Modeling brain deformations in Alzheimer disease by fluid registration of serial 3D MR images. *Journal of Computer Assisted Tomography*, **22** (5), 838–43.

Friston, K. J. (1997). Testing for anatomically specified regional effects. *Human Brain Mapping*, **5** (2), 133–6.

Friston, K. J., Passingham, R. E., Nutt, J. G., Heather, J. D., Sawle, G. V., and Frackowiak, R. S. J. (1989). Localization in PET images: direct fitting of the intercommissural (AC-PC) line. *Journal of Cerebral Blood Flow and Metabolism*, **9**, 690–5.

Friston, K. J., Frith, C. D., Liddle, P. F., and Frackowiak, R. S. J. (1991). Plastic transformation of PET images. *Journal of Computer Assisted Tomography*, **9** (1), 141–53.

Friston, K. J., Holmes, A. P., Worsley, K. J., Poline, J. P., Frith, C. D., and Frackowiak, R. S. J. (1995). Statistical parametric maps in functional imaging: A general linear approach. *Human Brain Mapping*, **2**, 189–210.

Gaser, C., Volz, H. P., Kiebel, S., Riehemann, S., and Sauer, H. (1999). Detecting structural changes in whole brain based on nonlinear deformations – application to schizophrenia research. *Neuroimage*, **10** (2), 107–13.

Gaser, C., Nenadic, I., Buchsbaum, B. R., Hazlett, E. A., and Buchsbaum, M. S. (2001). Deformation-based morphometry and its relation to conventional volumetry of brain lateral ventricles in MRI. *Neuroimage*, **13** (6 Pt 1), 1140–5.

Gee, J. C. and Bajcsy, R. K. (1998). Elastic matching: Continuum-mechanical and probabilistic analysis. In *Brain warping*, (ed. A. W. Toga). Academic Press, San Diego.

Gerig, G., Styner, M., Shenton, M. E., and Lieberman, J. A. (2001). Shape versus size: Improved understanding of the morphology of brain structures. *Proceedings MICCAI 2001, October,* LNCS 2208, pp. 24–32. Springer, Berlin.

Giedd, J. N., Jeffries, N. O., Blumenthal, J., Castellanos, F. X., Vaituzis, A. C., Fernandez, T. *et al.* (1999*a*). Childhood-onset schizophrenia: progressive brain changes during adolescence. *Biological Psychiatry*, **46** (7), 892–8.

Giedd, J. N., Blumenthal, J., Jeffries, N. O., Castellanos, F. X., Liu, H., Zijdenbos, A., *et al.* (1999*b*). Brain development during childhood and adolescence: a longitudinal MRI study. *Nature Neuroscience*, **2** (10), 861–3.

Gitelman, D. R., Ashburner, J., Friston, K. J., Tyler, L. K. and Price, C. J. (2001). Voxel-based morphometry of herpes simplex encephalitis. *Neuroimage*, **13** (4), 623–31.

Goldman-Rakic, P. S. and Selemon, L. D. (1998). Functional and anatomical aspects of prefrontal pathology in schizophrenia. *Schizophrenia Bulletin*, **23** (3), 437–58.

Goldszal, A. F., Davatzikos, C., Pham, D. L., Yan, M. X., Bryan, R. N., and Resnick, S. M. (1998). An image-processing' system for qualitative and quantitative volumetric analysis of brain images. *Journal of Computer Assisted Tomography*, **22** (5), 827–37.

Golland, P., Grimson, W. E. L., Shenton, M. E., and Kikinis, R. (2001). Deformation analysis for shaped based classification. *Proceedings IPMI'01: The 17th International Conference on Information Processing and Medical Imaging*, LNCS 2082, pp. 517–30. Springer-Verlag, Berlin.

Good, C. D., Ashburner, J., and Frackowiak, R. S. J. (2001*a*). Computational neuroanatomy: new perspectives for neuroradiology. *Revue Neurologique (Paris)*, **157** (8–9), 797–806.

Good, C. D., Johnsrude, I. S., Ashburner, J., Henson, R. N., Friston, K. J., and Frackowiak, R. S. J. (2001*b*). A voxel-based morphometric study of ageing in 465 normal adult human brains. *Neuroimage*, **14** (1), 21–36.

Haker, S., Angenent, S., Tannenbaum, A., and Kikinis, R. (1999). Nondistorting flattening maps and the 3-D visualization of colon CT images. *IEEE Transactions on Medical Imaging*, **19** (7), 665–70.

Haller, J. W., Banerjee, A., Christensen, G. E., Gado, M., Joshi, S., Miller, M. I. *et al.* (1997). Three-dimensional hippocampal MR morphometry with high-dimensional transformation of a neuro-anatomic atlas. *Radiology*, **202** (2), 504–10.

Han, X., Xu, C., Braga-Neto, U., and Prince, J. L. (2001). Graph-based topology correction for brain cortex segmentation. *Proceedings IPMI' 01: The 17th International Conference on Information Processing and Medical Imaging, LNCS 2082*, pp. 395–401.

Haney, S., Thompson, P. M., Cloughesy, T. F., Alger, J. R., Frew, A., Torres-Trejo, A. *et al.* (2001). Mapping response in a patient with malignant glioma. *Journal of Computer Assisted Tomography*, 25, 529–36.

Hayashi, K. M., Thompson, P. M., Mega, M. S., Zoumalan, C. I., Sowell, E. R., *et al.* (2002). Medial hemispheric surface gyral pattern delineation in 3D: Surface curve protocol. Available via Internet: http://www.loni.ucla.edu/~khayashi/Public/medial_surface/

Holmes, A. P., Blair, R. C., Watson, J. D. G., and Ford, I. (1996). Nonparametric analysis of statistic images from functional mapping experiments. *Journal of Cerebral Blood Flow and Metabolism*, **16** (1), 7–22.

Holmes, C. J., Hoge, R., Collins, L., Woods, R., Toga, A. W., and Evans, A. C. (1998). Enhancement of MR images using registration for signal averaging. *Journal of Computer Assisted Tomography*, **22** (2), 324–33.

Hulshoff Pol, H. E., Posthuma, D., Baare, W. F., De Geus, E. J., Schnack, H. G., van Haren, N. E. *et al.* (2002*a*). Twin-singleton differences in brain structure using structural equation modelling. *Brain,* **125** (2), 384–90.

Hulshoff Pol, H. E., Schnack, H. G., Bertens, M. G., van Haren, N. E., van der Tweel, I., Staal, W. G. *et al.* (2002*b*). Volume changes in gray matter in patients with schizophrenia. *American Journal of Psychiatry,* **159** (2), 244–50.

Jäncke, L., Staiger, J. F., Schlaug, G., Huang, Y., and Steinmetz, H. (1997). The relationship between corpus callosum size and forebrain volume. *Cerebral Cortex,* **7**(1), 48–56.

Janke, A. L., Zubicaray, G. D., Rose, S. E., Griffin, M., Chalk, J. B., and Galloway, G. J. (2001). 4D deformation modeling of cortical disease progression in Alzheimer's dementia. *Magnetic Resonance in Medicine,* **46** (4), 661–6.

Janssen, J. C., Scahill, R. I., Schott, J. M., Whitwell, J. L., Stevens, J. M., Cipolotti, L. *et al.* (2002). In vivo mapping of neurodegeneration in frontotemporal lobar degeneration. *8th International Conference of Alzheimer's Disease and Related Disorders* (abstract).

Jernigan, T. L., Archibald, S. L., Fennema-Notestine, C., Gamst, A. C., Stout, J. C., Bonner, J. *et al.* (2001). Effects of age on tissues and regions of the cerebrum and cerebellum. *Neurobiology of Aging,* **22** (4), 581–94.

Job, D. E., Whalley, H. C., McConnell, S., Glabus, M., Johnstone, E. C., and Lawrie, S. M. (2002). Structural gray matter differences between first-episode schizophrenics and normal controls using voxel-based morphometry. *NeuroImage,* **17**(2), 880–9.

Joshi, S., Grenander, U., and Miller, M. I. (1997). On the geometry and shape of brain sub-manifolds. *IEEE Transactions on Pattern Analysis and Machine Intelligence,* **11**, 1317–43.

Joshi, S., Lorenzen, P., Gerig, G., and Bullitt, E. (2001). Tumor-induced structural and radiometric asymmetry in brain images. *Mathematical Methods in Biomedical Image Analysis, IEEE Computer Society,* pp. 163–70.

Kennedy, D. N., Lange, N., Makris, N., Bates, J., Meyer, J., and Caviness, V. S., Jr (1998). Gyri of the human neocortex: an MRI-based analysis of volume and variance. *Cerebral Cortex,* **8** (4), 372–84.

Kikinis, R., Shenton, M. E., Gerig, G., Hokama, H., Haimson, J., O'Donnell, B. F., *et al.* (1994). Temporal lobe sulco-gyral pattern anomalies in schizophrenia: An *in vivo* MR three-dimensional surface rendering study. *Neuroscience Letters,* **182**, 7–12.

Kochunov, P., Lancaster, J., Thompson, P. M., Toga, A. W., Brewer, P., Hardies, J. *et al.* (2002). An optimized individual target brain in the Talairach coordinate system, *Neuroimage,* **17** (2), 922–7.

Krzanowski, W.J. (1988). *Principles of multivariate analysis: A user's perpective.* Clarendon Press, Oxford.

Laakso, M. P., Frisoni, G. B., Kononen, M., Mikkonen, M., Beltramello, A., Geroldi, C. *et al.* (2000). Hippocampus and entorhinal cortex in frontotemporal dementia and Alzheimer's disease: a morphometric MRI study. *Biological Psychiatry,* **47** (12), 1056–63.

Lange, N. (1996). Statistical approaches to human brain mapping by functional magnetic resonance imaging. *Statistics in Medicine,* **15**, 389–428.

Lawrie, S. M. and Abukmeil, S. S. (1998). Brain abnormality in schizophrenia. A systematic and quantitative review of volumetric magnetic resonance imaging studies. *British Journal of Psychiatry,* **172**, 110–20.

Lawrie, S. M., Whalley, H. C., Abukmeil, S. S., Kestelman, J. N., Miller, P., Best, J. J. *et al.* (2002). Temporal lobe volume changes in people at high risk of schizophrenia with psychotic symptoms. *British Journal of Psychiatry,* **181**, 138–43.

Lorensen, W. E. and Cline, H. E. (1987). Marching cubes: A high resolution 3D surface construction algorithm. *Computer Graphics (SIGGRAPH '87 Proceedings),* **21**(3),163–9.

MacDonald, D. (1998). *A method for identifying geometrically simple surfaces from three dimensional images.* PhD thesis, McGill University, Canada.

MacDonald, D., Kabani, N., Avis, D., and Evans, A. C. (2000). Automated 3-D extraction of inner and outer surfaces of cerebral cortex from MRI. *Neuroimage*, **12** (3), 340–56.

Maguire, E. A., Gadian, D. G., Johnsrude, I. S., Good, C. D., Ashburner, J., Frackowiak, R. S. *et al.* (2000). Navigation-related structural change in the hippocampi of taxi drivers. *Proceedings of the National Academy of Sciences USA*, **97** (8), 4398–403.

Mazziotta, J. C., Toga, A. W., Evans, A. C., Fox, P., and Lancaster, J. (1995). A probabilistic atlas of the human brain: Theory and rationale for its development. *Neuroimage*, **2**, 89–101.

Mazziotta, J. C., Toga, A. W., Evans, A. C., Fox, P. T., Lancaster, J., Zilles, K. *et al.* (2001). A probabilistic atlas and reference system for the human brain [invited paper]. *Journal of the Royal Society*, **356** (1412), 1293–1322.

McCarley, R. W., Niznikiewicz, M. A., Salisbury, D. F., Nestor, P. G., O'Donnell, B. F., Hirayasu, Y. *et al.* (1999). Cognitive dysfunction in schizophrenia: unifying basic research and clinical aspects. *European Archives of Psychiatry and Clinical Neuroscience*, **249** (suppl. 4), 69–82.

Mega, M. S., Thompson, P. M., Toga, A. W., and Cummings, J. L. (2000). Brain mapping in dementia. In *Brain mapping: the disorders*, (ed. A.W. Toga and J. C. Mazziotta). Academic Press, San Diego, CA.

Miller, M. I., Trouvé, A., and Younes, L. (2002). On the metrics and Euler–Lagrange equations of computational anatomy. *Annual Review of Biomedical Engineering*, **4**, 375–405.

Mummery, C. J., Patterson, K., Price, C. J., Ashburner, J., Frackowiak, R. S., and Hodges, J. R. (2000). A voxel-based morphometry study of semantic dementia: relationship between temporal lobe atrophy and semantic memory. *Annals of Neurology*, **47** (1), 36–45.

Narr, K. L., Thompson, P. M., Sharma, T., Moussai, J., Cannestra, A. F., and Toga, A. W. (2000). Mapping corpus callosum morphology in schizophrenia. *Cerebral Cortex*, **10** (1), 40–9.

Narr, K. L., Thompson, P. M., Sharma, T., Moussai, J., Blanton, R., Anvar, B. *et al.* (2001*a*). Three-dimensional mapping of temporo-limbic regions and the lateral ventricles in schizophrenia: gender effects. *Biological Psychiatry*, **50** (2), 84–97.

Narr, K. L., Thompson, P. M., Sharma, T., Moussai, J., Zoumalan, C. I., Rayman, J. *et al.* (2001*b*). 3D Mapping of gyral shape and cortical surface asymmetries in schizophrenia: Gender effects. *American Journal of Psychiatry*, **158** (2), 244–55.

Narr, K. L., Cannon, T. D., Woods, R. P., Thompson, P. M., Kim, S., Asunction, D. *et al.* (2002). Genetic contributions to altered callosal morphology in schizophrenia. *Journal of Neuroscience*, **22** (9), 3720–9.

Nichols, T. E. and Holmes, A. P. (2002). Nonparametric permutation tests for functional neuroimaging: a primer with examples. *Human Brain Mapping*, **15** (1), 1–25.

O'Brien, J. T., Paling, S., Barber, R., Williams, E. D., Ballard, C., McKeith, I. G. *et al.* (2001). Progressive brain atrophy on serial MRI in dementia with Lewy bodies, AD, and vascular dementia. *Neurology*, **56** (10), 1386–8.

Pitiot, A., Thompson, P. M., and Toga, A. W. (2002). Spatially and temporally adaptive elastic template matching. *IEEE Transactions on Medical Imaging*, **21**(8), 910–23.

Plomin, R. and Kosslyn, S. M. (2001). Genes, brain and cognition. *Nature Neuroscience*, **4** (12), 1153–4.

Posthuma, D., De Geus, E. J., Baare, W. F., Hulshoff Pol, H. E., Kahn, R. S. and Boomsma, D. I. (2002). The association between brain volume and intelligence is of genetic origin. *Nature Neuroscience*, **5** (2), 83–4.

Rapoport, J. L., Giedd, J., Kumra, S., Jacobsen, L., Smith, A., Lee, P. *et al.* (1997). Childhood-onset schizophrenia. Progressive ventricular change during adolescence [see comments]. *Archives of General Psychiatry*, **54**, 897–903.

Rapoport, J. L., Giedd, J. N., Blumenthal, J., Hamburger, S., Jeffries, N., Fernandez, T. *et al.* (1999). Progressive cortical change during adolescence in childhood-onset schizophrenia. A longitudinal magnetic resonance imaging study. *Archives of General Psychiatry*, **56** (7), 649–54.

Rasser, P. E., Johnston, P., Lagopoulos, J., Ward, P. B., Schall, U., Thienel, R. *et al.* (2003). Analysis of fMRI BOLD activation during the Tower of London Task using cortical pattern matching. *Proceedings of the International Congress on Schizophrenia Research (ICSR)* Colorado Springs, Co, March 29–April 2.

Ratnanather, J. T., Botteron, K. N., Nishino, T., Massie, A. B., Lal, R. M., Patel, S. G. *et al.* (2001). Validating cortical surface analysis of medial prefrontal cortex. *Neuroimage*, **14** (5), 1058–69.

Rex, D. E., Pouratian, N., Thompson, P. M., Cunanan, C. C., Sicotte, N. L., Collins, R. C. *et al.* (2000). Cortical surface warping applied to group analysis of fMRI of tongue movement in the left hemisphere. *Proceedings of the Society for Neuroscience*, Washington, DC.

Rosen, H. J., Gorno-Tempini, M. L., Goldman, W. P., Perry, R. J., Schuff, N., Weiner, M. *et al.* (2002). Patterns of brain atrophy in frontotemporal dementia and semantic dementia. *Neurology*, **58** (2), 198–208.

Salmond, C., Ashburner, J., Vargha-Khadem, F., Connelly, A., Gadian, D., and Friston, K. (2002). Distributional assumptions in voxel-based morphometry. *Neuroimage*, **17** (2), 1027–30.

Shattuck, D. and Leahy, R. M. (1999). Topological refinement of volumetric data. *SPIE Medical Imaging Conference Proceedings*, **3661**, 204–213.

Shattuck, D. W. and Leahy, R. M. (2001). Automated graph-based analysis and correction of cortical volume topology. *IEEE Transactions on Medical Imaging*, **20** (11), 1167–77.

Sled, J. G., Zijdenbos, A. P., and Evans, A. C. (1998). A non-parametric method for automatic correction of intensity non-uniformity in MRI data. *IEEE Transactions on Medical Imaging*, **17**, 87–97.

Smith, S. M., De Stefano, N., Jenkinson, M., and Matthews, P. M. (2002). Measurement of brain change over time. FMRIB Technical Report TR00SMS1, http://www.fmrib.ox.ac.uk/analysis/research/siena/siena/siena.html

Sowell, E. R., Levitt, J., Thompson, P. M., Holmes, C. J., Blanton, R. E., Kornsand, D. S. *et al.* (1999*a*). Brain abnormalities in early-onset schizophrenia spectrum disorder observed with statistical parametric mapping of structural magnetic resonance images. *American Journal of Psychiatry*, **157** (9), 1475–84.

Sowell, E. R., Thompson, P. M., Holmes, C. J., Jernigan, T. L., and Toga, A. W. (1999*b*). Progression of structural changes in the human brain during the first three decades of life: *In vivo* evidence for post-adolescent frontal and striatal maturation. *Nature Neuroscience*, **2** (10), 859–61.

Sowell, E. R., Thompson, P. M., Mega, M. S., Zoumalan, C. I., Lindshield, C., Rex, D. E. *et al.* (2000). Gyral pattern delineation in 3D: Surface curve protocol. Available via the Internet: http://www.loni.ucla.edu/~esowell/new_sulcvar.html

Sowell, E. R., Thompson, P. M., Tessner, K. D., and Toga, A. W. (2001). Accelerated brain growth and cortical gray matter thinning are inversely related during post-adolescent frontal lobe maturation. *Journal of Neuroscience*, **21** (22), 8819–29.

Stuart, G. W., Abdalla, A., Jenkinson, M. and Pantelis, C. (2001). Global variation in brain structure and its relation to head shape. *NeuroImage Human Brain Mapping 2002 Meeting*, Poster No. 10395, http://www.academicpress.com/www/journal/hbm2002/14982.html

Studholme, C., Cardenas, V., Schuff, N., Rosen, H., Miller, B., and Weiner, M. W. (2001). Detecting spatially consistent structural differences in Alzheimer's and frontotemporal dementia using deformation morphometry. *Proceedings of the International Conference on Medical Image Computing and Computer-Assisted Intervention*, pp. 41–8.

Styner, M. and Gerig, G. (2001). Medial models incorporating object variability for 3D shape analysis. *Proceedings on Information Processing in Medical Imaging (IPMI)*, *University of California Davis*, pp. 502–16.

Suzuki, M., Nohara, S., Hagino, H., Kurokawa, K., Yotsutsuji, T., Kawasaki, Y. *et al.* (2002). Regional changes in brain gray and white matter in patients with schizophrenia demonstrated with voxel-based analysis of MRI. *Schizophrenia Research,* **55** (1–2), 41–54.

Talairach, J. and Tournoux, P. (1988). *Co-planar stereotaxic atlas of the human brain.* Thieme, New York.

Taylor, J. E. and Adler, R. J. (2003). Euler characteristics for Gaussian fields on manifolds. *Annals of Probability,* **31** (2), 533–64.

Thirion, J.-P., Prima, S., and Subsol, S. (2000). Statistical analysis of dissymmetry in volumetric medical images. *Medical Image Analysis,* **4** (2), 111–21.

Thompson, P. M. and Toga, A. W. (1996). A surface-based technique for warping 3-dimensional images of the brain. *IEEE Transactions on Medical Imaging,* **15** (4), 402–17.

Thompson, P. M. and Toga, A. W. (1997). Detection, Visualization and animation of abnormal anatomic structure with a deformable probabilistic brain atlas based on random vector field transformations. *Medical Image Analysis,* **1** (4), 271–94.

Thompson, P. M. and Toga, A. W. (2000). Elastic image registration and pathology detection. In *Handbook of medical image processing,* (ed. I. Bankman, R. Rangayyan, A. C. Evans, R. P. Woods, E. Fishman, and H. K. Huang). Academic Press, San Diego, CA.

Thompson, P. M. and Toga, A. W. (2001). A framework for computational anatomy. *Computing and Visualization in Science,* **5,** 13–34.

Thompson, P. M., Schwartz, C., Lin, R. T., Khan, A. A., and Toga, A. W. (1996*a*). 3D Statistical analysis of sulcal variability in the human brain. *Journal of Neuroscience,* **16** (13), 4261–74.

Thompson, P. M., Schwartz, C., and Toga, A. W. (1996*b*). High-resolution random mesh algorithms for creating a probabilistic 3D surface atlas of the human brain. *NeuroImage,* **3,** 19–34.

Thompson, P. M., MacDonald, D., Mega, M. S., Holmes, C. J., Evans, A. C., and Toga, A. W. (1997). Detection and mapping of abnormal brain structure with a probabilistic atlas of cortical surfaces. *Journal of Computer Assisted Tomography,* **21** (4), 567–81.

Thompson, P. M., Moussai, J., Khan, A. A., Zohoori, S., Goldkorn, A., Mega, M. S. *et al.* (1998). Cortical variability and asymmetry in normal aging and Alzheimer's disease. *Cerebral Cortex,* **8** (6), 492–509.

Thompson, P. M., Giedd, J. N., Woods, R. P., MacDonald, D., Evans, A. C., and Toga, A. W. (2000*a*). Growth patterns in the developing brain detected by using continuum-mechanical tensor maps. *Nature,* **404,** 190–3.

Thompson, P. M., Mega, M. S., Narr, K. L., Sowell, E. R., Blanton, R. E., and Toga, A. W. (2000*b*). Brain image analysis and atlas construction. In *SPIE Handbook on Medical Image Analysis,* (ed. M. Fitzpatrick). Society of Photo-Optical Instrumentation Engineers (SPIE) Press.

Thompson, P. M., Mega, M. S., and Toga, A. W. (2000*c*). Disease-specific brain atlases. In *Brain mapping: The disorders,* (ed. A. W. Toga and J. C. Mazziotta). Academic Press, San Diego, CA.

Thompson, P. M., Woods, R. P., Mega, M. S., and Toga, A. W. (2000*d*). Mathematical/computational challenges in creating population-based brain atlases. *Human Brain Mapping,* **9** (2), 81–92.

Thompson, P. M., Cannon, T. D., Narr, K. L., van Erp, T., Khaledy, M., Poutanen, V.-P. *et al.* (2001*a*). Genetic influences on brain structure. *Nature Neuroscience,* **4** (12), 1253–8.

Thompson, P. M., Mega, M. S., Vidal, C., Rapoport, J. L., and Toga, A. W. (2001*b*). Detecting disease-specific patterns of brain structure using cortical pattern matching and a population-based probabilistic brain atlas. IEEE Conference on Information Processing in Medical Imaging (IPMI), University of California Davis. In *Lecture Notes in Computer Science (LNCS),* (ed. M. Insana and R. Leahy), vol. 2082, pp. 488–501. Springer-Verlag, Berlin.

Thompson, P. M., Mega, M. S., Woods, R. P., Blanton, R. E., Moussai, J., Zoumalan, C. I. *et al.* (2001*c*). Cortical change in Alzheimer's disease detected with a disease-specific population-based brain atlas. *Cerebral Cortex*, **11** (1), 1–16.

Thompson, P. M., Vidal, C. N., Giedd, J. N., Gochman, P., Blumenthal, J., Nicolson, R. *et al.* (2001*d*). Mapping adolescent brain change reveals dynamic wave of accelerated gray matter loss in very early-onset schizophrenia. *Proceedings of the National Academy of Sciences of the USA*, **98** (20), 11650–5.

Thompson, P. M., Hayashi, K. M., de Zubicaray, G., Janke, A. L., Rose, S. E., Dittmer, S. S. *et al.* (2003). Dynamics of gray matter loss in Alzheimer's disease, with video sequences at: http://www.loni.ucla.edu/~thompson/AD_4D/dynamic.html, *Journal of Neuroscience*, **23**, 994–1005.

Thompson, P. M., Narr, K. L., Blanton, R. E., and Toga, A. W. (2003). Mapping structural alterations of the corpus callosum during brain development and degeneration. In *The corpus callosum*, (ed. M. Iacoboni and E. Zaidel). MIT Press, Cambridge, MA.

Tisserand, D. L., Pruessner, J. C., Sanz Arigita, E. J., van Boxtel, M. P. J., Evans, A. C., Jolles, J., *et al.* (2002). Regional frontal cortical volumes decrease differentially in aging: an MRI study to compare volumetric approaches and voxel-based morphometry. *Neuroimage*, **17** (2), 657–69.

Toga, A. W. (1998). *Brain warping*. Academic Press, San Diego, CA.

Toga, A. W., Mazziotta, J. C. (2002). *Brain mapping: The methods*, (2nd edn). Academic Press, San Diego.

Toga, A. W., Rex, D. E., and Ma, J. (2001). A graphical interoperable processing pipeline. *International Conference on Human Brain Mapping, Brighton, UK*. Abstract No. 266.

Toga, A. W. and Thompson, P. M. (2003*a*). Mapping brain asymmetry. *Nature Reviews Neuroscience*, **4** (1), 37–48.

Toga, A. W. and Thompson, P. M. (2003*b*). Temporal dynamics of brain anatomy. *Annual Review of Biomedical Engineering*, **5**, 119–45.

Vidal, C., Rapoport, J. L., Giedd, J. N., Blumenthal, J., Gochman, P., Nicolson, R. *et al.* (2001). Dynamic patterns of accelerated gray matter loss are linked with clinical and cognitive change in childhood-onset schizophrenia. *Seventh Annual Meeting of the Organization for Human Brain Mapping, Brighton, UK, June*.

Viola, P. A. and Wells, W. M. (1995). Alignment by maximization of mutual information. *Fifth IEEE International Conference on Computer Vision, Cambridge, MA*, pp. 16–23.

Wang, L., Joshi, S. C., Miller, M. I., and Csernansky, J. G. (2001). Statistical analysis of hippocampal asymmetry in schizophrenia. *Neuroimage*, **14** (3), 531–45.

Warfield, S., Robatino, A., Dengler, J., Jolesz, F., and Kikinis, R. (1998). Nonlinear registration and template driven segmentation. In *Brain warping*, (ed. A. W. Toga), pp. 67–84. Academic Press.

Watkins, K. E., Paus, T., Lerch, J. P., Zijdenbos, A., Collins, D. L., Neelin, P. *et al.* (2001). Structural asymmetries in the human brain: a voxel-based statistical analysis of 142 MRI scans. *Cerebral Cortex*, **11** (9), 868–77.

Weinberger, D. R. and McClure, R. K. (2002). Neurotoxicity, neuroplasticity, and magnetic resonance imaging morphometry: what is happening in the schizophrenic brain? *Archives of General Psychiatry*, **59** (6), 553–8.

Weinberger, D. R., Egan, M. F., Bertolino, A., Callicott, J. H., Mattay, V. S., Lipska, B. K. *et al.* (2001). Prefrontal neurons and the genetics of schizophrenia. *Biological Psychiatry*, **50** (11), 825–44.

Wells, W. M., Viola, P., Atsumi, H., Nakajima, S., and Kikinis, R. (1997). Multi-modal volume registration by maximization of mutual information. *Medical Image Analysis*, **1** (1), 35–51.

Wilke, M., Schmithorst, V. J., and Holland, S. K. (2002). Assessment of spatial normalization of whole-brain magnetic resonance images in children. *Human Brain Mapping*, **17** (1), 48–60.

Witelson, S. F. (1989). Hand and sex differences in the isthmus and genu of the human corpus callosum. A postmortem morphological study. *Brain*, **112**, 799–835.

Woods, R. P., Cherry, S. R., and Mazziotta, J. C. (1992). Rapid automated algorithm for aligning and reslicing PET images. *Journal of Computer Assisted Tomography*, **16**, 620–33.

Woods, R. P., Mazziotta, J. C., and Cherry, S. R. (1993). MRI-PET registration with automated algorithm. *Journal of Computer Assisted Tomography*, **17**, 536–46.

Woods, R. P., Grafton, S. T., Watson, J. D. G., Sicotte, N. L., and Mazziotta, J. C. (1998). Automated image registration: II. Intersubject validation of linear and nonlinear models. *Journal of Computer Assisted Tomography*, **22**, (1), 139–52.

Woods, R. P., Dapretto, M., Sicotte, N. L., Toga, A. W., and Mazziotta, J. C. (1999). Creation and use of a Talairach-compatible atlas for accurate, automated, nonlinear intersubject registration, and analysis of functional imaging data. *Human Brain Mapping*, **8** (2–3), 73–9.

Worsley, K. J. (1994*a*). *Quadratic tests for local changes in random fields with applications to medical images*. Technical Report, Department of Mathematics and Statistics, McGill University, pp. 94–108.

Worsley, K. J. (1994*b*). Local maxima and the expected Euler characteristic of excursion sets of chi-squared, F and t fields. *Advances in Applied Probability*, **26**, 13–42.

Worsley, K. J., Marrett, S., Neelin, P., and Evans, A. C. (1996). Searching scale space for activation in PET images. *Human Brain Mapping*, **4**, 74–90.

Worsley, K. J., Andermann, M., Koulis, T., MacDonald, D., and Evans, A. C. (1999). Detecting changes in nonisotropic images. *Human Brain Mapping*, **8** (2–3), 98–101.

Wright, I. C., McGuire, P. K., Poline, J. B., Travere, J. M., Murray, R. M., Frith, C. D. *et al.* (1995). A voxel-based method for the statistical analysis of gray and white matter density applied to schizophrenia. *Neuroimage*, **2**, 244–52.

Zeineh, M. M., Engel, S. A., Thompson, P. M., and Bookheimer, S. (2001). Unfolding the human hippocampus with high-resolution structural and functional MRI. *The New Anatomist (Anatomical Record)*, **265** (2), 111–20.

Zhou, Y., Thompson, P. M., and Toga, A. W. (1999). Automatic extraction and parametric representations of cortical sulci. *Computer Graphics and Applications*, **19** (3), 49–55.

Chapter 7

Functional mapping with single-photon emission computed tomography and positron emission tomography

Andreas Heinz, Berenice Romero, and Daniel R. Weinberger

Introduction: history of SPECT brain imaging techniques

Single-photon emission computed tomography (SPECT) is a brain imaging method that allows the measurement of cerebral blood flow and radioligand binding sites such as neuroreceptors and transporters (e.g. Celsis *et al.* 1981; Eckelman *et al.* 1985; Kung *et al.* 1990). In this chapter, we will give an overview of the history of SPECT, describe the method, and discuss some of its research and clinical applications.

SPECT combines noninvasive techniques to measure blood flow with topographic techniques for localizing brain regions. Once psychiatric disorders were known to be characteristically associated with structural changes in the human brain, it became necessary to address how physiological and biochemical processes may be disrupted in pathophysiological models of these disorders.

Cerebral blood flow is coupled to cerebral metabolism through autoregulatory processes. This allows insight into neuronal function. Kety and Schmidt (1948) used nitrous oxide as a diffusible indicator of brain blood flow in humans. Brain perfusion was determined using the Fick principle, which requires monitoring the arterial input and the venous outflow of a freely diffusible and inert substance. The difference between these two showed the cellular uptake, which in turn was directly related to perfusion. These early measurements required carotid injection and jugular sampling to measure whole brain perfusion. Two disadvantages were the invasive technique and the impossibility of assessing regional blood flow. Chemically inert and free diffusible radioisotopes soon replaced nitrous oxide. Collimated detectors could then measure perfusion in specific brain areas.

One of the fist radioisotopes used for these measurements was xenon-133. ^{133}Xe emits gamma rays that can be detected though the skull. Multiple scintillation probes allowed the measurement of regional blood flow as well as the mathematical separation of flows in gray and white matter (Obrist *et al.* 1967; Risberg *et al.* 1975). Soon it was possible for intra-arterial injection to be replaced by either inhalation or intravenous injection of the radioisotope ^{133}Xe, making this imaging method more accessible and practical.

The reconstruction of three-dimensional images deriving from radiotracer distribution in the human brain was first achieved by Kuhl and Edwards (1963). This achievement gave birth to both SPECT and positron emission tomography (PET).

SPECT makes it possible to detect the three-dimensional distribution of a radiotracer in the human brain. There are two sorts of radiotracers, simple radioactive elements such as ^{133}Xe, and chemically more elaborate tracers such as labeled neurotransmitters. The radiopharmaceuticals used in SPECT differ from those used in PET in their radiation modus. While radiotracers used in PET emit a positron which is annihilated after collision with an electron, yielding two gamma rays simultaneously in exactly opposite directions, the radioligands used in SPECT emit single gamma rays.

Early SPECT instruments provided resolutions of 15–20 mm, and the imaging data were obtained after 20–60 min. Today SPECT images have a resolution of about 7–12 mm and can be acquired for some purposes within 10 min. In addition to blood flow, neuroreceptors and transporters can be imaged.

How does SPECT work?

SPECT functional imaging of the brain occurs in two steps: the radiotracer is administered and then the radiotracer's distribution is assessed by a topographic instrument. This measurement can occur instantly, as in ^{133}Xe tomography, or after a specific delay period. This is, for instance, the case when radiolabeled receptor ligands are used for measurement.

In studies measuring regional cerebral blood flow (rCBF), the fundamental idea is that the distribution of a chemical compound in the brain reflects physiology. The compound flows into the brain and so areas with high perfusion rates receive higher quantities of the radioactive compound, which can be measured accordingly.

What exactly is measured?

The radiotracers emit gamma rays. External detectors record the emitted rays. In order to construct an image, the origin of these rays must be determined. As gamma rays are emitted in all directions, it is difficult to trace their origin. A device is needed to filter all gamma rays that do not fall perpendicularly on the detector. This device is called a collimator.

A collimator is a lead sheet, which can stop gamma rays from penetrating the detector. The lead sheet has long apertures though which the perpendicular gamma rays can pass to the detector surface. The gamma rays that pass through are assumed to come from a part of the brain that lies directly beneath the detector. This is not completely accurate, as gamma rays may come from any place in the brain that lies on a line with the apertures of the collimator. Therefore the recorded radiation follows a line though the brain, but not a precise point. A series of lines representing radiation from the brain allow the reconstruction of two-dimensional pictures. If the detectors are moved around the brain, three-dimensional pictures can be calculated. The algorithm used is similar to that of X-ray computed tomography (CT) and PET (Andreasen 1989).

How is radiation transformed into a picture?

The gamma rays pass through the collimator to a detector. The detectors are made of sodium crystals, which respond to radiation by emitting light. An electronic circuit detects the light with photomultipliers and measures its intensity. The combination of both the information about the position and the energy (light intensity) are necessary to produce an image. The tissue under observation is reconstructed as a series of volume elements determined by the reconstruction algorithm and called a voxel.

Radiopharmaceuticals

Through the years many radiotracers have been developed to measure rCBF with SPECT, e.g. ^{133}Xe, [^{123}I]iodoamphetamine (IMP) and [^{99}Tc] hexamethyl propylene amine oxime (HMPAO). All these differ from each other in half-life, emitted energy and resolution (e.g. ^{133}Xe has a poor resolution and limited gray/white matter distinction), lipophilicity, distribution, and, last but not least, cost.

Data interpretation

The acquired data can be analyzed quantitatively and qualitatively. Quantitative analyses have been used infrequently because they involve invasive and relatively impractical techniques. Qualitative analysis must take mental activity into account, and changes in regional blood flow must be valued as relative (e.g. rCBF at rest and rCBF while performing a working memory task; see below). For spatial localization, regions of interest (ROIs) are determined, based on anatomical zones.

PET: assessment of glucose utilization

Like SPECT, PET can be used to measure cerebral blood flow. An advantage of PET is its improved spatial resolution and its capacity to more acutely correct for scattered radiation. In PET, positrons are annihilated with electrons. As a result, two gamma rays are emitted at a 180° angle, which can be detected by the PET camera. The camera is programmed so that—like a coincidence detector—it will only record gamma rays if two of them appear within a certain narrow time window at a 180° angle. Background radiation is thus effectively filtered out and spatial resolution is improved. Most modern PET cameras achieve a spatial resolution of about 4 mm.

Another way to assess brain activity with PET is to measure cerebral glucose utilization in regions of interest using a radiotracer called fluorodeoxyglucose (FDG). FDG enables researchers to explore directly the interactive organization of the brain, since neuronal activity is coupled to glucose utilization (Phelps *et al.*, 1979). The FDG PET technique to measure glucose utilization in the brain is well established and widely used. Many FDG studies have been performed on normal individuals, as well as in patients with different cerebral disorders. In Alzheimer's disease, for instance, local cerebral metabolic rate for glucose shows no abnormalities in primary sensorimotor, visual, and cerebellar metabolic activity, while parietal, temporal, and frontal glucose metabolism is diminished.

SPECT: perfusion studies

Studies on cerebral blood flow were first performed in 1948, in healthy individuals, using an inert gas wash-out technique (Kety and Schmidt 1948). Normal cerebral blood flow values were defined by different research groups (Scheinberg and Stead 1949; Heyman *et al.* 1951). Whole-brain blood-flow rates were reported that ranged between 50 and 60 ml/min/100 g of tissue. With ongoing technical progress, a multi-compartment model was developed that permitted deconvolution of blood flow values so that gray and white matter could be measured separately in specific brain regions. This made it possible to differentiate local changes in blood flow.

A large number of studies have been performed to assess changes in cerebral blood flow during sensory stimulation (e.g. visual, acoustic, somatosensory). The effects of visual hemi-field stimulation, or of acoustic stimulation, have been reported to enhance metabolic activity in the correspondingly activated areas (Greenberg *et al.* 1981). Also, many studies have focused on changes in brain perfusion while performing cognitive tasks, e.g. while solving visual/spatial problems (Risberg and Ingvar 1973; Halsey and Blauenstein 1975; Kraut *et al.*, 1995).

SPECT: receptor binding studies

Specific binding sites for various neurotransmitters can also be measured with SPECT, including various neuroreceptors (Eckelman *et al.* 1984, 1985; Kung *et al.* 1990; Lee *et al.* 1996; Chefer *et al.* 1998) and transporters (Laruelle *et al.* 1993, 1994). This research approach has been applied to study, for example, dopaminergic, serotonergic, and muscarinergic systems in various psychiatric and neurological disorders (Table 7.1). Some examples of how specific hypotheses and questions can be addressed with these methods follow.

Muscarinic receptors

Weinberger *et al.* (1990) carried out studies with (R,S)-3-quinuclidinyl-4-[^{123}I]iodobenzilate ([^{123}I]QNB). This radioligand showed high affinity to central muscarinic acetylcholine receptors (Weinberger *et al.* 1990). In control subjects [^{123}I]QNB was found to show a high binding in brain regions that were also implicated in post-mortem studies of muscarinic receptor distribution in humans. These findings demonstrated the feasibility of using SPECT to measure neuroreceptors in the context

Table 7.1 Radioligands used in neuropsychiatric research (after Heinz *et al.* 2000c)

Radioligand	Disorder	Reference
Dopamine D_2 receptors (striatum), [^{123}I]IBZM, ([^{123}I]iodobenzamide)	Schizophrenia, Tourette syndrome, Parkinson's disease, substance abuse	Kung *et al.* (1989, 1990), Daniel *et al.* (1991), Knable *et al.* (1995, 1997a, b), Heinz *et al.* (1996, 1998b, 1999), Pickar *et al.* (1996), Wolf *et al.* (1996), Bertolino *et al.* (1999), Raedler *et al.* (1999)
Monoamine transporters (dopamine: striatum, serotonin: midbrain, thalamus), [^{123}I]β-CIT, (2β-carbomethoxy-3β-(4-[^{123}I]iodophenyl)tropane)	Parkinson's disease, depression, ADHD, substance abuse, Tourette syndrome	Heinz *et al.* (1997, 1998a, c, d, 2000a, b), Jones *et al.* (1998), Laruelle *et al.* (1993, 1994)
Muscarinic acetylcholine receptors (cortex, striatum, thalamus, pons), [^{123}I]QBN, ((R,S)-3-quinuclidinyl-4-[^{123}I]iodobenzilate)	Alzheimer's disease, Pick's disease, other dementias, schizophrenia	Eckelman *et al.* (1984, 1985), Weinberger *et al.* (1990, 1991, 1992a, b), Sunderland *et al.* (1995), Lee *et al.* (1996), Raedler *et al.* (2000),
Nicotinic acetylcholine receptors (thalamus, cortex, striatum), 5-[^{123}I]iodo-A-85380, 5-[^{123}I]iodo-3-(2(S)-azetidinylmethoxy)pyridin)	Substance abuse, schizophrenia	Chefer *et al.* (1998)

ADHD, attention deficit/hyperactivity disorder.

of brain disease, e.g. in dementia research. A reduced availability of these receptors was found in patients with dementia, e.g. Alzheimer's disease (Weinberger *et al.* 1992a, b; Sunderland *et al.* 1995).

Dopaminergic receptors

The high affinity of radioligand [^{123}I] iodobenzamide ([^{123}I]IBZM) to D2/D3 receptors makes the investigation of extrapyramidal diseases possible (see Fig. 7.1). Knable *et al.* (1995) studied patients with Parkinson's disease and lateralized motor symptoms, and found an increase in [^{123}I]IBZM binding in the contralateral side. These findings could be due to either a receptor upregulation or a decreased competition between endogenous synaptic dopamine and the radioligand for binding at striatal D_2 receptors. In this case, the combination of radioligand binding and clinical symptoms increased our knowledge of Parkinson's disease. Another widely used approach in this research field is to measure the influence of antipsychotic drugs on radioligand binding, since all drugs used to treat schizophrenia block dopamine receptors.

Monoamine transporter radioligands

[^{123}I]β-CIT (2β-carbomethoxy-3β-(4-[^{123}I]iodophenyl)tropane) is a radioligand that binds to dopamine transporters in the striatum and to serotonin transporters in the

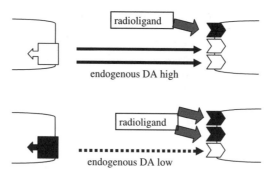

Fig. 7.1 Radioligand binding reflects intrasynaptic dopamine (DA) concentrations. If intrasynaptic dopamine concentrations are high, most postsynaptic dopamine D_2 receptors are occupied by endogenous dopamine, and radioligand binding to free receptor sites is low. If, on the other hand, intrasynaptic dopamine concentrations are low, this is reflected in high radioligand binding to unoccupied D_2 receptors.

midbrain and thalamus. Some studies tested the specificity of radioligand binding to certain monoamine transporters in a given brain region. For example, blockade of serotonin production with *p*-chlorophenylalanine (pCPA) increases serotonin transporter availability, probably as a result of reduced competition between the radioligand and endogenous serotonin for binding at the serotonin reuptake site. Administration of 5-hydroxytryptophane bypasses the pCPA-induced blockade of serotonin production and restores the intracellular serotonin concentration. The resulting increase in synaptic serotonin concentrations was reflected in a displacement of the radioligand [^{123}I]β-CIT from its binding site at the serotonin transporter (Jones *et al.* 1998).

Monoaminergic neurotransmitter systems have also been implicated in the development of major depression, alcohol-dependence, and Parkinson's disease. An animal study with non-human primates may serve as an example of the use of SPECT in addiction research. Rhesus monkeys that had experienced social isolation stress after birth displayed a persistent reduction in serotonin turnover during adulthood (as measured in the cerebro-spinal fluid; CSF). Low CSF serotonin concentrations were negatively correlated with the availability of serotonin transporters in the brainstem area, measured with [^{123}I]β-CIT and SPECT. The low serotonin turnover rate and the increased availability of brainstem serotonin transporters were correlated with a low reaction to alcohol, which predicts subsequent excessive alcohol intake in humans (Heinz *et al.* 1998*a*).

Methodological considerations and constraints

Several constraints have to be kept in mind when brain imaging studies with SPECT and PET are to be interpreted. How to quantify brain imaging data is of central importance.

Most perfusion studies of patients with neuropsychiatric disorders with SPECT show perfusion deficits compared with overall cerebral blood flow; however, it is difficult to distinguish hypoperfusion in certain brain areas from hyperperfusion in those brain areas that are used for comparison with the region of interest. This constraint is not a problem when using absolute methods, such as when FDG-PET or [^{15}O]water PET is used with arterial sampling, since methods to quantify glucose turnover and rCBF with these approaches have been established and validated (Andreasen 1988).

For receptor-binding studies, quantification depends on several factors. First, there should be a brain region that has no or very few neurotransmitter receptors or transporters, and which is strikingly similar to the region of interest. It can then be used to measure nonspecific uptake of a lipophilic radioligand, which has to be subtracted from total binding in the region of interest to measure the specific binding to neuroreceptors or transporters. Great care should be taken to assure that nonspecific binding in the control region is not systematically affected by disease-specific processes that are independent of those processes that change neuroreceptor density or availability. Nonspecific binding to brain tissue is often assessed by measuring radioactivity in a brain area that is mostly devoid of transporters or receptors. For example, there are few if any serotonin transporters in the cerebellum, which can thus be used to measure nonspecific uptake of β-CIT in the brain (Laruelle *et al.* 1993). However, chronic alcohol intoxication may be associated with cerebellar atrophy, which may then be an unreliable measure of nonspecific radioligand uptake (Heinz *et al.* 1998*c*). If a ratio between specific binding in the region of interest and nonspecific binding in the cerebellum is used to assess, for example, serotonin transporter availability in the brainstem (Laruelle *et al.* 1994), slight differences in unspecific uptake may greatly affect the measure of interest. Alternatively, the ratio of specific binding to the concentration of the free radioligand in plasma can be used to assess the binding potential, and is equivalent to B_{max}/K_d (e.g. the density of receptors/affinity) (Laruelle *et al.* 1994; Heinz *et al.* 1998*c*).

Secondly, pseudoequilibrium has to be established in the region of interest and in the control region. If this is not the case, then radioligand binding may still increase or decrease and measurements may depend upon blood flow or unspecific radioligand turnover rather then binding to neuroreceptors or other target structures (Heinz and Jones 2000). For example, β-CIT binding to serotonin transporters approaches equilibrium conditions about 3–4 h after injection (Laruelle *et al.* 1994; Pirker *et al.* 1995). If measurements are made too early, the studied system will not be in a near-equilibrium condition and will thus reflect radioligand delivery via brain perfusion and washout rather than transporter binding (Heinz and Jones 2000). Some radioligands never seem to reach an interindividually stable pseudoequilibrium during defined periods of time after bolus injection. Instead, maximum binding to target molecules varies between different subjects. In such situations, all study participants should be scanned continuously after radioligand application; however, this is often not feasible and may increase movement artifacts. The best solution may be to infuse the radioligand continuously and thus achieve a forced steady-state condition (Laruelle and Innis 1996; Laruelle *et al.* 1996).

Thirdly, there should be a reliable difference between total binding in a brain area rich in neuroreceptors or transporters, and nonspecific uptake in a control region. For example, the SPECT radioligand β-CIT binds to serotonin transporters all over the brain, but only the density in the brainstem and thalamus is high enough to give a reliable difference between specific binding to serotonin transporters and nonspecific uptake in brain areas mainly free of serotonin transporters, such as the cerebellum (Laruelle *et al.* 1993; Heinz *et al.* 1998c, Heinz and Jones 2000). One way to prove specific binding to receptors or transporters is *in vivo* displacement of radioligands by drugs that bind selectively to the receptor or transporter of interest. Laruelle *et al.* (1994) and Farde *et al.* (1994) demonstrated that, in humans β-CIT binding can be displaced selectively by selective serotonin reuptake inhibitors (SSRI) in the midbrain and thalamus, while in the basal ganglia, it can only be displaced by substances that bind specifically to dopamine transporters (see Fig. 7.2).

Fourthly, spatial resolution of PET and SPECT is limited. In PET, spatial resolution is at best about 4 mm, and in SPECT, resolution may be as good as 7 mm but usually ranges from 10 to 12 mm for most scanners. In neuroreceptor binding, as well as cerebral blood flow and glucose utilization studies, it is very helpful if individually coregistered magnetic resonance imaging (MRI) scans are used to place ROIs.

Fifthly, there is a considerable interindividual variance, which may even be enlarged if certain neuroreceptor or neurotransporter genotypes affect radioligand binding. For example, carrying a certain allele of the promoter for the serotonin transporter gene has been associated *in vitro* as well as *in vivo* with a twofold increase in serotonin transporter density and functional capacity (Lesch *et al.* 1996; Heinz *et al.* 2000b). If patients and control subjects are not matched for genotype, then accidental differences in the distribution of the genetic constitution of the serotonin transporter, e.g. between alcoholics and control subjects, may be mistaken for disease-associated differences in radioligand binding. Likewise, disease-specific differences may not be detected due to an accidental overrepresentation of certain genotypes with higher or lower bindings among control subjects or alcoholics.

If central glucose utilization or cerebral blood flow is measured during 'resting' conditions, patients may not be at rest but be anxious, tense, worried, tired, etc. Variance is greatly reduced if all subjects perform the same task. However, more variance can occur if task performance differs significantly between patients and control groups (Callicot *et al.* 1999), as is common. Reduced task performance may be associated with reduced activation of a certain brain region, while normal activation will be observed when subjects are matched for performance, e.g. if the subjects are able to complete the task successfully.

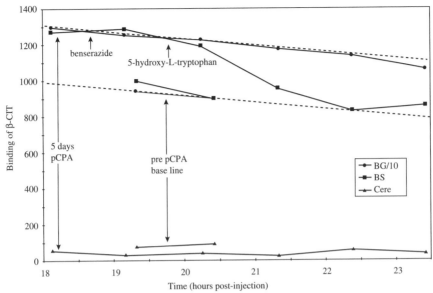

Fig. 7.2 Example of a neurotransmitter depletion and restoration study to assess intrasynaptic neurotransmitter concentrations (Jones *et al.* 1998). Binding of the radioligand β-CIT (2β-car-bomethoxy-3β-(4-[123I]iodophenyl)tropane) to serotonin transporters in the brainstem (BS) of a rhesus monkey was measured at baseline and again after 5 days of serotonin depletion induced by p-chlorophenylalanine (pCPA), which blocks serotonin production. A significant increase in β-CIT binding to serotonin transporters in the midbrain/brainstem reflected an increased availability of serotonin transporters after neurotransmitter depletion, which drastic-ally reduced competition between the radioligand and the endogenous neurotransmitter. When the blockade of serotonin production was bypassed by the application of 5-hydroxy-tryptophan, serotonin concentrations in the synapse were restored. The neurotransmitter serotonin could then compete with β-CIT for binding at serotonin transporters, and β-CIT binding was accordingly reduced to baseline levels (Original data provided by the authors, cf. Heinz *et al.* 2004). BG/10 = basal ganglia binding of β-CIT divided by 10. Cere = cerebellum binding of β–CIT. BS = brainstem binding of β-CIT.

In measuring neuroreceptors or transporters, one further potential limitation, that has recently been changed into an advantage, merits discussion. Radioligand binding competes with endogenous neurotransmitter concentrations in the synapse for bind-ing at the neuroreceptor or transport target site (Laruelle *et al.* 1993; Laruelle and Innis 1996; Abi-Dargham *et al.* 2000). This effect may limit data interpretation, since increased radioligand binding to receptors may be either due to a real increase in receptor density or to reduced release and concentration of neurotransmitters in the synapse. In any case, increased binding reflects low neurotransmitter concentrations relative to the binding sites. Systematic manipulation of neurotransmitters, e.g. via pharmacologically induced release or blockade of production, can be used to quantify changes in receptor binding, which reflect intrasynaptic neurotransmitter concentrations

(Laruelle and Innis 1996; Abi-Dargham *et al.* 2000). This procedure offers the unique opportunity to functionally assess *in vivo* neurotransmitter concentrations in different disease states and in normal control subjects, and is one of the currently most promising brain imaging techniques.

A conceptual framework for brain mapping in schizophrenia

Functional neuroimaging studies with PET and SPECT have demonstrated three patterns of abnormal cerebral blood flow in schizophrenia. First, abnormal blood flow and glucose utilization in the dorsolateral prefrontal cortex (DLPFC) have been associated with impaired executive functions and working memory (Weinberger and Lipska 1995). Secondly, dysfunction of temporal–limbic circuits has been associated with a disinhibition of subcortical dopamine release and the manifestation of positive symptoms (Laruelle *et al.* 1996; Heinz *et al.* 1999; Meyer-Lindenberg *et al.* 2002). Thirdly, positive symptoms such as auditory hallucinations have been associated with increased blood flow in subcortical, medial temporal, and limbic brain areas (Silbersweig *et al.*, 1995). The variety of symptoms and neuronal networks implied in the development of schizophrenia can best be understood if they are discussed in the light of a hypothesis that dates back to 1884, when Jackson (1927) distinguished between positive and negative symptoms. According to this hypothesis, the evolution of the brain renders complex brain centers, such as the frontal or temporolimbic cortex, more vulnerable to disease-associated dysfunction. The resulting loss of function causes negative symptoms, i.e. those clinical symptoms that reflect this loss of normal neuronal function. As a consequence of this primary loss of function, evolutionary older and more basic brain areas may be disinhibited, leading secondarily to the manifestation of positive symptoms, such as hallucinations or delusions.

The neurodevelopmental hypothesis of schizophrenia

A neurodevelopmental hypothesis of schizophrenia suggests that a dysfunction of the temporolimbic–frontal network, acquired early during individual development, may be associated with a disinhibition of subcortical neurocircuits, especially dopamine release in the striatum (Weinberger 1987; Marenco and Weinberger 2000; Hirsch and Weinberger 2003). A wide range of epidemiological and neuropathological findings have provided circumstantial evidence in support of the neurodevelopmental hypothesis of schizophrenia. However, the respective studies do not agree in all details, and questions remain as to which specific factors have to coincide to create a dysfunction of the frontal–temporolimbic network, which may interfere with subcortical dopamine release after puberty (Marenco and Weinberger 2000).

Brain imaging data have provided indirect support to some of the cornerstones of the neurodevelopmental hypothesis. Anatomical studies with CT and MRI allowed identification of structural abnormalities in specific brain regions. The most consistent findings are enlarged ventricles in the brain of schizophrenic patients and subtle changes in the temporal lobe. These changes appear to exist at the onset of illness and have been correlated with early developmental antecedents, such as obstetrical complications and neurological development (Marenco and Weinberger 2000). It has been speculated that the manifestation of psychotic symptoms after puberty may originate from the normal maturational processes of specific neuronal networks. Neuroimaging studies have provided some of the most consistent evidence that dysfunction of the prefrontal cortex is a characteristic of schizophrenia, and that the prefrontal cortex is among the latest maturing brain systems in primates.

Abnormal frontal cortex function: resting studies and studies during cognitive task performance

Because the frontal lobes are involved in executive function and because executive function deficits are characteristic of patients with schizophrenia, a series of cerebral blood flow or glucose utilization studies focused on dysfunctional frontal-lobe activation. A review of the literature shows that the so-called resting condition changes in frontal-lobe activity, while reported in many studies, are not consistent findings. It is likely that the inconsistency in this literature relates to the poorly controlled nature of the resting state. Furthermore, medication and clinical state can affect brain activity and add noise to resting blood flow data. For example, Miller *et al.* (1997) observed that antipsychotic medication significantly increased the mean relative cerebral perfusion in the left basal ganglia. Furthermore, different antipsychotic drugs may result in different effects on brain perfusion, and studies of the influence of neuroleptics on cortical metabolism have brought mixed results. None the less, most studies suggest that there is some decrease in frontal cerebral blood flow and glucose utilization that cannot be explained by medication alone (Table 7.2).

It is also unclear whether hypofrontality in the resting condition worsens during the course of the disease. Inconsistencies in the literature could be due to variation in patients' symptoms. Specifically, negative symptoms have been consistently associated with decreased frontal metabolism (Kotrla and Weinberger, 1995). Some authors have observed that distinctive patterns of cerebral blood flow are associated with different syndromes, such as psychomotor poverty, disorganization, and reality distortion (hallucinations and delusions). Liddle *et al.* (1992) observed that psychomotor poverty and disorganization, obtained from a psychopathology symptom rating scale, are associated with altered perfusion at different loci in the prefrontal cortex. Ratings taken to reflect reality distortion, on the other hand, were associated with altered perfusion in the medial temporal lobe. Altogether, the variety of results during resting functional studies in schizophrenia is most probably due to the heterogeneous symptoms present in this disease and the poor control of the differing aspects of the resting state between one individual and another.

More consistent results have been achieved when subjects were scanned while performing cognitive tasks. The advantage of this method is that it controls, to some degree, for mental state, and that hypotheses can be derived from studies in normals that indicate which brain circuits should be active during particular cognitive tasks.

Table 7.2 Selected SPECT and PET studies under resting conditions

Reference	Diagnosis, number of patients	Test	Brain imaging method	Hypofrontality	Other findings
Satoh et al. (1993)	Catatonia, n = 6; schizophrenia, n = 13; controls, n = 7	At rest	IMP-SPECT	↓ rCBF in the frontoparietal lobe in all schizophrenics.	–
Yuasa et al. (1995)	Schizophrenia (medicated), n = 26	At rest	IMP-SPECT	Psychomotor poverty syndrome was correlated with ↓ rCBF in bilateral superior frontal areas; disorganization syndrome was correlated with ↑ rCBF in bilateral anterior cingulate and ↓ rCBF in bilateral middle frontal areas; alienation syndrome was correlated with ↑ rCBF in the right inferior frontal area and parietal area	Psychomotor poverty correlated with ↑ rCBF in the left thalamus and right basal ganglia
O'Connell et al. (1995)	Schizophrenia, n = 21; mania, n = 11; controls, n = 15	At rest	IMP-SPECT	Both manic and schizophrenic patients showed cortical tracer uptake heterogeneity	Significant ↑ in tracer uptake in lobes was observed in both patient groups

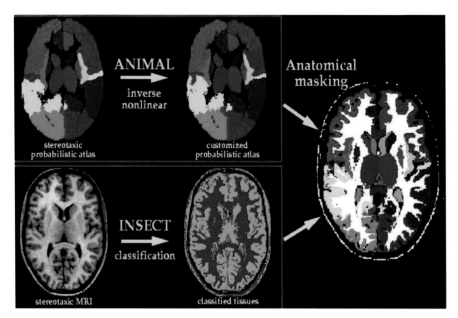

Plate 1(a). INSECT (intensity normalized stereotaxic environment for classification of tissue) is an automated program for classifying each voxel of a brain MR image into gray matter, white matter, or cerebrospinal fluid, based on the intensity of the voxel. ANIMAL (automatic nonlinear image matching and anatomical labeling) is also an automated approach that labels a voxel's location in space based on prior anatomic knowledge. The MNI (Montreal Neurological Institute) program is unique in that it combines the two techniques. This allows for an automated voxel-intensity and anatomically informed classification of the brain tissue (reproduced from Collins *et al.* 1999, with permission). See Chapter 3, Fig. 3.1.

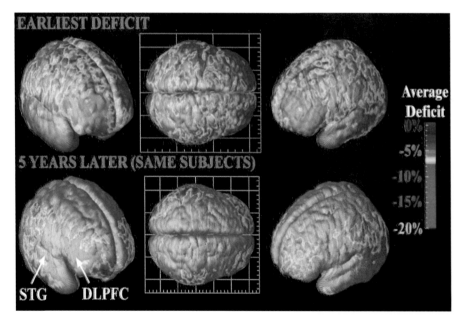

Plate 1(b). Progressive and region-specific loss of cortical gray matter in childhood-onset schizophrenia compared with age- and sex-matched community controls. STG, superior temporal sulcus; DLPFC, dorsolateral prefontal cortex. Loss of gray matter is shown as deficit per year (reproduced from Thompson *et al.* 2001, with permission). See Chapter 3, Fig. 3.6.

(a) (b) (c)

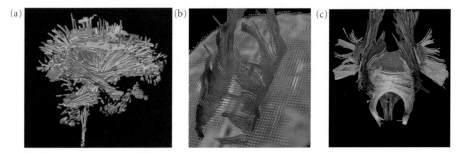

Plate 2(a). Examples of *in vivo* tracking of white matter fibre bundles from DT-MRI data. (a) The three-dimensional information contained within **D** can be visualized by identifying regions of linear (white matter tracts) and planar (crossing fibres) diffusion and representing them as red streamtubes and green stream-surfaces, respectively. This figure shows geometric models representing the diffusion metric data obtained from a 33-year-old female volunteer. Such methods provide a powerful way of tracking fibres throughout the entire brain. The number of linear, planar, and spherical diffusion voxels in a region can also be determined (Zhang *et al.* 2004). A more standard approach is to depict the direction of fastest diffusion ε_1 using streamlines. Such an analysis is shown for the same volunteer at the level of the centrum semiovale (b) and for the whole brain (c). See Chapter 5, Fig. 5.6.

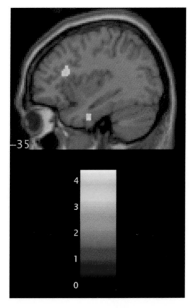

Plate 2(b). Statistical parametric map overlaid on a T_1-weighted image, showing FA reduction in the left uncinate fasciculus and left arcuate fasciculus for 30 schizophrenic patients compared with 30 matched controls (Burns *et al.* 2003). The threshold for the analysis was set at $P = 0.001$ (uncorrected). The colour bar shows Z values corresponding to colours in the figure. See Chapter 5. Fig. 5.7.

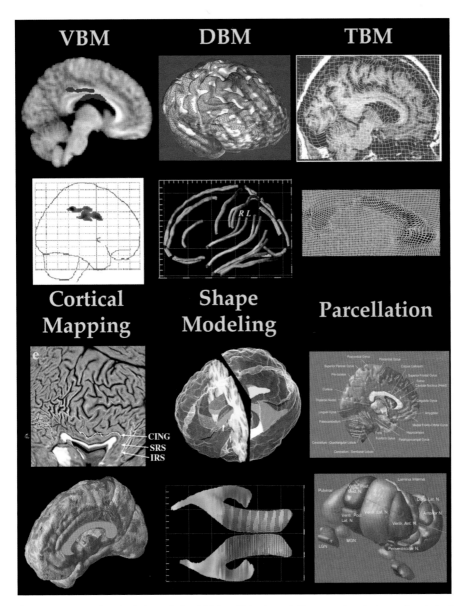

Plate 3. Taxonomy of methods for analyzing MRI data. This schematic illustrates six major types of analysis of structural images, showing some of the data used in each case (see Table 6.1 for the key concepts underlying each method). Voxel-based morphometry (VBM; top left panels) compares anatomy voxel by voxel to find voxels (shown here in blue) where the tissue classification (gray, white matter, CSF) depends on diagnosis or other factors. Results are typically plotted in stereotaxic space (lower panel), and their significance assessed using random field or permutation methods (see text for details). Deformation-based morphometry (DBM) can be used to analyze shape differences in the cortex, or brain asymmetries (colored sulci: red colors show regions of greatest asymmetry). Tensor-based morphometry (TBM) uses three-dimensional warping fields with millions of degrees of freedom (top) to recover and study local shape differences in anatomy across subjects or over time (red colors indicate growth rates in the corpus callosum of a young child). Other methods focus on structures such as the cerebral cortex, which can be flattened to assist the analysis (bottom left), or the lateral ventricles ('shape modeling'). If anatomic structures are represented as parametric surface meshes (Thompson *et al.* 2000*d*), their shapes can be compared, their variability can be visualized, or they can be used to show where gray matter is lost (e.g. in Alzheimer's disease: bottom left panel, red colors denote greatest gray matter loss in the limbic and entorhinal areas). Fine-scale anatomical parcellation (lower right) can be used compare structure volumes across groups, or to create hand-labeled templates that can be automatically warped onto new MRI brain datasets, creating regions of interest where analyses are performed. [VBM data courtesy of Elizabeth Sowell, Ph.D. (adapted from Sowell *et al.* 2000) and parcellation data courtesy of Jacopo Annese, Ph.D., UCLA Laboratory of Neuro Imaging]. See Chapter 6, Fig. 6.1.

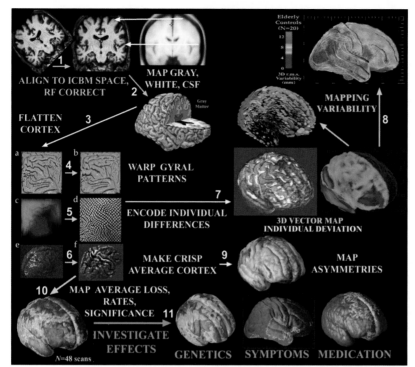

Plate 4. An image analysis pipeline. This schematic illustrates the sequence of analysis steps in an MRI study (Thompson *et al.* 2001*b*). By using several of these processing modules, aninvestigator can create maps that reveal how brain structure varies in large populations, differs in disease, and is modulated by genetic or therapeutic factors. See Chapter 6, Fig. 6.2. for full details.

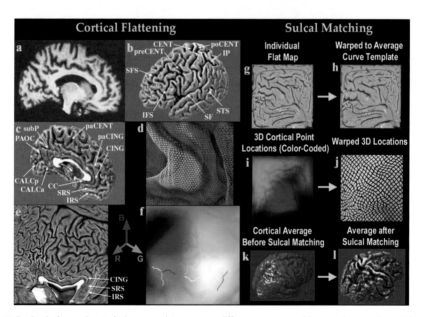

Plate 5. Cortical mapping techniques used to measure differences across subjects and across time. Using cortical flattening (a–f), and sulcal matching (g–l), an average model of the cortex (l) can be built for a group of subjects. Sulcal landmarks are defined on individual cortices, and this enables data to be averaged from corresponding regions of cortex across subjects, reinforcing systematic features. See text for details of this procedure. [Sulci shown in (b), (c) include the superior and inferior frontal (SFS, IFS), pre- and postcentral (preCENT, poCENT), central (CENT), intraparietal (IP), superior temporal (STS), Sylvian fissures (SF), paracentral (paCENT), cingulate (CING) and paracingulate (paCING), subparietal (subP), callosal (CC), superior and inferior rostral (SRS, IRS), parieto-occipital (PAOC), anterior and posterior calcarine (CALCa/p) sulci.]. See Chapter 6, Fig. 6.7.

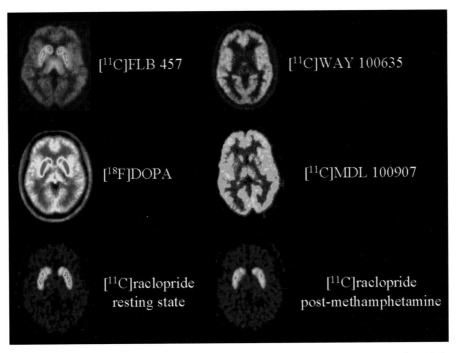

Plate 9. Transverse brain sections of PET scans using a variety of radioligands. The predominantly cortical signal of [^{11}C]MDL100907 and [^{11}C] WAY100635, representing 5-HT$_{2A}$ and 5-HT$_{1A}$ receptors, respectively, can be contrasted with the mainly striatal signal of the dopaminergic ligands. See Chapter 8, Fig. 8.1.

The 'Eyes' Task

Concerned/Angry

Male/Female

Wisconsin Card Sort Task

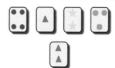

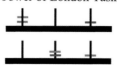

Tower of London Task

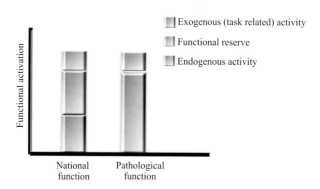

Plate 10(a). Examples of executive function tasks used in fMRI. All these tasks require judgements—as to the displayed emotion (versus a sex decision control), the matching card, and the minimum number of moves, respectively. See Chapter 9, Fig. 9.1.

█ Exogenous (task related) activity

█ Functional reserve

█ Endogenous activity

Functional activation

National function   Pathological function

Plate 10(b). Capacity model of normal and pathological function. See Chapter 9, Fig. 9.3.

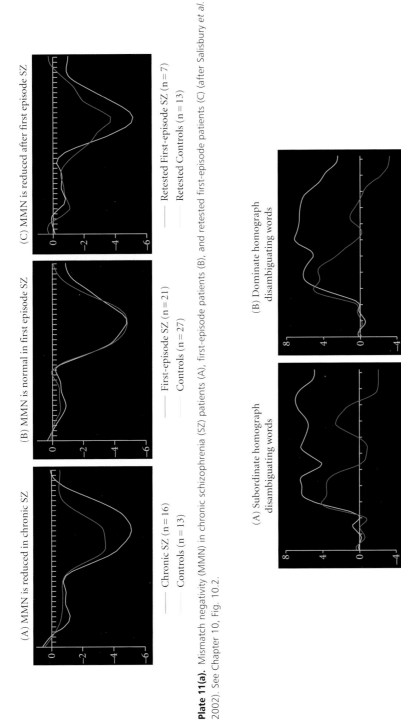

Plate 11(a). Mismatch negativity (MMN) in chronic schizophrenia (SZ) patients (A), first-episode patients (B), and retested first-episode patients (C) (after Salisbury et al. 2002). See Chapter 10, Fig. 10.2.

Plate 11(b). N400 in a homograph task in schizophrenic (SZ) and normal control individuals. See Chapter 10, Fig. 10.4.

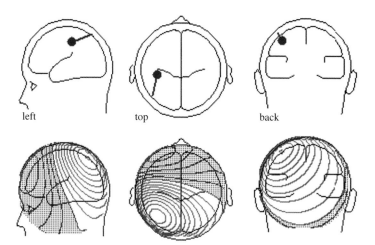

left   top   back

Plate 12(a). Brian electric field topography generated by a single model dipole source. The upper row shows the three-dimensional location of the dipole. The lower row shows the field generated by that dipole shown with equipotential field lines (shaded [blue] = negative, clear [red] = positive). Note that although a point-like source model has been used, the fields obtained extend over the entire scalp. Picture generated using the Dipole Simulator by Patrick Berg. See Chapter 12, Fig. 12.1.

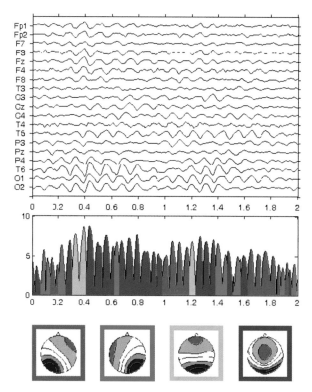

Plate 12(b). Example of a 2-second multichannel EEG segment (upper part) parsed into spatially defined microstates. The middle section of the figure shows the momentary field strength (Global Field Power, vertical), colour-scale coded with the microstate class identified as function of time (horizontal axis). The microstate topographies with their colour-scale code are shown in the lower part, they were constructed from a large normative population (Koenig et al. 2002). See Chapter 12, Fig. 12.4.

Ebmeier et al. (1995)	Schizophrenia, n = 70; schizophreniform psychosis, n = 60; controls, n = 20	At rest	[99Tcm] Exametazime	Active psychotic patients not taking drugs showed ↑ uptake in the frontal cortex; ↓ uptake occurred in the mesial frontal cortex of schizophrenic patients, particularly if taking drugs	–
Vita et al. (1995)	Schizophrenia (drug naive and drug free), n = 17; controls, n = 12	At rest	[99Tcm]-HMPAO-SPECT	Drug-naive patients showed a significant bilateral ↓ rCBF in the mesial, dorsolateral, and basal prefrontal cortex, in the temporal cortex, and in the subcortical gray structures; no hypofrontality in patients who had undergone various periods of pharmacological washout	↓ rCBF in the basal ganglia and thalamus of the drug-naive. but not the drug-free patients
Batista et al. (1995)	Schizophrenia (drug naive), n = 15	At rest	[99Tcm]-HMPAO-SPECT	Hypofrontality, especially in the left frontal lobe.	–
Holcomb et al. (1996)	Schizophrenia (teated with haloperidol), n = 12	Fixed dose of medication, after 5 days and after 30 days of pause	[18F]FDG PET	In the frontal cortex and in the anterior cingulate, metabolism increased 30 days after withdrawal, indicating that in those two cortical areas haloperidol depressed glucose metabolism	Decrease in glucose metabolism in the caudate and putamen 30 days after withdrawal

Table 7.2 (continued)

Reference	Diagnosis, number of patients	Test	Brain imaging method	Hypofrontality	Other findings
Klemm et al. (1996)	Schizophrenia, n = 17; depression n = 7	At rest	SPECT	↓ rCBF in five of the schizophrenic patients; Patients with ↓ rCBF showed higher severity of symptoms	Hypoperfusion of the left temporal lobe was observed in seven of the schizophrenic and five of the depressed patients; ↓ rCBF in the temporal cortex was significantly correlated with positive symptoms
Sabri et al. (1997)	Schizophrenia (drug free), n = 24; of these n = 22 controlled after medication	At rest before and after medication	[⁹⁹Tcm] HMPAO-SPECT	↓ rCBF in frontal cortex was associated with negative symptoms before and after medication; delusional ideas, hallucinatory behavior and suspiciousness were negatively correlated with bifrontal, cingulate, left temporal and left thalamic rCBF before medication	After therapy, only negative symptoms correlated to hypoperfusion in the bifrontal, bitemporal, cingulate, basal ganglia and thalamic ROIS.
Russell et al. (1997)	Schizophrenia, n = 22; controls n = 22	At rest	[⁹⁹Tcm] HMPAO-SPECT	No significant changes	↓ rCBF in the left temporal lobes of schizophrenics

Study	Sample	Condition	Technique	Result	Result
Sachdev et al. (1997)	Schizophrenia, n = 22 (n = 15 late onset, n = 7 early onset); controls n = 27	At rest	[^{99}Tc^m] HMPAO-SPECT	Late-onset schizophrenics showed ↓ rCBF in bilateral frontal and temporal lobes; early-onset subjects had ↓ rCBF in frontal cortex versus controls	↓ Left-to-right hemisphere blood flow ratios; ↓ rCBF in temporal lobe in late- but not early-onset schizophrenics versus controls temporal lobe perfusion correlated with mini-mental-scores and verbal memory measures
Min et al. (1999)	Schizophrenia (drug naive), n = 17	At rest	[^{99}Tc^m]ECD-SPECT	↑ rCBF in the left frontal region correlated with positive symptoms	Negative symptoms were correlated with ↓ rCBF in the left thalamic region, positive symptoms correlated with ↓ rCBF in the temporal region
Lauer M. et al. (2001)	Schizophrenia (chronic catatonic schizophrenia), n = 3	At rest	[^{18}F]FDG PET	Both patients with the simple speech-sluggish catatonia showed bilateral thalamic hypermetabolism and bilateral hypometabolism of the frontal cortex, especially on the left side	During their permanent hallucinations, all catatonic patients showed a clear bitemporal hypometabolism
Desco M et al. (2003)	Schizophrenia, n = 17 (recent onset); n = 34 (long-term treated); controls n = 18	At rest	[^{18}F]FDG PET	Certain degree of hypofrontality were observed in the long-term group when compared to recent-onset patients	Decreased activation of the visual cortex in recent-onset and long-term patients, when compared to healthy controls

ECD, ethyl cysteinate dimer; FDG, fluorodeoxyglucose; HMPAO, hexamethyl propylene amine oxime; IMP, iodoamphetamine; PET, positron emission tomography; rCBF, regional cerebral blood flow; ROI, region of interest; SPECT, single-photon emission computed tomography; ^{99}Tc^m, technetium-99m.

Table 7.3 Selected SPECT and PET studies during cognitive activation

Reference	Diagnosis, number of patients	Test	Brain imaging method	Frontal cortex	Other findings
Sagawa et al. (1990–91)	Schizophrenia, $n = 59$	Wisconsin Card Sorting Test (WCST) (at rest and during activation)	^{133}Xe-SPECT	↓ rCBF in frontal cortex correlated with the number of perseverative errors in WCST and moderately with anhedonia	—
Paulman et al. (1990)	Schizophrenia, $n = 40$ (including 20 unmedicated patients); mached controls, $n = 31$	WCST, Luria-Nebraska Battery (at rest and during activation)	Dynamic-SPECT	Bifrontal and bitemporal ↓ rCBF; frontal deficits were most prominent in paranoic patients; left frontal ↓ rCBF was associated with neuropsychological impairment in WCST and Luria-Nebraska Battery	Right temporal deficits were most prominent in non-paranoic patients; no medication effects; hemispheric ↑ rCBF was correlated with the presence of positive schizophrenic symptom
Sagawa et al. (1990)	Schizophrenia, $n = 57$	WCST, Word Fluency Test (WFT), Maze Test (at rest and during activation)	^{133}Xe-SPECT corrected by using PECO2	↓ rCBF in the frontal cortex correlated with ↓ performance in the WCST	—
Daniel et al. (1991)	Schizophrenia, $n = 10$	WCST, Sensorimotor Controls Task Test performed	^{133}Xe-SPECT + dextroamphetamine	Amphetamine produced modest, non-significant global ↓ rCBF; the amphetamine group	—

Study	Sample	Task	Method	Findings		
Andreasen et al. (1992)	Schizophrenia, n = 36; controls, n = 15	Tower of London, looking at ondulating colored shapes on a video monitor	133Xe-SPECT	Hypofrontality in correlation with negative symptoms	—	double-blind, placebo-controlled; showed task-dependent activation (↑ rCBF) in the left DLPFC.
Buchsbaum et al. (1992)	Schizoprenia, (drug naive), n = 18; controls, n = 20	Continuous Performance Test	[18F]FDG PET	Relative hypofrontality in schizophrenia.	Significantly reduced ratios of inferior and medial frontal regions to occipital cortex were found, together with diminished metabolism in the basal ganglia	
Kawasaki et al. (1993)	Schizoprenia, n = 10; controls, n = 10	WCST (at rest and during activation)	[99Tcm]HMPA O-SPECT	↓ rCBF during WCST in the left medial prefrontal cortex correlated possitively with the number of unique errors	↑ rCBF in the left hippocampus during resting conditions; ↑ rCBF in the fronto-parietal cortex in patients at rest and during WCST	
Rubin et al. (1994a)	Schizophrenia/sc hizophreniform disorder, n = 24; controls, n = 17	WCST (at rest and during activation)	[99Tcm] HMPAO-SPECT	At rest and during activation ↓ rCBF in the prefrontal regions	↑ rCBF in the left striatum during activation	
Parellada et al. (1994)	Schizophrenia (drug naive), n = 6; controls, n = 6	WCST (at rest and during activation)	[99Tcm] HMPAO-SPECT	At rest ↑ rCBF in PFC in schizophrenics; failure to increase rCBF during WCST in the PFC	Control group had lower prefrontal rCBF at rest and showed significant increase during WCST	

Table 7.3 (continued)

Reference	Diagnosis, number of patients	Test	Brain imaging method	Frontal cortex	Other findings
Rubin et al. (1994b)	Schizophrenia, $n = 50$; controls, $n = 25$	WCST (at rest and during activation)	[^{99}Tc^m] HMPA O-SPECT	↓ rCBF in the prefrontal cortex. Negative symptoms correlated with ↑ rCBF in the prefrontal cortex	Positive symptoms correlated positively with ↑ rCBF in the striatum during activation
Busatto et al. (1995)	Schizophrenia, $n = 18$	Memory-activation paradigm	[^{99}Tc^m]HMPA O-SPECT	No significant changes.	↑ rCBF during testing in the left basal ganglia
Andreasen et al. (1996)	Schizophrenia, $n = 14$; control, $n = 13$	Practiced recall	PET (75 mCi[^{15}O] water)	During the practiced task, the patients showed decreased flow in fronto-thalamic–cerebellar regions	Decreases are seen in the patients during the novel task in the anterior cingulate, mammillary bodies, bilateral anterior temporal regions, and bilateral lenticular nuclei
Katz M et al. (1996)	Schizophrenia (never medicated), $n = 18$; control, $n = 22$	Continuous performance test	[^{18}F]FDG PET	Schizophrenics showed correlation of glucose metabolic rate in the anterior thalamus with the frontal cortex	Correlations of the frontal lobe with other regions were more positive in normal controls than schizophrenics; controls had three correlational paths from the frontal cortex (to temporal cortex, ventral anterior thalamus, and dorsal medial thalamus) with significantly more positive correlations than schizophrenics

Study	Subjects	Task	Technique	Findings	Correlations/other
Steinberg et al. (1996)	Schizophrenia, n = 13 (including six drug naive patients); controls, n = 7	WCST, number matching (at rest and during activation)	[133Xe] D-SPECT	↓ rCBF during number matching and WCST and number matching task in first break patients compared to normals; less absolute and relative left middle frontal rCBF	↓ rCBF in chronic patients in the left middle frontal cortex
Gracia Marco et al. (1997)	Schizophrenia, n = 18; controls, n = 10	WCST (at rest and during activation)	[99Tcm] HMPAO-SPECT	Hypofrontality at rest and while performing WCST	–
Parellada et al. (1998)	Schizophrenia, n = 25; controls, n = 15	WCST (at rest and during activation)	[99Tcm]HMPAO-SPECT	During WCST patients failed to activate the frontal lobe	The left anterior temporal rCBF at rest correlated with the total score in the Scale for the Assesment of positive Symptoms
Blackwood et al. (1999)	Schizophrenia, n = 19; high risk asymtomatic relatives n = 36; controls, n = 34	Memory tasks, P300 event-related potential, Independent from brain imaging	[99Tcm]HMPAO-SPECT	↓ rCBF in the left inferior prefrontal and anterior cingulate cortex at rest; perfusion in the left inferior prefrontal cortex correlated positively with verbal memory and P300 amplitude	↑ rCBF bilaterally in subcortical regions at rest
Crespo-Fancorro et al. (1999)	Schizophrenia, n = 14; control, n = 13	Rey Auditory Verbal Learning Test	MR, PET (75 mCi[15 O]water	When recalling the practiced word lists, the patients showed decreased flow in the left dorsolateral prefrontal cortex, bilateral medial frontal cortex, left supplementary motor area, left thalamus, left cerebellar regions, anterior vermis, and right cuneus	During the novel memory task, the patients showed decreased flow in the right anterior cingulate, right thalamus, and bilateral cerebellum (left greater than right) relative to the control subjects

Table 7.3 (continued)

Reference	Diagnosis, number of patients	Test	Brain imaging method	Frontal cortex	Other findings
Chen et al. (2000)	Schizophrenia, $n = 1$	WCST, Semantic Verbal Fluency Test, logical memory in Weschler Memory Scale	[^{99}Tc^m]HMPA O-SPECT	Bilateral prefrontal metabolic under-activity was associated with negative symptoms	↓ rCBF in the temporal left area. After response to clozapine, the right prefrontal activity normalized
Toone et al. (2000)	Schizophrenia, $n = 72$	WCST	[^{99}Tc^m]HMPA O-SPECT	No significant changes	The poorly performing group showed a modest ↑ rCBF in the left anterior cingulate
Hazlett et al. (2000)	Schizophrenics (unmedicated patients), $n = 20$; controls, $n = 32$	California Verbal Learning Test	[^{18}F]FDG PET	Patients exhibited hypofrontality (lower ratio of frontal to occipital rGMR) compared with normal subjects, which associated with increased perseveration errors	Among patients, greater use of the serial-ordering strategy was associated with decreased regional glucose metabolic rates (rGMR) in frontal cortex and increased rGMR in temporal cortex
Clark et al. (2001)	Schizophrenia, $n = 26$; controls, $n = 32$	University of Pennsylvania Smell Identification Test	[^{18}F]FDG PET	Patients with schizophrenia had reduced rates of glucose metabolism in the right and left thalamus that reached significance if not corrected for multiple comparisons	

Reference	Subjects	Task	Method	Findings	
Liu et al. (2002)	Schizophrenia, n = 21; controls n = 12	WCST	[99Tcm]ECD-SPECT	Schizophrenics: ↓ rCBF in left frontal lobe during WCST as well as during resting conditions; executive function deficits correlated with ↓ rCBF in the left prefrontal cortex	Interhemispheric differences (↓ rCBF in left frontal lobe during WCST) were seen during WCST, but not under resting conditions in schizophrenics
Buchsbaum et al. (2002)	Schizophrenia, n = 10 (unremitting and severe course), n = 17 (remitting course)	California serial verbal learning task	[18F]FDG PET	Unremitting patients were characterized by lower metabolic rates in the temporal lobe and cingulate gyrus and lower fronto/occipital ratios than the remitting subtype patients	Lower metabolic rates in the right striatum in unremitting versus remitting patients

DLPFC, dorsolateral prefrontal cortex; ECD, ethyl cysteinate dimer ; FDG, fluorodeoxyglucose; HMPAO, hexamethyl propylene amine oxime; PECO2, end-tidal carbon dioxide concentration values; PET, positron emission tomography; PFC, prefrontal cortex; rCBF, regional cerebral blood flow; rGMR, regional glucose metabolic rate; SPECT, single-photon emission computed tomography; 99Tcm, technetium-99m; 133Xe, xenon-133.

Numerous studies have shown that schizophrenic patients displayed dysfunctional activation of their frontal lobes during frontally mediated tasks, regardless of antipsychotic treatment or of chronicity of illness (Table 7.3). Since a range of cognitive tasks are associated with frontal cortical function, the precise location of underactivated cortical areas depends on the task being performed.

A series of studies have centered on working memory, the ability to keep information 'online' and to manipulate it. Several studies used the Wisconsin Card Sorting Test (WCST), which in normal individuals activates a network involving the prefrontal, superior parietal, and medial temporal cortices. Most PET and SPECT studies observed that in schizophrenics who performed poorly on the test, the WCST failed to activate the dorsolateral prefrontal cortex (DLPFC) (Table 7.3). Reduced frontal activation has not been observed in Raven's Progressive Matrices Test, which requires similar abstract reasoning and problem solving as the WCST, but does not appear to be as dependent on prefrontal cortical processing. Raven's task primarily activates posterior cortical areas in control subjects and schizophrenic patients, and does not show specific prefrontal regional cerebral blood flow engagement. These studies indicate that not all abstract cognitive reasoning is associated with prefrontal activation. Similarly, studies during verbal fluency or motor control paradigms rarely find differences in prefrontal activation between schizophrenic patients and normal control subjects (Tables 7.4 and 7.5).

Several factors have been identified that interact with prefrontal activation in schizophrenics and normal control subjects. First, reduced medial temporal lobe volumes in schizophrenic patients, as detected with MRI, are correlated with reduced cerebral blood flow in the DLPFC during the WCST (Kotrla and Weinberger 1995). This finding indicates that the severity of temporolimbic dysfunction may interact with reduced frontal activation during certain cognitive tasks. Secondly, studies with functional MRI revealed that prefrontal activation depends upon the amount of information handled by the frontal cortices (Callicott et al. 1999). When a parametric n-back working memory task was used, normal controls increased prefrontal activation with increasing working memory load. However, when a certain capacity constraint was reached, further increase of working memory load was associated with a decrease in prefrontal activation and task performance. Brain areas within the DLPFC showed an 'inverted-U'-shaped neurophysiological response from lowest to highest cognitive load, indicating capacity constraints on the response of the prefrontal cortex. In schizophrenics, a strong activation of the frontal cortices was observed at a relatively low working memory load, while reduced activation was observed when memory load was increased. When schizophrenics and normal control subjects were compared during the performance of a task with a relatively high working memory load, hypofrontality was indeed observed. However, when subjects were matched for performance and the average working memory load was accordingly reduced in schizophrenic patients, no differences or increases in prefrontal activation were observed (Callicott et al. 1998, 1999; Manoach et al. 2000). Furthermore, when schizophrenic patients performed tasks with a high working memory load, they showed increased spatial heterogeneity of DLPFC activation and also activated the basal ganglia and thalamus, a finding that may reflect dysfunctional frontostriatal circuitry in schizophrenia (Manoach *et al.* 2000). Increased activation of the prefrontal cortex was also observed when schizophrenic patients performed a selective attention task with the same accuracy as healthy controls (Weiss *et al.* 2003).

Genotype effects on prefrontal brain activation

Another variable that may influence prefrontal function during working memory performance is genetic variation of the catechol-*O*-methyl-transferase (COMT) gene. In the prefrontal cortex, there is a scarcity of dopamine transporter, so that synaptic dopamine concentrations are not regulated by presynaptic dopamine reuptake. Instead, extracellular dopamine is metabolized by COMT, which thus plays a more important role in terminating the extracellular activity of dopamine at dopamine receptors. A common functional polymorphism in the COMT gene (Val[108/158]Met) accounts for a fourfold variation in enzyme activity and presumably dopamine catabolism. Patients who carry the genotype that metabolizes dopamine more slowly, and who presumably have higher prefrontal dopamine concentrations, had better performance on the WCST compared with subjects who carry a genotype that metabolizes extracellular dopamine rapidly (Egan *et al.*, 2001). A similar relationship was found in schizophrenic subjects, who altogether performed on a much lower level. Relatives of schizophrenics showed intermediate performance and may have additional protective factors that prevent the manifestation of psychotic symptoms (Egan *et al.*, 2001), but the effect of COMT on WCST performance was analogous.

In functional brain imaging, subjects carrying the genotype with lower dopamine concentrations showed increased activation of the dorsolateral prefrontal cortex and anterior cingulate, which was attributed to greater inefficiency of brain area recruitment. Altogether, these findings indicate that prefrontal activation in schizophrenia is subject to a multitude of influences, including the degree of disorganization in the temporolimbic cortex, metabolization of prefrontal dopamine, task difficulty with respect to capacity constraints in working memory, and the type of task used to activate the frontal cortex.

Brain mapping of the task-relevant activation of different fronto-striatal–thalamic neurocircuits

In a study by Hazlett *et al.* (2000), verbal memory performance and relative glucose metabolic utilization were simultaneously assessed in unmedicated schizophrenic patients. Similar to working memory tasks, a decreased frontal cortex glucose utilization rate was found. Patients also showed increased glucose utilization rates in the temporal cortex, which correlated with the use of an inefficient strategy (serial-ordering instead of semantic clustering) when patients tried to memorize a word list. When patients tried to recall novel word lists, they showed decreased blood flow in the anterior

Table 7.4 Verbal Fluency tests

Reference	Diagnosis, number of patients	Test	Brain imaging method	Hypofrontality	Other findings
Ford et al. (1992)	Schizophrenia, n = 25, right-handed	Word-fluency Task (at rest and during activation)	[^{99}Tc^{m}]HMPAO-SPECT	↑ Ventricular-brain ratio correlated with ↓ ratio of right medial frontal blood flow	
Busatto et al. (1994)	Schizophrenia, n = 10; controls, n = 10	Verbal memory task	[^{99}Tc^{m}]HMPAO-SPECT	No significant changes	No differences in activation of the medial temporal lobe
Scottish Schizophrenia Research Group (1998) pp. 440–9	Schizophrenia, n = 38; controls, n = 38	Verbal fluency task (before and after receiving antipsychotic drug treatment)	SPECT	Hypofrontality before and after drug-treatment	Increased blood flow in the putamen after drug treatment
Mellers et al. (1998)	Schizophrenia, n = 11; schizophrenia-like psychosis of epilepsy (SLPE), n = 12; epilepsy, n = 16	Verbal fluency task, word repetition task (at rest and during activation)	[^{99}Tc^{m}]HMPAO-SPECT	During the verbal fluency task, patients with primary schizophrenia showed a greater ↑ rCBF in the anterior cingulate than the other two groups	Patients with SLPE differed from both other groups by showing ↓ rCBF in the left superior temporal gyrus during performance of a verbal fluency task compared with a word repetition task

Study	Subjects	Technique	Task	Findings in patients	Findings in controls
Nohara et al. (2000)	Schizophrenia, n = 10; controls, n = 9	Verbal learnig task, Verbal repetition task (at rest and during activation)	[99Tcm]ECD-SPECT	No significant frontal lobe activation in left inferior and left anterior cingulate region during verbal learning task in patients as compared to controls	In normal controls, rCBF in the left inferior frontal and left anterior cingulate regions was significantly increased during the verbal learning task, compared with the verbal repetition task
Chen et al. (2000)	Schizophrenia, n = 1	WCST, semantic verbal fluency test, logical memory, Wechsler Memory Scale, WAIS-R verbal subscales	[99Tcm]HMPAO-SPECT	↓ rCBF in the bilateral prefrontal cortex correlated with negative symptoms, executive neurocognitive dysfunction and the treatment-resistant state; after response to clozapine, the right prefrontal activity returned to a normal level	–
Ashton et al. (2000)	Schizoprenia (drug naive), n = 39	Verbal fluency test	SPECT	↓ rCBF in the anterior cingulate during verbal fluency test PANSS negative scores correlate negatively with rCBF in the cingulate gyrus	–

ECD, ethyl cysteinate dimer; HMPAO, hexamethyl propylene amine oxide; PANSS, positive and negative syndrome scale; rCBF, regional cerebral blood flow; SLPE, schizophrenia-like psychosis of epilepsy; SPECT, single-photon emission tomography; 99Tcm, technetium-99m; WAIS-R, Wechsles Adult Intelligence Scale Revised; WCST, Wisconsin Card Sorting Test.

Table 7.5 Motor tasks

Reference	Diagnosis, number of patients	Test	Brain imaging method	Frontal cortex	Other
Gunther et al. (1991)	Schizophrenia, $n = 31$; controls, $n = 31$	Simple motor activation	[133Xe]SPECT	No significant changes	In controls, strictly contralatera activation after motor task, patients with positive symptoms showed diffuse ↑ rCBF, patients with negative symptoms showed no reaction
Crawford et al (1996)	Schizophrenia, $n = 18$	WCST, anti-saccade task (at rest and during activation)	[99 Tcm]HMPAO-SPECT	↓ rCBF in the high error group bilaterally in the anterior cingulate	↓ rCBF in the high error group bilaterally in the bilateral insula and left striattum
Matsui et al. (1997)	Schizophrenia, $n = 23$; controls, $n = 23$	Saccadic-eye-movements (simple stationary targets)	[99Tcm]HMPAO-SPECT	No significant changes	Some patients view the stationary targets too fast, which may be related to dysfunction in the limbic–parietal association area in the left hemisphere
Malaspina et al. (1999)	Schizophrenia, $n = 6$; controls, $n = 8$	Visual fixation	[99Tcm]HMPAO-SPECT	Left prefrontal hypoperfusion in schizophrenic compared with control subjects	Compared controls patients had medial temporal lobe hyperperfusion

HMPAO, hexamethyl propylene amine oxime; rCBF, regional cerebral blood flow; SPECT, single-photon emission computed tomography; 99Tcm, technetium-99m; WCST, Wisconsin Card Sorting Test; 133Xe, xenon-133.

cingulate and cerebellum (Crespo-Facorro *et al.* 1999). When they recalled a practiced word list, decreased flow was observed in the left dorsolateral prefrontal cortex, bilateral medial frontal cortex, left supplementary motor area, left thalamus, left cerebellar regions, anterior vermis, and right cuneus (Crespo-Facorro *et al.* 1999). These findings support the notion of prefrontal dysfunction during the performance of certain tasks in schizophrenia. Not surprisingly, because prefrontal cortex participates in diverse distributed processing of many cognitive behaviors, abnormalities of different fronto-striato–thalamic and cerebellar neurocircuits are implicated in the performance of specific cognitive tasks, and some of them are impaired in schizophrenia.

Overall, the majority of studies support the notion of dysfunctional frontal activation in schizophrenia. While most perfusion and glucose utilization studies pointed to hypofrontality, functional MRI studies revealed that schizophrenic patients do not show a simple underactivation of the frontal cortex, but rather show an inefficient use of their frontal cortices. Accordingly, several studies indicated that increased activity is associated with inefficient working memory performance at relatively low cognitive loads, while hypofrontality can be observed when subjects perform poorly due to an excess of working memory load (Weinberger *et al.* 2001). Under circumstances of excessive working memory load, additional brain areas such as the striatum or thalamus may be activated to compensate for functional constraints (Callicott *et al.* 1998, 1999; Manoach *et al.* 2000).

Measuring dopamine release in the striatum with radioligand infusion and its interaction with prefrontal dysfunction

A series of studies support the notion of a dysfunction in temporolimbic–frontal networks in schizophrenia, which is associated with negative symptoms, such as cognitive impairment, during the performance of working memory or verbal recall. Some results support the notion that the temporolimbic–prefrontal dysfunction observed in schizophrenia is associated with increased subcortical dopamine release and the manifestation of certain positive symptoms. Increased subcortical dopamine release in association with positive symptoms has long been postulated in schizophrenia (Weinberger 1987). However, it was not until the recent arrival of brain imaging techniques, which measure dopamine release under steady-state conditions and manipulate synaptic dopamine concentrations, that an increased dopamine release was demonstrated in the striatum of acutely psychotic patients. Laruelle *et al.* (1996, 1997) and Breier *et al.* (1997) demonstrated that amphetamine induces increased striatal dopamine release in schizophrenics compared with healthy control subjects. A decisive methodological step was the use of steady-state infusion paradigms (Laruelle and Innis 1996), which establish a stable baseline and abolish confounding effects of individual differences in peak radioligand binding. As a result, the degree of radioligand displacement by dopamine, which is released during amphetamine application, can be measured and reflects changes in intrasynaptic dopamine concentrations. The observation that schizophrenics release relatively higher amounts of dopamine compared with age-matched healthy control subjects is in accordance with a series of [^{18}F]DOPA PET studies, which showed that presynaptic dopamine production is increased in never-treated schizophrenic subjects (Reith *et al.* 1994; Dao-Castellana *et al.* 1997; Hietala *et al.* 1999).

Another test of this hypothesis was a study of Abi-\Dargham *et al.* (2000), which showed that blockade of dopamine production by α-methyl-*para*-tyrosine (AMPT) induced a relatively larger increase in radioligand binding to now unoccupied dopamine D$_2$ receptors. This increased radioligand binding reflects (originally) higher intrasynaptic dopamine concentrations in acutely psychotic schizophrenic patients.

Several studies have suggested that this increase in intrasynaptic dopamine concentrations in the striatum of acutely schizophrenic patients is due to a dysfunction of prefrontal–temporolimbic networks. In rodent and primate studies, an early developmental lesion of the temporolimbic cortices was associated with a pathological disinhibition of subcortical dopamine release after prefrontal cortical activation (Weinberger and Lipska 1995, Heinz *et al.* 1999). In humans, increased subcortical dopamine release is not only observed in schizophrenic subjects but also in normal control subjects who were medicated with ketamine, a potent antagonist at glutamatergic *N*-methyl-D-aspartate (NMDA) receptors (Kegeles *et al.* 2000). It has been suggested that the systematic application of ketamine may preferentially interfere with prefrontal cortical function, thus interfering with prefrontal control of subcortical dopaminergic neurotransmission and disinhibiting dopamine release.

Two studies tested directly the hypothesis that prefrontal cortical dysfunction is associated with increased striatal dopamine production. In the first, Bertolino *et al.* (2000) found that prefrontal *N*-acetyl-aspartate (NAA) concentration, an intraneuronal measure of synaptic abundance and integrity acquired with NMR spectroscopy, predicted amphetamine-induced dopamine (DA) release in the striatum in patients with schizophrenia. Meyer-Lindenberg *et al.* (2002) measured prefrontal activation during the performance of a working memory task simultaneously with presynaptic dopamine production using [^{18}F]DOPA and PET. A strong negative correlation was observed between reduced prefrontal activation during the memory task and increased subcortical dopamine production, supporting the hypothesis that a prefrontal deficit is associated with a disinhibition of subcortical dopaminergic neurotransmission.

Indicators of a dopamine deficit in the prefrontal cortex

There is some evidence that prefrontal dysfunction itself is at least partially caused by a deficit in tonic dopamine release. The first clinical evidence of this hypothesis came from a study in which prefrontal rCBF during the WCST was predicted by levels of homovanillic acid (HVA) in spinal fluid, which correlated with prefrontal DA turnover (Weinberger *et al.* 1988). Further indirect evidence of this hypothesis comes from the observation that the administration of amphetamine increases both working memory performance and signal to noise ratio in the prefrontal cortex (Daniel *et al.* 1991; Mattay *et al.*1996). Furthermore, changes in dopamine D1 receptor availability in the prefrontal cortex may reflect dysfunctional dopamine input (Okubo *et al.* 1997). A study that combined spectroscopy and functional brain imaging (with radioactively labeled water and PET) showed that reduced working memory performance was associated with a reduction in a marker of neuronal integrity, *N*-acetyl-aspartate, in the prefrontal cortex of schizophrenic patients (Bertolino *et al.* 2000).

Brain imaging reveals temporolimbic dysfunction in schizophrenia

Not all cognitive deficits associated with schizophrenia can be attributed to the prefrontal cortex. Some brain imaging studies support the hypothesis that there is hippocampal dysfunction during at least certain cognitive tasks in schizophrenia. The hippocampus is activated during conscious recollection in humans (Schacter *et al.* 1996). Perfusion studies with PET demonstrated that schizophrenics show reduced hippocampal activation during conscious recollection of studied words in a verbal episodic memory retrieval test (Heckers *et al.* 1998). In contrast, schizophrenic patients showed increased activation in the parietal and prefrontal cortices. Altogether, schizophrenic patients were less accurate when they were required to use more complex semantic encoding and search strategies, and did not show hippocampal recruitment during conscious recollection. Hofer *et al.* (2003) described impairments in activation of the lateral temporal cortices and the dorsolateral prefrontal cortex during word recognition. Adverse medication effects do not easily explain this finding, since withdrawal of the neuroleptic haloperidol induced significant decreases in recent verbal memory function (Gilbertson and van Kammen 1997). The hippocampus–amygdala complex was also less activated during facial affect discrimination in schizophrenics compared with healthy controls (Hempel *et al.* 2003).

Brain imaging of adverse antipsychotic effects on negative symptoms

It has been shown that antipsychotics do not appear to have marked positive or negative effects on working memory in schizophrenics (Goldberg and Weinberger 1996). However, there is evidence that they may increase the severity of some negative symptoms, particularly affective flattening, anhedonia, and avolition/apathy (Heinz *et al.* 1998*b*; Schmidt *et al.* 2001). In a brain imaging study that compared the degree of occupancy of dopamine D_2 receptors in the striatum with the severity of negative symptoms, a positive correlation was observed between increased blockade of striatal D_2 receptors and psychomotor slowing, as well as avolition and apathy.

The association between psychomotor slowing and dopamine D2 receptor blockade in the striatum is unsurprising, given the well-known role of dopamine in extrapyramidal neurocircuits that link the prefrontal and the premotor cortices with the thalamus. In the ventral striatum, which includes the nucleus accumbens, a core area of the brain reward system, dopamine release strongly reinforces behaviors that cause dopaminergic cell firing (Robinson and Berridge 1993). Dopamine release in this brain area is normally stimulated by primary reinforces such as food and sex, but a wide range of drugs of abuse can also stimulate dopamine release in the ventral striatum (Heinz 2002). In animal models, it has been shown that dopamine release attributes incentive salience to reward-indicating stimuli, which may thus induce a motivational state that facilitates reward-seeking behaviors (Schultz *et al.* 1993). Blockade of dopamine receptors in the brain reward system may thus induce a loss of motivation, i.e. apathy and avolition. Affective flattening may also result from a disinterest in environmental stimuli that indicate potential reward (Schmidt *et al.* 2001). Another prominent negative symptom, anhedonia, the loss of the ability to experience pleasure, may indirectly result from a loss of motivation and reward-seeking behavior due to dopamine receptor blockade in the ventral striatum. These observations indicate that not all negative symptoms may be due to prefrontal or cortical dysfunction, but that some negative symptoms, especially in association with negative affect and loss of motivation, may result from a dysfunction of the striatal parts of the dopaminergic reward system.

Brain mapping of neurocircuits associated with positive symptoms

It has long been surmised that dopaminergic hyperactivity in the striatum may play a decisive role in the development of positive symptoms. If increased dopaminergic activity in the ventral striatum attributes incentive salience to environmental cues, a chaotic or overactive dopaminergic system may mis-attribute salience to a wide range of stimuli, thus causing a breakdown of filter effects of fronto-striato–thalamic neurocircuits. Indirect support for this hypothesis was given in the study of Abi-Dargham *et al.* (2000), in which increased dopamine concentrations in the striatum of acutely psychotic schizophrenics were associated with positive symptoms. A functional brain activation study by Silbersweig *et al.* (1995) showed that acute auditory hallucinations are associated with activations in the thalamus and striatum, the hippocampus, and in paralimbic regions such as the parahippocampal and cingular gyri and the orbitofrontal cortex. The authors suggested that activity in deep brain structures such as the striatum may generate or modulate hallucinations, and that the particular neocortical regions entrained in individual patients may effect their specific perceptual content. These observations illustrate that functional brain imaging can map the specific neurocircuits associated with the development of positive and negative symptoms in schizophrenia.

PET and SPECT studies in other neuropsychiatric disorders

In patients suffering from obsessive–compulsive disorder, several SPECT and PET studies (Table 7.6) have found increased activation of the orbitofrontal cortex, caudate nuclei, and thalamus (Baxter *et al.* 1987; Perani *et al.* 1995). Orbitofrontal disinhibition may be associated with conflict and negative mood states, while basal ganglia activation may correlate with stereotypic behavior patterns (Heinz 1999). Orbitofrontal and striatal activation was reduced after successful behavioral therapy as well as after application of selective serotonin reuptake inhibitors (Baxter *et al.* 1992). In monozygotic (MZ) twins with Tourette's syndrome, differences in D_2 receptor binding in the caudate predicted virtually the entire difference in tic severity between twins of a pair (Wolf *et al.* 1996). Serotonin transporter function was also implicated in the manifestation of complex compulsive impulses such as vocal tics in Tourette's patients (Heinz *et al.* 1998*d*).

Reduced serotonin transporters in the raphe area, the center of origin of central serotonergic projections, were associated with clinical depression in patients suffering from seasonal affective disorder, major depression, and alcoholism (Heinz *et al.* 1998*c*; Malison *et al.* 1998; Willeit *et al.* 2000). In patients suffering from major depression, brain perfusion and glucose utilization studies showed hypofrontality, especially in the prefrontal cortex ventral to the genu of the corpus callosum (Drevets *et al.* 1997). Primary depression has also been associated with abnormal activation in the amygdala and the cingulate gyrus (George *et al.* 1993). Stimulation of these brain regions increases serotonin release via serotonergic neurons in the raphe area, so that dysfunctional activation of the medial prefrontal cortex may contribute to monoaminergic dysfunction in major depression (Juckel *et al.* 1999).

In currently drinking alcoholics, PET and SPECT studies showed frontal deficits that were associated with cognitive dysfunction and recovered within the first months of abstinence (Adams *et al.* 1993; Volkow and Fowler 2000). After detoxification, increases of frontal cerebral blood flow were associated with alcohol craving (Volkow and Fowler 2000). Frontal cortical activation and alcohol craving were also elicited when alcohol-associated visual cues were presented to alcoholics compared with control subjects (George *et al.* 2001). Current combined PET and fMRI studies assess neurobiological correlates of increased cue-reactivity in alcoholics (Heinz *et al.* 2002).

SPECT studies with the radioligand β-CIT showed reductions in striatal dopamine and brainstem serotonin transporters during early abstinence, which were associated with clinical depression (Heinz *et al.* 1998*b*; Laine *et al.* 1999). Other SPECT studies in detoxified alcoholics revealed low availability of GABA$_A$ receptors, which mediate the acute sedative effect of alcohol in the cerebellum (Abi-Dargham *et al.* 1998). Such studies may help to indicate dysfunctional neurotransmitter systems and their psychopathological correlates, and may point to target systems for additional relapse-reducing medication.

In dementia, brain perfusion and glucose utilization studies consistently revealed hypoperfusion and hypometabolism in temporo-parieto-occipital regions (Table 7.7). Abnormalities in cerebral blood flow detected with SPECT can be used routinely for differential diagnosis of dementia. The SPECT radioligand QNB binds with high affinity to muscarinic acetylcholine receptors and can be used to support the diagnosis of Alzheimer's disease (Weinberger *et al.* 1992*a,b*; Sunderland *et al.* 1995). Bilateral

Table 7.6 Fluorodeoxyglucose (FDG)-PET studies in obsessive compulsive disorder

Reference	Diagnosis, number of patients	Test	Brain imaging method	Frontal cortex	Other findings
Baxter et al. (1987)	OCD, n = 14; controls (patients with unipolar depression), n = 14	Clinical scales	[18F]FDG PET	In OCD, metabolic rates were significantly creased in the left orbital gyrus and bilaterally in the caudate nuclei; the right orbital gyrus showed a trend to an increased metabolic rate	
Baxter et al. (1992)	OCD, n = 20 (2 groups: 10 patients in behavioral therapy, 10 patients with both behavioral therapy and drug therapy); controls, n = 4	Before and after treatment with fluoxetin hydrochloride and/or behavior therapy, OCD symptom ratings	[18F]FDG PET	After treatment, rGMR in the head of the right caudate nucleus divided by glucose metabolic rate in the ipsilateral hemisphere (Cd/hem), was decreased significantly compared with pretreatment values in responders to both drug and behavior therapy	Percentage change in obsessive–compulsive disorder symptom ratings correlated significantly with the percent of right Cd/hem change in subjects receiving drug therapy and trendwise in subjects receiving behavior therapy
Schwartz et al. (1996)	OCD, n = 9	Before and after 10 weeks of structured exposure and response prevention behavioral and cognitive treatment	[18F]FDG PET	Before treatment, there were significant correlations of brain activity between the orbital gyri and the head of the caudate nucleus and the orbital gyri and the thalamus on the right; these correlations decreased significantly after effective treatment	Behavior therapy responders had significant bilateral decreases in caudate glucose metabolic rates that were greater than those seen in poor responders to treatment

Perani et al. (1995)	OCD, (unmedicated patients), n = 11; controls, n = 18	Before and after treatment with serotonin-specific reuptake inhibitors	[¹⁸F]FDG PET	Before treatment, rCMRglu values were significantly increased in the cingulate cortex, thalamus and pallidum/putamen complex	After treatment, a significant improvement in obsessive–compulsive symptoms was correlated with a significant bilateral decrease of metabolism in the cingulate cortex
Saxena et al. (1999)	OCD, n = 20	Before and after treatment with paroxetine	[¹⁸F]FDG PET	In patients who responded to paroxetine, glucose metabolism decreased significantly in right anterolateral OFC and right caudate nucleus; lower pretreatment metabolism in both left and right OFC predicted greater improvement in OCD severity with treatment	–
Saxena et al. (2003)	OCD, n = 27; major depression n = 27; concurrent OCD and major depression, n = 17	Before and after treatment with paroxetine	[¹⁸F]FDG PET	Improvement of major depressive disorder symptoms was significantly correlated and with higher pretreatment metabolism in the medial prefrontal cortex and rostral anterior cingulate gyrus	Improvement of OCD symptoms was significantly correlated with higher pretreatment glucose metabolism in the right caudate nucleus; Improvement of major depressive disorder symptoms was significantly correlated with lower pretreatment metabolism in the amygdala (partial r = 0.71) and thalamus (partial r = 0.34).

FDG, fluorodeoxyglucose; OCD, obsessive–compulsive disorder; OFC, orbitofrontal cortex; rGMR, regional glucose metabolic rate.

Table 7.7 SPECT studies in dementia

Dementia type	Patterns of rCBF and metabolism	Location of changes	References
Alzheimers disease	Hypoperfusion, hypometabolism	Frontal lobe, temporo-parieto-occipital region, posterior cingulate	Jagust *et al.* (1997); Cummings and McPherson (2001); Devous (2002)
Lewy body dementia	Hypoperfusion, hypometabolism, defects in the nigrostriatal dopamine pathways	Temporo-parieto-occipital region, greater degree in the occipital region	Talbot *et al.* (1998); Barber *et al.* (2001); Mirzaei *et al.* (2003)
Parkinson's disease	Hypoperfusion, hypometabolism, changes in dopaminergic neurotransmission	Temporo-parieto-occipital region	Kawabata *et al.* (1991); Jagust *et al.* (1995)
Chorea Huntington's disease	Hypoperfusion, hypometabolism	Nuclei caudati	Smith *et al.* (1988); Lang *et al.* (1990)
Pick's disease	Decrease of radiotracer activity	Frontal lobe	Kuwabara *et al.* (1990); Lang *et al.* (1990); Habert *et al.* (1991)

rCBF, Regional cerebral blood flow.

posterior CBF reductions were found to increase significantly the risk of a patient having Alzheimer's disease as opposed to vascular dementia or frontotemporal dementia, while bilateral anterior CBF abnormality increased the odds of a patient having frontotemporal dementia as opposed to Alzheimer's disease, vascular dementia or Lewy body disease (Talbot *et al.* 1998).

Summary

Within the past two decades, functional brain imaging has seen extremely rapid development, starting from relatively simple perfusion studies which showed large perfusion deficits in patients with gross anatomical lesions towards a fine mapping of neurocircuits associated with specific brain functions. A multimodal combination of different techniques, such as functional brain imaging with PET or fMRI, structural brain imaging of the integrity of certain brain areas with spectroscopy, and the assessment of neurotransmitter precursors, neuroreceptors and transporters with SPECT and PET, may be most promising in elucidating the complex biological correlates of mental disorders. However, the methodological limits of the techniques have to be observed. Binding to neuroreceptors or transporters has to be substantially higher than unspecific binding of lipophilic radioligands to brain tissue in areas mainly devoid of receptors or transporters. Genetic variance in neuroreceptor or transporter expression may affect radioligand binding to these transporters (Heinz *et al.* 2000*b*), and genotype differences may be mistaken for differences in diagnostic groups if patients and subjects are not matched for genotype. Finally, false-positive and false-negative findings may result from too liberal or too strict statistical thresholds.

Variance within diagnostic groups may be related to the heterogeneity of causes and consequences of mental disorders. It was this variance that Bleuler (1911) wanted to address when he did not speak of 'schizophrenia' as a single disease but named it the 'group of schizophrenias'. Therefore, the currently most promising research strategy may be to use brain imaging for the assessment of neurobiological correlates of so-called intermediate phenotypes, i.e. syndromes with defined neurobiological correlates. An example would be deficits in working memory, which are a prominent but non-specific symptom of schizophrenia, and which can be attributed to a dysfunction of a neuronal network that includes the prefrontal cortex.

Altogether, functional brain imaging is just starting to integrate the vast knowledge centered on environmental and genetic variance. We are just beginning to learn how brain imaging can increase our knowledge about the causes and consequences of mental disorders and the best ways of treatment.

References

Abi-Dargham, A., Rodenhiser, J., Printz, D., Zea-Ponce, Y., Gil, R., Kegeles, L. S. *et al.* (2000). From the cover: increased baseline occupancy of D2 receptors by dopamine in schizophrenia. *Proceedings of the National Academy of Sciences USA,* **97**, 8104–9.

Adams, K. M., Gilman, S., Koeppe, R. A., Kluin, K. J., Brunberg, J. A., Dede, D. *et al.* (1993). Neuropsychological deficits are correlated with frontal hypometabolism in positron emission tomography studies of older alcoholic patients. *Alcoholism, Clinical and Experimental Research,* **17**, 205–10.

Andreasen, N. C. (1988). Evaluation of brain imaging techniques in mental illness. *Annual Review of Medicine,* **39**, 335–45.

Andreasen, N. C. (1989). Brain *Imaging: Applications in psychiatry.* American Psychiatric Press Inc.

Andreasen, N. C., Rezai, K., Alliger, R., Swayze, V. W. 2nd, Flaum, M., Kirchner, P., *et al.* (1992). Hypofrontality in neuroleptic-naive patients and in patients with chronic schizophrenia. Assessment with xenon 133 single-photon emission computed tomography and the Tower of London. *Archives of General Psychiatry,* **49**, 943–58.

Andreasen, N. C., O'Leary, D. S., Cizadlo, T., Arndt, S., Rezai, K., Ponto, L. L. *et al.* (1996). Schizophrenia and cognitive dysmetria: a positron-emission tomography study of dysfunctional prefrontal-thalamic-cerebellar circuitry. *Proceedings of the National Academy of Sciences USA,* **93** (18), 9985–90.

Ashton, L., Barnes, A., Livingston, M., and Wyper, D. (2000). Cingulate abnormalities associated with PANSS negative scores in first episode schizophrenia. *Behavioural Neurology,* **12**, 93–101.

Batista, J. F., Galiano, M. C., Torres, L. A., Hernandez, M. C., Sosa, F., Perera, A., *et al.* (1995). Brain single-photon emission tomography with technetium-99m hexamethylpropylene amine oxime in adolescents with initial-stage schizophrenia. *European Journal of Nuclear Medicine,* **22**, 1274–7.

Barber, R., Panikkar, A., and McKeith, I. G. (2001). Dementia with Lewy bodies: diagnosis and management. *International Journal of Geriatric Psychiatry,* **16**, Suppl 1, S12–8.

Baxter, L. R. Jr, Phelps, M. E., Mazziotta, J. C., Guze, B. H., Schwartz, J. M., and Selin, C. E. (1987). Local cerebral glucose metabolic rates in obsessive-compulsive disorder. A comparison with rates in unipolar depression and in normal controls. *Archives of General Psychiatry*, **44** (3), 211–18.

Baxter, L. R., Schwartz, J. M., Bergman, K. S., Szuba, M. P., Guze, B. H., Mazziotta, J. C. *et al.* (1992). Caudate glucose metabolic rate changes with both drug and behavior therapy for obsessive–compulsive disorder. *Archives of General Psychiatry*, **49**, 681–9.

Bertolino, A., Knable, M. B., Saunders, R. C., Callicott, J. H., Kolachana, B., Mattay, V. S. *et al.* (1999). The relationship between dorsolateral prefrontal N-acetylaspartate measures and striatal dopamine activity in schizophrenia. *Biological Psychiatry*, **45**, 660–7.

Bertolino, A., Esposito, G., Callicott, J. H., Mattay, V. S., Van Horn, J. D., Frank, J. A. *et al.* (2000). Specific relationship between prefrontal neuronal N-acetylaspartate and activation of the working memory cortical network in schizophrenia. *American Journal of Psychiatry*, **157** (1), 26–33.

Blackwood, D. H., Glabus, M. F., Dunan, J., O'Carroll, R. E., Muir, W. J., and Ebmeier, K. P. (1999). Altered cerebral perfusion measured by SPECT in relatives of patients with schizophrenia. Correlations with memory and P300. *British Journal of Psychiatry*, **175**, 357–66.

Breier, A., Su, T. P., Saunders, R., Carson, R. E., Kolachana, B. S., de Bartolomeis, A. *et al.* (1997). Schizophrenia is associated with elevated amphetamine-induced synaptic dopamine concentrations: evidence from a novel positron emission tomography method. *Proceedings of the National Academy of Sciences USA*, **94**, 2569–74.

Buchsbaum, M. S., Haier, R. J., Potkin, S. G., Nuechterlein, K., Bracha, H. S., Katz, M. *et al.* (1992). Frontostriatal disorder of cerebral metabolism in never-medicated schizophrenics. *Archives of General Psychiatry*, **49** (12), 935–42.

Buchsbaum, M. S., Shihabuddin, L., Hazlett, E. A., Schroder, J., Haznedar, M. M., Powchik, P. *et al.* (2002). Kraepelinian and non-Kraepelinian schizophrenia subgroup differences in cerebral metabolic rate. *Schizophrenia Research*, **55** (1–2), 25–40.

Busatto, G. F., Costa, D. C., Ell, P. J., Pilowsky, L. S., David, A. S., Kerwin, R. W. (1994). Regional cerebral blood flow (rCBF) in schizophrenia during verbal memory activation: a 99mTc-HMPAO single photon emission tomography (SPET) study. *Psychological Medicine*, **24** (2), 463–72.

Busatto, G. F., David, A. S., Costa, D. C., Ell, P. J., Pilowsky, L. S., Lucey, J. V. *et al.* (1995). Schizophrenic auditory hallucinations are associated with increased regional cerebral blood flow during verbal memory activation in a study using single photon emission computed tomography. *Psychiatry Research*, **61** (4), 255–64.

Callicott, J. H., Ramsey, N. F., Tallent, K., Bertolino, A., Knable, M. B., Coppola, R. *et al.* (1998). Functional magnetic resonance imaging brain mapping in psychiatry: methodological issues illustrated in a study of working memory in schizophrenia. *Neuropsychopharmacology*, **18** (3), 186–96.

Callicott, J. H., Mattay, V. S., Bertolino, A., Finn, K., Coppola, R., Frank, J. A. *et al.* (1999). Physiological characteristics of capacity constraints in working memory as revealed by functional MRI. *Cerebral Cortex*, **9** (1), 20–6.

Celsis, P., Goldman, T., Henriksen, L., and Lassen, N. A. (1981). A method for calculating regional cerebral blood flow from emission computed tomography of inert gas concentrations. *Journal of Computer Assisted Tomography*, **5** (5), 641–5.

Chefer, S. I., Horti, A. G., Lee, K. S., Koren, A. O., Jones, D. W., Gorey, J. G. *et al.* (1998). In vivo imaging of brain nicotinic acetylcholine receptors with 5-[123I]iodo-A-85380 using single photon emission computed tomography. *Life Sciences*, **63**, PL355–60.

Chen, R. Y., Chen, E., and Ho, W. Y. (2000). A five-year longitudinal study of the regional cerebral metabolic changes of a schizophrenic patient from the first episode using Tc-99m HMPAO SPECT. *European Archives of Psychiatry and Clinical Neuroscience*, **250** (2), 69–72.

Clark, C., Kopala, L., Li, D. K., and Hurwitz, T. (2001). Regional cerebral glucose metabolism in never-medicated patients with schizophrenia. *Canadian Journal of Psychiatry*, **46** (4), 340–5.

Coppola, R., Marenco, S., Jones, D. W., Berman, K. F., and Weinberger, D. R. (1992). A comparison of xenon-133 and xenon-127 for the determination of regional cerebral blood flow measured by dynamic SPECT. *Psychiatry Research*, **45**, 187–200.

Crawford, T. J., Puri, B. K., Nijran, K. S., Jones, B., Kennard, C., and Lewis, S. W. (1996). Abnormal saccadic distractibility in patients with schizophrenia: a 99mTc-HMPAO SPET study. *Psychological Medicine*, **26** (2), 265–77.

Crespo-Facorro, B., Paradiso, S., Andreasen, N. C., O'Leary, D. S., Watkins, G. L., Boles Ponto, L. L. *et al.* (1999). Recalling word lists reveals 'cognitive dysmetria' in schizophrenia: a positron emission tomography study. *American Journal of Psychiatry*, **156** (3), 386–92.

Cummings, J. L. and McPherson, S. (2001). Neuropsychiatric assessment of Alzheimer's disease and related dementias. *Aging (Milano)*. **13**(3), 240–6.

Daniel, D. G., Weinberger, D. R., Jones, D. W., Zigun, J. R., Coppola, R., Handel, S. *et al.* (1991). The effect of amphetamine on regional cerebral blood flow during cognitive activation in schizophrenia. *Journal of Neuroscience*, **11** (7), 1907–17.

Dao-Castellana, M. H., Paillere-Martinot, M. L., Hantraye, P., Attar-Levy, D., Remy, P., Crouzel, C. *et al.* (1997). Presynaptic dopaminergic function in the striatum of schizophrenic patients. *Schizophrenia Research*, **23** (2), 167–74.

Desco, M., Gispert, J. D., Reig, S., Sanz, J., Pascau, J., Sarramea, F. *et al.* (2003). Cerebral metabolic patterns in chronic and recent-onset schizophrenia. *Psychiatry Research*, **122** (2), 125–35.

Devous, M. D. Sr. (2002). Functional brain imaging in the dementias: role in early detection, differential diagnosis, and longitudinal studies. *European Journal of Nuclear Medicine and Molecular Imaging*. **29**(12), 1685–96. Epub 2002 Sep 25.

Drevets, W. C., Price, J. L., Simpson, J. R. Jr, Todd, R. D., Reich, T., Vannier, M. *et al.* (1997). Subgenual prefrontal cortex abnormalities in mood disorders. *Nature*, **386** (6627), 824–7.

Ebmcicr, K. P., Lawric, S. M., Blackwood, D. H., Johnstone, E. C., and Goodwin, G. M. (1995). Hypofrontality revisited: a high resolution single photon emission computed tomography study in schizophrenia. *Journal of Neurology, Neurosurgery and Psychiatry*, **58** (4), 452–6.

Eckelman, W. C., Reba, R. C., Rzeszotarski, W. J., Gibson, R. E., Hill, T., Holman, B. L. *et al.* (1984). External imaging of cerebral muscarinic acetylcholine receptors. *Science*, **223** (4633), 291–3.

Eckelman, W. C., Eng, R., Rzeszotarski, W. J., Gibson, R. E., Francis, B., and Reba, R. C. (1985). Use of 3-quinuclidinyl 4-iodobenzilate as a receptor binding radiotracer. *Journal of Nuclear Medicine*, **26** (6), 637–42.

Egan, M. F., Goldberg, T. E., Kolachana, B. S., Callicott, J. H., Mazzanti, C. M., Straub, R. E. *et al.* (2001). Effect of COMT Val108/158 Met genotype on frontal lobe function and risk for schizophrenia. *Proceedings of the National Academy of Sciences USA*, **98** (12), 6917–22.

Farde, L., Halldin, C., Muller, L., Suhara, T., Karlsson, P., and Hall, H. (1994). PET study of [11C]beta-CIT binding to monoamine transporters in the monkey and human brain. *Synapse*, **16** (2), 93–103.

Ford, R. A., Lewis, S. W., Syed, G. M., Reveley, A., and Toone, B. K. (1992). Ventricular size and regional cerebral blood flow in schizophrenia: an attempted replication. *Psychiatry Research*, **45** (4), 209–13.

George, M. S., Ketter, T. A., and Post, R. M. (1993). SPECT and PET imaging in mood disorders. *Journal of Clinical Psychiatry*, **54** (suppl.), 6–13.

George, M. S., Anton, R. F., Bloomer, C., Teneback, C., Drobes, D. J., Lorberbaum, J. P. *et al.* (2001). Activation of prefrontal cortex and anterior thalamus in alcoholic subjects on exposure to alcohol-specific cues. *Archives of General Psychiatry*, **58**, 345–52.

Gilbertson, M. W. and van Kammen, D. P. (1997). Recent and remote memory dissociation: medication effects and hippocampal function in schizophrenia. *Biological Psychiatry,* **42** (7), 585–95.

Goldberg, T. E. and Weinberger, D. R. **(1996).** Effects of neuroleptic medications on the cognition of patients with schizophrenia: a review of recent studies. *Journal of Clinical Psychiatry,* **57** (suppl. 9), 62–5.

Gracia Marco, R., Aguilar Garcia-Iturrospe, E. J., Fernandez Lopez, L., Cejas Mendez, M. R., Herreros Rodriguez, O., and Diaz Ramirez, A. *et al.* (1997). Hypofrontality in schizophrenia: influence of normalization methods. *Progress in Neuro-Psychopharmacology and Biological Psychiatry,* **21** (8), 1239–56.

Greenberg, J. H., Reivich, M., Alavi, A., Hand, P., Rosenquist, A., Rintelmann, W. *et al.* (1981). Metabolic mapping of functional activity in human subjects with the [18F]fluorodeoxyglucose technique. *Science,* **212** (4495), 678–80.

Gunther, W., Petsch, R., Steinberg, R., Moser, E., Streck, P., Heller, H. *et al.* (1991). Brain dysfunction during motor activation and corpus callosum alterations in schizophrenia measured by cerebral blood flow and magnetic resonance imaging. *Biological Psychiatry,* **29** (6), 535–55.

Habert, M. O., Spampinato, U., Mas, J. L., Piketty, M. L., Bourdel, M. C., de Recondo, J. *et al.* (1991). A comparative technetium 99m hexamethylpropylene amine oxime SPET study in different types of dementia. *European Journal of Nuclear Medicine,* **18**(1), 3–11.

Halsey, J. H. Jr and Blauenstein, U. W. (1975). Hemispheric regional cerebral blood flow patterns during brain work in cases of left hemiparesis. *Transactions of the American Neurological Association,* **100**, 71–4.

Hazlett, E. A., Buchsbaum, M. S., Jeu, L. A., Nenadic, I., Fleischman, M. B., Shihabuddin, L. *et al.* (2000). Hypofrontality in unmedicated schizophrenia patients studied with PET during performance of a serial verbal learning task. *Schizophrenia Research,* **43** (1), 33–46.

Heckers, S., Rauch, S. L., Goff, D., Savage, C. R., Schacter, D. L., Fischman, A. J. *et al.* (1998). Impaired recruitment of the hippocampus during conscious recollection in schizophrenia. *Nature Neuroscience,* **1** (4), 318–23.

Heinz, A. (1999). Neurobiological and anthropological aspects of compulsions and rituals. *Pharmacopsychiatry,* **32** (6), 223–9.

Heinz, A. (2002). Dopaminergic dysfunction in alcoholism and schizophrenia/ psychopathological and behavioral correlates. *European Psychiatry,* **17** (1), 9–16.

Heinz, A. and Jones, D. W. (2000). Serotonin transporters in ecstasy users. *British Journal of Psychiatry,* **176**, 193–5.

Heinz, A., Knable, M. B., and Weinberger, D. R. (1996). Dopamine D2 receptor imaging and neuroleptic drug response. *Journal of Clinical Psychiatry,* **57** (suppl. 11), 84–8.

Heinz, A., Jones, D. W., Gorey, J. G., Knable, M. B., Lee, K. S., Saunders, R. C. *et al.* (1997). Analysis of the metabolites of [I-123] beta-CIT in plasma of human and nonhuman primates. *Synapse,* **25**, 306–8.

Heinz, A., Higley, J. D., Gorey, J. G., Saunders, R. C., Jones, D. W., Hommer, D. *et al.* (1998*a*). In vivo association between alcohol intoxication, aggression, and serotonin transporter availability in nonhuman primates. *American Journal of Psychiatry,* **155**, 1023–8.

Heinz, A., Knable, M. B., Coppola, R., Gorey, J. G., Jones, D. W., Lee, K. S. *et al.* (1998*b*). Psychomotor slowing, negative symptoms and dopamine receptor availability IBZM SPECT study in neuroleptic-treated and drug-free schizophrenic patients. *Schizophrenia Research,* **31** (1), 19–26.

Heinz, A., Ragan, P., Jones, D. W., Hommer, D., Williams, W., Knable, M. B. *et al.* (1998*c*). Reduced central serotonin transporters in alcoholism. *American Journal of Psychiatry,* **155**, 1544–9.

Heinz, A., Knable, M. B., Wolf, S. S., Jones, D. W., Gorey, J. G., Hyde, T. M. *et al.* (1998*d*).Tourette's syndrome: [I-123]beta-CIT SPECT correlates of vocal tic severity. *Neurology,* **51** (4), 1069–74.

Heinz, A., Saunders, R. C., Kolachana, B. S., Jones, D. W., Gorey, J. G., Bachevalier, J. *et al.* (1999). Striatal dopamine receptors and transporters in monkeys with neonatal temporal limbic damage. *Synapse,* **32** (2), 71–9.

Heinz, A., Goldman, D., Jones, D. W., Palmour, R., Hommer, D., Gorey, J. G. *et al.* (2000*a*). Genotype influences in vivo dopamine transporter availability in human striatum. *Neuropsychopharmacology,* **22**, 133–9.

Heinz, A., Jones, D. W., Mazzanti, C., Goldman, D., Ragan, P., Hommer, D. *et al.* (2000*b*). A relationship between serotonin transporter genotype and in vivo protein expression and alcohol neurotoxicity. *Biological Psychiatry,* **47** (7), 643–9.

Heinz, A., Jones, D. W., Raedler, T., Coppola, R., Knable, M. B., and Weinberger, D. R. (2000*c*). Neuropharmacological studies with SPECT in neuropsychiatric disorders. *Nuclear Medicine and Biology,* **27** (7), 677–82.

Heinz, A., Siessmeier, T., Wrase, J., Hermann, D., Klein, S., Bucholz, H. G. *et al.* (2002). Striatal D2 receptor availability is associated with cue-induced activation of the orbitofrontal cortex in FMRI and with alcohol craving. *Journal of Nuclear Medicine,* **43** (suppl.), 261P.

Heinz, A., Wilwer, M., and Gallinat, J. (2003). Pharmacogenetic insights to monoaminergic dysfunction in alcohol dependence. *Psychopharmacology,* in press.

Hempel, A., Hempel, E., Schonknecht, P., Stippich, C., and Schroder, J. (2003). Impairment in basal limbic function in schizophrenia during affect recognition. *Psychiatry Research,* **122** (2), 115–24.

Heyman, A., Patterson, J. L., and Jones, R. W. (1951). Cerebral circulation and metabolism in uremia. *Circulation,* **3**, 558–64.

Hietala, J., Syvalahti, E., Vilkman, H., Vuorio, K., Rakkolainen, V., Bergman, J. *et al.* (1999). Depressive symptoms and presynaptic dopamine function in neuroleptic-naive schizophrenia. *Schizophrenia Research,* **35** (1), 41–50.

Hirsch, S. R. and Weinberger, D. R. (2003). *Schizophrenia,* (2nd Rev). Blackwell Science Ltd., Oxford, UK.

Hofer, A., Weiss, E. M., Golaszewski, S. M., Siedentopf, C. M., Brinkhoff, C., Kremser, C. *et al.* (2003). An FMRI study of episodic encoding and recognition of words in patients with schizophrenia in remission. *American Journal of Psychiatry,* **160** (5), 911–18.

Holcomb, H. H., Cascella, N. G., Thaker, G. K., Medoff, D. R., Dannals, R. F., and Tamminga, C.A. (1996). Functional sites of neuroleptic drug action in the human brain: PET/FDG studies with and without haloperidol. *American Journal of Psychiatry,* **153** (1), 41–9.

Jackson, J. H. (1927). *Die Croon-Vorlesungen über Aufbau und Abbau des Nervensystems.* Berlin.

Jagust, W. J., Johnson, K. A., and Holman, B. L. (1995). SPECT perfusion imaging in the diagnosis of dementia. *Journal of Neuroimaging.* **Suppl 1**, S45–52.

Jagust, W. J., Eberling, J. L., Reed, B. R., Mathis, C. A., and Budinger, T. F. (1997). Clinical studies of cerebral blood flow in Alzheimer's disease. *Annals of the New York Academy of Sciences.* **826**, 254–62.

Jones, D. W., Gorey, J. G., Zajicek, K., Das, S., Urbina, R., Lee, K. S. *et al.* (1998). Depletion–restoration studies reveal the impact of endogenous dopamine and serotonin on [I-123]b-CIT SPECT imaging in primate brain. *Journal of Nuclear Medicine,* **39** (suppl.), 42.

Juckel, G., Mendlin, A., and Jacobs, B. L. (1999). Electrical stimulation of rat medial prefrontal cortex enhances forebrain serotonin output: implications for electroconvulsive therapy and transcranial magnetic stimulation in depression. *Neuropsychopharmacology,* **21** (3), 391–8.

Kanno, I. and Lassen, N. A. (1979). Two methods for calculating regional cerebral blood flow from emission computed tomography of inert gas concentrations. *Journal of Computer Assisted Tomography,* **3** (1), 71–6.

Katz, M., Buchsbaum, M. S., Siegel, B. V. Jr, Wu, J., Haier, R. J., and Bunney, W. E. Jr (1996). Correlational patterns of cerebral glucose metabolism in never-medicated schizophrenics. *Neuropsychobiology,* **33** (1), 1–11.

Kawabata, K., Tachibana, H., and Sugita, M. (1991). Cerebral blood flow and dementia in Parkinson's disease. *Journal of Geriatric Psychiatry and Neurology,* **4**(4), 194–203.

Kawasaki, Y., Maeda, Y., Suzuki, M., Urata, K., Higashima, M., Kiba, K. *et al.* (1993). SPECT analysis of regional cerebral blood flow changes in patients with schizophrenia during the Wisconsin Card Sorting Test. *Schizophrenia Research,* **10** (2), 109–16.

Kegeles, L. S., Abi-Dargham, A., Zea-Ponce, Y., Rodenhiser-Hill, J., Mann, J. J., Van Heertum, R. L. *et al.* (2000). Modulation of amphetamine-induced striatal dopamine release by ketamine in humans: implications for schizophrenia. *Biological Psychiatry,* **48** (7), 627–40.

Kety, S. S. and Schmidt, C. F. (1948). The nitrous oxide method for the quantitative determination of cerebral blood flow in man: theory, procedure and normal values. *Journal of Clinical Investigation,* **27**, 476–83.

Klemm, E., Danos, P., Grunwald, F., Kasper, S., Moller, H. J., and Biersack, H. J. (1996). Temporal lobe dysfunction and correlation of regional cerebral blood flow abnormalities with psycho-pathology in schizophrenia and major depression—a study with single photon emission computed tomography. *Psychiatry Research,* **68** (1), 1–10.

Knable, M. B., Jones, D. W., Coppola, R., Hyde, T. M., Lee, K. S., Gorey, J. *et al.* (1995). Lateralized differences in iodine-123-IBZM uptake in the basal ganglia in asymmetric Parkinson's disease. *Journal of Nuclear Medicine,* **36** (7), 1216–25.

Knable, M. B., Egan, M. F., Heinz, A., Gorey, J., Lee, K. S., Coppola, R. *et al.* (1997*a*). Altered dopaminergic function and negative symptoms in drug-free patients with schizophrenia. [123I]-iodobenzamide SPECT study. *British Journal of Psychiatry,* **171**, 574–7.

Knable, M. B., Heinz, A., Raedler, T., and Weinberger, D. R. (1997*b*). Extrapyramidal side effects with risperidone and haloperidol at comparable D2 receptor occupancy levels. *Psychiatry Research,* **75**, 91–101.

Kotrla, K. J. and Weinberger, D. R. (1995). Brain imaging in schizophrenia. *Annual Review of Medicine,* **46**, 113–22.

Kraut, M. A., Marenco, S., Sohler, B. J., Wong, D. F., and Bryan, R. N. (1995). Comparison of functional MR and H2 15O positron emission tomography in stimulation of the primary visual cortex. *American Journal of Neuroradiology,* **16**, 2101–7.

Kuhl, D. E. and Edwards, R. Q. (1963). Image separation radioisotope scanning. *Radiology* **80**, 653–62.

Kung, H. F., Alavi, A., Chang, W., Kung, M. P., Keyes, J. W. Jr, Velchik, M. G. *et al.* (1990). In vivo SPECT imaging of CNS D-2 dopamine receptors: initial studies with iodine-123-IBZM in humans. *Nuclear Medicine,* **31** (5), 573–9.

Kung, M. P. and Kung, H. (1989). Peracetic acid as a superior oxidant for preparation of I-123-IBZM, a potential dopamine D2 receptor imaging agent. *J Radiopharm Lab Comp,* **27**, 691–700.

Kuwabara, Y., Ichiya, Y., Otsuka, M., Tahara, T., Fukumura, T., Gunasekera, R. *et al.* (1990). Comparison of I-123 IMP and Tc-99m HMPAO SPECT studies with PET in dementia. *Annals of Nuclear Medicine,* **4**(3), 75–82.

Laine, T. P., Ahonen, A., Torniainen, P., Heikkilä, J., Pyhtinen, J., Räsänen, P. *et al.* (1999). Dopamine transporters increase in human brain after alcohol withdrawal. *Molecular Psychiatry,* **4**, 189–91.

Lang, C., Herholz, K., Huk, W., and Feistel, H. (1990). [Diagnostic differentiation of dementia diseases by modern imaging procedures]. *Fortschr Neurol Psychiatr.* **58**(10), 380–98.

Laruelle, M. and Innis, R. B. (1996). Images in neuroscience. SPECT imaging of synaptic dopamine. *American Journal of Psychiatry,* **153** (10), 1249.

Laruelle, M., Baldwin, R. M., Malison, R. T., Zea-Ponce, Y., Zoghbi, S. S., al-Tikriti, M. S. *et al.* (1993). SPECT imaging of dopamine and serotonin transporters with [123I]beta-CIT: pharmacological characterization of brain uptake in nonhuman primates. *Synapse,* **13** (4), 295–309.

Laruelle, M., Wallace, E., Seibyl, J. P., Baldwin, R. M., Zea-Ponce, Y., Zoghbi, S. S. *et al.* (1994). Graphical, kinetic, and equilibrium analyses of in vivo [123I] beta-CIT binding to dopamine transporters in healthy human subjects. *Journal of Cerebral Blood Flow and Metabolism,* **14** (6), 982–94.

Laruelle, M., Abi-Dargham, A., van Dyck, C. H., Gil, R., D'Souza, C. D., Erdos, J. *et al.* (1996). Single photon emission computerized tomography imaging of amphetamine-induced dopamine release in drug-free schizophrenic subjects. *Proceedings of the National Academy of Sciences USA,* **93** (17), 9235–40.

Laruelle, M., Iyer, R. N., al-Tikriti, M. S., Zea-Ponce, Y., Malison, R., Zoghbi, S. S. *et al.* (1997). Microdialysis and SPECT measurements of amphetamine-induced dopamine release in nonhuman primates. *Synapse,* **25** (1), 1–14.

Lauer, M., Schirrmeister, H., Gerhard, A., Ellitok, E., Beckmann, H., Reske, S. N. *et al.* (2001). Disturbed neural circuits in a subtype of chronic catatonic schizophrenia demonstrated by F-18-FDG-PET and F-18-DOPA-PET. *Journal of Neural Transmission,* **108** (6), 661–70.

Lee, K. S., He, X. S., Jones, D. W., Coppola, R., Gorey, J. G., Knable, M. B. *et al.* (1996). An improved method for rapid and efficient radioiodination of iodine-123-IQNB. *Journal of Nuclear Medicine,* **37**, 2021–4.

Lesch, K. P., Bengel, D., Heils, A., Sabol, S. Z., Greenberg, B. D., Petri, S. *et al.* (1996). Association of anxiety-related traits with a polymorphism in the serotonin transporter genes regulatory region. *Science,* **274**, 1527–31.

Liddle, P. F., Friston, K. J., Frith, C. D., Hirsch, S. R., Jones, T., and Frackowiak, R. S. (1992). Patterns of cerebral blood flow in schizophrenia. *Britain Journal of Psychiatry,* **160**, 179–86.

Little, K. Y., Duncan, G. E., Breese, G. R., and Stumpf, W. E. (1992). Beta-adrenergic receptor binding in human and rat hypothalamus. *Biological Psychiatry,* **32** (6), 512–22.

Malaspina, D., Storer, S., Furman, V., Esser, P., Printz, D., Berman, A. *et al.* (1999). SPECT study of visual fixation in schizophrenia and comparison subjects. *Biological Psychiatry,* **46** (1), 89–93.

Malison, R. T., Price, L. H., Berman, R., van Dyck, C. H., Pelton, G. H., and Carpenter, L. (1998). Reduced brain serotonin transporter availability in major depression as measured by [^{123}I]-2β-carboxy-3β-(4-iodophenyl)tropane and single photon emission computed tomography. *Biological Psychiatry,* **44**, 1090–8.

Manoach, D. S., Gollub, R. L., Benson, E. S., Searl, M. M., Goff, D. C., Halpern, E. *et al.* (2000). Schizophrenic subjects show aberrant fMRI activation of dorsolateral prefrontal cortex and basal ganglia during working memory performance. *Biological Psychiatry,* **48** (2), 99–109.

Marenco, S. and Weinberger, D. R. (2000). The neurodevelopmental hypothesis of schizophrenia: following a trail of evidence from cradle to grave. *Development and Psychopathology,* **12**, 501–27.

Matsui, M., Kurachi, M., Yuasa, S., Aso, M., Tonoya, Y., Nohara, S. *et al.* (1997). Saccadic eye movements and regional cerebral blood flow in schizophrenic patients. *European Archives of Psychiatry and Clinical Neuroscience,* **247** (4), 219–27.

Mattay, V. S., Berman, K. F., Ostrem, J. L., Esposito, G., Van Horn, J. D., Bigelow, L. B. *et al.* (1996). Dextroamphetamine enhances 'neural network-specific' physiological signals: a positron-emission tomography rCBF study. *Journal of Neuroscience,* **16** (15), 4816–22.

Mellers, J. D., Adachi, N., Takei, N., Cluckie, A., Toone, B. K., and Lishman, W. A. (1998). SPET study of verbal fluency in schizophrenia and epilepsy. *British Journal of Psychiatry,* **173**, 69–74.

Meyer-Lindenberg, A., Miletich, R. S., Kohn, P. D., Esposito, G., Carson, R. E., Quarantelli, M. *et al.*
(2002). Reduced prefrontal activity predicts exaggerated striatal dopaminergic function in
schizophrenia. *Nature Neuroscience,* **5** (3), 267–71.

Miller, D. D., Rezai, K., Alliger, R., and Andreasen, N. C. (1997). The effect of antipsychotic
medication on relative cerebral blood perfusion in schizophrenia: assessment with technetium-
99m hexamethyl-propyleneamine oxime single photon emission computed tomography.
Biological Psychiatry, **41** (5), 550–9.

Min, S. K., An, S. K., Jon, D. I., and Lee, J. D. (1999). Positive and negative symptoms and regional
cerebral perfusion in antipsychotic-naive schizophrenic patients: a high-resolution SPECT
study.*Psychiatry Research,* **90** (3), 159–68.

Mirzaei, S., Rodrigues, M., Koehn, H., Knoll, P., and Bruecke, T. (2003). Metabolic impairment of
brain metabolism in patients with Lewy body dementia. *European Journal of Neurology,* **10** (5),
573–5.

Nohara, S., Suzuki, M., Kurachi, M., Yamashita, I., Matsui, M., Seto, H. *et al.* (2000). Neural correlates of memory organization deficits in schizophrenia. A single photon emission computed
tomography study with 99mTc-ethyl-cysteinate dimer during a verbal learning task.
Schizophrenia Research, **42** (3), 209–22.

Obrist, W. D., Thompson, H. K. Jr, King, C. H., and Wang, H. S. (1967). Determination of
regional cerebral blood flow by inhalation of 133-Xenon. *Circulation Research,* **20** (1),
124–35.

O'Connell, R. A., Van Heertum, R. L., Luck, D., Yudd, A. P., Cueva, J. E., Billick, S. B. *et al.* (1995).
Single-photon emission computed tomography of the brain in acute mania and schizophrenia.
Journal of Neuroimaging, **5** (2), 101–4.

Okubo, Y., Suhara, T., Suzuki, K., Kobayashi, K., Inoue, O., Terasaki, O. *et al.* (1997). Decreased
prefrontal dopamine D1 receptors in schizophrenia revealed by PET. *Nature* **385,** 634–66.

Parellada, E., Catafau, A. M., Bernardo, M., Lomena, F., Gonzalez-Monclus, E., and Setoain, J.
(1994). Prefrontal dysfunction in young acute neuroleptic-naive schizophrenic patients: a resting
and activation SPECT study. *Psychiatry Research,* **55** (3), 131–9.

Parellada, E., Catafau, A. M., Bernardo, M., Lomena, F., Catarineu, S., and Gonzalez-Monclus, E.
(1998). The resting and activation issue of hypofrontality: a single photon emission computed
tomography study in neuroleptic-naive and neuroleptic-free schizophrenic female patients.
Biological Psychiatry, **44** (8), 787–90.

Paulman, R. G., Devous, M. D. Sr, Gregory, R. R., Herman, J. H., Jennings, L., and Bonte, F. J. (1990).
Hypofrontality and cognitive impairment in schizophrenia: dynamic single-photon tomography
and neuropsychological assessment of schizophrenic brain function. *Biological Psychiatry,* **27** (4),
377–99.

Perani, D., Colombo, C., Bressi, S., Bonfanti, A., Grassi, F., Scarone, S. *et al.* (1995). [F-18]FDG Pet
study in obsessive–compulsive disorder. A clinical/metabolite correlation study after treatment.
British Journal of Psychiatry **166,** 244–50.

Phelps, M. E., Huang, S. C., Hoffman, E. J., Selin, C., Sokoloff, L., and Kuhl, D. E. (1979).
Tomographic measurement of local cerebral glucose metabolic rate in humans with
(F-18)2-fluoro-2-deoxy-D-glucose: validation of method. *Annals of Neurology,* **6** (5), 371–88.

Pickar, D., Su, T. P., Weinberger, D. R., Coppola, R., Malhotra, A. K., Knable, M. B. *et al.* (1996).
Individual variation in D2 dopamine receptor occupancy in clozapine-treated patients. *American
Journal of Psychiatry,* **153,** 1571–8.

Pirker, W., Asenbaum, S., Kasper, S., Walter, H., Angelberger, P., Koch, G. *et al.* (1995). β-CIT SPECT
demonstrates blockade of 5H-uptake sites by citalopram in the human brain in vivo. *Journal of
Neural Transmission,* **100,** 247–56.

Raedler, T. J., Knable, M. B., Lafargue, T., Urbina, R. A., Egan, M. F., Pickar, D. *et al.* (1999). In vivo determination of striatal dopamine D2 receptor occupancy in patients treated with olanzapine. *Psychiatry Research,* **90,** 81–90.

Raedler, T. J., Knable, M. B., Jones, D. W., Lafargue, T., Urbina, R. A., Egan, M. F. *et al.* (2000). In vivo olanzapine occupancy of muscarinic acetylcholine receptors in patients with schizophrenia. *Neuropsychopharmacology,* **23,** 56–68.

Reith, J., Benkelfat, C., Sherwin, A., Yasuhara, Y., Kuwabara, H., Andermann, F. *et al.* (1994). Elevated dopa decarboxylase activity in living brain of patients with psychosis. *Proceedings National Academy of Sciences USA,* **91** (24), 11651–4.

Risberg, J. and Ingvar, D. H. (1973). Patterns of activation in the grey matter of the dominant hemisphere during memorizing and reasoning. A study of regional cerebral blood flow changes during psychological testing in a group of neurologically normal patients. *Brain,* **96,** 737–56.

Risberg, J., Ali, Z., Wilson, E. M., Wills, E. L., and Halsey, J. H. (1975). Regional cerebral blood flow by 133xenon inhalation. *Stroke,* **6** (2), 142–8.

Robinson, T. E. and Berridge, K. C. (1993). The neural basis of drug craving: an incentive-sensitization theory of addiction. *Brain Research. Brain Research Reviews,* **18** (3), 247–91.

Rubin, P., Holm, S., Madsen, P. L., Friberg, L., Videbech, P., Andersen, H. S. *et al.* (1994a). Regional cerebral blood flow distribution in newly diagnosed schizophrenia and schizophreniform disorder. *Psychiatry Research,* **53** (1), 57–75.

Rubin, P., Hemmingsen, R., Holm, S., Moller-Madsen, S., Hertel, C., Povlsen, U. J. *et al.* (1994b). Relationship between brain structure and function in disorders of the schizophrenic spectrum: single positron emission computerized tomography, computerized tomography and psychopathology of first episodes. *Acta Psychiatrica Scandinavica,* **90** (4), 281–9.

Russell, J. M., Early, T. S., Patterson, J. C., Martin, J. L., Villanueva-Meyer, J., and McGee, M. D. (1997). Temporal lobe perfusion asymmetries in schizophrenia. *Journal of Nuclear Medicine,* **38** (4), 607–12.

Sabri, O., Erkwoh, R., Schreckenberger, M., Cremerius, U., Schulz, G., Dickmann, C. *et al.* (1997). Regional cerebral blood flow and negative/positive symptoms in 24 drug-naiveschizophrenics. *Journal of Nuclear Medicine,* **38** (2), 181–8.

Sachdev, P., Brodaty, H., Rose, N., and Haindl, W. (1997). Regional cerebral blood flow in late-onset schizophrenia: a SPECT study using 99mTc-HMPAO. *Schizophrenia Research,* **27** (2-3), 105–17.

Sagawa, K., Kawakatsu, S., Shibuya, I., Oiji, A., Morinobu, S., Komatani, A. *et al.* (1990). Correlation of regional cerebral blood flow with performance on neuropsychological tests in schizophrenic patients. *Schizophrenia Research,* **3** (4), 241–6.

Sagawa, K., Kawakatsu, S., Komatani, A., and Totsuka, S. (1990–1). Frontality, laterality, and cortical-subcortical gradient of cerebral blood flow in schizophrenia : relationship to symptoms and neuropsychological function. *Neuropsychobiology,* **24** (1), 1–7.

Satoh, K., Suzuki, T., Narita, M., Ishikura, S., Shibasaki, M., Kato, T. *et al.* (1993). Regional cerebral blood flow in catatonic schizophrenia. *Psychiatry Research,* **50** (4), 203–16.

Saxena, S., Brody, A. L., Maidment, K. M., Dunkin, J. J., Colgan, M., Alborzian, S. *et al.* (1999). Localized orbitofrontal and subcortical metabolic changes and predictors of response to paroxetine treatment in obsessive–compulsive disorder. *Neuropsychopharmacology,* **21** (6), 683–93.

Saxena, S., Brody, A. L., Ho, M. L., Zohrabi, N., Maidment, K. M., and Baxter, L. R. Jr. (2003). Differential brain metabolic predictors of response to paroxetine in obsessive–compulsive disorder versus major depression. *American Journal of Psychiatry,* **160** (3), 522–32.

Schacter, D. L., Alpert, N. M., Savage, C. R., Rauch, S. L., and Albert, M. S. (1996). Conscious recollection and the human hippocampal formation: evidence from positron emission tomography. *Proceedings of the National Academy of Sciences USA,* **93** (1), 321–5.

Scheinberg, P. and Stead, E. A. (1949). The cerebral blood flow in male subjects as measures by the nitrous oxide technique: normal values for blood flow, oxygen utilization, glucose utilization and peripheral resistance, with observations on the effect of tilting and anxiety. *Journal of Clinical Investigation,* **28,** 1163–71.

Schmidt, K., Nolte-Zenker, B., Patzer, J., Bauer, M., Schmidt, L. G., and Heinz, A. (2001). Psychopathological correlates of reduced dopamine receptor sensitivity in depression schizophrenia, and opiate and alcohol dependence. *Pharmacopsychiatry,* **34** (2), 66–72.

Schultz, W., Apicella, P., and Ljungberg, T. (1993). Responses of monkey dopamine neurons to reward and conditioned stimuli during successive steps of learning a delayed response task. *J Neurose,* **13,** 900–13.

Schwartz, J. M., Stoessel, P. W., Baxter, L. R. Jr, Martin, K. M., and Phelps, M. E. (1996). Systematic changes in cerebral glucose metabolic rate after successful behavior modification treatment of obsessive–compulsive disorder. *Archives of General Psychiatry,* **53** (2), 109–13.

Scottish Schizophrenia Research Group (1998). Regional cerebral blood flow in first-episode schizophrenia patients before and after antipsychotic drug treatment. *Acta Psychiatrica Scandinavica,* **97** (6), 440–9.

Silbersweig, D. A., Stern, E., Frith, C., Cahill, C., Holmes, A., Grootoonk, S. *et al.* (1995). A functional neuroanatomy of hallucinations in schizophrenia. *Nature,* **378,** 176–9.

Smith, F. W., Gemmell, H. G., Sharp, P. F., and Besson, J. A. (1988). Technetium-99m HMPAO imaging in patients with basal ganglia disease. *British Journal of Radiology,* **61** (730), 914–20.

Steinberg, J. L., Devous, M. D. Sr, and Paulman, R. G. (1996). Wisconsin card sorting activated regional cerebral blood flow in first break and chronic schizophrenic patients and normal controls. *Schizophrenia Research,* **19** (2-3), 177–87.

Sunderland, T., Esposito, G., Molchan, S. E., Coppola, R., Jones, D. W., Gorey, J. *et al.* (1995). Differential cholinergic regulation in Alzheimer's patients compared to controls following chronic blockade with scopolamine: a SPECT study. *Psychopharmacology,* **121,** 231–41.

Talbot, P. R., Lloyd, J. J., Snowden, J. S., Neary, D., and Testa, H. J. (1998). A clinical role for 99mTc-HMPAO SPECT in the investigation of dementia. *Journal of Neurology, Neurosurgery and Psychiatry,* **64** (3), 306–13.

Vita, A., Bressi, S., Perani, D., Invernizzi, G., Giobbio, G. M., Dieci, M. *et al.* (1995). High-resolution SPECT study of regional cerebral blood flow in drug-free and drug-naive schizophrenic patients. *American Journal of Psychiatry,* **152** (6), 876–82.

Volkow, N. D. and Fowler, J. S. (2000). Addiction, a disease of compulsion and drive: involvement of the orbitofrontal cortex. *Cerebral Cortex,* **10,** 318–25.

Weinberger, D. R. (1987). Implications of normal brain development for the pathogenesis of schizophrenia. *Archives of General Psychiatry,* **44** (7), 660–9.

Weinberger, D. R. (1996). On the plausibility of 'the neurodevelopmental hypothesis' of schizophrenia. *Neuropsychopharmacology,* **14** (3 suppl.), 1S–11S.

Weinberger, D. R. and Lipska, B. K. (1995). Cortical maldevelopment, anti-psychotic drugs, and schizophrenia: a search for common ground. *Schizophrenia Research,* **16,** 87–110.

Weinberger, D. R., Bergman, K. F., and Illowsky, B. P. (1988). Physiological dysfunction of dorsolateral prefrontal cortex in schizophrenia. III. A new cohort and evidence for a monoaminergic mechanism. *Archives of General Psychiatry,* **45,** 605–15.

Weinberger, D. R., Mann, U., Gibson, R. E., Coppola, R., Jones, D. W., Braun, A. R. *et al.* (1990). Cerebral muscarinic receptors in primary degenerative dementia as evaluated by SPECT with iodine-123-labeled QNB. *Advances in Neurology, 51,* 147–50.

Weinberger, D. R., Gibson, R., Coppola, R., Jones, D. W., Molchan, S., Sunderland, T. *et al.* (1991). The distribution of cerebral muscarinic acetylcholine receptors in vivo in patients with dementia. A controlled study with 123IQNB and single photon emission computed tomography. *Archives of Neurology, 48,* 169–76.

Weinberger, D. R., Jones, D., Reba, R. C., Mann, U., Coppola, R., Gibson, R. *et al.* (1992*a*). A comparison of FDG PET and IQNB SPECT in normal subjects and in patients with dementia. *Journal of Neuropsychiatry and Clinical Neuroscience, 4,* 239–48.

Weinberger, D. R., Jones, D. W., Sunderland, T., Lee, K. S., Sexton, R., Gorey, J. *et al.* (1992*b*). In vivo imaging of cerebral muscarinic receptors with I-123 QNB and SPECT: studies in normal subjects and patients with dementia. *Clinical Neuropharmacology, 15* (suppl. 1 Pt A), 194A–5A.

Weinberger, D. R., Egan, M. F., Bertolino, A., Callicot, J. H., Mattay, V. S., Lipska, B. K. *et al.* (2001). Prefrontal neurons and the genetics of schizophrenia. *Biological Psychiatry, 50,* 825–44.

Weiss, E. M., Golaszewski, S., Mottaghy, F. M., Hofer, A., Hausmann, A., Kemmler, G. *et al.* (2003). Brain activation patterns during a selective attention test-a functional MRI study in healthy volunteers and patients with schizophrenia. *Psychiatry Research, 123* (1), 1–15.

Willeit, M., Praschak-Rieder, N., Neumeister, A., Pirker, W., Asenbaum, S., and Vitouch, O. (2000). [123I]-beta-CIT SPECT imaging shows reduced brain serotonin transporter availability in drug-free depressed patients with seasonal affective disorder. *Biological Psychiatry, 47,* 482–9.

Wolf, S. S., Jones, D. W., Knable, M. B., Gorey, J. G., Lee, K. S., Hyde, T. M. *et al.* (1996). Tourette syndrome: prediction of phenotypic variation in monozygotic twins by caudate nucleus D2 receptor binding. *Science, 273,* 1225–7.

Yuasa, S., Kurachi, M., Suzuki, M., Kadono, Y., Matsui, M., Saitoh, O. *et al.* (1995). Clinical symptoms and regional cerebral blood flow in schizophrenia. *European Archives of Psychiatry and Clinical Neuroscience, 246* (1), 7–12.

Chapter 8

Neuroreceptor mapping with PET and SPECT

R. A. Bantick, A. J. Montgomery, and P. M. Grasby

Introduction

Neurochemical techniques can help to identify the underlying biochemical mechanisms involved in schizophrenia and its pharmacological treatment. Post-mortem neurochemistry, although highly sensitive, is limited by tissue changes after death, additional pathologies that have led to death and the use of generally elderly subjects who have had lengthy durations of illness and treatment. In contrast, neurochemical imaging, in addition to permitting comparisons of patients (including the drug naïve) and controls, also enables a wealth of within-subject comparisons (see below). The modalities of *in vivo* neuroreceptor imaging comprise positron emission tomography (PET), single-photon emission computerized tomography (SPECT) and magnetic resonance spectroscopy (MRS). PET and SPECT enable specific and highly sensitive (nanomolar to picomolar) delineation of *in vivo* neurochemistry. MRS is less sensitive (millimolar to micromolar) but non-invasive and without the exposure to ionizing radiation that limits subjects' involvement in PET/SPECT studies. All three techniques have expanding applications within schizophrenia research.

This chapter describes briefly the methodologies of PET and SPECT, and then reviews neurochemical imaging studies of schizophrenia and its pharmacological treatment. In particular, recent work supporting the hyperdopaminergic theory of schizophrenia, insights into neuroleptic dose–response relationships, and mechanisms of atypicality are discussed.

Methodology

PET and SPECT can be used to generate quantitative brain maps of neurochemical targets such as receptors, neurotransmitter transporters, and enzymes. Some examples of scans in transverse section using different radioligands are shown in Fig. 8.1.

Production of radionuclides

PET and SPECT use a limited number of short-lived, proton-rich radionuclides (Table 8.1). PET radionuclides are produced using a cyclotron that accelerates small,

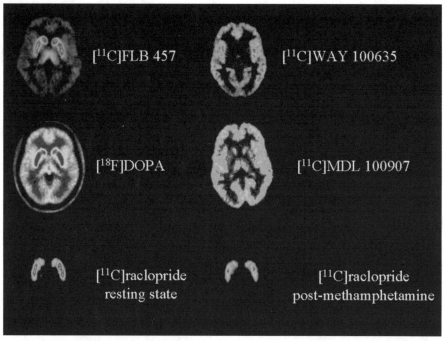

Fig. 8.1 Transverse brain sections of PET scans using a variety of radioligands. The predominantly cortical signal of [^{11}C]MDL100907 and [^{11}C] WAY100635, representing 5-HT$_{2A}$ and 5-HT$_{1A}$ receptors, respectively, can be contrasted with the mainly striatal signal of the dopaminergic ligands. See Plate 9 of the plate section at the centre of this book.

positively charged particles (e.g. protons, deuterons) at target atoms. SPECT radionuclides are either produced in cyclotrons (e.g. ^{123}I) or reactors (e.g. ^{99}Mo, the parent of shorter-lived ^{99m}Tc employed in the blood flow ligand [^{99m}Tc]HMPAO). The radionuclides used for PET scanning are particularly suitable for inclusion in biologically active molecules without changing their function, for example ^{11}C can substitute for normal carbon atoms in many organic molecules. Although SPECT radionuclides are somewhat less amenable, [^{123}I]radioligands are now available for imaging several neurotransmitter systems. PET and SPECT radionuclides differ in their mode of radioactive decay. PET radionuclides decay by emitting a positron (antimatter—a positively charged electron) which travels a short distance (for example 2 mm for ^{11}C) before undergoing an annihilation reaction with an electron. Matter is converted to energy in the form of two high-energy (511 keV) gamma photons travelling at 180° to each other. The maximal resolution of PET is limited to 2–3 mm because of the distance that positrons travel from their source before annihilation, and also because the angle between photons may vary slightly from 180°. In contrast, the proton-rich nuclei of SPECT radionuclides undergo electron capture with release of single gamma photons.

Table 8.1 A comparison of PET and SPECT

	PET	**SPECT**
Radionuclides available (and their half-lives in minutes, hours or days)	^{11}C (20 min) ^{15}O (2.0 min) ^{18}F (110 min) ^{76}Br (16 h)	^{99m}Tc (6.0 h) ^{123}I (13.0 h) ^{133}Xe (5.3 days)
Range of radioligands available	Greater	Narrower
Sensitivity	Higher	Lower
Maximum resolution	2.5–4 mm	6–8 mm
On-site cyclotron	Required	Not required: ligand synthesis elsewhere
Infrastructure and staff requirements	Greater	Lesser
Availability	Restricted	More widespread

Incorporation of radionuclides into radioligands

Simple molecules containing the radionuclides generated above are reacted with radioligand precursors to form radioligands, and purified using automated radiochemistry techniques. For example [^{11}C]raclopride is prepared by methylation of the desmethyl precursor using [^{11}C]methyl iodide. The radioligands used for receptor scans are nearly always selective antagonists and are administered in tracer concentrations (typically occupying ≤ 1% of receptors), thus they do not produce any pharmacological effect. Prior to administration, careful quality control checks are made to ensure purity of the radiotracer. The properties of an ideal radioligand are as follows:

- ease of synthesis and quality control given short half-lives;
- high specific activity (ideally > 2000 Ci/mmol) and purity (>95%);
- high-affinity selective binding to neurochemical target;
- blood–brain barrier penetration;
- absence of labelled lipophilic metabolites;
- accurate modelling;
- absence of toxicity.

The dynamic emission scan

The radiotracer is administered intravenously. The dose of radioactivity used is a compromise between the need to minimize subjects' exposure to ionizing radiation, while ensuring sufficient counts for good scan quality, given the statistical variability associated with radioactive decay. Data from the emission scan are separated into time frames. Arterial blood sampling may be required to provide an input function (see below), and plasma radiotracer levels may also be required to ensure that there is no difference in radiotracer metabolism between groups. The difference in radionuclide decay between PET and SPECT necessitates quite different camera design. In both cases, gamma photons are detected using scintillation detectors made of dense crystalline material that convert the gamma photons into light. The light is then converted into an electrical pulse by a photomultiplier tube. For PET, coincidences (simultaneous pairs of 511 keV photons) are detected by crystal blocks on opposite sides (180°) of the scanner. Blocks are arranged into rings, and multiple adjacent rings surround the scanner's field of view. The source of a coincidence will lie along a line connecting the blocks. For SPECT, the camera relies on collimators—narrow channels in lead overlying the detector crystals that only permit entry of aligned photons. Plates of these are usually rotated around the field of view during a scan, stopping to record at regular intervals. For both PET and SPECT, the sources of individual photons can be backprojected to lines, and point sources identified where these overlap. The residual artefactual line traces are filtered out mathematically. Correction needs to be made for scatter and attenuation of PET and SPECT gamma photons. Compton scatter is deviation of photon course as a result of collisions with electrons. The consequent loss of energy allows such photons to be identified to a certain degree (scatter correction). Attenuation is due to scatter and absorption of photons by tissue and is related to the thickness and density of tissue that the photon passes through. The correction required for attenuation can be determined by performing a transmission scan measuring absorption of photons using an external radioactive source as it rotates around the field of view. The resolution of scans is the limit at which two point sources can be discriminated, and is generally described in terms of full width at half maximum, referring to the count frequency distribution curve obtained from a point source. The resolution is in the order of millimetres, leading to scans appearing blurred. More detailed general reviews of PET and SPECT are given by Bailey and Parker (1998) and Meikle and Dahlbom (1998). For a comparison of PET and SPECT, see Table 8.1.

Modelling

Scan data are in the form of maps of counts during different time frames and require processing in order to obtain useful physiochemical parameters—most importantly a quantitative map of the density of the radioligand target. In the following description, the target type discussed is the receptor, but the principles can be extended to other types of target. Most simply, a ratio of the activity in a region of interest (ROI) and a reference region over a given time period is sometimes adequate for quantification (empirical method). With this method it is assumed that the reference region contains similar levels of non-specifically bound and free radioligand to the ROI, but lacks radioligand specifically bound to receptors. More often, mathematical modelling is required (model-based methods). A model is a representation of radiotracer distribution *in vivo*. More specifically, it describes the biochemical compartments (plasma, free, non-specifically bound and specifically bound) available to the radiotracer and the radiotracer's movement between

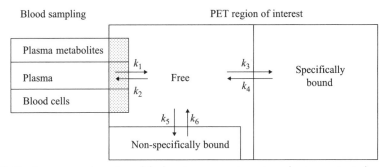

Fig. 8.2 The four-compartment model: showing compartments and rate constants k_{1-6} (adapted from Cunningham and Lammertsma 1994).

them (see Fig. 8.2). Provided certain assumptions are met, simplifications of this otherwise unwieldy four-compartment model can sometimes be made (for example, combining the free and non-specific binding compartments). The radiotracer concentrations in the different compartments vary over time, passing through an uptake phase then a washout phase in the specifically bound compartment after a bolus of a reversibly binding radiotracer. The concentrations and the rate constants for the movements of radiotracer between the compartments can be brought together with receptor density in mathematical expressions derived from the model. These formulae can be rearranged to expresses radioactivity in the target tissue in relation to an 'input function'. The input function is usually the arterial plasma level of parent radiotracer over time. In some cases an indirect input function, the time activity curve (TAC) from a reference tissue (lacking specific binding) can be used after careful experimental validation. Experimentally obtained activity data over the scan time points are substituted into the model equations and parameters estimated. When equilibrium is reached during the time course of the study, the receptor density parameter is binding potential (BP) or volume of distribution (V_D). These are composite measures: BP is related to B_{max}/k_D where B_{max} is the receptor density and k_D the apparent receptor dissociation constant. In some cases when equilibrium is reached during a study, it can be sustained using a constant infusion of the radiotracer after the initial bolus, enabling a simplification of the modelling and the possibility of two experimental conditions within one study (for example, baseline then intravenous drug). The results obtained with any model depend on the goodness of fit of the model to the complex biological system it describes. Models of a radioligand's behaviour must be carefully validated experimentally before being applied to clinical studies. For more information about modelling, the interested reader is referred to Cunningham and Lammertsma (1994) and Slifstein and Laruelle (2001).

Data analysis

There are two principal methods of data analysis:

◆ Region of interest (ROI) analysis. Anatomical regions are defined either using the detailed structural information of an MRI image coregistered to the PET/SPECT image, or using an integrated PET/SPECT image of the time frames that best show the structure of interest. Regions may be defined by hand on images according to algorithms, or on the basis of image intensity boundaries using imaging software, or by normalizing a standard anatomical map drawn on an MRI to the individual's PET/SPECT image. The first method is labour intensive and requires consistent region definition over all scans by the operator, while the latter two methods are rapid and completely reproducible (automated). Usually regions are applied to the dynamic image (set of images at different times) to generate time–activity curves, and the model then used to determine the parameters sought. An alternative is to produce a map of the receptor density measure using the model on a voxel-by-voxel basis, and then to sample this map using the regions. The resolution of PET/SPECT means that at the borders of regions, a given voxel (volume element) is an averaged signal from adjacent regions. This 'partial volume effect' is particularly important for small regions of high activity within a low-activity background (underestimation of activity) or of low activity within a high-activity background (overestimation). Techniques are available to correct for the effect.

◆ Voxel-by-voxel statistical mapping. In this method, ROIs are not defined, rather images are interrogated on a voxel-by-voxel basis. Typically, receptor density maps are normalized (linear and non-linear spatial transformation) into a standard anatomical space (e.g. Montreal Neurological Institute space) using an averaged radioligand binding template map already in standard space. The anatomically normalised images are then smoothed—voxel values are adjusted towards neighbouring voxel values in order principally to improve the signal to noise ratio. Groups of scans can be compared statistically on a voxel-by-voxel basis, as each voxel represents an identical anatomical location. This comparison generates statistical maps. Clusters of voxels significantly different between groups are identified. Corrections can be made for multiple comparisons and for the likelihood of clusters arising by chance. The anatomical identity of a cluster can be determined using an anatomical atlas which contains anatomically segmented brain slices with a spatial coordinates system (e.g. Talairach and Tournoux 1988).

ROI versus voxel-by-voxel statistical mapping

The ROI method is used to detect differences in readily defined anatomical structures. It will fail to detect changes outside those regions. If there are changes in only part of the region, these may be missed as data is averaged over the region. By contrast, voxel-by-voxel statistical mapping uses information from the entire brain and is not constrained by structural anatomy, which may differ from functional anatomy. It is important that the statistical thresholds selected are sufficiently rigorous. In practice, the two methods are often complementary, with an a priori regional hypothesis being tested first, then a statistical parametric mapping (SPM) analysis performed to confirm the ROI analysis and detect any changes in other areas.

Applications of PET and SPECT receptor imaging in schizophrenia research

Many experimental designs are possible, including:

- comparisons of neurochemical target (e.g. receptor) densities between patients and healthy controls;
- within-subject (or between-subject) observation of changes in receptor density during the course of an illness;
- within-subject (or between-subject) studies measuring radioligand blocking by an *exogenous* compound (drug). Drug occupancy can be correlated with drug levels and rating scales, and is usually defined as follows:

$$\text{Occupancy} = \{[(\text{Receptor})_{\text{drug free}} - (\text{Receptor})_{\text{drug treated}}] / (\text{Receptor})_{\text{drug free}}\} \times 100\%;$$

- within-subject studies measuring radioligand displacement by an *endogenous* compound (neurotransmitter) in response to a pharmacological or psychological challenge.

Receptor studies

The main focus in schizophrenia research has been on the monoaminergic systems—particularly the dopaminergic and serotononergic systems. This reflects the history of receptor identification and the known pharmacology of antipsychotic drugs.

Dopamine D$_2$ receptor

Many PET and SPECT studies have estimated striatal dopamine D$_2$ receptor number. Initially, Wong and colleagues, using [^{11}C] N-methylspiperone as a radiotracer, reported a two- to threefold raised striatal D$_2$ receptor number in drug-naïve schizophrenic patients (Wong *et al.* 1986). However, subsequently Farde *et al.* (1987) and other investigators (Hietala *et al.* 1994; Pilowsky *et al.* 1994; Nordstrom *et al.* 1995a), using [^{11}C]raclopride, [^{11}C] N-methylspiperone, and [^{123}I]iodobenzamide, respectively, failed to show such elevations of striatal dopamine D$_2$ receptor number. The suggestion that these conflicting results arose from the different radiotracer methodologies employed is less convincing now that Farde's group has used [^{11}C] N-methylspiperone, in addition to [^{11}C]raclopride, to show no elevation of D$_2$ receptor number (Nordstrom *et al.* 1995a). Further studies have been performed and two meta-analyses provide an overview (Laruelle 1998; Zakzanis and Hansen 1998). Both conclude that dopamine D$_2$ receptor expression is elevated, but with a significant degree of overlap with healthy controls. Post-mortem studies have generally found larger increases in dopamine D$_2$ receptor density in neuroleptic-treated and drug-naïve patients, but *in vivo* studies are subject to the influence that endogenous dopamine may have on estimates of radioligand binding in patients (Gjedde and Wong 2001).

Two studies have examined extra-striatal D_2 receptor density. Receptor densities are considerably lower in cortical and limbic regions than in the striatum, so that to achieve adequate signal to noise ratios, radiotracers of very high affinity (picomolar) are needed. Such tracers are available but are technically challenging to implement and model successfully. However, using the high-affinity radiotracer [^{11}C]FLB457, Suhara et al. (2002b) found reduced D_2 receptor binding in the anterior cingulate cortex (ACC) in a group of 11 drug-naïve male patients with schizophrenia, although inspection of the data suggests that there may be a generalized decrease. Interestingly, the ACC BP was negatively correlated with positive symptom scores. A recent study examining the thalamus in drug-naïve patients with schizophrenia has reported a significant reduction in D_2 receptor binding in the right medial thalamus, using both [^{11}C]raclopride in a group of 19 patients and [^{11}C]FLB457 in a group of 9 patients (Talvik et al. 2003).

Dopamine D_1 receptor

The D_1 receptor is of interest in schizophrenia because it is highly expressed in the prefrontal cortex, and appears to have an important role in working memory, which is impaired in schizophrenia. However, most post-mortem studies have found no change in frontal or striatal D_1 receptor density. There have now been three PET studies of the D_1 receptor in neuroleptic-free or -naïve patients. The radioligands do not distinguish between D_1 receptors and the lower-density D_5 receptors. The first two studies (Okubo et al. 1997; Karlsson et al. 2002) used [^{11}C]SCH23390, which has a relatively high level of non-specific binding and appreciable affinity for the 5-HT$_{2A}$ receptor. The studies were of 17 and 10 patients, respectively. The most recent study (Abi-Dargham et al. 2002) used the more optimal ligand [^{11}C]NNC 112 and involved 17 patients. None of the studies found any change in D_1 receptor density in the striatum, or in cortical regions, with the exception of the prefrontal cortex, where a reduction, no change, and an increase were reported, respectively. On tasks of prefrontal function, Abi-Dargham et al. (2002) found an inverse correlation between D_1 receptor density and performance using the n-back task, while, in contrast, Okubo et al. (1997) found reduced binding to be associated with poor performance in the Wisconsin Card Sorting Test. Opposite directions of association were reported between D_1 receptor density and severity of negative symptoms when comparing the Okubo and Karlsson studies. Clearly, further studies are needed to resolve these discrepancies. In this regard, an ex vivo dissection study has recently been performed in rats, using subchronic depletion of dopamine with reserpine to model the deficit in prefrontal dopaminergic function seen in schizophrenia. Interestingly, this manipulation significantly increased the binding of [^{11}C]NNC 112 in the prefrontal cortex, but left that of [^{3}H]SCH23390 unchanged (Guo et al. 2003).

5-HT$_{2A}$ receptor

A majority of post-mortem studies report a reduction of 5-HT$_{2A}$ receptor density in the prefrontal cortex in schizophrenic patients. Thus there is a clear hypothesis to be investigated *in vivo*. The first available PET radioligand for 5-HT$_{2A}$ receptors, [^{11}C]NMSP, was limited by modelling problems and its appreciable affinity for 5-HT$_{2C}$ receptors, D$_2$ receptors (although these are at low density in the cortex) and α_1 adrenoreceptors. The development of the highly selective PET radiotracer [^{18}F]setoperone has facilitated the examination of the post-mortem-derived hypothesis. Two studies using large cortical regions of interest (including frontal) did not find significant reductions of 5-HT$_{2A}$ receptor binding potential (BP) in drug-naïve/drug-free schizophrenic patients (Trichard *et al.* 1998; Lewis *et al.* 1999). The latter study was reanalysed on a voxel-by-voxel basis to confirm the absence of any specific localized changes (Verhoeff *et al.* 2000). The possible origins of discrepancies between the neuroimaging and post-mortem data are many—in this case, previous treatment or differential ageing effects are the most likely candidates. A further, smaller, voxel-by-voxel [^{18}F]setoperone study (Ngan *et al.* 2000) found a significant decrease in 5-HT$_{2A}$ receptor BP in the frontal cortex of patients with schizophrenia (16% age-adjusted reduction). Further studies using the novel radioligand [^{11}C]MDL-100907 may help to clarify matters, as it is more selective and more readily modelled.

5-HT$_{1A}$ receptor

The majority of post-mortem studies in schizophrenia have found an increase of prefrontal 5-HT$_{1A}$ receptor density, and those that have not, have usually found non-significant increases. In addition, the 5-HT$_{1A}$ receptor may be a suitable target for antipsychotic drugs (reviewed in Bantick *et al.* 2001). The development of the highly selective radioligand [^{11}C]WAY-100635 has permitted PET examination *in vivo*. Two studies using this radioligand in drug-naïve/drug-free schizophrenic patients have been published. One found small increases in cortical 5-HT$_{1A}$ receptor binding potential in patients with schizophrenia that reached regional significance in the left medial temporal cortex only (Tauscher *et al.* 2002*b*). The other found a reduction of 5-HT$_{1A}$ BP in cortical areas that reached significance in the anterior cingulate, although not surviving Bonferroni correction (Lombardo *et al.* 2002, and personal communication). Our own study of drug-treated schizophrenic patients using [^{11}C]WAY-100635 has not identified any change in frontal 5-HT$_{1A}$ receptor density (Bantick *et al.* 2004).

GABA receptor

The γ-aminobutyric acid (GABA) deficit hypothesis of schizophrenia has received mixed support from post-mortem studies. *In vivo* studies have used SPECT and the GABA$_A$/benzodiazepine receptor ligand [^{123}I]iomazenil in mixed groups of neuroleptic-treated and neuroleptic-free schizophrenic patients. No regional differences in benzodiazepine receptor binding have been identified in schizophrenia, using either ROI analysis (Busatto *et al.* 1997, using a semi-quantitative method with 15 patients), statistical parametric mapping (Verhoeff *et al.* 1999, using a constant infusion method with

25 patients), or both techniques combined (Abi-Dargham *et al.* 1999, using a constant infusion method with 16 patients). The first of these studies reported that positive symptom severity correlated inversely with left medial temporal [^{123}I]iomazenil uptake, whereas negative symptom severity correlated inversely with medial frontal uptake, although these did not survive Bonferroni correction. Using the same patients, a later analysis suggested a relationship between reduced uptake and poorer cognitive functioning involving memory and visual attention processes, although again results did not survive Bonferroni correction (Ball *et al.* 1998). Another semi-quantitative study involving 20 patients but no control group found [^{123}I]iomazenil uptake in the medial frontal cortex to be correlated with Brief Psychiatric Rating Scale total score (Schröder *et al.* 1997). However, the two equilibrium method studies failed to find any correlations between clinical rating scales and benzodiazepine receptor levels (Abi-Dargham *et al.* 1999; Verhoeff *et al.* 1999).

Dopaminergic transmission

The dopaminergic system is uniquely accessible to PET and SPECT imaging. Not only can receptor density be quantified (see above), so too can DOPA metabolism and dopamine release and reuptake.

DOPA metabolism

The formation and storage of dopamine in presynaptic terminals can be imaged using [^{18}F]DOPA, a radioactive analogue of DOPA—the precursor of dopamine. [^{18}F]DOPA is taken up by presynaptic monoaminergic neurons and metabolized by DOPA decarboxylase to [^{18}F]dopamine. This is stored within vesicles in the nerve terminals and effectively trapped, as turnover is slow relative to the duration of a PET scan. [^{18}F]DOPA uptake, quantified as the influx constant, K_i, measures DOPA decarboxylase activity and vesicular storage capacity. High values for [^{18}F]DOPA K_i are observed in areas of dense dopamine nerve terminal innervation (e.g. the striatum).

To date, six studies using [^{18}F]DOPA and one using [^{11}C]DOPA have been reported in patients with schizophrenia. These contain 5-12 patients per study and approximately 50 patients in total. Five of the studies describe elevated DOPA metabolism in the striatum (Reith *et al.* 1994; Hietala *et al.* 1995, 1999; Lindstrom *et al.* 1999; Meyer-Lindenberg *et al.* 2002) whereas one found no difference (Dao-Castellana *et al.* 1997) and one reported reduced [^{18}F]DOPA striatal uptake (Elkashef *et al.* 2000). The two studies of Hietala *et al.* used largely overlapping patient samples. Elevations of [^{18}F]DOPA and [^{11}C]DOPA in the striatum were observed in both medication-naïve and medication-free patients. Our own studies using medicated patients have confirmed elevations of [^{18}F]DOPA K_i (McGowan *et al.* 2004). Unfortunately, quantification of cortical [^{18}F]DOPA uptake had not been attempted or achieved in the majority of studies due to the small signal magnitude in cortical areas and the limited sensitivity of the PET cameras.

Dopamine release

An assessment of the functional activity of the dopamine system is possible because of a particular property of two chemically related dopamine radiotracers, [^{123}I] IBZM and [^{11}C]raclopride, binding of which is sensitive to endogenous levels of dopamine. Thus pre-treatment with amphetamine (which releases dopamine and blocks its reuptake) reduces the binding of [^{123}I] IBZM and [^{11}C]raclopride (Volkow *et al.* 1994; Laruelle *et al.* 1995), while the dopamine-depleting drug α-methyl-*para*-tyrosine (AMPT) (Laruelle *et al.* 1997), and tyrosine and phenylalanine depletion (Montgomery *et al.* 2003) increase radiotracer binding. Increased levels of synaptic dopamine reduce the number of binding sites available to the radiotracer.

Using an amphetamine challenge approach, patients with schizophrenia displayed an exaggerated amphetamine-induced release of dopamine compared to normal controls (Laruelle *et al.* 1996; Breier *et al.* 1997; Abi-Dargham *et al.* 1998). Although the increase in positive symptoms after amphetamine challenge correlated with reduction in radiotracer binding, baseline symptom severity did not (Laruelle *et al.* 1999). Interestingly, the only demographic or clinical variable that distinguished patients with an exaggerated response was their clinical state: those who were experiencing an exacerbation of symptoms necessitating admission to hospital had an enhanced response, while stable patients were not significantly different from controls (Laruelle *et al.* 1999). This appears unlikely to represent a non-specific effect of psychiatric illness as non-psychotic unipolar depressed patients do not show such exaggerated responses to amphetamine challenge (Parsey *et al.* 2001). However, interpretation of amphetamine challenge studies is complicated by the wide range of mechanisms by which the drug increases dopamine concentrations in the synapse, including blockade of the reuptake site and promotion of dopamine synthesis and release (Kuczenski and Segal 1997). In the future it may be possible to use more specific pharmacological challenges such as methylphenidate, which reduces [^{11}C]raclopride binding to a similar degree as amphetamine (Volkow *et al.* 1994) but is thought to act purely by blocking the reuptake site (Kuczenski and Segal 1997).

Using the complementary technique of AMPT to measure the relative occupancy of D_2 receptors by dopamine, patients with schizophrenia were found to have significantly increased baseline striatal dopamine levels (Abi-Dargham *et al.* 2000). Interestingly, those patients with the lowest basal levels of dopamine (i.e. smallest increase of [^{11}C]raclopride binding after AMPT) had the least favourable response to treatment with antipsychotic drugs, suggesting that a subgroup of patients may experience positive symptoms due to non-dopaminergic mechanisms.

Dopamine reuptake

Recently, analogues of cocaine have been developed as radioligands for imaging the dopamine transporter (DAT). DATs are located on presynaptic terminals and are considered markers of the density of dopaminergic terminals. Two SPECT studies have

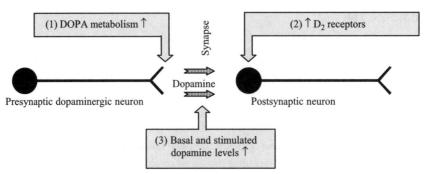

Fig. 8.3 The hyperdopaminergic hypothesis of schizophrenia—positive PET and SPECT findings. Studies of dopamine transporter density and D_1 receptor density have produced negative and conflicting results, respectively.

been performed in mixed groups of drug-naïve, free and treated schizophrenic patients, using $[^{123}I]\beta$-CIT (Laruelle *et al.* 2000) and $[^{123}I]$FP-CIT (Lavalaye *et al.* 2001). In keeping with the post-mortem data, neither study found any change in specific radioligand binding in the striatum in schizophrenic patients. These studies suggest that the changes in DOPA metabolism and dopamine release above are not secondary to an increased density of dopaminergic terminals. Indeed, the former study used patients from their amphetamine challenge study and did not find any association between amphetamine-induced dopamine release and the DAT equilibrium uptake ratio. Antipsychotic drugs did not affect DAT density-this is consistent with *in vitro* studies. Ratings of symptoms did not correlate significantly with the measures of DAT density, although Laruelle *et al.* reported a *trend* level inverse correlation with negative symptom severity.

Overall, DOPA metabolism and release studies provide some of the most direct evidence to date that schizophrenia may be associated with dysfunction of presynaptic striatal dopaminergic function (Fig. 8.3), although the extent to which this abnormality represents the core pathophysiological deficit is uncertain.

It is not clear how presynaptic striatal dopaminergic dysfunction in schizophrenia is related, if at all, to activity in cortical areas such as the prefrontal cortex. Prefrontal lesions modulate striatal dopaminergic function in some, but not all, studies (reviewed in Grace 1991; Carlsson *et al.* 1999). Some recent PET studies are pertinent to this issue. The latest $[^{18}F]$DOPA study demonstrated a negative correlation between striatal $[^{18}F]$DOPA K_i and prefrontal activation in patients with schizophrenia (Meyer-Lindenberg *et al.* 2002). In another study, dorsolateral prefrontal cortical *N*-acetyl-aspartate (NAA) concentration was measured by proton MRS in patients with schizophrenia and found to correlate inversely with amphetamine-induced $[^{11}C]$raclopride displacement (Bertolino *et al.* 2000). While these studies support the hypothesis of prefrontal pathology giving rise to enhanced striatal dopamine release, they do not discriminate between the prefrontal corticostriatal glutamatergic projections and the dopaminergic and GABA-ergic neurons that regulate them. Interestingly, healthy volunteers given the N-methyl-D-aspartate (NMDA) receptor antagonist ketamine show an exaggerated response to amphetamine (Kegeles *et al.* 2000), suggesting that an underlying NMDA receptor hypofunction could account for the exaggerated amphetamine response seen in schizophrenia.

PET and SPECT in the investigation of antipsychotic drugs

All antipsychotic drugs block dopamine D_2 receptors, with affinities closely correlated with clinical potency (Creese *et al.* 1976; Seeman *et al.* 1976). PET and SPECT have proven invaluable tools for measuring drug occupancy at D_2 and other receptors in the living brain, and exploring relationships between occupancy and clinical measures. They complement *in vitro* studies, as they are influenced by plasma binding, metabolism and metabolites, the blood–brain barrier, and, of course, the dynamic biochemical complexity of the brain (including the presence of neurotransmitters competing for receptors). However, PET and SPECT are limited at the present time by being unable to determine the functional effect on receptors (e.g. agonism). D_2 receptor ligands do bind to additional receptors—even the highly selective benzamides (such as raclopride and epidepride) also bind to D_3 receptors. It is important to note how occupancy is calculated and the assumptions made (see Methodology section). Single/brief-dosing, within-subject study designs in patients that would minimize assumptions and errors are rarely possible for practical or ethical reasons: for example, the delays between starting drug administration and responses usually prevent brief dosing studies. Between-subject studies should employ a carefully matched (including usually for illness) control group. When occupancy values are given for individuals in a between-subject study, these are only estimates, as a mean control group receptor density measure is used rather than the individual's true pre-treatment value. When drug treatment is chronic, it may underestimate occupancy if receptor upregulation occurs. In addition, increases in dopamine release may occur following neuroleptics, and could theoretically reduce radioligand binding. However, such effects are of small magnitude (compared to amphetamine-induced dopamine release for example) and therefore unlikely to influence calculated occupancy (see, for example, Farde *et al.* 1992). This section will describe PET and SPECT research in this extensive field, along with the implications for clinical practice and theories of atypicality.

Striatal D_2 occupancy and clinical effects

Three [^{11}C]raclopride PET studies have been of particular importance in elucidating the relationship between D_2 receptor occupancy and clinical response. In an open study by Farde *et al.* (1992) striatal D_2 receptor occupancy was 70–89% in schizophrenic patients treated with a range of chemically distinct classical neuroleptics titrated to a dose to which they responded. Interestingly, occupancy was only 38–63% in patients treated with clozapine. Furthermore, patients with extrapyramidal side-effects (EPS) had a higher mean D_2 receptor occupancy (82% ± 4% SD) than those without (74% ± 4% SD). Two double-blind randomized treatment studies have subsequently investigated the relationship between typical neuroleptic D_2 receptor occupancy and outcome measures at different doses of neuroleptics, with similar results. Nordström *et al.* (1993), treating patients with pharmacological doses of raclopride, found a significant relationship between D_2 receptor occupancy and both clinical improvement and EPS. Three out of the four poor responders had D_2 occupancy below 50%, suggesting a threshold effect for response. In a later extension of the analysis, prolactin elevation (an effect on D_2 receptors outside the blood–brain barrier) occurred in eight of nine patients with a striatal D_2 occupancy above 50%, but none of those with lower occupancies, suggesting a threshold at around 50% for prolactin elevation with raclopride (Nordstrom and Farde 1998). Kapur *et al.* (2000*b*), treating patients with haloperidol doses of 1 or 2.5 mg/day, found that striatal D_2 occupancy predicted antipsychotic response, EPS and akathesia, and prolactin elevation. A threshold of 65% occupancy best separated treatment responders from non-responders, and above this threshold there was no relationship between clinical response and D_2 occupancy. Although the numbers were small, the patients who had extrapyramidal side-effects or akathisia all had higher occupancies (mean 81%), while none of the patients below 78% occupancy showed extrapyramidal side-effects or akathisia. Prolactin elevation became prominent above 72% occupancy. The concept of thresholds of striatal D_2 occupancy for different clinical effects is illustrated in Fig. 8.4. Clinical doses of atypical antipsychotics also produce occupancies above the 65% threshold for clinical response, with the exceptions of clozapine and quetiapine (see below). Intriguingly, Nyberg *et al.* have suggested that once psychosis is in remission, relapse prevention may be possible with lower occupancy levels (Nyberg *et al.* 1995).

The above results strongly suggest that drug treatment with typical neuroleptics should aim for striatal D_2 receptor occupancy that is above the antipsychotic threshold but below the EPS threshold. Above the antipsychotic threshold, higher doses do not improve antipsychotic efficacy. One important clinical implication of the above studies was that typical neuroleptics were being used at excessive doses both clinically and in trials against atypical drugs (Nyberg and Farde 2000).

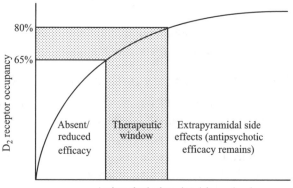

Fig. 8.4 D_2 receptor occupancy plotted against dose for a typical antipsychotic drug, showing the therapeutic threshold (shown as 65%, although various values between 50 and 70% have been proposed) and the theshold for extrapyramidal side-effects (quite consistently located at around 80%).

Notwithstanding the above, there are at least three major limitations to the dopaminergic occupancy model of antipsychotic drug efficacy:

- although D_2 occupancy appears necessary for clinical response, it is not always sufficient (Pilowsky *et al.* 1993);

- antipsychotic response occurs at least 10 to 14 days after D_2 blockade has been established;

- relapse after discontinuation of an antipsychotic may take months.

Investigating proposed mechanisms of atypicality

PET and SPECT have been valuable in evaluating hypotheses about mechanism(s) of atypicality (here defined as a low liability to EPS in the clinical dose range):

Low striatal D_2 occupancy

Following the report of low striatal D_2 occupancy at clinically effective doses of clozapine (Farde *et al.* 1992), the patient group was extended by Nordstrom and Farde. Over the range of usual UK clinical doses (200–900 mg/day), the study by Nordstrom *et al.* (1995b) found 33–67% occupancy, while a later independent study found a similar range of 47–68% occupancy (Kapur *et al.* 1999). Dose-occupancy curves for clozapine in these studies indicated a theoretical maximal striatal D_2 binding around 70%—suggesting a unique mechanism for clozapine's atypicality. However, subsequent PET studies in primates, using higher doses of clozapine than would be tolerated in humans, have demonstrated that occupancies of up to 89% can be achieved (Nyberg *et al.* 2002; Suhara *et al.* 2002a). Interestingly, quetiapine also has low striatal D_2 occupancy: 0–50% at 2 h (Gefvert *et al.* 2001) falling to 0–27% after 12–14 h (Kapur *et al.* 2000a). This low striatal D_2 occupancy is not shared by the atypical antipsychotic drug risperidone, which has an occupancy of 53–85% in the 2–8 mg/day dose range (Kapur *et al.* 1999; Nyberg *et al.* 1999), nor by olanzapine, with an occupancy of 43–80% over the 5–20 mg/day dose range (Nyberg *et al.* 1997; Kapur *et al.* 1999). At lower striatal D_2 occupancies, theoretically, sufficient dopamine can reach postsynaptic receptors to avoid EPS (Strange 2001). The low-affinity drugs clozapine and quetiapine do not reach the occupancy threshold for EPS over their clinical dose ranges. Interestingly, they may also possess additional kinetic protection from EPS by having unusually high k_{off} rates (Kapur and Seeman 2001). In the dynamic environment of the synapse, equilibrium is not reached, thus it is more appropriate to consider k_{on} (similar between antipsychotics) and k_{off} (markedly variable) rather than the affinity constant for the drug-receptor complex ($k_D = k_{off}/k_{on}$). A high k_{off} rate leads to loose binding, enabling rapid displacement of clozapine and quetiapine from the D_2 receptor by endogenous dopamine. As a result, phasic dopaminergic release can be at least partially transmitted (Seeman and Tallerico 1999). The high k_{off} rates of clozapine and quetiapine are also consistent with their relatively short brain half-lives compared to those of other antipsychotic drugs (Jones *et al.* 2000; Kapur *et al.* 2000a; Tauscher *et al.* 2002a).

Limbic selectivity

This concept takes into consideration both striatal and limbic D_2 occupancy to account for clozapine's antipsychotic activity despite low striatal D_2 occupancy. Blockade of the mesolimbic pathways is believed to underlie the therapeutic response to antipsychotic drugs, while blockade of the nigrostriatal pathway is responsible for EPS. The limbic selectivity theory posits that a neuroleptic is atypical when it produces a relatively high limbic D_2 receptor occupancy (thus antipsychotic efficacy) but a relatively low striatal occupancy (thus low liability to EPS). This hypothesis was difficult to test until high-affinity (picomolar) ligands capable of detecting low-density extrastriatal D_2 receptors became available. Using [^{123}I]epidepride SPECT, Pilowsky et al. (1997) found that clozapine produced high D_2 occupancy (90% mean) in a temporal cortex region that included limbic regions, despite significantly lower striatal occupancy (58% mean), while typical antipsychotics produced high occupancy in both regions (96% and 90% respectively). The mechanism of limbic selectivity is unclear. It may arise because higher striatum dopamine levels displace atypical antipsychotic drugs with high k_{off} rates. Levels of dopamine in the temporal cortex are lower, thus atypical and typical antipsychotic drugs behave similarly (Kapur and Seeman 2002). Limbic selectivity has also been identified for quetiapine, olanzapine, sertindole, and amisulpride (Bigliani et al. 2000; Stephenson et al. 2000; Xiberas et al. 2001a, b), but results are mixed for risperidone [selectivity was identified by Xiberas et al. (2001b) and Bressan et al. (2003), but not by Yasuno et al. (2001)]. However, at low doses, typical neuroleptics may also show limbic selectivity (see individual patient data in Bigliani et al. 1999; Kopecek et al. 2002). A comprehensive study examining limbic selectivity of atypical over typical drugs at comparable striatal occupancies is awaited.

In contrast to Pilowsky et al. (1997) and Xiberas et al. (2001b), two recent studies have not replicated clozapine's limbic selectivity: a study in humans found *low* occupancy in striatal and extrastriatal regions (Talvik et al. 2001), while in monkeys *moderate* occupancy occurs in both regions at peak clozapine levels (Mukherjee et al. 2001). These discrepancies may reflect differences between the ligands or their modelling. For example, if radiotracer equilibrium is not attained in high-signal areas (striatum) compared to low-signal areas (cortex), occupancy values may be underestimated in striatal areas. The use of the cerebellum as a reference region is controversial when using high-affinity D_2 radioligands, as they detect displaceable specific binding.

5-HT$_{2A}$ antagonism

Clozapine, quetiapine, olanzapine, and risperidone have relatively high affinities for the 5-HT$_{2A}$ receptor *in vitro*. PET and SPECT have been used to explore whether this may reduce the liability to EPS *in vivo*. Using PET, it has been found that, despite saturation of 5-HT$_{2A}$ receptors, both risperidone (Kapur et al. 1995; Nyberg et al. 1999) and olanzapine (Kapur et al. 1998) can produce EPS at higher doses when striatal D_2 occupancy exceeds 80%, in a manner similar to conventional antipsychotics.

Furthermore, a SPECT study comparing risperidone and haloperidol at similar striatal D_2 occupancies, using [^{123}I]IBZM, did not find any difference in EPS (Knable *et al.* 1997). Although 5-HT$_{2A}$ receptor blockade does not appear to have a major role in generating atypicality, that does not exclude possible utility in other areas, such as mood, negative, and cognitive symptoms. That 5-HT$_{2A}$ antagonism is not in itself antipsychotic is indicated by the high levels of 5-HT$_{2A}$ receptor occupancy by doses of clozapine below the therapeutic range (Nordstrom *et al.* 1995*b*; Kapur *et al.* 1999).

D$_2$ receptor partial agonism

Therapeutic doses of the novel atypical antipsychotic drug aripiprazole are reported to produce a low incidence of EPS in patients (reviewed in McGavin and Goa 2002). In an [^{11}C]raclopride within-subject PET study in healthy volunteers, therapeutic doses of aripiprazole were found to produce average striatal occupancies in excess of 80% without producing EPS (Yokoi *et al.* 2002). This striking result is probably accounted for by aripiprazole being a *partial agonist* at the D_2 receptor (Shapiro *et al.* 2003), although partial agonist effects at the 5-HT$_{1A}$ receptor (Jordan *et al.* 2002) and antagonist effects at the 5-HT$_{2A}$ receptor may also be of relevance.

Current and future use of PET and SPECT scanning with antipsychotic drugs

Striatal D_2 occupancy measures central drug activity and is, in general, well correlated with both therapeutic effects and EPS. Thus PET and SPECT are vital tools for determining the dose and dosing interval required for novel antipsychotic drugs. Other receptors may be useful targets for antipsychotic drugs (e.g. 5-HT$_{2C}$, 5-HT$_{1A}$, α_2-adrenoceptor, glutamatergic) but, in the majority of cases, are awaiting selective radioligands for full investigation.

Conclusions

PET and SPECT are powerful techniques that enable exploration of the neurochemistry of the living human brain. They have been instrumental in developing and testing the hyperdopaminergic theory of schizophrenia and the dopaminergic occupancy theory of antipsychotic drugs. Although receptor density studies have been somewhat disappointing, overactivity of striatal dopaminergic neurons has been demonstrated in schizophrenic patients. Occupancy of D_2 receptors has been found to be a necessary, but not sufficient, condition for antipsychotic drug efficacy. Plausible explanations of atypicality have been investigated. Clearly these theories are only part of a broader neurochemical understanding of schizophrenia that remains to be fully developed. Currently the number of available radiotracers is very small in relation to the increasing number of receptor and other radioligand targets so far characterized. Work on the effect of cognitive challenges on striatal dopamine levels has demonstrated that links between cognitive processes and neurochemistry can be explored. Interactions between different transmitter systems can be explored using highly selective pharmacological probes and radiotracers (see Kegeles *et al.* 2000 discussed above).Within a broader research context, combinations of PET and SPECT with other imaging modalities, animal and *in vitro* work offer much greater investigative power than any single technique, and further fruitful collaborations are awaited.

References

Abi-Dargham, A., Gil, R., Krystal, J., Baldwin, R. M. Seibyl, J. P., Bowers, M. *et al.* (1998). Increased striatal dopamine transmission in schizophrenia: confirmation in a second cohort. *American Journal of Psychiatry,* **155,** 761–7.

Abi-Dargham, A., Laruelle, M., Krystal, J., D'Souza, C., Zoghbi, S., Baldwin, R. M. *et al.* (1999). No evidence of altered in vivo benzodiazepine receptor binding in schizophrenia. *Neuropsychopharmacology,* **20,** 650–61.

Abi-Dargham, A., Rodenhiser, J., Printz, D., Zea-Poncce, Y., Gil, R., Kegeles, L. *et al.* (2000). Increased baseline occupancy of D2 receptors by dopamine in schizophrenia. *Proceedings of the National Academy of Sciences USA,* **97,** 8104–9.

Abi–Dargham, A., Mawlawi, O., Lombardo, I., Gil, R., Martinez, D., Huang, Y. *et al.* (2002). Prefrontal dopamine D1 receptors and working memory in schizophrenia. *Journal of Neuroscience,* **22,** 3708–19.

Bailey, D. L. and Parker, J. A. (1998). Single photon emission computed tomography. In *Nuclear medicine in clinical diagnosis and treatment,* (ed. P. J. Ell), (2nd edn), pp. 1589–1601. Churchill Livingstone, Edinburgh.

Ball, S., Busatto, G. F., David, A. S. Jones, S.H., Hemsley, D.R., Pilowsky, L. S. *et al.* (1998). Cognitive functioning and $GABA_A$/benzodiazepine receptor binding in schizophrenia: a 123I-iomazenil SPET study. *Biological Psychiatry,* **43,** 107–17.

Bantick, R. A., Deakin, J. F., and Grasby, P. M. (2001). The $5-HT_{1A}$ receptor in schizophrenia: a promising target for novel atypical neuroleptics? *Journal of Psychopharmacology,* **15,** 37–46.

Bantick, R. A., Montgomery, A. J., Bench, C. J., Choudhry, T., Malek, N., Mckenna, P. J. (2004). A PET study of the $5-HT_{1A}$ receptor in schizophrenia and during clozapine treatment. *Journal of Psychopharmacology,* **18** (3), 346–54.

Bertolino, A., Breier, A., Callicott, J. H., Adler, C., Mattay, V. S., Shapiro, M. *et al.* (2000). The relationship between dorsolateral prefrontal neuronal N- acetylaspartate and evoked release of striatal dopamine in schizophrenia. *Neuropsychopharmacology,* **22,** 125–32.

Bigliani, V., Mulligan, R. S., Acton, P. D., Visvikis, D., Ell, P. J., Stephenson, C. *et al.* (1999). In vivo occupancy of striatal and temporal cortical D2/D3 dopamine receptors by typical antipsychotic drugs. [^{123}I]epidepride single photon emission tomography (SPET) study. *British Journal of Psychiatry,* **175,** 231–8.

Bigliani, V., Mulligan, R. S., Acton, P. D., Ohlsen, R. I., Pike, V. W., Ell, P. J. *et al.* (2000). Striatal and temporal cortical D2/D3 receptor occupancy by olanzapine and sertindole *in vivo*: a [^{123}I]epidepride single photon emission tomography (SPET) study. *Psychopharmacology (Berlin),* **150,** 132–40.

Breier, A., Su, T. P., Saunders, R., Carson, R. E., Kolachana, B. S., de Bartolomeis, A. *et al.* (1997). Schizophrenia is associated with elevated amphetamine-induced synaptic dopamine concentrations: evidence from a novel positron emission tomography method. *Proceedings of the National Academy of Sciences USA,* **94,** 2569–74.

Bressan, R. A., Erlandsson, K., Jones, H. M., Mulligan, R. S., Ell, P. J., and Pilowsky, L. S. (2003). Optimizing limbic selective D_2/D_3 receptor occupancy by risperidone: a [^{123}I]-epidepride SPET study. *Journal of Clinical Psychopharmacology,* **23,** 5–14.

Busatto, G. F., Pilowsky, L. S., Costa, D. C., Ell, P. J., David, A. S., Lucey, J. V. *et al.* (1997). Correlation between reduced in vivo benzodiazepine receptor binding and severity of psychotic symptoms in schizophrenia. *American Journal of Psychiatry*, **154**, 56–63.

Carlsson, A., Waters, N., and Carlsson, M. L. (1999). Neurotransmitter interactions in schizophrenia–therapeutic implications. *Biological Psychiatry*, **46**, 1388–95.

Creese, I., Burt, D. R., and Snyder, S. H. (1976). Dopamine receptor binding predicts clinical and pharmacological potencies of antischizophrenic drugs. *Science*, **192**, 481–3.

Cunningham, V. J. and Lammertsma, A. A. (1994). Radioligand studies in brain: kinetic analysis of PET data. *Med Chem Research*, **5**, 79–96.

Dao-Castellana, M. H., Paillere-Martinot, M. L., Hantraye, P., Attar-Levy, D., Remy, P., Crouzel, C. *et al.* (1997). Presynaptic dopaminergic function in the striatum of schizophrenic patients. *Schizophrenia Research*, **23**, 167–74.

Elkashef, A. M., Doudet, D., Bryant, T., Cohen, R. M., Li, S. H., and Wyatt, R. J. (2000). 6-(18) F-DOPA PET study in patients with schizophrenia. Positron emission tomography. *Psychiatry Research*, **100**, 1–11.

Farde, L., Wiesel, F. A., Hall, H., Halldin, C., Stone-Elander, S., and Sedvall, G. (1987). No D2 receptor increase in PET study of schizophrenia. *Archives of General Psychiatry*, **44**, 671–2.

Farde, L., Nordstrom, A. L., Wiesel, F. A., Pauli, S., Halldin, C., and Sedvall, G. (1992). Positron emission tomographic analysis of central D1 and D2 dopamine receptor occupancy in patients treated with classical neuroleptics and clozapine. Relation to extrapyramidal side effects. *Archives of General Psychiatry*, **49**, 538–44.

Gefvert, O., Lundberg, T., Wieselgren, I. M., Bergstrom, M., Langstrom, B., Wiesel, F. *et al.* (2001). D(2) and 5HT(2A) receptor occupancy of different doses of quetiapine in schizophrenia: a PET study. *European Neuropsychopharmacology*, **11**, 105–10.

Gjedde, A. and Wong, D. F. (2001). Quantification of neuroreceptors in living human brain v. endogenous neurotransmitter inhibition of haloperidol binding in psychosis. *Journal of Cerebral Blood Flow and Metabolism*, **21**, 982–94.

Grace, A. A. (1991). Phasic versus tonic dopamine release and the modulation of dopamine system responsivity: a hypothesis for the etiology of schizophrenia. *Neuroscience*, **41**, 1–24.

Guo, N., Hwang, D. R., Lo, E. S., Huang, Y. Y., Laruelle, M., and Abi-Dargham, A. (2003). Dopamine depletion and *in vivo* binding of PET D_1 receptor radioligands: implications for imaging studies in schizophrenia. *Neuropsychopharmacology*, **28**, 1703–11.

Hietala, J., Syvalahti, E., Vuorio, K., Nagren, K., Lehikoinen, P., Ruotsalainen, U. *et al.* (1994). Striatal D2 dopamine receptor characteristics in neuroleptic-naive schizophrenic patients studied with positron emission tomography. *Archives of General Psychiatry*, **51**, 116–23.

Hietala, J., Syvalahti, E., Vuorio, K., Rakkolainen, V., Bergman, J., Haaparanta, M. *et al.* (1995). Presynaptic dopamine function in striatum of neuroleptic-naive schizophrenic patients. *Lancet*, **346**, 1130–1.

Hietala, J., Syvalahti, E., Vilkman, H., Vuorio, K., Rakkolainen, V., Bergman, J. *et al.* (1999). Depressive symptoms and presynaptic dopamine function in neuroleptic-naive schizophrenia. *Schizophrenia Research*, **35**, 41–50.

Jones, C., Kapur, S., Remington, G., and Zipursky, R. B. (2000). Transient D_2 dopamine receptor occupancy in low EPS-incidence drugs: PET evidence [abstract]. *Biological Psychiatry*, **47**, 112S.

Jordan, S., Koprivica, V., Chen, R., Tottori, K., Kikuchi, T., and Altar, C. A. (2002). The antipsychotic aripiprazole is a potent, partial agonist at the human 5-HT_{1A} receptor. *European Journal of Pharmacology*, **441**, 137–40.

Kapur, S. and Seeman, P. (2001). Does fast dissociation from the dopamine d(2) receptor explain the action of atypical antipsychotics?: A new hypothesis. *American Journal of Psychiatry*, **158**, 360–9.

Kapur, S. and Seeman, P. (2002). Atypical antipsychotics, cortical D_2 receptors and sensitivity to endogenous dopamine: letter. *British Journal of Psychiatry*, **180**, 465–6.

Kapur, S., Remington, G., Zipursky, R. B., Wilson, A. A., and Houle, S. (1995). The D2 dopamine receptor occupancy of risperidone and its relationship to extrapyramidal symptoms: a PET study. *Life Science*, **57**, PL103–7.

Kapur, S., Zipursky, R. B., Remington, G., Jones, C., Dasilva, J., Wilson, A. A. et al. (1998). 5-HT2 and D2 receptor occupancy of olanzapine in schizophrenia: a PET investigation. *American Journal of Psychiatry*, **155**, 921–8.

Kapur, S., Zipursky, R. B., and Remington, G. (1999). Clinical and theoretical implications of 5-HT2 and D2 receptor occupancy of clozapine, risperidone, and olanzapine in schizophrenia. *American Journal of Psychiatry*, **156**, 286–93.

Kapur, S., Zipursky, R., Jones, C., Shammi, C. S., Remington, G., and Seeman, P. (2000a). A positron emission tomography study of quetiapine in schizophrenia: a preliminary finding of an antipsychotic effect with only transiently high dopamine D2 receptor occupancy. *Archives of General Psychiatry*, **57**, 553–9.

Kapur, S., Zipursky, R., Jones, C., Remington, G., and Houle, S. (2000b). Relationship between dopamine D_2 occupancy, clinical response, and side effects: a double-blind PET study of first-episode schizophrenia. *American Journal of Psychiatry*, **157**, 514–20.

Karlsson, P., Farde, L., Halldin, C., and Sedvall, G. (2002). PET study of D(1) dopamine receptor binding in neuroleptic-naive patients with schizophrenia. *American Journal of Psychiatry*, **159**, 761–7.

Kegeles, L. S., Abi-Dargham, A., Zea-Ponce, Y., Rodenhiser-Hill, J., Mann, J. J., Van Heertum, R. L. et al. (2000). Modulation of amphetamine-induced striatal dopamine release by ketamine in humans: implications for schizophrenia. *Biological Psychiatry*, **48**, 627–40.

Knable, M. B., Heinz, A., Raedler, T., and Weinberger, D. R. (1997). Extrapyramidal side effects with risperidone and haloperidol at comparable D2 receptor occupancy levels. *Psychiatry Research*, **75**, 91–101.

Kopecek, M., Hoschl, C., and Hajek, T. (2002). Regional selectivity of novel antipsychotics [letter]. *British Journal of Psychiatry*, **181**, 254–5.

Kuczenski, R. and Segal, D. S. (1997). Effects of methylphenidate on extracellular dopamine, serotonin, and norepinephrine: comparison with amphetamine. *Journal of Neurochemistry*, **68**, 2032–7.

Laruelle, M. (1998). Imaging dopamine transmission in schizophrenia. A review and meta-analysis. *Quarterly Journal of Nuclear Medicine*, **42**, 211–21.

Laruelle, M., Abi-Dargham, A., van Dyck, C. H., Rosenblatt, W., Zea-Ponce, Y., Zoghbi, S. S. et al. (1995). SPECT imaging of striatal dopamine release after amphetamine challenge *Journal of Nuclear Medicine*, **36**, 1182–90.

Laruelle, M., Abi-Dhargam, A., van Dyck, C., Gil, R., D'Souza, C., Erdos, J. et al. (1996). Single photon emission computerized tomography imaging of amphetamine-induced dopamine in drug-free schizophrenic subjects. *Proceedings of the National Academy of Sciences USA*, **93**, 9235–40.

Laruelle, M., D'Souza, C. D., Baldwin, R. M., Abi-Dargham, A., Kanes, S. J., Fingado, C. L. et al. (1997). Imaging D2 receptor occupancy by endogenous dopamine in humans. *Neuropsychopharmacology*, **17**, 162–74.

Laruelle, M., Abi-Dargham, A., Gil, R., Kegeles, L., and Innis, R. (1999). Increased dopamine transmission in schizophrenia: relationship to illness phases. *Biological Psychiatry*, **46**, 56–72.

Laruelle, M., Abi-Dargham, A., Van Dyck, C., Gil, R., D'Souza, D. C., Krystal, J. et al. (2000). Dopamine and serotonin transporters in patients with schizophrenia: an imaging study with [(123)I]beta-CIT. *Biological Psychiatry*, **47**, 371–9.

Lavalaye, J., Linszen, D. H., Booij, J., Dingemans, P. M., Reneman, L., Habraken, J. B. *et al.* (2001). Dopamine transporter density in young patients with schizophrenia assessed with [123]FP-CIT SPECT. *Schizophrenia Research*, **47**, 59–67.

Lewis, R., Kapur, S., Jones, C., Dasilva, J., Brown, G. M.,Wilson, A. A. *et al.* (1999). Serotonin 5-HT2 receptors in schizophrenia: a PET study using [18F]setoperone in neuroleptic-naive patients and normal subjects. *American Journal of Psychiatry*, **156**, 72–8.

Lindstrom, L. H., Gefvert, O., Hagberg, G., Lundberg, T., Bergstrom, M., Hartvig, P. *et al.* (1999). Increased dopamine synthesis rate in medial prefrontal cortex and striatum in schizophrenia indicated by L-(beta-11C) DOPA and PET. *Biological Psychiatry*, **46**, 681–8.

Lombardo, I., Slifstein, M., Fullerton, C., Gil, R., Hwang, D., Martin, J. *et al.* (2002). Imaging the 5-HT1A receptor in patients with schizophrenia and healthy controls using [^{11}C]WAY-100635 [abstract]. *Neuroimage*, **16**, S106.

McGavin, J. K. and Goa, K. L. (2002). Aripiprazole. *CNS Drugs,* **16**, 779–86; discussion 787–8.

McGowan, S., Lawrence, A. D., Sales, T., Quested, D. and Grasby, P. (2004). Presynaptic dopaminergic dysfunction in schizophrenia: a positron emission tomographic [^{18}F] fluorodopa study. *Archives of General Psychiatry*, **61**,134-42.

Meikle, S. R. and Dahlbom, M. (1998). Positron emission tomography. In *Nuclear medicine in clinical diagnosis and treatment,* (ed. P. J. Ell), (2nd edn), pp. 1603–16. Churchill Livingstone,

Meyer-Lindenberg, A., Miletich, R. S., Kohn, P. D., Esposito, G., Carson, R. E., Quarantelli, M. *et al.* (2002). Reduced prefrontal activity predicts exaggerated striatal dopaminergic function in schizophrenia. *Nature Neuroscience*, **5**, 267-71.

Montgomery, A. J., McTavish, S. F. B., Cowen, P. J., and Grasby, P. M. (2003). Reduction of brain dopamine concentration with dietary tyrosine plus phenylalanine depletion: an [^{11}C]raclopride PET study. *American Journal of Psychiatry*, **160**, 1887–9.

Mukherjee, J., Christian, B. T., Narayanan, T. K., Shi, B., and Mantil, J. (2001). Evaluation of dopamine D-2 receptor occupancy by clozapine, risperidone, and haloperidol in vivo in the rodent and nonhuman primate brain using 18F-fallypride. *Neuropsychopharmacology*, **25**, 476–88.

Ngan, E. T., Yatham, L. N., Ruth, T. J., and Liddle, P. F. (2000). Decreased serotonin 2A receptor densities in neuroleptic-naive patients with schizophrenia: A PET study using [(18)F]setoperone. *American Journal of Psychiatry*, **157**, 1016–18.

Nordstrom, A. L. and Farde, L. (1998). Plasma prolactin and central D2 receptor occupancy in antipsychotic drug-treated patients. *Journal of Clinical Psychopharmacology*, **18**, 305–10.

Nordstrom, A. L., Farde, L., Wiesel, F. A. Forslund, K., Pauli, S., Halldin, C. *et al.* (1993). Central D2-dopamine receptor occupancy in relation to antipsychotic drug effects: a double-blind PET study of schizophrenic patients. *Biological Psychiatry*, **33**, 227–35.

Nordstrom, A. L., Farde, L., Eriksson, L., and Halldin, C. (1995*a*). No elevated D2 dopamine receptors in neuroleptic-naive schizophrenic patients revealed by positron emission tomography and [11C]N-methylspiperone. *Psychiatry Research*, **61**, 67–83.

Nordstrom, A. L., Farde, L., Nyberg, S., Karlsson, P., Halldin, C., and Sedvall, G. (1995*b*). D1, D2, and 5-HT2 receptor occupancy in relation to clozapine serum concentration: a PET study of schizophrenic patients. *American Journal of Psychiatry*, **152**, 1444–9.

Nyberg, S. and Farde, L (2000). Non-equipotent doses partly explain differences among antipsychotics–implications of PET studies. *Psychopharmacology (Berlin)*, **148**, 22–3.

Nyberg, S., Farde, L., Halldin, C., Dahl, M. L., and Bertilsson, L. (1995). D2 dopamine receptor occupancy during low-dose treatment with haloperidol decanoate. *American Journal of Psychiatry*, **152**, 173–8.

Nyberg, S., Farde, L., and Halldin, C. (1997). A PET study of 5-HT2 and D2 dopamine receptor occupancy induced by olanzapine in healthy subjects. *Neuropsychopharmacology*, **16**, 1–7.

Nyberg, S., Eriksson, B., Oxenstierna, G., Halldin, C., and Farde, L. (1999). Suggested minimal effective dose of risperidone based on PET-measured D2 and 5-HT2A receptor occupancy in schizophrenic patients. *American Journal of Psychiatry*, **156**, 869–75.

Nyberg, S., Chou, Y. H., and Halldin, C. (2002). Saturation of striatal D2 dopamine receptors by clozapine. *International Journal of Neuropsychopharmacology*, **5**, 11–16.

Okubo, Y., Suhara, T., Suzuki, K., Kobayashi, K., Inoue, O., Terasaki, O. *et al.* (1997). Decreased prefrontal dopamine D1 receptors in schizophrenia revealed by PET. *Nature*, **385**, 634–6.

Parsey, R. V., Oquendo, M. A., Zea-Ponce, Y., Rodenhiser, J., Kegeles, L. S., Pratap, M. *et al.* (2001). Dopamine D(2) receptor availability and amphetamine-induced dopamine release in unipolar depression. *Biological Psychiatry*, **50**, 313–22.

Pilowsky, L. S., Costa, D. C., Ell, P. J., Murray, R. M., Verhoeff, N. P., and Kerwin, R. W. (1993). Antipsychotic medication, D2 dopamine receptor blockade and clinical response: a 123I IBZM SPET (single photon emission tomography) study. *Psychological Medicine*, **23**, 791–7.

Pilowsky, L. S., Costa, D. C., Ell, P. J., Verhoeff, N. P., Murray, R. M., and Kerwin, R. W. (1994). D2 dopamine receptor binding in the basal ganglia of antipsychotic-free schizophrenic patients. An 123I-IBZM single photon emission computerised tomography study. *British Journal of Psychiatry*, **164**, 16–26.

Pilowsky, L. S., Mulligan, R. S., Acton, P. D., Ell, P. J., Costa, D. C., and Kerwin, R. W. (1997). Limbic selectivity of clozapine. *Lancet*, **350**, 490–1.

Reith, J., Benkelfat, C., Sherwin, A., Yasuhara, Y., Kuwabara, H., Andermann, F. *et al.* (1994). Elevated dopa decarboxylase activity in living brain of patients with psychosis. *Proceedings of the National Academy of Sciences USA*, **91**, 11651–4.

Seeman, P. and Tallerico, T. (1999). Rapid release of antipsychotic drugs from dopamine D2 receptors: an explanation for low receptor occupancy and early clinical relapse upon withdrawal of clozapine or quetiapine. *American Journal of Psychiatry*, **156**, 876–84.

Seeman, P., Lee, T., Chau-Wong, M., and Wong, K. (1976). Antipsychotic drug doses and neuroleptic/dopamine receptors. *Nature*, **261**, 717–19.

Shapiro, D. A., Renock, S., Arrington, E., Chiodo, L. A., Liu, L. X., Sibley, D. R. *et al.* (2003). Aripiprazole, a novel atypical antipsychotic drug with a unique and robust pharmacology. *Neuropsychopharmacology*, **28**, 1400–11.

Slifstein, M. and Laruelle, M. (2001). Models and methods for derivation of in vivo neuroreceptor parameters with PET and SPECT reversible radiotracers. *Nuclear Medicine and Biology*, **28**, 595–608.

Stephenson, C. M., Bigliani, V., Jones, H. M., Mulligan, R. S., Acton, P. D., Visvikis, D. *et al.* (2000). Striatal and extra-striatal D(2)/D(3) dopamine receptor occupancy by quetiapine in vivo. [(123)I]-epidepride single photon emission tomography(SPET) study *British Journal of Psychiatry*, **177**, 408–15.

Strange, P. G. (2001). Antipsychotic drugs: importance of dopamine receptors for mechanisms of therapeutic actions and side effects. *Pharmacological Reviews*, **53**, 119–33.

Suhara, T., Okauchi, T., Sudo, Y., Takano, A., Kawabe, K., Maeda, J. *et al.* (2002*a*). Clozapine can induce high dopamine D(2) receptor occupancy in vivo. *Psychopharmacology (Berlin)*, **160**, 107–12.

Suhara, T., Okubo, Y., Yasuno, F., Inoue, M., Ichimiya, T., Nakashima, Y. *et al.* (2002*b*). Decreased dopamine D2 receptor binding in the anterior cingulate cortex in schizophrenia. *Archives of General Psychiatry*, **59**, 25–30.

Talairach, P. and Tournoux, J. (1988). *A stereotactic coplanar atlas of the human brain*. Thieme, Stuttgart.

Talvik, M., Nordstrom, A. L., Nyberg, S., Olsson, H., Halldin, C., and Farde, L. (2001). No support for regional selectivity in clozapine-treated patients: a PET study with [(11)C]raclopride and [(11)C]FLB 457. *American Journal of Psychiatry*, **158**, 926–30.

Talvik, M., Nordstron, A., and Farde, L. (2002). Decreased dopamine D2 receptor binding in the thalalmus in drug-naive schizophrenia patients. *International Journal of Neuropsychopharmcology*, **5**, S185.

Talvik, M., Nordstrom, A. L., Olsson, H., Halldin, C., and Farde, L. (2003). PET examinations of thalamic D2 receptors in schizophrenic patients (Abstract). *European Neuropsychopharmacology*, **13**, S330.

Tauscher, J., Jones, C., Remington, G., Zipursky, R. B., and Kapur, S. (2002*a*). Significant dissociation of brain and plasma kinetics with antipsychotics. *Molecular Psychiatry*, **7**, 317–21.

Tauscher, J., Kapur, S., Verhoeff, N. P., Hussey, D. F., Daskalakis, Z. J., Tauscher-Wisniewski, S. *et al.* (2002*b*). Brain serotonin 5-HT(1A) receptor binding in schizophrenia measured by positron emission tomography and [^{11}C]WAY-100635. *Archives of General Psychiatry*, **59**, 514–20.

Trichard, C., Paillere-Martinot, M. L., Attar-Levy, D., Blin, J., Feline, A., and Martinot, J. L. (1998). No serotonin 5-HT2A receptor density abnormality in the cortex of schizophrenic patients studied with PET. *Schizophrenia Research*, **31**, 13–17.

Verhoeff, N. P., Soares, J. C., D'Souza, C. D., Gil, R., Degen, K., Abi-Dargham, A. *et al.* (1999). [^{123}I]Iomazenil SPECT benzodiazepine receptor imaging in schizophrenia. *Psychiatry Research*, **91**, 163–73.

Verhoeff, N. P., Meyer, J. H., Kecojevic, A., Hussey, D., Lewis, R., Tauscher, J. *et al.* (2000). A voxel-by-voxel analysis of [^{18}F]setoperone PET data shows no substantial serotonin 5-HT(2A) receptor changes in schizophrenia. *Psychiatry Research*, **99**, 123–35.

Volkow, N. D., Wang, G. J., Fowler, J. S., Logan, J., Schlyer, D., Hitzemann, R. *et al.* (1994). Imaging endogenous dopamine competition with [^{11}C]raclopride in the human brain. *Synapse*, **16**, 255–62.

Wong, D. F., Wagner, H. N. Jr, Tune, L. E., Dannals, R. F., Pearlson, G. D., Links, J. M. *et al.* (1986). Positron emission tomography reveals elevated D2 dopamine receptors in drug-naive schizophrenics. *Science*, **234**, 1558–63.

Xiberas, X., Martinot, J. L., Mallet, L., Artiges, E., Canal, M., Loc, H. C. *et al.* (2001*a*). In vivo extrastriatal and striatal D2 dopamine receptor blockade by amisulpride in schizophrenia. *Journal of Clinical Psychopharmacology*, **21**, 207–14.

Xiberas, X., Martinot, J. L., Mallet, L., Artiges, E., Loc, H. C., Maziere, B. *et al.* (2001*b*). Extrastriatal and striatal D(2) dopamine receptor blockade with haloperidol or new antipsychotic drugs in patients with schizophrenia. *British Journal of Psychiatry*, **179**, 503–8.

Yasuno, F., Suhara, T., Okubo, Y, Sudo, Y., Inoue, M., Ichimiya, T. *et al.* (2001). Dose relationship of limbic-cortical D2-dopamine receptor occupancy with risperidone. *Psychopharmacology (Berlin)*, **154**, 112–14.

Yokoi, F., Grunder, G., Biziere, K., Stephane, M., Dogan, A. S., Dannals, R. F. *et al.* (2002). Dopamine D2 and D3 receptor occupancy in normal humans treated with the antipsychotic drug aripiprazole (OPC 14597): a study using positron emission tomography and [^{11}C]raclopride. *Neuropsychopharmacology*, **27**, 248–59.

Zakzanis, K. K. and Hansen, K. T. (1998). Dopamine D2 densities and the schizophrenic brain. *Schizophrenia Research*, **32**, 201–6.

Chapter 9

Functional magnetic resonance imaging (fMRI)

Garry D. Honey, Phillip K. McGuire, and Edward T. Bullmore

Introduction

The first report of localized changes in cerebral blood oxygenation in the occipital cortex following visual stimulation in humans (Belliveau *et al.* 1991) was of seminal importance to neuropsychiatric research. Only 3 years following this technological development, which enabled non-invasive visualization of *in vivo* human brain function, the application of the technique was first reported in psychiatric patients (Renshaw *et al.* 1994; Wenz *et al.* 1994). This ushered in a new era in functional neuroimaging, and provided a powerful tool in cognitive neuroscience to explore both normal and abnormal brain function, complementing earlier techniques such as positron emission tomography (PET), single-photon emission computed tomography (SPECT), and non-topographic electrophysiological procedures such as electroencephalography (EEG) and evoked response potentials (ERPs). Following the initial application of fMRI to schizophrenia research, the technique has been reported with increasing frequency over the past decade, with almost 100 full papers published to date in a range of scientific periodicals.

Here we consider the impact that fMRI has had on our understanding of the neurocognitive basis of schizophrenia, and its future potential to directly inform clinical management in psychiatry. We begin by reviewing the methodological principles that underpin the fMRI signal, and consider the advantages and disadvantages of the technique for scanning psychiatric populations, compared to other imaging modalities. We then review the current literature on the basis of the cognitive and clinical aspects of schizophrenia, and aim to identify progress and developments that have emerged within the field, and in the context of the application of fMRI to other psychiatric conditions. Finally, we conclude by considering a number of issues that remain to be addressed by future studies.

fMRI data acquisition and analysis

The blood oxygen level dependent (BOLD) signal

Coupling of neuronal activity to vascular response

The most common form of fMRI data acquisition is blood oxygenation level dependent (BOLD) imaging, first reported in humans by Ogawa *et al.* (1990). This is based on the differential magnetic susceptibility of oxyhaemoglobin and deoxyhaemoglobin (Pauling and Coryell 1936), which accordingly have different MR signal decay rates (Thulborn *et al.* 1982). Oxyhaemoglobin is diamagnetic, that is, it does not greatly disturb local magnetic field gradients. In contrast, deoxyhaemoglobin is paramagnetic, and will therefore affect the local magnetic field, by increasing the magnetic susceptibility, and causing a loss of image intensity. Deoxyhaemoglobin, present only in red blood cells, thus provides a particularly good paramagnetic endogenous contrast agent, being present in the bloodstream at high concentrations. Neuronal activity leads to an initial transient (100–200 ms) increase in oxygen consumption and concomitant increased deoxyhaemoglobin concentration. This is followed by increased local capillary blood flow and oxygen delivery to the activated region lasting several seconds, but oxygen consumption does not increase proportionately with hyperoxemia. This causes a marked decrease in the ratio of deoxyhaemoglobin compared to oxyhaemoglobin concentration in that region, and consequently produces an increase in the MR signal, due to increased T_2^* relaxation time. With the use of ultra-fast imaging techniques, such as echo-planar imaging (EPI) (Mansfield 1977), which are sensitive to changes in T_2^*, multiple slices covering the whole brain can be collected rapidly (for a full account of the basic physical principles of magnetization and nuclear magnetic resonance, see Bullmore and Suckling 2000, 2001). A vast range of physiological, sensory, and cognitive stimuli have since been used to examine the consequent changes in cerebral blood oxygenation, and thus indirectly, brain function.

The haemodynamic delay

The change in the local vasculature which is initiated by neuronal activity does not reach its peak instantaneously, but takes several seconds to develop and decay (Bandettini *et al.* 1993). The BOLD response measured in fMRI therefore provides an indirect measure of the temporospatial pattern of neuronal activity, in the context of a haemodyanmic lag, which smoothes and delays the signal. It is generally the underlying neuronal activity which is of interest in fMRI research, and thus statistical procedures must be used to account for the haemodynamic delay.

Advantages of functional MRI

Non-invasive methodology

The primary advantage of fMRI is that it is non-invasive, and does not involve exposure to ionizing radiation. This is a critical advantage in relation to other imaging techniques, such as PET and SPECT, particularly given the parity of results obtained from direct comparisons of fMRI and PET (Baumann *et al.* 1995; Paulesu *et al.* 1995; Dettmers *et al.* 1996). The absence of exposure to radiation also facilitates the scanning of subjects not previously amenable to functional imaging studies, such as women during pregnancy and children. Moreover, individuals can be scanned repeatedly, which is a particularly important feature in clinical research, allowing investigators to perform longitudinal studies to monitor changes in brain function associated with the progression of a disease state, and also in response to clinical interventions, particularly pharmacological treatments.

Reduced financial cost

A further advantage of the capacity to perform functional imaging without the requirement of short-life radioisotopes is the reduced financial cost, as the substantial expense associated with the requirement of an on-site cyclotron necessary for PET is circumvented. This has important practical implications for research expenditure and the potential of fMRI for future routine clinical applications.

Spatial and temporal resolution

fMRI has the advantage of optimal spatial resolution of the imaging modalities, with a full-width-at-half-maximum (FWHM) of 1 mm, compared to 4 mm for PET. fMRI data can be mapped directly and precisely on to high-resolution anatomical scans. Temporal resolution is also considerably improved in fMRI compared to PET. The temporal resolution of fMRI is restricted by the vascular phenomenon involved, rather than technological constraints. The haemodynamic delay between the onset of stimulus presentation and the latency of peak fMRI signal is in the range of several seconds. While this is considerably slower than the electrophysiological response recorded using EEGs and ERPs, imaging epochs using ^{15}O PET are typically between 40 and 120 s, thus providing little opportunity to study the temporal dynamics of functional response, which occur at considerably shorter periods.

Sensitivity

fMRI is capable of identifying reliable signal changes in a single individual in response to cognitive and sensory stimuli. Inter-subject averaging can therefore be avoided. In practice, inter-subject averaging is frequently used in fMRI, in order that the observed results be representative of a particular population.

Disadvantages of fMRI

The scanning environment

There are a number of practical challenges with fMRI, and particularly in its application to psychiatric populations. The high magnetic field-strength (typically 1.5 Tesla in the clinical setting, although higher field strengths are increasingly being used for research purposes) clearly precludes introduction of patients with metallic implants or cardiac pacemakers, for example. The narrow enclosure inside the bore of the magnet in which subjects lie is restrictive in terms of the types of tasks that can be performed, and can occasionally elicit feelings of claustrophobia. This problem frequently subsides as the subject acclimatizes to the unfamiliar environment of the MR scanner; however, occasionally unacceptable levels of anxiety can require the scan to be terminated, or may affect the subject's performance or emotional response to affective stimuli.

The enclosed and restrictive scanning environment also hinders observation of the patient, thus limiting the type of behavioural responses that can be monitored in the scanner. Customized MR-compatible apparatus is necessary for the monitoring of physiological responses during scanning, though rapid progress has been made in this area: for example, the recording of psychophysiological data, such as eye movements and EEG is now possible during scanning in some centres (Lemieux *et al.* 1997, 2001). Motor responses are limited within the scanner, and may cause head motion (see below). Overt verbal responses can also be problematic, in that they have been shown to cause artefacts due to movement of air in the pharynx and of the head during articulation (Wu *et al.* 1997; Fu *et al.* 2002). The environment also restricts the presentation of stimuli: visually presented material is typically presented via a prismatic mirror above the patient's head, allowing viewing of projected stimuli.

Acoustic noise

The high level of acoustic noise during image acquisition, caused by the gradient switching, can exceed 90 dB. This can be limited with active sound-suppression, such as the use of shielded headphones, but problems may remain with the use of aurally presented stimuli and tasks involving auditory perception in the scanner. Novel and inventive approaches are currently being developed for this purpose, such as the use of compressed pulse sequences, in which images are acquired in brief bursts, allowing auditory stimuli to be presented during the intervening silent periods (Amaro *et al.* 2002).

Signal-to-noise ratio

At 1.5 Tesla, signal change associated with visual stimulation is between 2 and 4%, despite 50–100% change in regional cerebral blood flow (rCBF). Thus there is a low signal-to-noise ratio; that is, the signal change related to neuronal activation can be only marginally greater than that produced by other, non-specific events, such as respiration.

Cognitive activity is associated with smaller changes in signal, with only 5–20% changes in CBF. Increasing the field strength can improve this to some extent, with an increase of signal up to three times larger being observed at 4 T (Turner *et al.* 1993). At lower field strengths, it is often necessary to average over repeated image acquisition to obtain significant results, analogous to that applied to ERPs. Sophisticated statistical analysis is therefore required to identify signal related to brain function (Bullmore *et al.* 1996a, b, 1999b, 2001; Brammer *et al.* 1997; Brammer 1998) (see below).

Subject movement

Perhaps the most difficult challenge for fMRI studies involves the changes in signal intensity that can be caused by slight subject movement within the millimetre range. This is due to the high spatial resolution of MRI and the high intrinsic contrast. Head motion can reduce the signal-to-noise ratio, but can also induce spurious 'activation', particularly at the periphery of the image. This problem has been confronted both at the point of acquisition, using various types of head restraint/support, and using post-processing image realignment (Friston *et al.* 1996; Bullmore *et al.* 1999*a*).

Statistical analysis of fMRI time series data

The statistical analysis of fMRI data is central to the transformation of large quantities of 'raw' data (typically 32 Mb per scan) into visually intelligible maps of brain activation by a task, or between-group differences of functional activation, e.g. hypofrontality. The procedures used for this purpose vary somewhat from lab to lab, and are still an active focus of research development: a good introduction is Lange (1999). However, the process may very broadly be subdivided into the following stages:

- Pre-processing: the time series of observations at each voxel is corrected for the effects of head movement during scanning. Additional components of noise may be removed and the data may be temporally filtered.

- Time series analysis: a linear model is fitted to the pre-processed time series to estimate effects of experimental interest, e.g. the variance attributable to the contrast between baseline and activation conditions. Time series regression in fMRI is typically complicated by the fact that the residuals are not serially independent white noise.

- Spatial co-registration and second level analysis: the pre-processed time series data or the statistic maps derived from them are co-registered in a standard anatomical space and second-level modelling of group activation or between-group differences can then be conducted at each voxel (volume element) of the images.

- Hypothesis testing: typically investigators wish to map brain regions that are significantly activated or show a significant between-group difference. This can be done by referring the appropriate test statistics estimated at each voxel to a null distribution ascertained by asymptotic theory or data resampling. An important general point is that because there will usually be 10 000+ voxels per maps, stringent *P*-values are required to retain control over type 1 (false-positive) error in the context of multiple comparisons, and this imperative naturally mitigates the power of the study [or increases the risk of type 2 (false-negative) errors].

Summary of fMRI research findings in schizophrenia

Experimental design

Neuroimaging research in schizophrenia has explored a broad range of cognitive functioning, encompassing primarily executive function, attention, working memory, psychomotor function, and basic sensory processing. In order to examine the neurobiological basis of dysfunction within these cognitive domains, a case-control design has typically been adopted, involving the comparison of patient groups with healthy volunteers. Given the heterogeneity of psychiatric disorders, and variability over the course of the illness, this design may not be optimal. Longitudinal within-subjects assessments, to which fMRI is ideally suited, may provide a more powerful approach to identify dynamic changes in brain function over periods of relapse and remission in schizophrenia.

A further advantage of the application of fMRI within psychiatry, is the use of event-related designs: this has the benefit of improved psychological validity (avoiding the need to artificially block similar trials together), *post-hoc* selection of individual trial types (for example, selecting only trials for which correct or incorrect task performance was observed), and examining the temporal dynamics of the BOLD response. Event-related fMRI is therefore clearly of particular use in psychiatric research, where behavioural task performance is a crucial consideration, and disease processes may affect not only the response amplitude of a given brain region, but also the dynamic properties of the signal. Finally, a methodological caveat to note is that the majority of studies to date have involved small sample sizes (see Tables 9.1–9.6), and therefore must be treated with some caution at this stage, until robust findings have emerged from replication.

Executive function

Executive functioning is a somewhat elusive concept, which is generally used to refer to 'higher' cognitive functions, often used synonymously with functions critically involving the prefrontal cortex. Green (1998) provides the following definition: 'Executive functioning refers to a host of neurocognitive abilities that are associated with the prefrontal cortex, such as planning, problem solving, shifting cognitive set, and alternating between two or more tasks'.

Functional imaging studies have incorporated a correspondingly wide range of tasks to investigate executive function in schizophrenia. fMRI studies have recently begun to be reported (see Table 9.1), and it is interesting to note that a 'hypofrontal' response has often been observed in schizophrenic patients, as frequently reported in studies using other imaging techniques. Volz *et al.*, (1997) found reduced activation of the right prefrontal cortex during performance of the Wisconsin Card Sort Test (WCST) (see Fig. 9.1). This has subsequently been demonstrated in neuroleptic-naïve patients, indicating that the frontal deficit associated with executive dysfunction is not confounded by medication, and is present early in the illness (Riehemann *et al.* 2001). Yurgelun-Todd *et al.* (1996) also showed reduced frontal activation when patients performed a verbal fluency task; additionally, they showed increased left temporal activity, replicating previous findings using PET (Dolan *et al.* 1995; Frith *et al.* 1995; Fletcher *et al.* 1996, 1999). Studies using fMRI have further refined the notion of hypofrontality during the performance of executive tasks; for example, reduced frontal activation was evident when patients

Table 9.1 Functional magnetic resonance imaging (fMRI) studies of executive function and attention in schizophrenia

Reference	Sample	Cognitive task(s)	Aims/hypotheses	Main findings
Yurgelun-Todd et al. (1996)	12 pts, 11 ctrls	Verbal fluency	To test the feasibility of using functional magnetic resonance imaging (fMRI) to examine changes in cortical activation in response to verbal tasks	Reduced frontal activation and greater left temporal activation in pts
Volz et al. (1997)	13 pts, 31 ctrls	WCST	To compare frontal activation during the WCST with previous studies using PET and SPECT	Reduced right frontal activation, and a trend towards increased left temporal activity
Curtis et al. (1998)	5 pts, 5 ctrls	Paced orthographic verbal fluency	To study changes in activation in scz pts performing a verbal fluency task	Pts demonstrated decreased frontal and increased parietal activation; fronto-parietal activation was negatively correlated in both groups
Curtis et al. (1999)	5 pts, 5 ctrls	Paced orthographic verbal fluency, and semantic categorization	To investigate whether prefrontal deficits in scz represent a fixed deficit, or depend on the cognitive task	Reduced prefrontal activation evident during verbal fluency was not seen during the semantic decision task
Volz et al. (1999)	14 pts, 20 ctrls	CPT	To investigate whether hypofrontality, observed using PET, is also evident using fMRI	Pts showed reduced activation in medial PFC, thalamus and cingulate

Table 9.1 (continued)

Reference	Sample	Cognitive task(s)	Aims/hypotheses	Main findings
Russell et al. (2000)	5 pts, 7 ctrls	The 'eyes' test of mental state attribution	To investigate the hypothesis that patients with schizophrenia have a dysfunction in brain regions responsible for mental state attribution	Pts demonstrated an impaired 'theory of mind', which was associated with reduced activation of the left inferior frontal gyrus
Carter et al. (2001)	17 pts, 16 ctrls	CPT	To test the hypothesis that error-related activity in the anterior cingulate cortex is impaired in patients with schizophrenia	Pts failed to show the error-related activity in the anterior cingulate observed in ctrls
Curtis et al. (2001)	5 bipolar, 5 scz pts, 5 ctrls	Paced orthographic verbal fluency, and semantic categorization	To determine whether task-specific attenuation of activation of frontal cortex is specific to scz	Bipolar pts showed increased frontal activation compared to ctrls during verbal fluency; no between-group differences during semantic decision
Riehemann et al. (2001)	9 pts, 9 ctrls	WCST	Investigate frontal response to WCST in neuroleptic-naïve patients	Reduced activity in right frontal and left temporal lobe, and left cerebellum was observed in pts
Rubia et al. (2001)	6 pts, 7 ctrls	'Stop' and go/no-go tests of motor inhibition	To investigate the hypothesis that schizophrenia is associated with a dysfunction of prefrontal brain regions during motor responseinhibition	No between-group differences in task performance; reduced anterior cingulated activation in pts during both tasks; reduced activity in DLPFC, thalamus, and putamen during the 'stop' task.
Sommer et al. (2001)	12 pts, 12 ctrls	Verb generation Semantic decision	To determine whether reduced lateralization is the result of decreased language activity	Language processing was less lateralized in patients than in controls, which was due to increased right hemisphere activity,

Study	Sample	Task	Aim	Findings
			of the left hemisphere or whether it is the consequence of increased language-related activity in the right hemisphere	but not decreased left hemisphere activity. Reduced lateralization correlated with severity of hallucinations
Volz et al. (2001)	9 pts, 15 ctrls	Auditory time estimation and pitch estimation	To investigate neural basis of deficits in time estimation in scz	Reduced cortical and caudate activation during time estimation versus rest; timing versus pitch elicited deficits in cortico-striato-thalamic activity
Gur (2002)	14 pts, 14 ctrls	Facial affect processing	To test the hypothesis of reduced limbic activation related to emotional valence of facial stimuli	In judging emotional valence, patients showed reduced activity in amygdale and hippocampus
Kosaka et al. (2002)	12 pts, 12 ctrls	Facial affect processing	To investigate the involvement of the amygdala in schizophrenia during facial affect processing	Increased activation of right amygdala in pts during processing of positive emotions
Lawrie et al. (2002)	8 pts, 10 ctrls	Sentence completion	To investigate the fronto-temporal dysconnectivity hypothesis of schizophrenia	No difference in regional brain response; correlation between frontal and temporal activity significantly reduced in patients
Raemaekers et al. (2002)	16 pts, 17 ctrls	Prosaccadic, anti-saccadic and fixation eye movements	To investigate the hypothesis that abnormal eye movements in schizophrenia involve impaired oculomotor control over brainstem systems	Pts failed to activate the striatum during the inhibition of saccades, but no group difference was observed in supplementary motor and frontal eye-field regions

Table 9.1 (continued)

Reference	Sample	Cognitive task(s)	Aims/hypotheses	Main findings
Zorrilla et al. (2002)	9 pts, 10 ctrls	Viewing novel pictures compared to repeated picture presentation	To compare the brain response to novel picture encoding in schizophrenic patients and healthy volunteers	ROI analyses detected reduced activation in the hippocampal and fusiform gyri in schizophrenic patients
Hempel et al. (2003)	9 pts, 10 ctrls	Facial affect discrimination and labelling	To investigate performance related to changes in brain function during facial affect processing	Patients showed reduced activation of anterior cingulate during facial discrimination and reduced amygdale/hippocampus during labelling
Laurens et al. (2003)	10 pts, 16 ctrls	Go/No go task	To localise error negativity deficits associated with errors of commission in scz.	Reduced anterior cingulate and also limbic regions in pts, with increased parietal activation.
Paulus et al. (2003)	15 pts, 15 ctrls	Two-choice prediction task at varying error rates	To investigate the neural correlates of the degree of success and uncertainty on decision making in scz	Increased parietal activation in controls when outcome was most uncertain; parietal activation was not modulated by degree of uncertainty in patients
Quintana et al. (2003a)	2 × 6 pts, 2 × 6 ctrls	Facial affect with and without semantic processing; facial identity discrimination task; working memory task involving facial expressions	To investigate whether fusiform deficits are invariant to the adjunctive cognitive processes required of the task	Patients failed to activate the right lateral fusiform gyrus during facial information processing, irrespective of the associated cognitive requirements of the task

Study	Sample	Task	Aim	Findings
Sommer et al. (2003)	12 female pts, 12 female ctrls	Verb generation and reading words spelt backwards	To test the hypothesis of gender-specific reduction of lateralized linguistic function	Consistent with previous studies in male patients, female patients showed reduced lateralization, with increased right hemispheric activation compared to controls
Spaniel et al. (2003)	Monozygotic twin pair discordant for scz	Verbal fluency	To determine lateralization of language in twins discordant for schizophrenia	Reduced lateralization in affected twin compared to healthy sibling
Weiss, E. M. et al. (2003)	13 pts, 13 ctrls	Modified Stroop task	To investigate abnormal function in schizophrenia during selective attention	Increased activation of bilateral inferior frontal cortex and anterior cingulate

CPT, continuous performance test; ctrls, controls; PET, positron emission tomography; PFC, prefrontal cortex; pts, patients; ROI, region of interest; scz, schizophrenia; SPECT, single-photon emission computed tomography; WCST, Wisconsin Card Sort Test.

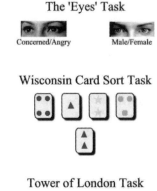

Fig. 9.1 Examples of executive function tasks used in fMRI. All these tasks require judgements—as to the displayed emotion (versus a sex decision control), the matching card, and the minimum number of moves, respectively. See Plate 10(a) of the plate section at the centre of this book.

performed a paced verbal fluency task (Curtis *et al.* 1998), but not during the performance of semantic categorization, which also recruited prefrontal activity (Curtis *et al.* 1999), and was not seen in patients with bipolar illness (Curtis *et al.* 2001). Further work indicates that the presence or absence of hypofrontality in schizophrenia during verbal fluency depends on both the severity of psychotic symptoms at the time of scanning and on the demands of the task (Fu *et al.* 2002). Attenuated frontal activation has been observed in a range of other executive tasks, including mental state attribution (Russell *et al.* 2000), and motor response inhibition (Rubia *et al.* 2001). Hypofrontality is also often referred to in terms of hypofunction of the lateral frontal region; however, medial frontal hypoactivity has also been observed during facial affect processing (Hempel *et al.* 2003), and the continuous performance test (Volz *et al.* 1999; Carter *et al.* 2001), which Carter and co-workers suggest may indicate a failure of internal monitoring of performance—an evaluative component of executive functioning. This was supported by a recent study by Laurens *et al.* (2003), showing reduced anterior cingulate activity during error processing. It is also worth noting that under certain conditions, patients with schizophrenia can show equivalent or *greater* prefrontal activation than controls (Arcuri *et al.* 2001; Walter *et al.* 2003; E. M. Weiss *et al.* 2003) (see below). It appears from these studies that the issue of between-group differences in task performance remains an important confound in the interpretation of frontal deficits in schizophrenia. Future studies will provide a more precise identification of regional deficits within the frontal cortex in schizophrenia, and the relationship to focused aspects of executive cognitive function.

Episodic and working memory

The concept of 'working memory' is a hypothetical construct in cognitive psychology that refers to a limited-capacity system that facilitates the simultaneous storage and processing of information, which can then be utilized to guide subsequent behaviour (Baddeley and Hitch 1974; Baddeley 1986, 1992;). It is suggested to comprise a central executive that organizes the allocation and co-ordination of processing resources to utilize stored representations, and modality-specific short-term 'slave stores' (e.g. a speech-based, 'phonological loop' verbal storage system and a 'visuospatial scratchpad' for storage of non-verbal information). Working memory is considered to be funda-mental to a broad range of cognitive processes, including reasoning, language compre-hension, and problem solving (Jonides 1995).

Accordingly, working memory deficits have consistently been demonstrated in patients with schizophrenia (Weinberger and Cermak 1973; Park and Holzman 1992; Fleming *et al.* 1995; Keefe *et al.* 1995; Morris *et al.* 1997; Park and McTigue 1997; Spindler *et al.* 1997; Park *et al.* 1999), and also first-degree asymptomatic relatives (Conklin *et al.* 2000), with evidence of disproportionate impairment relative to other domains of cognitive dysfunction (Saykin *et al.* 1991, 1994), and for prognostic implications of such deficits in psychosocial rehabilitation programmes (Green 1996). Deficient working memory is thus central to many contemporary cognitive psycho-logical models of schizophrenic symptoms (Goldman-Rakic 1990, 1994; Cohen and Servan-Schreiber 1992; Weinberger 1993).

Working memory paradigms have been used in conjunction with fMRI to character-ize the neurobiological basis of deficits in schizophrenia (Fig. 9.2). Consistent with the hypofrontal response to executive tasks described earlier, several studies have demon-strated hypofrontality during the performance of working memory tasks (Callicott *et al.* 1998; Stevens *et al.* 1998; Menon *et al.* 2001*b*; Barch *et al.* 2002, 2003) (Table 9.2).

Imaging research using graded levels of working memory demands have suggested that the term 'hypofrontality' may be too simplistic to describe the complex functional pathology evident in schizophrenia. Cognitive load can be parametrically manipulated in working memory paradigms in order to investigate the nature of the 'dose–response'. Using this design, several studies have shown that patients exhibit normal or, indeed, exaggerated frontal activation in response to working memory tasks, until the physio-logical capacity of the prefrontal cortex to respond to task-related requirements is exceeded by the cognitive load (Manoach *et al.* 1999, 2000; Callicott *et al.* 2000; Perlstein *et al.* 2001; Walter *et al.* 2003). Similar findings were also observed in two cohorts of non-schizophrenic siblings of patients with schizophrenia (Callicott *et al.* 2003). Callicot *et al.* (2000) noted that this increased prefrontal response in patients to a working memory task was predicted by reduced *N*-acetyl-aspartate (NAA) concen-trations in dorsolateral prefrontal cortex, supporting the assumption of the relation-ship to neuronal pathology. In reconciling apparently discrepant findings of both increased and decreased frontal function in schizophrenia during working memory performance, Manoach *et al.* (2000) noted a negative correlation between error rate and prefrontal activation in the patients, suggesting that activation increases with demand, until cognitive capacity is exceeded. As they noted, this leads to the intriguing

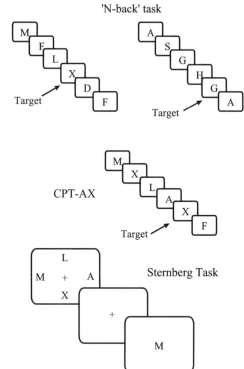

Fig. 9.2 Examples of working memory tasks used in fMRI. The diagrams show a 'two-back' task, 'X' following 'A' (but not 'non A') Continuous Performance Test (CPT) targets, and a Sternberg item location stimulus

speculation that further increases in load may have resulted in a hypofrontal response in the patients, whereas this increase may have remained within the performance capacity of the controls, and therefore resulted in increased activation in line with demand, thus reversing the between-group comparison they observed at lower cognitive loads. The hypofrontal response variably reported in schizophrenia is thus not a static phenomenon, but dynamically related to task requirements and subjects' capacity range to perform the task. Alternatively, based on findings in non-human primates, Quintana *et al.* (2003) hypothesized that discrepant findings regarding increased or decreased prefrontal activation in schizophrenia may be explained as compensatory responses depending on the precise cognitive processes engaged by the working memory task. In support of this hypothesis, they showed that decreased prefrontal (and increased parietal) activation occurred during a working memory task when the task requirements involved anticipatory responses, whereas increased prefrontal activation was observed when the task involved mnemonic working memory performance.

Episodic memory refers to the encoding, storage, and retrieval of information in long-term memory, with reference to personal incidents or events, and can be distinguished from semantic memory, involving conceptual and factual knowledge (Tulving 1983). There is evidence that encoding processes may be primarily affected in schizophrenia,

Table 9.2 Functional magnetic resonance imaging (fMRI) studies of episodic and working memory in schizophrenia

Reference	Sample	Cognitive task(s)	Aims/hypotheses	Main findings
Callicot et al. (1998)	10 pts, 10 ctrls	Verbal 2-back	To investigate methodological issues in the analysis of fMRI data in psychiatric populations	Pts demonstrated a failure to activate DLPFC, even when subjects were matched for signal variance on motor activation as an internal standard
Stevens et al. (1998)	12 pts, 12 ctrls	Word and Tone serial position tasks	To study the neural basis of the dissociation between verbal and non-verbal working memory	Pts showed reduced activation in inferior frontal, premotor, and anterior temporal regions in both tasks
Honey et al. (1999)	10 pts (typs), 10 pts (switched to atyps), 10 ctrls	2-back in ctrls and pts switched from typs to risp	Effects of atypical anti-psychotics on PFC function	Patients switched from typical anti-psychotics to risperidone showed increased PFC activation
Manoach et al. (1999)	12 pts, 10 ctrls	Sternberg Item Recognition Task	To investigate the relationship between working memory performance and prefrontal activation	No difference in activation of right DLPFC between groups, but increased activation of left DLPFC, which was inversely correlated with performance in the pts
Callicott et al. (2000)	13 pts, 18 ctrls	Graded n-back	To characterize PFC function to increasing cognitive demand in scz, and relate it to measures of neuronal integrity	Pattern of PFC response in pts across cognitive loads suggests exaggerated and inefficient physiological response, predicted by a measure of neuronal integrity (NAA)
Manoach et al. (2000)	9 pts, 9 ctrls	Sternberg Item Recognition Task	To investigate whether pts recruit different brain regions during performance of working memory tasks	Pts showed deficient working memory performance with equal magnitude of right DLPFC activation reduced left DLPFC, and uniquely recruited subcortical regions, even following performance matching

Table 9.2 (continued)

Reference	Sample	Cognitive task(s)	Aims/hypotheses	Main findings
Barch et al. (2001)	14 pts, 12 ctrls	CPT-AX	To test the hypothesis that WM deficits in schizophrenia reflect impaired context processing due to a disturbance in DLPFC	Pts showed specific deficits of dorsolateral PFC, but not ventrolateral PFC, or other components of the working memory system
Egan et al. (2001)	11 pts, 16 unaffected siblings, 11 unaffected siblings (group 2)	n-back	To evaluate the effect of the COMT genotype on efficiency of prefrontal function	Val allele load is related to inefficiency of performance of PFC during working memory, whereas the Met allele predicts improved function
Menon et al. (2001b)	11 pts, 13 ctrls	Auditory 2-back	To investigate the neural basis of auditory working memory, and its relationship to specific symptoms	Reduced lateralization, and decreased fronto-parietal activation in pts. Negative symptoms inversely correlated with frontal activation
Manoach et al. (2001)	7 pts, 7 ctrls	Sternberg Item Recognition Task	To quantify test (retest reliability in psychiatric imaging studies of working memory	Task performance was reliable in both groups; however, functional activation was not reliable in individual pts, with reasonable reliability in ctrls
Perlstein et al. (2001)	17 pts, 16 ctrls	n-back verbal working memory	To test the hypotheses that DLPFC dysfunction is seen in scz only during performance deficits, and may be related to cognitive disorganization	Dysfunction of DLPFC was observed in pts only when performance was lower than that of ctrls; DLPFC dysfunction was associated with disorganization symptoms
Barch et al. (2002)	38 pts, 48 ctrls	2-back verbal and non-verbal (faces) working memory, verbal and non-verbal encoding and retrieval	To test the hypothesis that DLPFC deficits contribute to both working memory and long-term memory disturbances in scz, and if these are domain-specific	Disturbed DLPFC activation was found in pts in both tasks, and also medial temporal deficits. Some evidence for more severe deficits with verbal, compared to non-verbal stimuli

Study	Sample	Task	Aim	Findings
Honey et al. (2002)	20 pts, 20 ctrls	2-back verbal working memory	Investigation of relationship between response latency and parietal activation	Phonological storage disrupted as indicated by breakdown of parietal activation association with response latency evident in controls
Wykes et al. (2002)	6 pts (CRT), 6 pts (ctrl), 6 ctrls	2-back verbal working memory	To determine whether there are concomitant brain activation changes as a result of engaging in cognitive remediation therapy	Frontal activation decreased in ctrls over time, but was increased in the pts receiving CRT
Honey et al. (2003)	27 ctrls, 30 pts	2-back working memory and psychomotor sequencing	To investigate associations between sub-syndromal structures of five factors of the PANSS and cognitive activation	Task-specific (working memory task) modulation of functional response associated with symptom expression; no relationship with psychomotor task
Leube et al. (2003)	10 pts, 10 ctrls	Facial encoding task	Investigate neurobiological basis of memory deficits in scz	Reduced right hippocampal and cerebellar activation in patients during facial encoding
Jessen et al. (2003)	12 pts, 12 ctrls	Semantic association during verbal encoding; recognition task	Investigate fronto-hippocampal deficits in scz during episodic memory, while controlling for recognition success	Reduced right and bilateral hippocampal in patients during encoding and retrieval, respectively
Eyler-Zorrilla et al. (2003)	9 pts, 10 ctrls	Visual encoding of complex photographs	To compare brain response during novel picture encoding in scz pts and ctrls	Increased hippocampal and parahippocampal activation in controls during encoding; increased hippocampal activation in pts during the control condition compared to ctrls
Schlosser et al. (2003)	6 ctrls, 6 pts (typs), 6 pts (atyps)	2-back working memory task	To investigate dysfunctional connectivity during working memory, and its modulation by typical and atypical treatment	Reduced prefronto-cerebellar and cerebellar-thalamic circuits in pts; enhanced inter-hemispheric connectivity in atypically treated patients

Table 9.2 (continued)

Reference	Sample	Cognitive task(s)	Aims/hypotheses	Main findings
Barch et al. (2003)	38 scz pts, 14 pts (major depression)	2-back working memory task	To test whether frontal deficits during working memory in schizophrenia are seen in other psychiatric illnesses	Reduced activation of right frontal cortex evident in the schizophrenic patients was not evident in patients with major depression
Callicott ?? (2003)	23 siblings, 18 ctrls, 25 siblings, 15 ctrls	n-back working memory task	To determine whether increased frontal response to working memory tasks previously reported in schizophrenic patients is also evident in unaffected siblings	2 separate groups of non-schizophrenic siblings of patients with schizophrenia showed exaggerated right prefrontal response during the working memory task in comparison to their matching control groups
Perlstein et al. (2003)	16 pts, 15 ctrls	n-back working memory task and CPT-AX	To investigate the hypothesis that deficits in working memory and inhibition of prepotent responding have overlapping localization and dysfunction in schizophrenia	Schizophrenic patients showed reduced right prefrontal activation with increasing working memory load and prepotent response inhibition
Quintana et al. (2003)	8 pts, 8 ctrls	Working memory task requiring responses based either on anticipation or retention	To determine whether increased or reduced activation during working memory in scz pts is related to the requirements of response anticipation or remembering cues	Patients showed decreased prefrontal and increased parietal activation during anticipatory working memory peformance, and increased prefrontal activation during mnemonic working memory performance
Walter et al. (2003)	15 pts, 15 ctrls	2-back verbal and spatial working memory tasks	To investigate hypofrontality and abnormal lateralization in in schizophrenia during working memory	Hypofrontality was not observed for either task. A failure to show left and right lateralization for verbal and spatial tasks was observed for patients; inverse correlation between performance and right prefrontal activation

atyps, atypical antipsychotics; COMT, catechol-o-methyltransferase; CPT, continuous performance test; CPT-AX, continuous performance test; CRT, cognitive remediation therapy; ctrls, controls; DLPFC, dorsolateral prefrontal cortex; NAA, N-acetyl-aspartate; PANSS, Positive and Negative Syndrome Scale; PFC, prefrontal cortex; pts, patients; risp, risperidone; scz, schizophrenia; typs, typical antipsychotics; WM, working memory.

due to a failure of semantic organization strategies (McClain 1983; Gold *et al.* 1992; Brebion *et al.* 1997; Chan *et al.* 2000), although others have argued for a retrieval deficit (Calev 1984*a, b*). fMRI studies have recently been reported showing evidence of fronto-hippocampal dysfunction during the encoding of verbal (Hofer *et al.* 2003; Jessen *et al.* 2003) and visual (Eyler Zorrilla *et al.* 2003; Leube *et al.* 2003) episodic information. Fronto-hippocampal deficits have previously been reported during episodic retrieval tasks using PET (Heckers *et al.* 1998; Ragland *et al.* 2001; A. P. Weiss *et al.* 2003), raising the question of whether disruptions of fronto-hippocampal function observed at retrieval may reflect a primary deficit that occurs during the encoding phase.

Sensorimotor function

Minor motor and sensory deficits, or neurological soft signs (NSS), are prevalent in schizophrenia, and have been shown to be independent of the effects of neuroleptic medication (King *et al.* 1991; Schroder *et al.* 1992). NSS are significantly correlated with psychotic symptoms, but not with extrapyramidal side-effects (Schroder *et al.* 1992). Accordingly, numerous studies have examined the neurobiological basis of these deficits using functional imaging (Table 9.3).

Several studies have found that activation of the supplementary motor area (SMA) and sensorimotor cortex during the performance of simple motor tasks is attenuated in patients with schizophrenia (Wenz *et al.* 1994; Schroder *et al.* 1995, 1999), though others have failed to find this effect (Buckley *et al.* 1997; Braus *et al.* 2000). Schroder *et al.* (1995) observed sensorimotor and SMA dysfunction in response to a motor task: in healthy volunteers, activation of SMA and sensorimotor cortices was observed bilaterally, with a more pronounced response contralaterally to the hand performing a thumb-to-digit task (left > right); patients with schizophrenia exhibited reversed sensorimotor lateralization, and attenuation of both SMA and sensorimotor regions. Wenz *et al.* (1994) studied subjects performing the thumb-to-digit task using both hands sequentially; activation was observed in sensorimotor cortex bilaterally, with increased activation associated with performance with the non-dominant hand. Patients demonstrated attenuated activation in comparison to the control group. While the patients showed impaired task performance, the control group data demonstrated that reduced performance is associated with increased, rather than decreased, activation (that is, in the comparison between left- compared to right-handed performance), suggesting that impaired performance may not account for the attenuated response in patients. Buckley *et al.* (1997) using a region-of-interest (ROI) approach to study the motor cortex, found no differences in sensorimotor activation between patients and controls, and suggest that this is consistent with the lack of post-mortem data to implicate the primary motor cortex as a pathomorphological site for NSS (Bogerts 1993).

Previous studies had included chronic patients treated with antipsychotic medication; however, Braus *et al.* (2000) found no difference in intensity or lateralization of

Table 9.3 Functional magnetic resonance imaging (fMRI) studies of sensorimotor function in schizophrenia

Reference	Sample	Cognitive task(s)	Aims/hypotheses	Main findings
Renshaw et al. (1994)	8 pts, 9 ctrls	Photic stimulation	To investigate the neural response to sensory stimulation in scz	Increased signal intensity in primary visual cortex
Wenz et al. (1994)	10 pts, 10 ctrls	Finger movement	To investigate motor activation in pts with scz	Reduced activation in pts, and disrupted laterality
Schroder et al. (1995)	10 pts, 7 ctrls	Finger/thumb opposition	Investigate cerebral changes underlying neurological soft signs	Reduced activation of SMA and sensorimotor cortices, and reversed lateralization
Wenz et al. (1995)	10 pts, 10 ctrls	Finger/thumb opposition	Investigate cerebral changes underlying neurological soft signs	Reduced activation of SMA and sensorimotor cortices, and reversed lateralization
Buckley et al. (1997)	9 pts, 9 ctrls	Finger tapping	Evaluate differential activation of motor cortex	No difference between pts and ctrls
Braus et al. (1999)	14 Dg-N, 13 typs, 13 atyps, 15 ctrls	Sequential finger opposition	Evaluate drug effects on motor cortex activation in schizophrenia	Similar PM ctx and SMA activation in FE pts and ctrls; reduced PM activation in typ pts; reduced SMA activation in both typ and atyp pts
Schroder et al. (1999)	12 pts, 12 ctrls	Pronation/supination at slow, medium and fast rates	Investigate motor ctx activation in scz, and relationship to motor performance.	Increased activation with increased motor speed in pts and ctrls; reduced activation in PM ctx in pts, and similar trend in SMA; similar performance in pts, but increased variability
Northoff et al. (1999)	2 pts, 2 ctrls	Finger/thumb opposition	Investigate neural basis of catatonia	Reduced activation of motor cortex, but not SMA; disrupted lateralization

Study	Subjects	Task	Aim	Findings
Braus et al. (2000)	12 Dg-N, 12 ctrls	Sequential finger opposition	To examine the motor system in never-medicated FE subjects to rule out medication and chronicity effects	No difference in cortical activation between pts and ctrls.
Kiehl and Liddle (2001)	11 pts, 11 ctrls	Auditory oddball stimulus detection	To characterize the spatial location of neural processes underlying auditory oddball target detection demonstrated using electrophysiological methods	Reduced extent and strength of activation observed throughout a widespread network of association cortex and thalamus
Kodama et al. (2001)	9 pts, 10 ctrls	Complex motor sequence learning before and after training	Investigate neural correlates of motor skill learning deficits in scz	Reduced premotor activation before training in pts; training increased activation in pts, but decreased in ctrls
Menon et al. (2001a)	8 pts, 12 ctrls	Motor sequencing task	Investigate basal ganglia dysfunction in scz	Reduced activation in putamen, pallidum and thalamus in pts; striatal and thalamic deficits were correlated
Stephan et al. (2001)	6 pts, 6 ctrls	Finger tapping task before and after olanzapine treatment	Investigate the effects of olanzapine on cerebellar connectivity	Olanzapine resulted in changes in connectivity between cerebellum and prefrontal cortex and thalamus
Wible et al. (2001)	10 pts, 10 ctrls	Auditory mismatch (oddball) stimuli	Investigate early acoustic processing	Decreased activation of the superior temporal gyrus in pts during mismatch processing
Kumari et al. (2002)	10 pts, 10 ctrls	Motor sequence learning	Investigate neural correlates of implicit learning deficits in scz	Cortico-striato-thalamic activation observed in ctrls who showed procedural learning, but not in pts, who failed to learn

Table 9.3 (continued)

Reference	Sample	Cognitive task(s)	Aims/hypotheses	Main findings
Braus et al. (2002)	11 pts, 11 ctrls	Visual checkboard and auditory drum beats	To determine which stages of the input processing network are disturbed in first-episode schizophrenic patients	Reduced activation in the right thalamus, right prefrontal cortex, parietal lobe and primary auditory cortex in pts
McDowell et al. (2002)	13 pts, 14 ctrls	Refixation and anti-saccade tasks	Investigate cortical involvement in abnormal saccadic inhibition	Increased prefrontal activation during saccades in ctrls, but not pts, despite normal activation in frontal eye fields and parietal cortex
Muller et al. (2002)	10 olz pts, 10 hal pts, 10 drug-free pts, 10 ctrls	Finger tapping	Investigate cortical and subcortical activation to motor performance in drug-treated and untreated pts	Untreated pts showed increased pallidal activation
Kumari et al. (2003)	7 pts, 7 ctrls	Somatosensory pre-pulse inhibition	To investigate the neural correlates of somatosensory PPI in controls and patients with schizophrenia	Increased activation was observed in controls in cortico-striato-thalamic circuitry, and related areas

atyps, atypical antipsychotics; ctrls, controls; ctx, cortex; Dg-N, drug-naive; FE, first episode; hal, haloperidol; olz, olanzapine; PM ctx, primary motor cortex; PPI, pre-pulse inhibition; pts, patients; SMA, supplementary motor area; scz, schizophrenia; typs, typical antipsychotics.

activation in motor regions in neuroleptic-naïve first-episode patients compared to healthy volunteers. In a cross-sectional comparison, Braus *et al.* (1999) also observed that attenuated response in SMA and bilateral sensorimotor cortex was evident in patients treated with typical neuroleptics, but not in patients treated with clozapine. These studies indicate that chronic neuroleptic treatment may be of critical significance in interpreting deficits observed using functional neuroimaging. This is supported by Stephan *et al.* (2001), who demonstrated modulation of cerebellar connectivity with prefrontal cortex and the thalamus during a finger-tapping task following treatment with olanzapine. Similarly, Muller *et al.* (2002) reported increased subcortical activation in untreated patients, compared to healthy volunteers, and patients treated with haloperidol or olanzapine (see also below).

fMRI has also been used to investigate activation of the cortico-striato-thalamic circuit engaged during motor sequence learning, and several studies have reported functional deficits within this system (Kodama *et al.* 2001; Menon *et al.* 2001*a*; Kumari *et al.* 2002). As reported by Kumari *et al.* (2002), schizophrenic patients fail to learn an implicit motor sequence. Interestingly, however, as performance improves following training on the task, functional activation remains abnormal: Kodama *et al.* (2001) demonstrated increased activation in patients following training, but decreased activation in controls.

Symptomatology

Functional imaging research in schizophrenia has demonstrated widespread deficits affecting multiple regions distributed throughout the brain, underpinning a range of cognitive functions. However, a pattern of brain dysfunction that would serve as a biological trait marker or predict treatment response has not emerged to date. There are a number of possible reasons why this may be (see below). Perhaps most fundamentally, equivocal findings may relate to historical difficulties in psychiatric nosology, which has attempted to categorize an heterogeneous disorder in the absence of pathognomonic symptoms, such that two patients diagnosed with the illness may have no symptoms at all in common (Bentall *et al.* 1988*a, b*; Bentall 1993). In recognition of this, a number of studies have focused on patients exhibiting individual psychotic symptoms, and comparing these patients to those with schizophrenia, but who do not display the specific symptom of interest (Table 9.4). This has proved to be a powerful approach, and much progress has been made in the study of auditory hallucinations in particular.

In using functional imaging to study psychotic symptoms, there are two broad experimental approaches (Fu and McGuire 1999). One involves the measurement of brain activity while the symptom of interest is being experienced. The second involves the assessment of neural activation during the performance of tasks that engage the cognitive processes which are putatively impaired in patients with the symptom of interest. These can be applied to the investigation of any phenomenon, but in schizophrenia have been especially employed in the study of auditory hallucinations and of formal thought disorder.

Table 9.4 Functional magnetic resonance imaging (fMRI) studies of symptomatology in schizophrenia

Reference	Sample	Cognitive task(s)	Aims/hypotheses	Main findings
David et al. (1996)	2 state + pts	Listening to external speech; visual checkerboard; on and off medication	To examine localized changes in activity in response to actual as well as imagined sensory stimulation	Attenuation of temporal cortical response to external speech during hallucinations, consistently both on and off medication
Woodruff et al. (1997)	8 trait + pts, 7 trait − pts, 7 state ± pts, 8 ctrls	Listening to external speech	To investigate whether abnormal functional lateralization of temporal cortical language areas in schizophrenia was associated with a predisposition to auditory hallucinations and whether the auditory hallucinatory state would reduce the temporal cortical response to external speech	Compared to ctrls, as a group the pts showed reduced activity in the left STG, but increased right MTG activation; no difference in the comparing the trait-positive and trait-negative patients; reduced right temporal response to speech in the state-positive patients, compared to when they were not hallucinating
Northoff et al. (1999)	2 pts, 2 ctrls	Finger/thumb opposition	Investigate neural basis of catatonia	Reduced activation of motor cortex, but not SMA; disrupted lateralization
Phillips et al. (1999)	5 state + pts, 5 state − pts, 5 ctrls	Viewing facial expressions of fear, anger, disgust or mild happiness	To compare the neural correlates of facial expression perception in paranoid and non-paranoid patient subgroups	Non-paranoid subjects categorized disgust as either anger or fear more frequently than paranoids, and demonstrated in response to disgust expressions activation in the amygdala

Reference	Subjects	Task	Aim	Findings
Lennox et al. (2000)	4 state + pts	Periods of hallucination compared to non-hallucinating	To map the cerebral activation associated with auditory hallucinations in four subjects with schizophrenia	Activation of left and right STG, left inferior parietal cortex and left middle frontal gyrus
Shergill et al. (2000a)	8 state + pts, 6 ctrls	Generating inner speech or imagining external speech	To investigate the functional neuroanatomy of inner speech and auditory verbal imagery in schizophrenic patients predisposed to auditory hallucinations	No between-group difference while subjects generated inner speech; auditory verbal imagery elicited deficits in activation of cerebellum, thalamus, hippocampus, and temporal cortex in pts with auditory hallucinations
Shergill et al. (2000b)	6 state + pts	Periods of hallucination (identified retrospectively) compared to non-hallucinating	To employ a novel method for acquiring imaging data during hallucinations, by irregularly acquiring scans, and questioning the patient for hallucinatory activity immediately after the period of acquisition	Periods of hallucinations associated with increased activation in inferior frontal, anterior cingulate, and temporal cortex bilaterally, right thalamus and left hippocampus
Kircher et al. (2001a)	6 state + pts, 6 state – pts, 7 ctrls	Subjects completed a sentence with a word which was either generated, selected or read	To investigate the neural correlates of processing linguistic context in schizophrenic patients with formal thought disorder.	Sentence completion with self-generated or self-selected words elicited reduced right temporal activation in pts with formal thought disorder, compared to pts without thought disorder.

Table 9.4 (continued)

Reference	Sample	Cognitive task(s)	Aims/hypotheses	Main findings
Kircher et al. (2001b)	6 pts, 6 ctrls	Rorschach ink blots	To investigate the pathophysiology of formal thought disorder	Severity of formal thought disorder negatively correlated with left STG and MTG, and correlated positively with activity in the caudate, cerebellum and pre-central gyrus
Shergill et al. (2001)	1 pt (case report)	Retrospective description of experiences during scanning	To compare the neurobiological substrate of somatic compared to auditory hallucinations	Somatic hallucinations associated with activation of somatosensory and parietal cortex; auditory hallucinations were associated with activation of STG and MTG
Surguladze et al. (2001)	7 state + pts, 7 state pts, 7 ctrls	Listening to auditory speech, silent lip-reading, and perception of meaningless lip movements	To examine abnormalities in the integration of auditory and visual language inputs as a mechanism for features of scz	Reduced activation in temporal cortex to silent lip-reading; pts also increased activation in fronto-striatal regions in response to the visual non-speech condition
Bentaleb et al. (2002)	1 patient with auditory hallucinations which disappeared when presented with loud external speech, 1 ctrl	Listening to external speech	To test the hypotheses that auditory hallucinations result from misinterpreted inner speech, or from aberrant activation of the primary auditory cortex	Auditory hallucinations were associated with increased activation of left primary auditory cortex and right MTG

Study	N	Task	Aim	Findings
Kircher et al. (2002)	6 pts, 7 ctrls	Rorschach ink blots	To investigate the pathophysiology of formal thought disorder	The amount of speech produced correlated with activation in left STG in ctrls, but right STG in pts
Honey et al. (2003a)	27 ctrls, 30 pts	2-back working memory and psychomotor sequencing	To investigate associations between sub-syndromal structures of five factors of the PANSS and cognitive activation	Task-specific (working memory task) modulation of functional response associated with symptom expression
Shergill et al. (2003)	8 ctrls, 8 pts	Subvocalization of the word 'rest' at 2 different frequencies	To investigate whether patient with auditory hallucinations show similar fronto-temporal deficits to increased rate of inner speech as previously identified to external speech	Attenuated response in right temporal, parietal and parahippocampal regions in pts when inner speech generation was increased

ctrls, controls; MTG, middle temporal gyrus; PANSS, Positive and Negative Symptom Scale; pts, patients; SMA, supplementary motor area; STG, superior temporal gyrus.

Using fMRI, Lennox *et al.* (2000) and Shergill *et al.* (2000*b*) showed that when patients experience auditory hallucinations, there is evidence of increased activation of inferior frontal and temporal cortex, supporting previous work using SPECT (McGuire *et al.* 1993). Further work contrasting auditory and somatic hallucinations has indicated areas are involved in mediating hallucinations in the auditory modality and which are modality-independent (Shergill *et al.* 2001). These studies have been complemented by work focused on the generation and monitoring of inner speech, which have been engaged by the varying the rate of covert articulation (Shergill *et al.* 2003), requiring subjects to imagine external speech (Shergill *et al.* 2000*a*), and manipulating the source and pitch of auditory verbal feedback during speech (Fu *et al.* 2001). This research indicates that patients who are prone to experience auditory hallucinations show reduced activation in temporal, parahippocampal, and cerebellar cortex, consistent with previous PET data (McGuire *et al.* 1995) and cognitive psychological models of auditory hallucinations (Frith 1992) implicating defective monitoring of inner speech. It is interesting, therefore, that some of these regions may also exhibit an attenuated response to exogenous stimulation: Woodruff *et al.* (1997) showed that independent of medication, activation in the temporal cortex to external speech was reduced during periods of auditory hallucinations. Other PET and fMRI data suggest that patients who are prone to experience auditory hallucinations show reduced temporal activation when required to monitor inner speech, suggesting this may be a cognitive mechanism by which auditory hallucinations occur (McGuire *et al.* 1995; Shergill *et al.* 2001).

fMRI has also been used to examine the brain areas active when patients are articulating thought-disordered speech. Kircher *et al.* (2001*b*) provoked disorganized speech by asking patients to describe ambiguous pictures, and correlated the severity of thought disorder over time with changes in BOLD response. They found that there was an inverse correlation between the severity of thought disorder and left superior temporal gyral activity, consistent with an earlier PET study which used a similar design (McGuire *et al.* 1998). Other work has sought to relate thought disorder to impairments in sentence processing. Kuperberg *et al.* (2000) used fMRI to examine the neural correlates of linguistic anomalies in sentences, while Kircher *et al.* (2001*a*) and Arcuri *et al.* (2001) have found that patients who are prone to thought disorder show attenuated activation in the inferior frontal and superior temporal cortex when completing sentence stems or making judgements about the meaning of sentences.

Although the individual symptoms of schizophrenia are not pathognomonic, certain features tend to co-occur. For example, delusional beliefs are frequently observed in patients who also exhibit hallucinations, constituting a 'positive' subsyndrome of the illness; similarly, negative symptoms are also often co-expressed. The co-occurrence of symptoms can be assessed formally using factor analysis, and the resulting subsyndromes correlated with neurobiological measures. This approach was first pioneered by Liddle *et al.* (1992), using PET to investigate the resting physiological substrate of a three-syndrome model, involving psychomotor poverty, disorganization, and reality distortion. This was recently extended by Honey *et al.* (2003*a*) to determine the pattern of cognitive activation associated with the five subsyndromes identified using factor analysis of the Positive and Negative Symptom Scale (PANSS) (Kay *et al.* 1987). A positive correlation was observed between overall severity of psychosis, and brain regions associated with language processing. Negative symptoms were associated with increased lateral and medial frontal response during the working memory task, and positive symptoms with reduced fronto-temporal response. These patterns were observed to be task-specific, since no relationship was observed between symptom structure and a psychomotor task. Intriguingly, a simple comparison of the patient group compared to controls, irrespective of symptom configuration, showed a pattern of hypofrontality in the patients. The authors noted that hypo-activated regions were not located in the same regions of frontal cortex that demonstrated psychophysiological associations with subsyndrome scores, suggesting that the observed hypofrontality may simply reflect the difference in behavioural performance between the two groups.

Some of these observations are consistent with a capacity model of cortical function (Just and Carpenter 1992; Just *et al.* 1996) (Fig. 9.3). Briefly, this suggests that different cognitive tasks may compete for common, capacity-limited neural resources. As the demands on processing resources increase, there is increasing functional activation of the brain regions specialized to perform the relevant tasks until a capacity limit is reached, at which point activation by one or more of the competing tasks is attenuated. Perturbations of endogenous or baseline activity may also compete for neural resources with exogenous or experimentally administered cognitive tasks; for example, a negative correlation between focal activation during visual stimulation and baseline rCBF has been demonstrated in healthy volunteers (Kastrup *et al.* 1999). In extending this model to the psychopathological literature, psychotic symptoms such as auditory hallucinations may represent an endogenous demand on fronto-temporal cortical processing resources which may be competitive with exogenous demands, such as processing external speech.

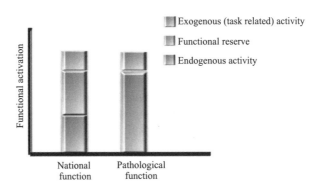

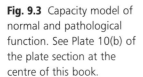

Fig. 9.3 Capacity model of normal and pathological function. See Plate 10(b) of the plate section at the centre of this book.

Effects of treatment

A fundamental consideration in any functional imaging study involving psychiatric patients is the potentially confounding effect of antipsychotic medication. However, the effects of pharmacotherapeutic interventions are frequently overlooked in experimental designs involving psychiatric patients, and have been specifically investigated in few studies (Table 9.5). In such circumstances it may be intractable to dissociate the effects of illness and treatment in the interpretation of any observed group differences. This is particularly problematic in functional imaging studies, in which drug treatment may affect outcome measures on several levels:

- *psychological*: antipsychotics may induce cognitive impairment, or exacerbate existing deficits associated with the illness (Green and Braff, 2001);

- *neural*: electrophysiological studies have demonstrated direct effects of antipsychotics on the regulation of neuronal firing (Dick *et al.* 1987);

- *neurovascular*: dopaminergic terminals form synapses in close proximity to the cerebral vasculature and dopamine agonists have been shown to cause vasoconstriction (Krimer *et al.* 1998) and a global reduction in cerebral perfusion (Gollub *et al.* 1998).

Honey *et al.* (1999) investigated the effect of the atypical antipsychotic, risperidone, on prefrontal function using fMRI. Atypical antipsychotics were predicted to enhance prefrontal function during performance of a working memory task, hypothetically via increased dopaminergic drive to the prefrontal cortex, on the basis of the following a priori evidence:

- patients with schizophrenia perform poorly on tests of working memory, and exhibit a hypofrontal response to such tasks (Callicott *et al.* 1998);

- hypofrontality can be reversed by administration of dopamine agonists (Daniel *et al.* 1989).

- atypical antipsychotics have been shown to increase prefrontal dopaminergic activity in animal models (Hertel *et al.* 1996).

Patients treated with typical antipsychotics were scanned using fMRI during performance of a working memory task, and then switched to risperidone for 6 weeks' treatment, following which patients were re-scanned. These patients were compared to a group of patients scanned at the same interval, but treated with typical antipsychotics throughout the period of study. Treatment with risperidone was associated with increased activation of prefrontal cortex, independent of symptomatic change. Using a cross-sectional design, Braus *et al.* (1999) also noted differences in functional activation between patients treated with typical and atypical antipsychotics in motor cortex. The neurobiological mechanism by which psychological and pharmacological therapeutics strategies may overlap, or have convergent effects on prefrontal dopaminergic function, remains an intriguing issue for future study.

Table 9.5 Functional magnetic resonance imaging (fMRI) studies of antipsychotic medication in schizophrenia

References	Sample	Study design	Cognitive task(s)	Aims/hypotheses	Main findings
Braus et al. (1999)	14 Dg-N, 13 typs, 13 atyps, 15 ctrls	Cross-sectional design	Sequential finger opposition	Evaluate drug effects on motor cortex activation in schizophrenia	Similar PM ctx and SMA activation in FE pts and ctrls; reduced PM activation in typ pts; reduced SMA activation in both typ and atyp pts
Honey et al. (1999)	20 pts, 10 ctrls	10 pts treated with typs throughout; 10 pts treated with typs at baseline, then switched to risperidone for 6 weeks; all pts scanned at baseline and 6 weeks	Verbal working memory (2-back)	To investigate the effects of atypical antipsychotics on PFC function.	Patients switched from typical antipsychotics to risperidone showed increased PFC activation
Stephan et al. (2001)	6 pts, 6 ctrls	Drug-naive or drug-free at baseline; then switched to olanzapine	Sequential finger opposition	To investigate the effects of olanzapine on cerebellar functional connectivity	Olanzapine treatment associated with changed connectivity of the cerebellum with frontal cortex and thalamus
Nahas et al. (2003)	6 pts	Treated with atypicals at baseline, and then 12 weeks of donepezil	Verbal fluency	To investigate whether a cognitive enchancer would normalize fronto-cinglate modulation of temporal cortex	Increased left frontal and cingulate activity compared to baseline

atyps, atypical antipsychotics; ctrls, controls; Dg-N, drug-naive; FE, first episode; PFC, prefrontal cortex; PM ctx, primary motor cortex; pts, patients; SMA, supplementary motor area.

Schizophrenia is viewed increasingly as a disconnection syndrome, in which the inter-regional communication in the brain is compromised, as opposed to a localized deficit in any one region (Friston and Frith 1995; McGuire and Frith 1996; Bullmore *et al.* 1997; Fletcher *et al.* 1999; Buchel *et al.* 2000; Lawrie *et al.* 2002; Schlosser *et al.* 2003). Accordingly, the mechanism of action of antipsychotic treatments presumably involves the modulation of inter-regional functional connectivity. Recent studies have begun to characterize the effects of pharmacological treatment on integrative brain function: functional connections between the cerebellum and prefrontal cortex have been shown to be significantly affected by treatment with olanzapine (Stephan *et al.* 2001), and fronto-temporal disconnectivity normalized by treatment with the acetylcholinesterase inhibitor, donepezil (Nahas *et al.* 2003). The integration of psychopharmacological experimental designs with multivariate assessments of inter-regional communication is likely to be of critical importance in future psychiatric drug development, and a recent study demonstrated that acute pharmacological effects on functional connectivity can be detected in healthy volunteers (Honey *et al.* 2003*b*).

Other neuropsychiatric conditions

In recent years, fMRI has begun to be applied to a wide range of neuropsychiatric disorders (Table 9.6) in an attempt to elucidate the neurobiological basis of these conditions. Clearly the application of the technique to non-schizophrenic psychoses is currently in the early stages of development, with only a small number of studies reported for any particular condition. A clear pattern of findings has therefore yet to emerge.

With this caution in mind, a number of studies of depressed patients are beginning to support the involvement of limbic regions, including the cingulate cortex and amydala/hippocampal complex, in major depression. Beauregard *et al.* (1998) and Elliott *et al.* (2002) found that depressed patients exhibit an increased functional activation of the anterior cingulate in response to viewing affective stimuli. Abnormal activation of the amygdala has also been reported in depressed patients during affective processing (Sheline *et al.* 2001; Siegle *et al.* 2002). Response dynamics of the amygdala have also been shown to be abnormal, with prolonged activation evident during presentation of emotional stimuli, extending throughout subsequent presentation of non-emotional stimuli; this anomalous response pattern in the amygdala was further shown to be associated with self-reports of rumination (Siegle *et al.* 2002). The critical involvement of the amygdala in depression was further demonstrated by its abnormal response even when affective stimuli are processed in the absence of conscious awareness (Sheline *et al.* 2001); moreover, this was shown to resolve following treatment with antidepressant medication.

One of the key advantages of fMRI is the non-invasive assessment of brain function. This facility is exploited most effectively in studies involving psychiatric conditions in childhood, previously unamenable to imaging technologies associated with exposure to radiation. fMRI can also be used to investigate neurodevelopmental trajectories using repeated assessment over the course of the illness from an early age. Reduced

Table 9.6 Functional magnetic resonance imaging (fMRI) studies of other psychiatric disorders

References	Condition	Sample	Cognitive task(s)	Aims/hypotheses	Main findings
Kalin et al. (1997)	Depression	2 pts (before and 2 weeks after venlafaxine), 2 ctrls	Viewing positively and negatively valenced stimuli	To identify the neural circuitry underlying emotional processing in control and depressed subjects	No activation to positive images in pts at baseline; following sympto-matic improvement after 2 weeks' treatment, activation was evident in secondary visual areas to positive stimuli; activation decreased to negative stimuli in ctrls and patients
Beauregard et al. (1998)	Depression	7 pts, 7 ctrls	Viewing of neutral film clips, and clips aimed at inducing sadness	To determine whether the functional brain changes associated with the affect disturbance seen in this syndrome are similar to those that accompany transient sadness in normal subjects	Increased activation of left medial prefrontal cortex and right cingulate in pts in response to emo tionally laden film clips
Sheline et al. (2001)	Depression	11 pts, 11 ctrls	Subliminal presen-tation of emotional faces, followed by conscious viewing of neutral faces	To investigate the involvement of the amygdala in depressed patients during affective processing, in the absence of conscious perseveration on emotional stimuli, and to examine the effects of antidepressant treatment	Increased activation of the left amygdala was observed in depressed patients in response to fearful faces, even in the absence of conscious awareness; this resolved with antidepressant treatment

Table 9.6 (continued)

References	Condition	Sample	Cognitive task(s)	Aims/hypotheses	Main findings
Elliott et al. (2002)	Depression	10 pts, 10 ctrls	Emotional go /no-go task	To determine whether mood-congruent processing biases are associated with specific neural substrates in depression	Depressed pts showed reduced neural response to emotional stimuli in ventral cingulate and orbitofrontal cortex; activation was increased in rostral anterior cingulate in response to sad emotional stimuli
Siegle et al. (2002)	Depression	7 pts, 10 ctrls	Valence identification and Sternberg tasks	To examine whether brain activity in response to emotional stimuli is sustained in depressed pts, even following subsequent distracting stimuli	Amygdala activation to emotional stimuli decayed within 10 s; in depressed pts, emotion-related amygdala activation lasted throughout subsequent non-emotional trials, 25 s later, and correlated with self-reported rumination
Smith et al. (2002)	Depression	10 pts (remitted), 8 ctrls	Noxious hot, or non-noxious warm stimuli presented, preceded by coloured lights to indicate onset of stimuli	To investigate whether abnormal brain activity is evident in remitted depressed patients in anticipation of a noxious stimulus	Similar patterns of activation were observed in patients and control subjects, but increased cerebellar activation was observed in pts
Thomas et al. (2001)	Childhood anxiety/ depression	12 children with panic disorder, 12 children without panic disorder, 5 girls with depression, 5 girls with anxiety disorder, 5 healthy girls	Viewing photographs of fearful and neutral facial expressions	To test the hypothesis that children with anxiety and depression may show atypical amygdala responses to emotional stimuli	Children with anxiety disorders showed increased amygdala activation to fearful faces, whereas depressed children showed reduced amygdala activation. Amygdala activation correlated with children's symptomatic self-reports

Study	Condition	n	Task	Purpose	Findings
Bystritsky et al. (2001)	Panic disorder	6 pts, 6 ctrls	Directed imagery of neutral, moderate and high idiosyncratic anxiety situations.	To examine brain regions associated with the experience of panic disorder	Pts demonstrated increased activation of frontal, hippocampal, and cingulate cortices
Maas et al. (1998)	Cocaine addiction	6 pts, 6 ctrls	Viewing pictures of neutral and drug-related scenes	To test whether brain activation was detectable in regions previously associated with cocaine cue-induced craving	Increased activation observed in pts with history of crack cocaine use in anterior cingulate and left DLPFC, which correlated with self-reports of drug craving
Li et al. (2000)	Cocaine addiction	7 pts	At rest following no injection, saline injection, and cocaine injection	To observe the effects of cocaine administration on the physiological fluctuations of fMRI signal in two brain regions	Reduction in activity in primary visual and motor cortex following cocaine administration
Garavan et al. (2000)	Cocaine addiction	17 pts, 14 ctrls	Viewing video images of cocaine smoking, neutral scenes or erotic images	To investigate the functional neuroanatomy of craving induced by drug-related cues	Frontal, parietal and limbic cortex showed increased activation to cocaine-craving cues, greater than that seen in the neutral and sexual images
Wexler et al. (2001)	Cocaine addiction	8 pts	Viewing videotapes designed to elicit happy feelings, sad feelings, or the desire to use cocaine	Identification of brain activity associated with craving	Activation of the anterior cingulate was observed in pts during drug craving, but not other emotional responses; activation preceded subject's report of craving, and was evident in pts who did not report craving

Table 9.6 (continued)

References	Condition	Sample	Cognitive task(s)	Aims/hypotheses	Main findings
Gollub et al. (1998)	Cocaine addiction	17 pts	Visual stimulation	To determine whether cocaine would cause changes in focal activation following visual stimulation	Visual stimulation resulted in comparable signal changes before and after cocaine
George et al. (2001)	Alcoholism	10 pts, 10 ctrls	Viewing pictures of neutral and drug-related scenes	To examine the neural basis of craving in alcoholic subjects	Increased activation in left DLPFC and thalamus in alcoholic subjects following brief exposure to alcohol and picture rating
Schneider et al. (2001)	Alcoholism	10 pts, 10 ctrls	Exposure to ethanol odour before and after therapy	To examine the functional cerebral correlates of craving in alcoholic patients	Cue-induced craving associated with amygdala/hippocampal activation before treatment; after treatment activation of superior temporal sulcus was evident
Curtis et al. (2001)	Schizophrenia/bipolar disorder	5 bipolar, 5 scz pts, 5 ctrls	Paced orthographic verbal fluency, and semantic categorization	To determine whether task-specific attenuation of activation offrontal cortex is specific to scz	Bipolar pts showed increased frontal activation compared to ctrls during verbal fluency; no between-group differences during semantic decision
Shin et al. (2001)	Post-traumatic stress disorder	8 combat veterans with PTSD, 8 combat veterans without PTSD	Emotional Counting Stroop	To test the functional integrity of anterior cingulate cortex in PTSD	Non-PTSD combat veterans activated anterior cingulate in response to combat-related words, compared to negative non-combat words; anterior cingulate activation was not evident in the PTSD pts
Lanius et al. (2002)	Post-traumatic stress disorder	7 pts with sexual-abuse-related PTSD, 7 pts with experience of traumatic history, but not PTSD	Script-driven imagery of traumatic events	To investigate the neural circuitry associated with dissociative responses in PTSD	PTSD pts showed increased response during dissociation throughout the cortex, involving middle temporal, occipital, parietal and lateral/medial frontal regions

Breiter *et al.* (1996)	OCD	10 pts, 5 ctrls	Symptom provocation	To investigate the neurobiological basis of OCD	Increased activation observed in patients in orbitofrontal, lateral frontal, anterior temporal, anterior cingulate, and insular cortex, as well as caudate, lenticulate, and amygdala
Phillips *et al.* (2000)	OCD	7 OCD pts with washing rituals, 7 OCD pts with checking rituals, 14 ctrls	Viewing disgusting, washing-related and neutral scenes	To identify the neural correlates of the urge to ritualize in washing and checking symptoms in OCD	Insula activation was observed in all groups in response to disgust stimuli, and only in OCD pts with washing symptoms in response to the washing-related stimuli; pts with checking rituals activated frontostriatal regions, associated with the urge to ritualize
Phillips *et al.* (2001)	OCD and depersonalization disorder	10 OCD pts, 6 DP pts, 6 ctrls	Viewing pictures of aversive and neutral scenes	To investigate the neural basis of emotional detachment in depersonalization disorder	In response to aversive stimuli, DP pts demonstrated reduced activation of insula and occipito-temporal cortex, and increased activation of right ventral prefrontal cortex
Seeger *et al.* (2002)	Anorexia nervosa	3 pts, 3 ctrls	Viewing pictures of idiosyncratic distortion of self- and other-body image	To examine the involvement of the amygdala in abnormal body image perception in anorexic patients	Activation of amygdala, brainstem and fusiform gyrus was observed in anorexic patients while they viewed distorted self-body images
Herpertz *et al.* (2001)	Borderline personality disorder	6 pts, 6 pts	Viewing emotionally aversive slides and neutral slides	To identify brain regions associated with affective processing in borderline personality disorder	Increased activation of amygdala bilaterally, and medial and ventrolateral prefrontal cortex

Table 9.6 (continued)

References	Condition	Sample	Cognitive task(s)	Aims/hypotheses	Main findings
Kiehl et al. (2001)	Criminal psychopathy	8 criminal psychopaths, 8 criminal non-psychopaths	Verbal episodic memory recognition task	To investigate the neurobiological basis of abnormal affective processing associated with psychopathy	Reduced activation of limbic regions: amygdala/hippocampus, parahippocampal gyrus, ventral striatum and cingulate cortex; increased activation of bilateral fronto-temporal cortex
Rubia et al. (1999)	Attention deficit hyperactivity disorder	7 boys with ADHD, 7 ctrls	Motor inhibition task, and a motor timing task	To investigate the hypothesis that ADHD is associated with a dysfunction of prefrontal brainregions during motor response inhibition and motor timing	ADHD pts showed reduced activation of right DLPFC in response to both tasks, and right inferior frontal cortex and caudate in response to the motor inhibition task
Bush et al. (1999)	Attention deficit hyperactivity disorder	8 pts, 8 ctrls	Emotional counting Stroop	To test the hypothesis that anterior cingulate dysfunction might contribute to core features of ADHD, namely inattention and impulsivity	Pts showed reduced activation of the anterior cingulate
Baron-Cohen et al. (1999)	Autism	6 pts, 12 ctrls	'Eyes' test of emotional attribution	To test Brother's theory of the network underlying the 'social brain': orbitofrontal cortex, STG and amygdala	Activation of regions associated with Brother's theory of the social brain were observed in ctrls during mental state attribution; pts with autism activated fronto-temporal regions, but not amygdala

Study	Condition	N	Task	Aim	Findings
Ring et al. (1999)	Autism	6 pts, 12 ctrls	Embedded figures task	To investigate the hypothesis that autistic subjects would engage different brain regions during a task which patients demonstrate improved performance	Despite an absence of behavioural differences, prefrontal activation was greater in the control subjects, while ventral occipito-temporal activation was evident in the patients
Critchley et al. (2000)	Autism	9 pts, 9 ctrls	Explicit and implicit facial affect processing	To investigate the neurobiological correlates of deficits in processing facial expression in autistic subjects	Patients showed dysfunctional activation of the 'fusiform face area' during explicit processing of facial emotions, and left amygdala and cerebellum during implicit facial processing
Schultz et al. (2000)	Autism and Asperger's syndrome	14 pts, 2 × 14 ctrls	Face and object processing tasks	To investigate the neural correlates of face recognition in autistic patients	Decreased activation of right fusiform gyrus and increased activation in right inferior temporal gyrus during face, but not object, recognition; in a replication analysis, increased activation of (left) inferior temporal gyrus was observed in the autistic group
Muller et al. (2001)	Autism	8 pts, 8 ctrls	Visually paced finger movement	To investigate neural dysfunction in autism in the absence of performance deficits	Decreased activation of peri-rolandic cortex and SMA, and increased activation of prefrontal cortex was observed in pts
Pierce et al. (2001)	Autism	7 pts, 8 ctrls	Facial (gender) and shape processing	To investigate structure–function relationships in autistic patients during facial processing	Reduced volume of the amygdala was observed in pts; functional deficits were observed in the amygdala, inferior occipital gyrus and superior temporal sulcus

Table 9.6 (continued)

References	Condition	Sample	Cognitive task(s)	Aims/hypotheses	Main findings
Luna (2002)	Autism	11 pts, 6 ctrls	Oculomotor spatial working memory and visual saccadic task	To test the hypothesis that deficits in spatial working working memory in autism are due to abnormalities in prefrontal circuitry	Autistic subjects showed normal activation to the saccadic task, but reduced activation of prefrontal and posterior cingulate cortices during the spatial working memory task
Berthoz et al. (2002)	Alexithymia	8 males with high scores on Alexithymia scale, 8 males with low scores on Alexithymia scale	Viewing pictures with validated positive or negative arousal capabilities	To investigate involve ment of the anterior cingulated in response to emotional stimuli in patients with alexithymia	Pts with alexithymia showed reduced activation in the left mediofrontal-paracingulate cortex in response to highly negative stimuli and more activation in the anterior cingulate, mediofrontal cortex, and middle frontal gyrus in response to highly positive stimuli
Howard (1997)	Lewy body dementia	1 state + pt	Photic stimulation. on and off medication	To investigate the visual cortex response to photic stimulation during and in the absence of continuous visual hallucinations	Attenuation of occipital activation from photic stimulation when patient experienced visual hallucinations, compared to non-hallucinating state
Ffytche et al. (1998)	Charles Bonnet syndrome	8 pts, 5 non-hallucinating ctrls with impaired vision	Pts signal onset/offset of hallucinations (expt 1) Viewing visual 'noise'	Investigate neural substrate of visual consciousness	Visual hallucinations were associated with increased occipital activation, in regions in which the regional specialization corresponded to the content of the experience

ADHD, attention deficit hyperactivity disorder; ctrls, controls; DLPFC, dorsolateral prefrontal cortex; DP, depersonalization; pts, patients; OCD, obsessive–compulsive disorder; PTSD, post-traumatic stress disorder; scz, schizophrenia; SMA, supplementary motor area; STG, superior temporal gyrus.

activation of fronto-striatal regions (Rubia *et al.* 1999) and anterior cingulate cortex (Bush *et al.* 1999) has been demonstrated in children with attention deficit hyperactivity disorder (ADHD) in which impaired response inhibition is evident.

A deficit in facial affect processing is a key feature of autism and related conditions in childhood, and fMRI has been used in a number of studies in order to investigate the pathophysiological mechanisms that may mediate abnormal facial affect recognition. In the first study to report the application of fMRI in autistic subjects, Baron-Cohen *et al.* (1999) demonstrated a failure to engage amygdala activation during mental state attribution from images of eye gaze. Amygdala dysfunction in autistic subjects during facial affect processing was replicated by Critchley *et al.* (2000) and Pierce *et al.* (2001). Pierce and coworkers also showed that the volume of the amygdala was reduced in autistic patients. Abnormal functional response in the 'fusiform face area' has also been reported (Critchley *et al.* 2000; Schultz *et al.* 2000; Pierce *et al.* 2001), suggesting that a network of regions that mediate social intelligence in the normal brain may be dysfunctional in these disorders (Baron-Cohen *et al.* 2000). In order to investigate brain function in the absence of potentially confounding behavioural deficits, Ring *et al.* (1999) and Muller *et al.* (2001) examined activity during the performance of behaviourally matched tasks; both studies reported abnormal activation of prefrontal cortex, which may reflect alternative strategies engaged by autistic subjects.

At present it is premature to assess the pattern of deficits emerging in other psychiatric disorders in relation to those seen in schizophrenia, in terms of diagnostic specificity. Few fMRI studies of schizophrenia have incorporated a non-schizophrenic psychiatric group. This is an important methodological issue, as one cannot categorically relate current findings to schizophrenia *per se*, but only to psychosis in general. Initial indications suggest that differential patterns of abnormal function may indeed be associated with different diagnostic categories. Curtis *et al.* (2001) found that patients with bipolar illness showed a pattern of frontal function distinct from that of patients with schizophrenia, exhibiting a hyperfrontal response compared to the hypofrontal activity observed in schizophrenics. Similarly, frontal deficits in schizophrenic patients, widely reported during working memory tasks, were not evident in patients with major depression (Barch *et al.* 2003). These studies allude to the intriguing possibility that fMRI may, in future, offer a means by which to aid diagnosis, or indeed reformulate diagnostic categories (Callicott and Weinberger 2003), though this remains a potential to be realized at present, and work specifically aimed at this is only beginning to emerge.

Future pitfalls and potential of fMRI research in psychiatry

Functional imaging research in schizophrenia has demonstrated widespread deficits affecting a range of cognitive functions distributed throughout the brain. However, a pattern of brain dysfunction that would serve as a biological trait marker or predict treatment response has not emerged to date. There are a number of possible reasons why this may be, which are summarized in Table 9.7 (see also Honey *et al.* 2002*b*).

Table 9.7 Issues in the application of fMRI to schizophrenia

Issue	Description
Heterogeneity of the disorder	Psychiatric conditions are, in reality, extremely difficult to define as discrete and homogeneous entities. The poor validity and reliability of schizophrenia as a concept means that non-replicable findings may frequently emerge, given the variability of the patient group in any given study, and between research centres
Clinical confounds	At present potentially confounding effects of gender, age of illness onset, duration of illness chronicity, medication status, age and symptom profile are frequently overlooked in psychiatric imaging studies
Cognitive subtraction	The identification of regional activation to a given cognitive process is typically made on the basis of reference to a baseline task, with the assumption that the subtraction of the two tasks identifies the process of interest. This is a potentially flawed approach, and the extension of this methodology to psychiatric phenomena is equally controversial: the subtraction of activity associated with a given symptom from a state in which the symptom is absent may not be a pure manipulation of the process of interest
Pathological baseline activity	Resting state studies have shown that endogenous baseline activity is associated with regionally specific increases in relation to pathology. Cognitive activation studies must therefore aim to identify and incorporate the change in the relationship between endogenous and exogenous activity in psychiatric patients
Functional connectivity	To date, psychiatric imaging studies have primarily been predicated on a segregationist perspective of brain function, whereby discrete cognitive functions can be mapped on to circumscribed brain regions. However, there is increasing evidence that psychiatric conditions represent a disorder of functional connectivity, rather than a focal functional abnormality.

An exciting development in functional imaging research is the quantitative assessment of the functional relationship between multiple brain regions, using multivariate methods such as path analysis and structural equation modelling (McIntosh *et al.* 1994; Buchel and Friston 1997; Bullmore *et al.* 2000) and multi-dimensional scaling (Welchew *et al.* 2002). This is a particularly important development in psychiatric imaging research, as schizophrenia is increasingly conceptualized as a disorder of functional connectivity, as originally proposed by Wernicke, and this has become a renewed focus of interest. A full description of psychiatric processes in neuronal terms is therefore likely to demand an appreciation of inter-regional integration (Friston and Frith

1995; McGuire and Frith 1996; Bullmore *et al.* 1997; Fletcher *et al.* 1999). Developments in the analysis of functional connectivity in imaging data may shed further light on this issue (Bullmore *et al.* 2000).

PET studies have demonstrated a relative decrease in activity of the temporal lobe during tasks that engage the frontal cortex, which implies functional connectivity between frontal and temporal cortices. Fronto-temporal connectivity has been shown to be abnormal in patients with schizophrenia (Fletcher *et al.* 1999; Lawrie *et al.* 2002), although other studies using PET suggest that patients in remission of psychotic illness, including both schizophrenia and bipolar disorder, do not exhibit a failure of temporal deactivation, indicating that fronto-temporal disconnectivity, like hypofrontality, may be state-related (Dye *et al.* 1999; Spence *et al.* 2000). However, these studies suggest that the *level* of activation of a given brain region may not be so critical as the inter-regional functional *integration* that exists within a neurocognitive network. For example, Honey *et al.* (2002c) have recently demonstrated increased inter-hemispheric communication between prefrontal regions and increased fronto-parietal connectivity in response to graded working memory load in healthy volunteers. Given the importance of working memory deficits in schizophrenia, this suggests that disordered systems-level responses to cognitive processing, such as working memory, may represent the neural substrate of such deficits in schizophrenia. This was recently supported by a study using structural equation modelling, in which patients treated with atypical antipsychotics showed increased inter-hemispheric connectivity (Schlosser *et al.* 2003), perhaps relating to the improvement in working memory function associated with treatment with atypical antipsychotics.

In conclusion, the application of fMRI to schizophrenia and other psychiatric disorders over the past decade has provided an indication of the widespread pathophysiology associated with such conditions. Considerable refinement of these findings and successful confrontation of the specific challenges associated with psychiatric imaging will be necessary before direct clinical application can be expected. The latter half of the twentieth century witnessed rapid technological advances which provided psychiatry with the capability to visualize human brain function in living patients-a remarkable tool in cognitive neuroscience, which the founders of modern neuropsychiatry surely could never have envisaged. The ultimate success of functional imaging in contributing to current clinical practice will depend on our success in meeting the scientific challenge of applying this technology appropriately in the twenty-first century.

References

Amaro, E., Williams, S., Shergill, S. S., Fu, C. H., MacSweeney, M., Picchioni, M. M. *et al.* (2002). Acoustic noise and functional magnetic resonance imaging: current strategies and future prospects. *Journal of Magnetic Resonance Imaging*, **16**, 497–510.

Arcuri, S. M., Morris, R., Rabe-Hesketh, S., Broome, M., Andrew, C., Menzes, C. *et al.* (2001). What a difference a symptom makes? Specific and non-specific cognitive correlates of thought disorder in schizophrenia. *Schizophrenia Research*, **49**, 128–9.

Baddeley, A. (1986). *Working memory*. Clarendon Press, Oxford.

Baddeley, A. (1992). Working memory. *Science*, **256**, 556–9.

Baddeley, A. and Hitch, G. (1974). Working memory. In *The psychology of learning and motivation*, Vol. 8, (ed. G. Bower), pp. 47–90. Academic Press, New York.

Bandettini, P. A., Jesmanowicz, A., Wong, E. C., and Hyde, J. S. (1993). Processing strategies for time-course data sets in functional MRI of the human brain. *Magnetic Resonance in Medicine*, **30** (2), 161–73.

Barch, D. M., Carter, C. S., Braver, T. S., Sabb, F. W., MacDonald, A., 3rd, Noll, D. C. *et al.* (2001). Selective deficits in prefrontal cortex function in medication-naive patients with schizophrenia. *Archives of General Psychiatry*, **58** (3), 280–8.

Barch, D. M., Csernansky, J. G., Conturo, T., and Snyder, A. Z. (2002). Working and long-term memory deficits in schizophrenia: is there a common prefrontal mechanism? *Journal of Abnormal Psychology*, **111** (3), 478–94.

Barch, D. M., Sheline, Y. I., Csernansky, J. G., and Snyder, A. Z. (2003). Working memory and prefrontal cortex dysfunction: specificity to schizophrenia compared with major depression. *Biolological Psychiatry*, **53**, 376–84.

Baron-Cohen, S., Ring, H. A., Wheelwright, S., Bullmore, E. T., Brammer, M. J., Simmons, A. *et al.* (1999). Social intelligence in the normal and autistic brain: an fMRI study. *European Journal of Neuroscience*, **11** (6), 1891–8.

Baron-Cohen, S., Ring, H. A., Bullmore, E. T., Wheelwright, S., Ashwin, C., and Williams, S. C. (2000). The amygdala theory of autism. *Neuroscience and Biobehavioral Reviews*, **24** (3), 355–64.

Baumann, S. B., Noll, D. C., Kondziolka, D. S., Schneider, W., Nichols, T. E., Mintun, M. A. *et al.* (1995). Comparison of functional magnetic resonance imaging with positron emission tomography and magnetoencephalography to identify the motor cortex in a patient with an arteriovenous malformation. *Journal of Image Guided Surgery*, **1** (4), 191–7.

Beauregard, M., Leroux, J. M., Bergman, S., Arzoumanian, Y., Beaudoin, G., Bourgouin, P. *et al.* (1998). The functional neuroanatomy of major depression: an fMRI study using an emotional activation paradigm. *Neuroreport*, **9** (14), 3253–8.

Belliveau, J., Kennedy, D., McKinstry, R., Buchbinder, B., Weisskoff, R., Cohen, M. *et al.* (1991). Functional mapping of the human visual cortex by magnetic resonance imaging. *Science*, **254**, 716–19.

Bentaleb, L. A., Beauregard, M., Liddle, P., and Stip, E. (2002). Cerebral activity associated with auditory verbal hallucinations: a functional magnetic resonance imaging case study. *Journal of Psychiatry and Neuroscience*, **27** (2), 110–15.

Bentall, R. (1993). Deconstructing the concept of schizophrenia. *Journal of Mental Health*, **2**, 223–38.

Bentall, R. P., Jackson, H. F., and Pilgrim, D. (1988*a*). The concept of schizophrenia is dead: long live the concept of schizophrenia? *British Journal of Clinical Psychology*, **27**, 329–31.

Bentall, R. P., Jackson, H. F., and Pilgrim, D. (1988*b*). Abandoning the concept of 'schizophrenia': some implications of validity arguments for psychological research into psychotic phenomena. *British Journal of Clinical Psychology*, **27**, 303–24.

Berthoz, S., Artiges, E., Van De Moortele, P. F., Poline, J. B., Rouquette, S., Consoli, S. M. *et al.* (2002). Effect of impaired recognition and expression of emotions on frontocingulate cortices: an fMRI study of men with alexithymia. *American Journal of Psychiatry*, **159** (6), 961–7.

Bogerts, B. (1993). The neuropathology of schizophrenia. *Schizophrenia Bulletin*, **19**, 68–75.

Brammer, M. J. (1998). Multidimensional wavelet analysis of functional magnetic resonance images. *Human Brain Mapping*, **6** (5–6), 378–82.

Brammer, M. J., Bullmore, E. T., Simmons, A., Williams, S. C., Grasby, P. M., Howard, R. J. *et al.* (1997). Generic brain activation mapping in functional magnetic resonance imaging: a nonparametric approach. *Magnetic Resonance Imaging*, **15** (7), 763–70.

Braus, D. F., Ende, G., Weber-Fahr, W., Sartorius, A., Krier, A., Hubrich-Ungureanu, P. *et al.* (1999). Antipsychotic drug effects on motor activation measured by functional magnetic resonance imaging in schizophrenic patients. *Schizophrenia Research*, **39** (1), 19–29.

Braus, D. F., Ende, G., Hubrich-Ungureanu, P., and Henn, F. A. (2000). Cortical response to motor stimulation in neuroleptic-naive first episode schizophrenics. *Psychiatry Research*, **98** (3), 145–54.

Braus, D. F., Weber-Fahr, W., Tost, H., Ruf, M., and Henn, F. A. (2002). Sensory information processing in neuroleptic-naive first-episode schizophrenic patients: a functional magnetic resonance imaging study. *Archives of General Psychiatry*, **59** (8), 696–701.

Brebion, G., Amador, X., Smith, M. J., and Gorman, J. M. (1997). Mechanisms underlying memory impairment in schizophrenia. *Psychological Medicine*, **27**, 383–93.

Breiter, H. C., Rauch, S. L., Kwong, K. K., Baker, J. R., Weisskoff, R. M., Kennedy, D. N. *et al.* (1996). Functional magnetic resonance imaging of symptom provocation in obsessive–compulsive disorder. *Archives of General Psychiatry*, **53** (7), 595–606.

Buchel, C. and Friston, K. J. (1997). Modulation of connectivity in visual pathways by attention: cortical interactions evaluated with structural equation modelling and fMRI. *Cerebral Cortex*, **7** (8), 768–78.

Buchel, C., Lawrie, S., Frith, C., and Friston, K. (2000). Fronto-temporal functional connectivity in schizophrenics is correlated with psychopathology. *Journal of Cognitive Neuroscience*, **4E**.

Buckley, P. F., Friedman, L., Wu, D., Lai, S., Meltzer, H. Y., Haacke, E. M. *et al.* (1997). Functional magnetic resonance imaging in schizophrenia: initial methodology and evaluation of the motor cortex. *Psychiatry Research*, **74** (1), 13–23.

Bullmore, E. T. and Suckling, J. (2000). Functional magnetic resonance imaging. In *New Oxford textbook of psychiatry*, Vol. 1, (ed. M. G. Gelder, J. J. Lopez-Ibor, and N. C. Andreasen), pp. 218–223. Oxford University Press, New York.

Bullmore, E. T. and Suckling, J. (2001). Functional magnetic resonance imaging. *International Review of Psychiatry*, **13**, 24–33.

Bullmore, E., Brammer, M., Williams, S. C., Rabe-Hesketh, S., Janot, N., David, A. *et al.* (1996a). Statistical methods of estimation and inference for functional MR image analysis. *Magnetic Resonance in Medicine*, **35** (2), 261–77.

Bullmore, E. T., Rabe-Hesketh, S., Morris, R. G., Williams, S. C., Gregory, L., Gray, J. A. *et al.* (1996b). Functional magnetic resonance image analysis of a large-scale neurocognitive network. *Neuroimage*, **4** (1), 16–33.

Bullmore, E. T., Frangou, S., and Murray, R. M. (1997). The dysplastic net hypothesis: an integration of developmental and dysconnectivity theories of schizophrenia. *Schizophrenia Research*, **28**, 143–56.

Bullmore, E. T., Brammer, M. J., Rabe-Hesketh, S., Curtis, V. A., Morris, R. G., Williams, S. C. *et al.* (1999a). Methods for diagnosis and treatment of stimulus-correlated motion in generic brain activation studies using fMRI. *Human Brain Mapping*, **7** (1), 38–48.

Bullmore, E. T., Suckling, J., Overmeyer, S., Rabe-Hesketh, S., Taylor, E., and Brammer, M. J. (1999b). Global, voxel, and cluster tests, by theory and permutation, for a difference between two groups of structural MR images of the brain. *IEEE Transactions in Medical Imaging*, **18** (1), 32–42.

Bullmore, E., Horwitz, B., Honey, G., Brammer, M., Williams, S., and Sharma, T. (2000). How good is good enough in path analysis of fMRI data? *Neuroimage*, **11** (4), 289–301.

Bullmore, E., Long, C., Suckling, J., Fadili, J., Calvert, G., Zelaya, F. *et al.* (2001). Colored noise and computational inference in neurophysiological (fMRI) time series analysis: resampling methods in time and wavelet domains. *Human Brain Mapping*, **12** (2), 61–78.

Bush, G., Frazier, J. A., Rauch, S. L., Seidman, L. J., Whalen, P. J., Jenike, M. A. *et al.* (1999). Anterior cingulate cortex dysfunction in attention-deficit/hyperactivity disorder revealed by fMRI and the Counting Stroop. *Biological Psychiatry*, **45** (12), 1542–52.

Bystritsky, A., Pontillo, D., Powers, M., Sabb, F. W., Craske, M. G., and Bookheimer, S. Y. (2001). Functional MRI changes during panic anticipation and imagery exposure. *Neuroreport*, **12** (18), 3953–7.

Calev, A. (1984a). Recall and recognition in mildly disturbed schizophrenics: the use of matched tasks. *Psychological Medicine*, **14**, 425–9.

Calev, A. (1984b). Recall and recognition in chronic nondemented schizophrenics: use of matched tasks. *Journal of Abnormal Psychology*, **93**, 172–7.

Callicott, J. H. and Weinberger, D. R. (2003). Brain imaging as an approach to phenotype characterization for genetic studies of schizophrenia. *Methods in Molecular Medicine*, **77**, 227–47.

Callicott, J. H., Ramsey, N. F., Tallent, K., Bertolino, A., Knable, M. B., Coppola, R. *et al.* (1998). Functional magnetic resonance imaging brain mapping in psychiatry: methodological issues illustrated in a study of working memory in schizophrenia. *Neuropsychopharmacology*, **18** (3), 186–96.

Callicott, J. H., Bertolino, A., Mattay, V. S., Langheim, F. J., Duyn, J., Coppola, R. *et al.* (2000). Physiological dysfunction of the dorsolateral prefrontal cortex in schizophrenia revisited. *Cerebral Cortex*, **10** (11), 1078–92.

Callicott, J. H., Egan, M. F., Mattay, V. S., Bertolino, A., Bone, A. D., Verchinksi, B. *et al.* (2003). Abnormal fMRI response of the dorsolateral prefrontal cortex in cognitively intact siblings of patients with schizophrenia. *American Journal of Psychiatry*, **160**, 709–19.

Carter, C. S., MacDonald, A. W., 3rd, Ross, L. L., and Stenger, V. A. (2001). Anterior cingulate cortex activity and impaired self-monitoring of performance in patients with schizophrenia: an event-related fMRI study. *American Journal of Psychiatry*, **158** (9), 1423–8.

Chan, A. S., Kwok, I. C., Chiu, H., Lam, L., Pang, A., and Chow, L. Y. (2000). Memory and organizational strategies in chronic and acute schizophrenic patients. *Schizophrenia Research*, **41**, 431–45.

Cohen, J. D. and Servan-Schreiber, D. (1992). Context, cortex, and dopamine: a connectionist approach to behavior and biology in schizophrenia. *Psychological Review*, **99** (1), 45–77.

Conklin, H., Curtis, C., Katsanis, J., and Iacono, W. (2000). Verbal working memory impairment in schizophrenia patients and their first-degree relatives: evidence from the digit span task. *American Journal of Psychiatry*, **157**, 275–7.

Critchley, H. D., Daly, E. M., Bullmore, E. T., Williams, S. C., Van Amelsvoort, T., Robertson, D. M. *et al.* (2000). The functional neuroanatomy of social behaviour: changes in cerebral blood flow when people with autistic disorder process facial expressions. *Brain*, **123** (Pt 11), 2203–12.

Curtis, V. A., Bullmore, E. T., Brammer, M. J., Wright, I. C., Williams, S. C., Morris, R. G. *et al.* (1998). Attenuated frontal activation during a verbal fluency task in patients with schizophrenia. *American Journal of Psychiatry*, **155** (8), 1056–63.

Curtis, V. A., Bullmore, E. T., Morris, R. G., Brammer, M. J., Williams, S. C., Simmons, A. *et al.* (1999). Attenuated frontal activation in schizophrenia may be task dependent. *Schizophrenia Research*, **37** (1), 35–44.

Curtis, V. A., Dixon, T. A., Morris, R. G., Bullmore, E. T., Brammer, M. J., Williams, S. C. *et al.* (2001). Differential frontal activation in schizophrenia and bipolar illness during verbal fluency. *Journal of Affective Disorders*, **66** (2–3), 111–21.

Daniel, D. G., Berman, K. F., and Weinberger, D. R. (1989). The effect of apomorphine on regional cerebral blood flow in schizophrenia. *Journal of Neuropsychiatry and Clinical Neurosciences*, 1 (4), 377–84.

David, A. S., Woodruff, P. W., Howard, R., Mellers, J. D., Brammer, M., Bullmore, E. *et al.* (1996). Auditory hallucinations inhibit exogenous activation of auditory association cortex. *Neuroreport*, 7 (4), 932–6.

Dettmers, C., Connelly, A., Stephan, K. M., Turner, R., Friston, K. J., Frackowiak, R. S. *et al.* (1996). Quantitative comparison of functional magnetic resonance imaging with positron emission tomography using a force-related paradigm. *Neuroimage*, 4 (3 Pt 1), 201–9.

Dick, J., Cantell, R., Bruma, O., Giox, M., Beneck, R., Day, B. *et al.* (1987). The Bereitschaftspotential, L-DOPA and Parkinson's disease. *Electroencephalography and Clinical Neurophysiology*, 66 (3), 263–74.

Dolan, R. J., Fletcher, P., Frith, C. D., Friston, K. J., Frackowiak, R. S., and Grasby, P. M. (1995). Dopaminergic modulation of impaired cognitive activation in the anterior cingulate cortex in schizophrenia. *Nature*, 378 (6553), 180–2.

Dye, S. M., Spence, S. A., Bench, C. J., Hirsch, S. R., Stefan, M. D., Sharma, T. *et al.* (1999). No evidence for left superior temporal dysfunction in asymptomatic schizophrenia and bipolar disorder. PET study of verbal fluency. *British Journal of Psychiatry*, 175, 367–74.

Egan, M. F., Goldberg, T. E., Kolachana, B. S., Callicot, J. H., Mazzanti, C. M., Straub, R. E. *et al.* (2001) Effect of COMT Val[108/158] Met genotype on frontal lobe function and risk for schizophrenia. *Proceedings of the National Academy of Sciences USA*, 98 (12), 6917–22.

Elliott, R., Rubinsztein, J. S., Sahakian, B. J., and Dolan, R. J. (2002). The neural basis of mood-congruent processing biases in depression. *Archives of General Psychiatry*, 59 (7), 597–604.

Eyler Zorrilla, L. T., Jeste, D. V., Paulus, M., and Brown, G. G. (2003). Functional abnormalities of medial temporal cortex during novel picture learning among patients with chronic schizophrenia. *Schizophrenia Research*, 59, 187–98.

Ffytche, D. H., Howard, R. J., Brammer, M. J., David, A., Woodruff, P., and Williams, S. (1998). The anatomy of conscious vision: an fMRI study of visual hallucinations. *Nature Neuroscience*, 1 (8), 738–42.

Fleming, K., Goldberg, T. E., Gold, J. M., and Weinberger, D. R. (1995). Verbal working memory dysfunction in schizophrenia: use of a Brown–Peterson paradigm. *Psychiatry Research*, 56 (2), 155–61.

Fletcher, P. C., Frith, C. D., Grasby, P. M., Friston, K. J., and Dolan, R. J. (1996). Local and distributed effects of apomorphine on fronto-temporal function in acute unmedicated schizophrenia. *Journal of Neuroscience*, 16 (21), 7055–62.

Fletcher, P., McKenna, P. J., Friston, K. J., Frith, C. D., and Dolan, R. J. (1999). Abnormal cingulate modulation of fronto-temporal connectivity in schizophrenia. *Neuroimage*, 9 (3), 337–42.

Friston, K. J. and Frith, C. D. (1995). Schizophrenia: a disconnection syndrome? *Clinical Neuroscience*, 3 (2), 89–97.

Friston, K. J., Williams, S., Howard, R., Frackowiak, R. S., and Turner, R. (1996). Movement-related effects in fMRI time-series. *Magnetic Resonance in Medicine*, 35 (3), 346–55.

Frith, C. D. (1992). *The cognitive neuropsychology of schizophrenia*. Lawrence Earlbaum Associates, Hove.

Frith, C. D., Friston, K. J., Herold, S., Silbersweig, D., Fletcher, P., Cahill, C. *et al.* (1995). Regional brain activity in chronic schizophrenic patients during the performance of a verbal fluency task. *British Journal of Psychiatry*, 167 (3), 343–9.

Fu, C. and McGuire, P. K. (1999). Functional neuroimaging in psychiatry. *Philosophical Transactions of the Royal Society*, 346, 1–12.

Fu, C., Vythelingum, N., Andrew, C., Brammer, M., Amaro, E., Jr, Williams, S. *et al.* (2001). Alien voices . . . who said that? Neural correlates of impaired verbal self-monitoring in schizophrenia. *Neuroimage*, **13**, s1052.

Fu, C., Morgan, K., Suckling, J., Williams, S., Andrew, C., Vythelingum, N. *et al.* (2002). An fMRI study of overt verbal fluency using a clustered acquisition sequence: greater anterior cingulate activation with increased task demand. *Neuroimage* **17**, 871–9.

Garavan, H., Pankiewicz, J., Bloom, A., Cho, J. K., Sperry, L., Ross, T. J. *et al.* (2000). Cue-induced cocaine craving: neuroanatomical specificity for drug users and drug stimuli. *American Journal of Psychiatry*, **157** (11), 1789–98.

George, M. S., Anton, R. F., Bloomer, C., Teneback, C., Drobes, D. J., Lorberbaum, J. P. *et al.* (2001). Activation of prefrontal cortex and anterior thalamus in alcoholic subjects on exposure to alcohol-specific cues. *Archives of General Psychiatry*, **58** (4), 345–52.

Gold, J. M., Randolph, C., Carpenter, C. J., Goldberg, T. E., and Weinberger, D. R. (1992). Forms of memory failure in schizophrenia. *Journal of Abnormal Psychology*, **101**, 487–94.

Goldman-Rakic, P. (1990). Prefrontal cortical dysfunction in schizophrenia: the relevance of working memory. In *Psychopathology and the Brain*, (ed. B. Carroll and J. Bartrett), pp. 1–23. Raven Press, New York.

Goldman-Rakic, P. S. (1994). Working memory dysfunction in schizophrenia. *Journal of Neuropsychiatry and Clinical Neurosciences*, **6** (4), 348–57.

Gollub, R. L., Breiter, H. C., Kantor, H., Kennedy, D., Gastfriend, D., Mathew, R. T. *et al.* (1998). Cocaine decreases cortical cerebral blood flow but does not obscure regional activation in functional magnetic resonance imaging in human subjects. *Journal of Cerebral Blood Flow and Metabolism*, **18** (7), 724–34.

Green, M. F. (1996). What are the functional consequences of neurocognitive deficits in schizophrenia? *American Journal of Psychiatry*, **153** (3), 321–30.

Green, M. F. (1998). *Schizophrenia from a neurocognitive perspective: probing the impenetrable darkness*. Allyn and Bacon, Boston.

Green, M. F. and Braff, D. L. (2001). Translating the basic and clinical cognitive neuroscience of schizophrenia to drug development and clinical trials of antipsychotic medications. *Biological Psychiatry*, **49** (4), 374–84.

Gur, R. E., McGrath, C., Chan, R. M., Schroeder, L., Turner, T., Turetsky, B. I. *et al.* (2002). An fMRI study of facial emotion processing in patients with schizophrenia. *American Journal of Psychiatry*. **159**, 1992–9.

Heckers, S., Rauch, S. L., Goff, D., Savage, C. R., Schacter, D. L., Fischman, A. J. *et al.* (1998). Impaired recruitment of the hippocampus during conscious recollection in schizophrenia. *Nature Neuroscience*, **1**, 318–23.

Hempel, A., Hempel, E., Schonknecht, P., Stippich, C., and Schroder, J. (2003). Impairment in basal limbic function in schizophrenia during affect recognition. *Psychiatry Research*, **122**, 115–24.

Herpertz, S. C., Dietrich, T. M., Wenning, B., Krings, T., Erberich, S. G., Willmes, K. *et al.* (2001). Evidence of abnormal amygdala functioning in borderline personality disorder: a functional MRI study. *Biological Psychiatry*, **50** (4), 292–8.

Hertel, P., Nomikos, G. G., Iurlo, M., and Svensson, T. H. (1996). Risperidone: regional effects in vivo on release and metabolism of dopamine and serotonin in the rat brain. *Psychopharmacology*, **124** (1–2), 74–86.

Hofer, A., Weiss, E. M., Golaszewski, S. M., Siedentopf, C. M., Brinkhoff, C., Kremser, C. *et al.* (2003). An FMRI study of episodic encoding and recognition of words in patients with schizophrenia in remission. *American Journal of Psychiatry*, **160**, 911–18.

Honey, G. D., Bullmore, E. T., Soni, W., Varatheesan, M., Williams, S. C., and Sharma, T. (1999). Differences in frontal cortical activation by a working memory task after substitution of risperidone for typical antipsychotic drugs in patients with schizophrenia. *Proceedings of the Nationl Academy of Sciences USA*, **96** (23), 13432–7.

Honey, G. D., Fletcher, P. C., and Bullmore, E. T. (2002a). Functional brain mapping of psychopathology. *Journal of Neurology, Neurosurgery and Psychiatry*, **72** (4), 432–9.

Honey, G. D., Bullmore, E. T., and Sharma, T. (2002b). De-coupling of cognitive performance and cerebral functional response during working memory in schizophrenia. *Schizophrenia Research*, **53** (1–2), 45–56.

Honey, G. D., Fu, C. H. Y., Kim, J., Brammer, M. J., Croudace, T. J., Suckling, J. *et al.* (2002c). Effects of verbal working memory on corticocortical connectivity modelled by path analysis of functional magnetic resonance imaging data. *Neuroimage*, **17** (2), 573–82.

Honey, G. D., Sharma, T., Suckling, J., Giampietro, V., Soni, W., Williams, S. C. *et al.* (2003a). The functional neuroanatomy of schizophrenic subsyndromes. *Psychological Medicine*, **33**, 1007–18.

Honey, G. D., Suckling, J., Zelaya, F., Long, C., Routledge, C., Jackson, S. *et al.* (2003b). Dopaminergic drug effects on physiological connectivity in a human cortico-striato-thalamic system. *Brain*, **126**, 1767–81.

Howard, R., David, A., Woodruff, P., Mellers, I., Wright, J., Brammer, M., *et al.* (1997). Seeing visual hallucinations with functional magnetic resonance imaging. *Dementia and Geriatric Cognitive Disorders*, **8**, 73–7.

Jessen, F., Scheef, L., Germeshausen, L., Tawo, Y., Kockler, M., Kuhn, K. U. *et al.* (2003). Reduced hippocampal activation during encoding and recognition of words in schizophrenia patients. *American Journal of Psychiatry*, **160**, 1305–12.

Jonides, J. (1995). Working memory and thinking. In *Invitation to cognitive science: Thinking*, Vol. 3, (ed. E. Smith and D. Osherson), pp. 215–65. MIT Press, Cambridge.

Just, M. A. and Carpenter, P. A. (1992). A capacity theory of comprehension: individual differences in working memory. *Psychological Review*, **99** (1), 122–49.

Just, M. A., Carpenter, P. A., and Keller, T. A. (1996). The capacity theory of comprehension: new frontiers of evidence and arguments [comment]. *Psychological Review*, **103** (4), 773–80.

Kalin, N. H., Davidson, R. J., Irwin, W., Warner, G., Orendi, J.L., Sutton, S. K. *et al.* (1997). Functional magnetic resonance imaging studies of emotional processing in normal and depressed patients: effects of venlafaxine. *Journal of Clinical Psychiatry*, **58** (suppl. 16), 32–9.

Kastrup, A., Li, T. -Q., Kruger, G., Glover, G., and Moseley, M. (1999). Relationship between cerebral blood flow changes during visual stimulation and baseline flow levels investigated with functional MRI. *Neuroreport*, **10**, 1751–6.

Kay, S. R., Fiszbein, A., and Opler, L. A. (1987). The positive and negative syndrome scale (PANSS) for schizophrenia. *Schizophrenia Bulletin*, **13**, 261–76.

Keefe, R. S., Roitman, S. E., Harvey, P. D., Blum, C. S., DuPre, R. L., Prieto, D. M. *et al.* (1995). A pen-and-paper human analogue of a monkey prefrontal cortex activation task: spatial working memory in patients with schizophrenia. *Schizophrenia Research*, **17** (1), 25–33.

Kiehl, K. A. and Liddle, P. F. (2001). An event-related functional magnetic resonance imaging study of an auditory oddball task in schizophrenia. *Schizophrenia Research*, **48** (2–3), 159–71.

Kiehl, K. A., Smith, A. M., Hare, R. D., Mendrek, A., Forster, B. B., Brink, J. *et al.* (2001). Limbic abnormalities in affective processing by criminal psychopaths as revealed by functional magnetic resonance imaging. *Biological Psychiatry*, **50** (9), 677–84.

King, D. J., Wilson, A., Cooper, S. J., and Waddington, J. L. (1991). The clinical correlates of neurological soft signs in chronic schizophrenia. *British Journal of Psychiatry*, **158**, 770–5.

Kircher, T. T., Bulimore, E. T., Brammer, M. J., Williams, S. C., Broome, M. R., Murray, R. M. *et al.* (2001*a*). Differential activation of temporal cortex during sentence completion in schizophrenic patients with and without formal thought disorder. *Schizophrenia Research*, **50** (1–2), 27–40.

Kircher, T. T., Liddle, P. F., Brammer, M. J., Williams, S. C., Murray, R. M., and McGuire, P. K. (2001*b*). Neural correlates of formal thought disorder in schizophrenia: preliminary findings from a functional magnetic resonance imaging study. *Archives of General Psychiatry*, **58** (8), 769–74.

Kircher, T. T., Liddle, P. F., Brammer, M. J., Williams, S. C., Murray, R. M., and McGuire, P. K. (2002). Reversed lateralization of temporal activation during speech production in thought disordered patients with schizophrenia. *Psychological Medicine*, **32** (3), 439–49.

Kodama, S., Fukuzako, H., Fukuzako, T., Kiura, T., Nozoe, S., Hashiguchi, T. *et al.* (2001). Aberrant brain activation following motor skill learning in schizophrenic patients as shown by functional magnetic resonance imaging. *Psychological Medicine*, **31** (6), 1079–88.

Kosaka, H., Omori, M., Murata, T., Iidaka, T., Yamada, H., Okada, T. *et al.* (2002). Differential amygdala response during facial recognition in patients with schizophrenia: an fMRI study. *Schizophrenia Research*, **57** (1), 87.

Krimer, L., Muly, E., Williams, G., and Goldman-Rakic, P. (1998). Dopaminergic regulation of cerebral cortical microcirculation. *Nature Neuroscience*, **1** (4), 286–9.

Kumari, V., Gray, J., Honey, G., Soni, W., Bullmore, E., Williams, S. *et al.* (2002). Procedural learning in schizophrenia: a functional magnetic resonance imaging investigation. *Schizophrenia Research*, **57** (1), 97–107.

Kumari, V., Gray, J. A., Geyer, M. A., ffytche, D., Soni, W., Mitterschiffthaler, M. T. *et al.* (2003). Neural correlates of tactile prepulse inhibition: a functional MRI study in normal and schizophrenic subjects. *Psychiatry Research*, **122**, 99–113.

Kuperberg, G., McGuire, P. K., Bullmore, E. T., Brammer, M. J., Wright, I. C., Lythgoe, D. *et al.* (2000). Common and distinct neural substrates for pragmatic, semantic, and syntactic processing of spoken sentences: an fMRI study. *Journal of Cognitive Neuroscience*, **12**, 321–41.

Lanius, R., Williamson, P., Boksman, K., Densmore, M., Gupta, M., Neufeld, R. *et al.* (2002). Brain activation during script-driven imagery induced dissociative responses in PTSD: a functional magnetic resonance imaging investigation. *Biological Psychiatry*, **52** (4), 305–11.

Laurens, K. R., Ngan, E. T., Bates, A. T., Kiehl, K. A., and Liddle, P. F. (2003). Rostral anterior cingulate cortex dysfunction during error processing in schizophrenia. *Brain*, **126**, 610–22.

Lawrie, S. M., Buechel, C., Whalley, H. C., Frith, C. D., Friston, K. J., and Johnstone, E. C. (2002). Reduced frontotemporal functional connectivity in schizophrenia associated with auditory hallucinations. *Biological Psychiatry*, **51**, 1008–11.

Lemieux, L., Allen, P. J., Franconi, F., Symms, M. R., and Fish, D. R. (1997). Recording of EEG during fMRI experiments: patient safety. *Magnetic Resonance in Medicine*, **38**, 943–52.

Lemieux, L., Salek-Haddadi, A., Josephs, O., Allen, P., Toms, N., Scott, C. *et al.* (2001). Event-related fMRI with simultaneous and continuous EEG: description of the method and initial case report. *Neuroimage*, **14**, 780–7.

Lennox, B. R., Park, S. B., Medley, I., Morris, P. G., and Jones, P. B. (2000). The functional anatomy of auditory hallucinations in schizophrenia. *Psychiatry Research*, **100** (1), 13–20.

Leube, D. T., Rapp, A., Erb, M., Grodd, W., Buchkremer, G., Bartels, M. *et al.* (2003). Hippocampal dysfunction during episodic memory encoding in patients with schizophrenia—an fMRI study. *Schizophrenia Research*, **64**, 83–5.

Li, S. J., Biswal, B., Li, Z., Risinger, R., Rainey, C., Cho, J. K. *et al.* (2000). Cocaine administration decreases functional connectivity in human primary visual and motor cortex as detected by functional MRI. *Magnetic Resonance in Medicine*, **43** (1), 45–51.

Liddle, P. F., Friston, K. J., Frith, C. D., Hirsch, S. R., Jones, T., Frackowiak, R. S. (1992). Patterns of cerebral blood flow in schizophrenia. *British Journal of Psychiatry*, **160**, 179–86.

Luna, B., Minshew, N. J., Garver, K. E., Lazar, N. A., Thulborn, K. R., Eddy, W. F. *et al.* (2002). Neocortical system abnormalities in autism: an fMRI study of spatial working memory. *Neurology*, **59**, 834–40.

Maas, L. C., Lukas, S. E., Kaufman, M. J., Weiss, R. D., Daniels, S. L., Rogers, V. W. *et al.* (1998). Functional magnetic resonance imaging of human brain activation during cue-induced cocaine craving. *American Journal of Psychiatry*, **155** (1), 124–6.

Manoach, D.-S., Press, D.-Z., Thangaraj, V., Searl, M.-M., Goff, D.-C., Halpern, E. *et al.* (1999). Schizophrenic subjects activate dorsolateral prefrontal cortex during a working memory task, as measured by fMRI. *Biological Psychiatry*, **45** (9), 1128–37.

Manoach, D. S., Gollub, R. L., Benson, E. S., Searl, M. M., Goff, D. C., Halpern, E. *et al.* (2000). Schizophrenic subjects show aberrant fMRI activation of dorsolateral prefrontal cortex and basal ganglia during working memory performance. *Biological Psychiatry*, **48** (2), 99–109.

Manoach, D. S., Halpern, E. F., Kramer, T. S., Chang, Y., Goff, D. C., Rauch, S. L. *et al.* (2001). Test—retest reliability of a functional MRI working memory paradigm in normal and schizophrenic subjects. *American Journal of Psychiatry*, **158** (6), 955–8.

Mansfield, P. (1977). Multiplanar image formation using NMR spin echoes. *Journal of Physics*, **10**, L55–8.

McClain, L. (1983). Encoding and retrieval in schizophrenics' free recall. *Journal of Nervous and Mental Disease*, **171**, 471–9.

McDowell, J. E., Brown, G. G., Paulus, M., Martinez, A., Stewart, S. E., Dubowitz, D. J. *et al.* (2002). Neural correlates of refixation saccades and antisaccades in normal and schizophrenia subjects. *Biological Psychiatry*, **51** (3), 216–23.

McGuire, P. K. and Frith, C. D. (1996). Disordered functional connectivity in schizophrenia. *Psychological Medicine*, **26**, 663–7.

McGuire, P. K., Shah, G. M., and Murray, R. M. (1993). Increased blood flow in Broca's area during auditory hallucinations in schizophrenia. *Lancet*, **342** (8873), 703–6.

McGuire, P. K., Silbersweig, D. A., Wright, I., Murray, R. M., David, A. S., Frackowiak, R. S. *et al.* (1995). Abnormal monitoring of inner speech: a physiological basis for auditory hallucinations. *Lancet*, **346** (8975), 596–600.

McGuire, P. K., Silbersweig, D. A., and Frith, C. D. (1996). Functional neuroanatomy of verbal self-monitoring. *Brain*, **119**, 907–17.

McGuire, P. K., Quested, D. J., Spence, S. A., Murray, R. M., Frith, C. D., and Liddle, P. F. (1998). Pathophysiology of 'positive' thought disorder in schizophrenia. *British Journal of Psychiatry*, **173**, 231–5.

McIntosh, A. R., Grady, C. L., Ungerleider, L. G., Haxby, J. V., Rapoport, S. I., and Horwitz, B. (1994). Network analysis of cortical visual pathways mapped with PET. *Journal of Neuroscience*, **14** (2), 655–66.

Menon, V., Anagnoson, R. T., Glover, G. H., and Pfefferbaum, A. (2001*a*). Functional magnetic resonance imaging evidence for disrupted basal ganglia function in schizophrenia. *American Journal of Psychiatry*, **158** (4), 646–9.

Menon, V., Anagnoson, R. T., Mathalon, D. H., Glover, G. H., and Pfefferbaum, A. (2001*b*). Functional neuroanatomy of auditory working memory in schizophrenia: relation to positive and negative symptoms. *Neuroimage*, **13** (3), 433–46.

Morris, S. K., Granholm, E., Sarkin, A. J., and Jeste, D. V. (1997). Effects of schizophrenia and aging on pupillographic measures of working memory. *Schizophrenia Research*, **27** (2–3), 119–28.

Muller, J. L., Roder, C., Schuierer, G., and Klein, H. E. (2002). Subcortical overactivation in untreated schizophrenic patients: A functional magnetic resonance image finger-tapping study. *Psychiatry and Clinical Neuroscience*, **56** (1), 77–84.

Muller, R. A., Pierce, K., Ambrose, J. B., Allen, G., and Courchesne, E. (2001). Atypical patterns of cerebral motor activation in autism: a functional magnetic resonance study. *Biological Psychiatry*, **49** (8), 665–76.

Nahas, Z., George, M. S., Horner, M. D., Markowitz, J. S., Li, X., Lorberbaum, J. P. *et al.* (2003). Augmenting atypical antipsychotics with a cognitive enhancer (donepezil) improves regional brain activity in schizophrenia patients: a pilot double-blind placebo controlled BOLD fMRI study. *Neurocase*, **9**, 274–82.

Northoff, G., Braus, D. F., Sartorius, A., Khoram-Sefat, D., Russ, M., Eckert, J. *et al.* (1999). Reduced activation and altered laterality in two neuroleptic-naive catatonic patients during a motor task in functional MRI. *Psychological Medicine*, **29** (4), 997–1002.

Ogawa, S., Lee, T. M., Kay, A. R., and Tank, D. W. (1990). Brain magnetic resonance imaging with contrast dependent on blood oxygenation. *Proceedings of the National Academy of Sciences USA*, **87** (24), 9868–72.

Park, S. and Holzman, P. S. (1992). Schizophrenics show spatial working memory deficits. *Archives of General Psychiatry*, **49** (12), 975–82.

Park, S. and McTigue, K. (1997). Working memory and the syndromes of schizotypal personality. *Schizophrenia Research*, **26** (2–3), 213–20.

Park, S., Puschel, J., Sauter, B. H., Rentsch, M., and Hell, D. (1999). Spatial working memory deficits and clinical symptoms in schizophrenia: a 4-month follow-up study. *Biological Psychiatry*, **46** (3), 392–400.

Paulesu, E., Connelly, A., Frith, C. D., Friston, K. J., Heather, J., Myers, R. *et al.* (1995). Functional MR imaging correlations with positron emission tomography. Initial experience using a cognitive activation paradigm on verbal working memory. *Neuroimaging Clinics of North America*, **5** (2), 207–25.

Pauling, L. and Coryell, C. (1936). The magnetic properties and structure of hemoglobin, oxyhaemoglobin and carbonmonoxyhemoglobin. *Proceedings of the National Academy of Sciences USA*, **232**, 210–16.

Paulus, M. P., Frank, L., Brown, G. G., and Braff, D. L. (2003). Schizophrenia subjects show intact success-related neural activation but impaired uncertainty processing during decision-making. *Neuropsychopharmacology*, **28**, 795–806.

Perlstein, W. M., Carter, C. S., Noll, D. C., and Cohen, J. D. (2001). Relation of prefrontal cortex dysfunction to working memory and symptoms in schizophrenia. *American Journal of Psychiatry*, **158** (7), 1105–13.

Perlstein, W. M., Dixit, N. K., Carter, C. S., Noll, D. C., and Cohen, J. D. (2003). Prefrontal cortex dysfunction mediates deficits in working memory and prepotent responding in schizophrenia. *Biological Psychiatry*, **53**, 25–38.

Phillips, M. L., Williams, L., Senior, C., Bullmore, E. T., Brammer, M. J., Andrew, C. *et al.* (1999). A differential neural response to threatening and non-threatening negative facial expressions in paranoid and non-paranoid schizophrenics. *Psychiatry Research*, **92** (1), 11–31.

Phillips, M. L., Marks, I. M., Senior, C., Lythgoe, D., O'Dwyer, A. M., Meehan, O. *et al.* (2000). A differential neural response in obsessive–compulsive disorder patients with washing compared with checking symptoms to disgust. *Psychological Medicine*, **30** (5), 1037–50.

Phillips, M. L., Medford, N., Senior, C., Bullmore, E. T., Suckling, J., Brammer, M. J. *et al.* (2001). Depersonalization disorder: thinking without feeling. *Psychiatry Research*, **108** (3), 145–60.

Pierce, K., Muller, R. A., Ambrose, J., Allen, G., and Courchesne, E. (2001). Face processing occurs outside the fusiform 'face area' in autism: evidence from functional MRI. *Brain*, **124** (10), 2059–73.

Raemaekers, M., Jansma, J. M., Cahn, W., Van der Geest, J. N., van der Linden, J. A., Kahn, R. S. *et al.* (2002). Neuronal substrate of the saccadic inhibition deficit in schizophrenia investigated with 3-dimensional event-related functional magnetic resonance imaging. *Archives of General Psychiatry*, **59** (4), 313–20.

Quintana, J., Wong, T., Ortiz-Portillo, E., Kovalik, E., Davidson, T., Marder, S. R. *et al.* (2003*a*). Prefrontal–posterior parietal networks in schizophrenia: primary dysfunctions and secondary compensations. *Biological Psychiatry*, **53**, 12–24.

Quintana, J., Wong, T., Ortiz-Portillo, E., Marder, S. R., and Mazziotta, J. C. (2003*b*). Right lateral fusiform gyrus dysfunction during facial information processing in schizophrenia. *Biological Psychiatry*, **53**, 1099–112.

Ragland, J. D., Gur, R. C., Raz, J., Schroeder, L., Kohler, C. G., Smith, R. J. *et al.* (2001). Effect of schizophrenia on frontotemporal activity during word encoding and recognition: a PET cerebral blood flow study. *American Journal of Psychiatry*, **158**, 1114–25.

Renshaw, P. F., Yurgelun-Todd, D. A., and Cohen, B. M. (1994). Greater hemodynamic response to photic stimulation in schizophrenic patients: an echo planar MRI study. *American Journal of Psychiatry*, **151** (10), 1493–5.

Riehemann, S., Volz, H. P., Stutzer, P., Smesny, S., Gaser, C., and Sauer, H. (2001). Hypofrontality in neuroleptic-naive schizophrenic patients during the Wisconsin Card Sorting Test—a fMRI study. *European Archives of Psychiatry and Clinical Neuroscience*, **251** (2), 66–71.

Ring, H. A., Baron-Cohen, S., Wheelwright, S., Williams, S. C., Brammer, M., Andrew, C. *et al.* (1999). Cerebral correlates of preserved cognitive skills in autism: a functional MRI study of embedded figures task performance. *Brain*, **122** (7), 1305–15.

Rubia, K., Overmeyer, S., Taylor, E., Brammer, M., Williams, S. C., Simmons, A. *et al.* (1999). Hypofrontality in attention deficit hyperactivity disorder during higher-order motor control: a study with functional MRI. *American Journal of Psychiatry*, **156** (6), 891–6.

Rubia, K., Russell, T., Bullmore, E. T., Soni, W., Brammer, M. J., Simmons, A. *et al.* (2001). An fMRI study of reduced left prefrontal activation in schizophrenia during normal inhibitory function. *Schizophrenia Research*, **52** (1–2), 47–55.

Russell, T. A., Rubia, K., Bullmore, E. T., Soni, W., Suckling, J., Brammer, M. J. *et al.* (2000). Exploring the social brain in schizophrenia: left prefrontal underactivation during mental state attribution. *American Journal of Psychiatry*, **157** (12), 2040–2.

Saykin, A. J., Gur, R. C., Gur, R. E., Mozley, P. D., Mozley, L. H., Resnick, S. M. *et al.* (1991). Neuropsychological function in schizophrenia. Selective impairment in memory and learning. *Archives of General Psychiatry*, **48** (7), 618–24.

Saykin, A. J., Shtasel, D. L., Gur, R. E., Kester, D. B., Mozley, L. H., Stafiniak, P. *et al.* (1994). Neuropsychological deficits in neuroleptic naive patients with first-episode schizophrenia. *Archives of General Psychiatry*, **51** (2), 124–31.

Schlosser, R., Gesierich, T., Kaufmann, B., Vucurevic, G., Hunsche, S., Gawehn, J. *et al.* (2003). Altered effective connectivity during working memory performance in schizophrenia: a study with fMRI and structural equation modeling. *Neuroimage*, **19**, 751–63.

Schneider, F., Habel, U., Wagner, M., Franke, P., Salloum, J. B., Shah, N. J. *et al.* (2001). Subcortical correlates of craving in recently abstinent alcoholic patients. *American Journal of Psychiatry*, **158** (7), 1075–83.

Schroder, J., Geider, F. J., Binkert, M., Reitz, C., Jauss, M., and Sauer, H. (1992). Subsyndromes in chronic schizophrenia: do their psychopathological characteristics correspond to cerebral alterations? *Psychiatry Research*, **42** (3), 209–20.

Schroder, J., Wenz, F., Schad, L. R., Baudendistel, K., and Knopp, M. V. (1995). Sensorimotor cortex and supplementary motor area changes in schizophrenia. A study with functional magnetic resonance imaging. *British Journal of Psychiatry*, **167** (2), 197–201.

Schroder, J., Essig, M., Baudendistel, K., Jahn, T., Gerdsen, I., Stockert, A. *et al.* (1999). Motor dysfunction and sensorimotor cortex activation changes in schizophrenia: A study with functional magnetic resonance imaging. *Neuroimage*, **9** (1), 81–7.

Schultz, R. T., Gauthier, I., Klin, A., Fulbright, R. K., Anderson, A. W., Volkmar, F. *et al.* (2000). Abnormal ventral temporal cortical activity during face discrimination among individuals with autism and Asperger syndrome. *Archives of General Psychiatry*, **57** (4), 331–40.

Seeger, G., Braus, D. F., Ruf, M., Goldberger, U., and Schmidt, M. H. (2002). Body image distortion reveals amygdala activation in patients with anorexia nervosa—a functional magnetic resonance imaging study. *Neuroscience Letters*, **326** (1), 25–8.

Sheline, Y. I., Barch, D. M., Donnelly, J. M., Ollinger, J. M., Snyder, A. Z., and Mintun, M. A. (2001). Increased amygdala response to masked emotional faces in depressed subjects resolves with antidepressant treatment: an fMRI study. *Biological Psychiatry*, **50** (9), 651–8.

Shergill, S. S., Bullmore, E., Simmons, A., Murray, R., and McGuire, P. (2000*a*). Functional anatomy of auditory verbal imagery in schizophrenic patients with auditory hallucinations. *American Journal of Psychiatry*, **157** (10), 1691–3.

Shergill, S. S., Brammer, M. J., Williams, S. C., Murray, R. M., and McGuire, P. K. (2000*b*). Mapping auditory hallucinations in schizophrenia using functional magnetic resonance imaging. *Archives of General Psychiatry*, **57** (11), 1033-8.

Shergill, S., Bullmore, E., Williams, S., Brammer, M., Murray, R. M., and McGuire, P. K. (2001). A functional magnetic resonance imaging study of auditory verbal imagery. *Psychological Medicine*, **31**, 241–53.

Shergill, S. S., Brammer, M. J., Fukuda, R., Williams, S. C., Murray, R. M., and McGuire, P. K. (2003). Engagement of brain areas implicated in processing inner speech in people with auditory hallucinations. *British Journal of Psychiatry*, **182**, 525–31.

Shin, L. M., Whalen, P. J., Pitman, R. K., Bush, G., Macklin, M. L., Lasko, N. B. *et al.* (2001). An fMRI study of anterior cingulate function in posttraumatic stress disorder. *Biological Psychiatry*, **50** (12), 932–42.

Siegle, G. J., Steinhauer, S. R., Thase, M. E., Stenger, V. A., and Carter, C. S. (2002). Can't shake that feeling: event-related fMRI assessment of sustained amygdala activity in response to emotional information in depressed individuals. *Biological Psychiatry*, **51** (9), 693–707.

Smith, K. A., Ploghaus, A., Cowen, P. J., McCleery, J. M., Goodwin, G. M., Smith, S. *et al.* (2002). Cerebellar responses during anticipation of noxious stimuli in subjects recovered from depression: Functional magnetic resonance imaging study. *British Journal of Psychiatry*, **181** (5), 411–15.

Sommer, I. E., Ramsey, N. F., and Kahn, R. S. (2001). Language lateralization in schizophrenia, an fMRI study. *Schizophrenia Research*, **52** (1–2), 57–67.

Sommer, I. E., Ramsey, N. F., Mandl, R. C., and Kahn, R. S. (2003). Language lateralization in female patients with schizophrenia: an fMRI study. *Schizophrenia Research*, **60**, 183–90.

Spaniel, F., Hajek, T., Tintera, J., Harantova, P., Dezortova, M., and Hajek, M. (2003). Differences in fMRI and MRS in a monozygotic twin pair discordant for schizophrenia (case report). *Acta Psychiatrica Scandinavica*, **107**, 155–8.

Spence, S. A., Crimlisk, H. L., Cope, H., Ron, M. A., and Grasby, P. M. (2000). Discrete neurophysio-logical correlates in prefrontal cortex during hysterical and feigned disorder of movement. *Lancet*, **355** (9211), 1243–4.

Spindler, K. A., Sullivan, E. V., Menon, V., Lim, K. O., and Pfefferbaum, A. (1997). Deficits in multiple systems of working memory in schizophrenia. *Schizophrenia Research*, **27** (1), 1–10.

Stephan, K. E., Magnotta, V. A., White, T., Arndt, S., Flaum, M., O'Leary, D. S. *et al.* (2001). Effects of olanzapine on cerebellar functional connectivity in schizophrenia measured by fMRI during a simple motor task. *Psychological Medicine*, **31** (6), 1065–78.

Stevens, A. A., Goldman-Rakic, P. S., Gore, J. C., Fulbright, R. K., and Wexler, B. E. (1998). Cortical dysfunction in schizophrenia during auditory word and tone working memory demonstrated by functional magnetic resonance imaging. *Archives of General Psychiatry*, **55** (12), 1097–103.

Surguladze, S. A., Calvert, G. A., Brammer, M. J., Campbell, R., Bullmore, E. T., Giampietro, V. *et al.* (2001). Audio-visual speech perception in schizophrenia: an fMRI study. *Psychiatry Research*, **106** (1), 1–14.

Thomas, K. M., Drevets, W. C., Dahl, R. E., Ryan, N. D., Birmaher, B., Eccard, C. H. *et al.* (2001). Amygdala response to fearful faces in anxious and depressed children. *Archives of General Psychiatry*, **58** (11), 1057–63.

Thulborn, K., Waterton, J., Matthews, P., and Radda, G. (1982). Oxygenation dependence of the transverse relaxation time of water protons in the whole blood at high field. *Biochem Biophys Acta*, **714**, 265–70.

Tulving, E. (1983). *Elements of episodic memory*. Clarendon Press, Oxford.

Turner, R., Jezzard, P., Wen, H., Kwong, K., LeBihan, D., Zeffiro, T. *et al.* (1993). Functional mapping of the human visual cortex at 4 and 1.5 Tesla using deoxygenation contrast EPI. *Magnetic Resonance in Medicine*, **29**, 277–9.

Volz, H. P., Gaser, C., Hager, F., Rzanny, R., Mentzel, H. J., Kreitschmann-Andermahr, I. *et al.* (1997). Brain activation during cognitive stimulation with the Wisconsin Card Sorting Test—a functional MRI study on healthy volunteers and schizophrenics. *Psychiatry Research*, **75** (3), 145–57.

Volz, H., Gaser, C., Hager, F., Rzanny, R., Ponisch, J., Mentzel, H. *et al.* (1999). Decreased frontal activation in schizophrenics during stimulation with the continuous performance test—a functional magnetic resonance imaging study. *European Psychiatry*, **14** (1), 17–24.

Volz, H. P., Nenadic, I., Gaser, C., Rammsayer, T., Hager, F., and Sauer, H. (2001). Time estimation in schizophrenia: an fMRI study at adjusted levels of difficulty. *Neuroreport*, **12** (2), 313–16.

Walter, H., Wunderlich, A. P., Blankenhorn, M., Schafer, S., Tomczak, R., Spitzer, M. *et al.* (2003). No hypofrontality, but absence of prefrontal lateralization comparing verbal and spatial working memory in schizophrenia. *Schizophrenia Research*, **61**, 175–84.

Weinberger, D. R. (1993). A connectionist approach to the prefrontal cortex. *Journal of Neuropsychiatry and Clinical Neurosciences*, **5** (3), 241–53.

Weinberger, E. and Cermak, L. S. (1973). Short-term retention in acute and chronic paranoid schizophrenics. *Journal of Abnormal Psychology*, **82** (2), 220–5.

Weiss, A. P., Schacter, D. L., Goff, D. C., Rauch, S. L., Alpert, N. M., Fischman, A. J., Heckers, S. (2003). Impaired hippocampal recruitment during normal modulation of memory performance in schizophrenia. *Biological Psychiatry*, **53**, 48–55.

Weiss, E. M., Golaszewski, S., Mottaghy, F. M., Hofer, A., Hausmann, A., Kemmler, G. *et al.* (2003). Brain activation patterns during a selective attention test—a functional MRI study in healthy volunteers and patients with schizophrenia. *Psychiatry Research*, **123**, 1–15.

Welchew, D. E., Honey, G. D., Sharma, T., Robbins, T. W., and Bullmore, E. T. (2002). Multidimensional scaling of integrated neurocognitive function and schizophrenia as a disconnexion disorder. *Neuroimage*, **17**, 1227–39.

Wenz, F., Schad, L. R., Knopp, M. V., Baudendistel, K. T., Flomer, F., Schroder, J. *et al.* (1994). Functional magnetic resonance imaging at 1.5 T: activation pattern in schizophrenic patients receiving neuroleptic medication. *Magnetic Resonance Imaging*, **12** (7), 975–82.

Wenz, F., Baudendistel, K., Knopp, M. V., Schad, L. R., Schroder, J., Flomer, F. *et al.* (1995). Functional magnetic resonance tomography of movement disorders in patients with schizophrenia. *Radiologe*, **35** (4), 267–71.

Wexler, B. E., Gottschalk, C. H., Fulbright, R. K., Prohovnik, I., Lacadie, C. M., Rounsaville, B. J. *et al.* (2001). Functional magnetic resonance imaging of cocaine craving. *American Journal of Psychiatry*, **158** (1), 86–95.

Wible, C. G., Kubicki, M., Yoo, S. S., Kacher, D. F., Salisbury, D. F., Anderson, M. C. *et al.* (2001). A functional magnetic resonance imaging study of auditory mismatch in schizophrenia. *American Journal of Psychiatry*, **158** (6), 938–43.

Woodruff, P. W., Wright, I. C., Bullmore, E. T., Brammer, M., Howard, R. J., Williams, S. C. *et al.* (1997). Auditory hallucinations and the temporal cortical response to speech in schizophrenia: a functional magnetic resonance imaging study. *American Journal of Psychiatry*, **154** (12), 1676–82.

Wu, D., Lewin, J., and Duerk, J. (1997). Inadequacy of motion correction algorithms in functional MRI: role of susceptibility-induced artefacts. *Journal of Magnetic Resonance Imaging*, **7** (2), 365–70.

Wykes, T., Brammer, M., Mellers, J., Bray, P., Reeder, C., Williams, C. *et al.* (2002). Effects on the brain of a psychological treatment: cognitive remediation therapy: functional magnetic resonance imaging in schizophrenia. *British Journal of Psychiatry*, **181**, 144–52.

Yurgelun-Todd, D. A., Waternaux, C. M., Cohen, B. M., Gruber, S. A., English, C. D., and Renshaw, P. F. (1996). Functional magnetic resonance imaging of schizophrenic patients and comparison subjects during word production. *American Journal of Psychiatry*, **153** (2), 200–5.

Zorrilla, L. T., Jeste, D. V., and Brown, G. G. (2002). Functional MRI and novel picture-learning among older patients with chronic schizophrenia: abnormal correlations between recognition memory and medial temporal brain response. *American Journal of Geriatric Psychiatry*, **10** (1), 52–61.

Chapter 10

Event related potentials

Margaret A. Niznikiewicz, Kevin M. Spencer,
Dean F. Salisbury, and Robert W. McCarley

Introduction

From a historical perspective, the realization that schizophrenia is a brain disorder has
been fairly recent (Kraepelin, 1899); even more recent has been the development of the
tools and methodologies that have allowed investigations into the nature of brain
dysfunction in schizophrenia. In this review, we are going to focus on event related
potential (ERP) methodology as a way of characterizing functional abnormality in
schizophrenia, and the progress that has occurred in this area in both methodological
and theoretical approaches to the study of this disease.

Much of the ERP research has been motivated by the belief that schizophrenia is a
disorder of cognition, and thus ERP methodology, with its excellent time resolution
and sensitivity to cognitive manipulations, provides a useful index of abnormal
processes that may contribute to the clinical presentation of schizophrenia. The characteristic symptoms include fragmentation of, and distortions in, thought processes,
often resulting in profound communication disturbances, including loose, discon-
nected speech, aberrant associations, and lack of discourse coherence. In addition, the
sensory experiences of schizophrenic persons often include a sense of being
overwhelmed with sensations. While not an exhaustive list, these were the symptoms
that inspired much of the ERP research on cognition in schizophrenia.

ERP methodology has been also employed in understanding the genetics of schizophrenia, as well as its neurochemistry and neural substrate. In addition, there has been
an ongoing interest in using ERPs as indexes to subtype schizophrenia. As will be
reviewed below, certain paradigms have served these different interests better than
others. Finally, various methodological approaches have been aimed at more faithful
representation and analysis of electrical/neural events as they happened, as well as
more accurate localization of the neural substrates from which they originated.

Over the years, researchers have studied abnormal processes of attention, sensory
memory and sensory filtering, short-term and working memory, as well as language
processes, with a variety of ERP components. In this review, we will discuss progress
that occurred in each of these areas starting from temporally the earliest, and
historically, the oldest, component, P50, and ending with measures of gamma-band

synchronization, which are the most recently discovered types of neural activity, and a burgeoning field of study in electrophysiology of schizophrenia. For each of the types of processes, and the components thought to index them, we will discuss their significance to the field of schizophrenia research.

The P50 sensory gating response

The initial motivation for the development of the P50 sensory gating paradigm had much to do with a model of an attentional system, where the initial stages of processing were devoted to selecting relevant pieces of information and filtering out or gating irrelevant pieces of information (e.g. Broadbent 1971). The mechanism for such a selective gating was believed to be a 'bottom-up' mechanism whereby events of high frequency might be less relevant, and thus gated out, while the events of low frequency were allowed to pass through. It has been proposed that many of the schizophrenic symptoms result from this inability to gate high-frequency events. Thus, the P50 paradigm was developed to explore defective gating mechanisms in schizophrenia. The preponderance of experimental P50 designs has been in the auditory modality.

The P50 is a middle-latency component of the auditory evoked potential, a small positive wave that peaks ~50 ms after stimulus onset. Davis et al. (1966) first observed the phenomenon that has come to be known as 'P50 suppression': when an auditory stimulus such as a click is followed by an identical stimulus about 500 ms later, and there is a relatively long interval between stimulus pairs (typically up to 10 s) to allow for the system to recover, the P50 evoked by the second stimulus (S2) is reduced in amplitude compared to the P50 evoked by the first stimulus (S1). The ratio of S2/S1 is interpreted as a measure of 'gating' or inhibitory mechanisms within the auditory system (Fig. 10.1). Dysfunction in this system has been proposed to underlie many of the clinical symptoms of schizophrenia resulting from poor filtering of external stimuli, leading possibly to delusions, hallucinations, and a sense of sensory inundation (e.g. McGhie and Chapman 1961; Venables 1964; Adler et al. 1982; Freedman et al. 1991). As discussed below, these initial interpretations have been modified recently to include proposals that the abnormality in P50 suppression in schizophrenia may index aspects of attention dysfunction.

The abnormal suppression of the P50 to the second stimulus has been reported in a number of studies in chronic schizophrenia patients, both medicated and unmedicated (e.g. Freedman et al. 1982, 1983; Leonard et al. 1996; Adler et al. 1998), first-episode patients (e.g. Yee et al. 1998), and first-degree relatives of schizophrenics (Clementz et al. 1998), as well as schizotypal individuals (e.g. Croft et al. 2001; Cadenhead et al. 2002; Cadenhead and Braff 2002).

Neurochemistry

The initial interest in examining 'gating' deficits in schizophrenia has been supplemented by the interest in neurochemical mediation of the P50 response. It has been

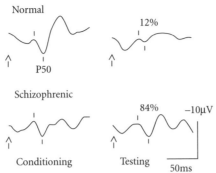

Fig. 10.1 Examples of gating of the P50-evoked potential in a normal subject and a subject with schizophrenia. The evoked potentials show the averaged responses from 32 presentations of paired auditory stimuli, with 0.5 s between the conditioning and testing stimuli. The arrows indicate when the stimuli were presented. The P50 wave (shown by the line below the tracing) was selected by a computer algorithm and measured relative to the preceding negative trough (shown by the line above the tracing). The percent ratio of test to conditioning wave amplitude is shown for each subject. (p. 181). (From Freedman *et al.* 1994.)

suggested that the auditory processes related to stimulus comparison and detection indexed by P50 may be modulated by dopamine (Pekkonen *et al.* 2002*a*). For example, Oranje *et al.* (2002) found that the combination of haloperidol and ketamine can disrupt P50 in healthy volunteers. Also, Light *et al.* (1999) found that amphetamine disrupts P50 suppression in healthy subjects. Along the same lines, Johnson and Adler (1993) found that normal individuals subjected to a stressful situation such as cold-pressor task showed a temporary abnormality in P50 suppression, as this task is associated with increased noradrenergic transmission. However, the role of dopamine in the generation of the P50 is not clear-cut (Adler *et al.* 1998), and other neurochemical mechanisms have been proposed.

The role of nicotinic receptors and cholinergic innervation has been explored in a number of studies (Leonard *et al.* 1996; Adler *et al.* 1998; Griffith *et al.* 1998; Olincy *et al.* 2000). For example, a short-lived (30 min) improvement in the P50 gating deficit was observed in schizophrenic patients allowed to smoke cigarettes before the ERP recording session (Adler *et al.* 1998). A similar response was noted by Adler *et al.* (1992) in first-degree relatives of schizophrenia patients. High (6 mg) but not low (2 mg) dose nicotine delivered in chewing gum normalized the P50 gating response in this group of subjects who shared a P50 gating deficit with their schizophrenic relatives. In fact, there are reports that smoking rates among schizophrenia patients are much higher than among general population (e.g. Goff *et al.* 1992), leading to a speculation that this maladaptive behavior may, in fact, be an attempt at self-medication. In addition, a temporary normalization of the P50 response was observed after a brief period of sleep (Griffith *et al.* 1993). Finally, the P50 gating deficit has also been reported to be improved with clozapine treatment (Nagamoto *et al.* 1996, 1999; Light *et al.* 2000). The exact nature of the clozapine effect is less clear, although it has been suggested that part of its action may be related to its role in dopaminergic regulation.

Functional significance

The functional significance of the P50 gating deficit has perhaps been most specifically articulated by Adler *et al.* (1998) as reflecting cholinergic innervation of the areas CA3 of the hippocampus, and which, if abnormal, may lead to faulty input processing along the lines articulated by the Hasselmo *et al.* (1995) model. Most recent studies relate P50 abnormality to aspects of attention, especially its inhibitory function.

One of the major difficulties in framing P50 deficits in terms of the construct of attention is the meaning of the construct itself, as operationalized and conceptualized across different studies. For example, White and Yee (1997) suggested that P50 is not responsive to direct manipulations of selective attention, and that, rather, it represents a pre-attentive process (Jerger *et al.* 1992). On the other hand, Cullum *et al.* (1993) found that the P50 abnormality correlated with measures of sustained attention, and Erwin *et al.* (1998) found relationships between the P50 gating deficit and neuropsychological measures of attention, especially vigilance. Also, Vinogradov *et al.* (1996) reported that semantic priming effects at short stimulus–onset asynchronies (SOAs), which reflect automatic aspects of semantic activation, were correlated with the size of the P50 gating deficit in schizophrenia patients. Furthermore, some studies suggest that the P50 gating abnormality does not seem to be related to the subjective sense of sensory overload or flooding as reflected in patients' self-reports (Jin *et al.* 1998). In schizotypy, though, perceptual features of unreality were reported to be related to less effective P50 suppression (Croft *et al.* 2001).

Progress has been also made in relating P50 to gene expression. Several studies demonstrated that the inhibitory dysfunction as indexed by the P50 abnormality was associated with the $\alpha7$ nicotinic acetylcholine receptor subunit gene (CHRNA7) at 15q13–14 (Freedman *et al.* 1997, 2001; Adler *et al.* 1999; Leonard *et al.* 2002).

Clinical specificity

The issue of the functional specificity of P50 abnormality is closely related to the issue of its clinical specificity. For example, Olincy *et al.* (2000) found higher P50 amplitude to the second stimulus but not to the first or conditioning stimulus, in schizophrenia relative to attention deficit disorder individuals, even though both groups suffer from attentional deficits, thus suggesting that different neurochemical abnormalities underlie attention abnormalities in these two disorders. Decreased P50 suppression was observed in acute mania and was related to a noradrenergic mechanism: the P50 gating deficit correlated with lower levels of 3-methoxy, 4-hydroxyphenylglycol (MHPG) which, when normalized with treatment, brought P50 suppression within a normal range (Franks *et al.* 1983; Adler *et al.* 1989, 1990). Similar dysfunction was found in cocaine addicts (Fein *et al.* 1996; Olincy *et al.* 2000). Baker *et al.* (1987) suggested that decreased P50 suppression is a trait deficit in schizophrenia, but a state deficit in other several mental illnesses with psychotic symptoms, again suggesting that different neurochemical action may underlie these deficits. Also, post-traumatic stress disorder can cause abnormal P50 gating (Adler *et al.* 1991; Gilette *et al.* 1997). Finally, as mentioned above, moderate stress can contribute to abnormal P50 gating.

Regarding the optimal method of measuring P50 suppression, studies have examined such issues as the recording site, inter-click interval, sound pressure level, filtering and its consequences for the morphology of the P50, as well as methods of measuring the component (Griffith *et al.* 1995; Freedman *et al.* 1996, 1998; Cardenas *et al.* 1997; Clementz *et al.*, 1997*b*, 1998; Boutros *et al.* 1999). The P50 is typically recorded from Cz, where it shows the largest group separation (Nagamoto *et al.* 1991), and magnetoencephalography (MEG) studies indicate that the sources of the P50 may reside in the bilateral planum temporale (Reite *et al.* 1988). Abnormal gating in schizophrenia is observed with the S1–S2 intervals of 150–2000 ms (Adler *et al.* 1982; Nagamoto *et al.* 1991), with the largest group separation at 500 ms, the value that Adler *et al.* (1998) speculate may be related to optimal temporal distance between two stimuli in learning.

Summary

In summary, the study of P50 suppression was one of the earliest experimental ERP approaches to the study of the biological bases of schizophrenia. Initially inspired by the observations of Venables (1964), and McGhie and Chapman (1961) of schizophrenic deficits in the filtering of irrelevant information, complex interactions among neurochemical systems and brain areas, as delineated by Adler *et al.* (1998) and Olincy *et al.* (2000), are likely to account for the P50 abnormality in schizophrenia and related clinical disorders. Much of the P50 research has been devoted to the role of neurotransmitters in P50 suppression and, by extension, to identifying the neurochemical and neural systems that are involved in mediating the neuro-cognitive phenomena indexed by this effect. It appears that both catecholaminergic and cholinergic contributions play a role in modulating P50 suppression, and progress is being made in identifying the genetic contribution to this effect. It has also been demonstrated that P50 suppression is a good candidate biological marker of schizophrenia, as the dysfunction indexed by this component was identified not only in chronic schizophrenia, but also in relatives of schizophrenic patients, and individuals with schizophrenia spectrum disorder diagnosis. It will be the task of future research to incorporate animal models, neurochemical challenge studies, and behavioral and clinical observations, to describe with a higher degree of specificity the neural substrates of P50 gating deficits and their relationships to psychiatric disorders.

Mismatch negativity

Mismatch negativity (MMN) is an ERP component that reflects the representation of auditory stimuli in sensory memory. The MMN is a negative wave that appears within 200 ms after stimulus onset, and is elicited by stimuli that deviate in some manner from the preceding stimuli (Näätänen *et al.* 1989; Näätänen 1992). This component is most commonly studied in an unattended 'oddball' paradigm, in which frequently occurring 'standard' stimuli are interspersed with infrequent 'deviants' which differ from the standards along an acoustic dimension such as duration (Shelley *et al.* 1991), frequency (Javitt *et al.* 1993, Hirayasu *et al.* 1998*a*), or phonemic, language-specific attributes (Näätänen 1992). While this component is elicited automatically by deviant stimuli that are not at the focus of attention, the amplitude of the MMN can be increased if attention is directed to the stimuli (Woldorff *et al.* 1998).

In the first report of MMN abnormalities in schizophrenia, Shelley *et al.* (1991) found that MMN amplitude was reduced in schizophrenia patients compared to controls in a paradigm employing duration deviants. This finding was subsequently replicated in numerous studies (Lembreghts and Timsit-Berthier 1993; Catts *et al.* 1995; Schall *et al.* 1995; Kasai *et al.* 1999; Mitchie *et al.* 2000). In addition, reductions in MMNs elicited by frequency deviants have been reported in schizophrenia (Javitt *et al.* 1993, 1995, 1998; Alain *et al.* 1998; Hirayasu *et al.* 1998*a*; Umbricht *et al.* 1998), although some studies failed to find this difference (O'Donnell *et al.* 1994; Kathmann *et al.* 1995). There is also a report of reduced MMN in a paradigm with speech sounds (Kasai *et al.* 2002*a*).

Functional significance

Evidence from studies of scalp topography and dipole models suggest that the generators of the MMN are located in the auditory cortex (Hari *et al.* 1984; Csëpe *et al.* 1992; Tiitinen *et al.* 1993; Alho *et al.* 1995; Pekkonen *et al.* 2002*b*). An additional source in the right prefrontal cortex has been proposed, based on scalp current density analysis (Giard *et al.* 1990). Functional and structural neuroimaging methods are also beginning to be used to examine the MMN. In an fMRI study comparing schizophrenia patients and healthy individuals, Wible *et al.* (2001) found a reduced mismatch effect in Heschl's gyrus and posterior superior temporal gyrus in schizophrenic patients. In correlating cortical volumes as measured by structural MRI with ERP data, Salisbury *et al.* (2001*a*) found that the amplitude of the MMN in first-episode schizophrenia patients was correlated with the volume of Heschl's gyrus.

It is believed that the MMN reflects a pre-attentive process within auditory echoic sensory memory (Cowan 1984, 1988; Javitt *et al.* 1995, 1998; Shelley *et al.* 1999). Shelley *et al.* (1999) view the echoic memory operations indexed by MMN as part of the acoustic slave memory system within working memory, and suggest that its abnormal amplitude in schizophrenia reflects dysfunction in echoic memory. Javitt *et al.* (1995) suggest that the impairment in the early pre-attentive processes indexed by

MMN may underlie later, attention-dependent processes indexed by the P300 component. In their study, Javitt *et al.* (1995) found that schizophrenic reductions in MMN amplitude were correlated with reductions in P300 amplitude. In a study of the MMN in a tone-matching task (Javitt *et al.* 2000), schizophrenic patients showed deficits in both the MMN and behavioral measures of acoustic memory, and the two measures highly correlated with each other. Furthermore, the MMN abnormality correlated most robustly with negative symptoms. The authors interpreted this result as suggesting the involvement of the *N*-methyl-D-aspartate (NMDA) neurotransmitter. Abnormalities in NMDA neurotransmission have been proposed to underlie the clinical symptoms of schizophrenia (Javitt and Zukin 1991; Krystal *et al.* 1994; Tsai *et al.* 1995).

Methodological considerations

Studying the stimulus parameters that influence MMN amplitude, and that distinguish best between healthy and schizophrenic individuals has been important not only on methodological grounds but also in the context of better characterizing the auditory sensory deficits in schizophrenia. In separate parametric studies involving both schizophrenia patients and normal controls, separately, Javitt *et al.* (1998) and Shelley *et al.* (1999) demonstrated that MMN amplitude was largest when the deviant probability was lowest (i.e. when the memory trace for the standard stimulus was the strongest) and when the pitch deviance was the largest; thus, the decrease in deviant probability and increase in pitch deviance resulted in the most negative MMN in both groups of subjects. In addition, the largest difference between the schizophrenic and control groups was obtained with the stimulus parameters that maximized MMN amplitude. Based on these results, the authors argued that the schizophrenic MMN deficit results not from a volume reduction in the auditory cortex, but from NMDA receptor abnormalities.

However, Michie *et al.* (2000) have argued that the large group difference between patients and controls at large pitch disparities may stem from contributions of the N1 component, although the findings of Shelley *et al.* (1999) regarding the N1 did not seem to support this view. Michie *et al.* suggest that the reduced duration MMN is a more robust finding than the reduced frequency MMN in schizophrenia, and suggested that both their results and previous findings indicate that there are separate neural generators for duration and frequency attributes (Giard *et al.* 1995; Frodl-Bauch *et al.* 1997; Baldweg *et al.* 1999).

Clinical associations

The diagnostic specificity of the MMN abnormality has been addressed in several studies. As already mentioned, both duration and frequency MMN were found to be reduced in chronic schizophrenia patients on traditional antipsychotics, and also in unmedicated chronic schizophrenic patients (Javitt *et al.* 1995), and in remitted

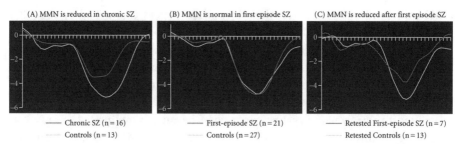

(A) MMN is reduced in chronic SZ   (B) MMN is normal in first episode SZ   (C) MMN is reduced after first episode SZ

—— Chronic SZ (n = 16)   —— First-episode SZ (n = 21)   —— Retested First-episode SZ (n = 7)
---- Controls (n = 13)   ---- Controls (n = 27)   ---- Retested Controls (n = 13)

Fig. 10.2 Mismatch negativity (MMN) in chronic schizophrenia (SZ) patients (A), first-episode patients (B), and retested first-episode patients (C) (after Salisbury *et al.* 2002). See Plate 11(a) of the plate section at the centre of this book.

schizophrenia patients (Catts *et al.* 1994). Pitch MMNs in first-episode patients were found within a normal range (Salisbury *et al.* 2001, 2002; Umbricht *et al.* 2002), suggesting that the subsequent amplitude reduction may be the effect of ongoing neuro-degenerative changes characterizing the disease (Salisbury *et al.* 2002).

Furthermore, there is recent evidence that first-episode patients studied longitudi-nally show a reduced MMN 2 years after presenting with normal MMN amplitude at first hospitalization (Salisbury *et al.* 2002, 2003) (Fig. 10.2). A strong trend to a reduced MMN in recent-onset schizophrenics was also reported by Javitt *et al.* (2000). On the other hand, the duration MMN was found to be reduced in both schizophrenic and first-degree relatives (Michie *et al.* 2002). These divergent results likely point to differ-ent ways in which frequency and duration deviants challenge the auditory system, with the duration MMN being more 'robust' or sensitive to abnormalities within this system (see Michie *et al.* 2000, 2002, for a discussion). At the very least, it appears that auditory pre-attentive processing is compromised already in individuals carrying a genetic risk for schizophrenia, and that this dysfunction becomes more apparent with frank psychosis and length of the illness.

The effects of treatment with typical compared to atypical (clozapine or risperidone) antipsychotics were addressed by Umbricht *et al.* (1998, 1999). The results of these studies suggest that neither typical nor atypical antipsychotics improve MMN ampli-tude. In addition, in the Umbricht *et al.* (1999) study, clozapine improved P300 ampli-tude. There is, however, one study (Kirino and Inoue 1999) that reported the presence of two groups of drug-naïve patients: one group whose MMNs were larger than those of normal controls and another other group whose MMNs were smaller. The respect-ive MMN amplitudes of the two groups were altered by neuroleptic treatment, resulting in the reduction of the MMN in the high MMN group and in the increase of MMN amplitude in the low MMN group. The lack of normalizing effects of clozapine on the MMN contrasts with those reported for another component marking 'pre-attentive processing', the P50. Also, Murakami *et al.* (2002) and Kasai *et al.* (2002*b*) sug-gest that the MMN elicited by both tones and phonemes is not sensitive to the effects of either high or low doses of anxiolytics or hypnotics, both with affinity to $GABA_A$ receptors.

MMN is typically reported from fronto-central electrode sites, typically referenced to a nose electrode (either on-line or off-line). Even though multiple electrode sites were used in most studies, data have typically been reported from the Fz electrode. More recent studies (Kasai *et al.* 2002*a*) used high-density electrode recordings to construct scalp current density maps, to better characterize subcomponents of the MMN in the phoneme and pure tone duration tasks. For both phoneme duration and across-phoneme conditions, both the left temporal component and the right frontal/temporal component were found to be active in the phoneme condition. As a further development of identifying brain sources of EEG scalp-recorded potentials, Park *et al.* (2002) used the low-resolution electromagnetic tomography (LORETA) technique in conjunction with individually registered MRI data and 128-channel EEG. The voxel-based statistical comparison used in that study showed a significant reduction of MMN current density in the left superior temporal gyrus (STG) and left inferior temporal lobule. Both of these structures are implicated in the reduced MMN by previous reports (e.g. Hirayasu *et al.* 1998*a*). Also, in a more recent development, functional magnetic resonance imaging (fMRI) 'translational' studies, using paradigms as close to the ones used in ERP research as technically possible, have been pursued (Opitz *et al.* 1999; Wible *et al.* 2001; Mathiak *et al.* 2002). Mathiak and co-workers used randomized gradient switching noises as deviants to study the blood oxygenation level dependent (BOLD) fMRI correlates of the MMN, in an attempt to control for the effects of MR scanner noise. Erwin and Rao (2000) reported the use of a 'mock' scanner, a device that is capable of generating real scanner noise, to obtain the MMN in an environment identical to that of an fMRI protocol, and thus were able to compare sources of data with high temporal and spatial resolution.

Summary

Like the P50, the MMN indexes pre-attentive processes. It is probably an index of auditory echoic memory and, as such, a part of the auditory working memory system (Näätänen *et al.* 1989; Cowan *et al.* 1993; Javitt *et al.*, 1995; Michie *et al.*, 2000). Thus, the reduction of MMN amplitude in schizophrenia indicates dysfunction at a level of sensory processing which might be brought about by an abnormal anatomical substrate, as indicated by correlations between MMN and Heschl gyrus volume (Salisbury *et al.* 2002), a neurochemical abnormality, or both. Again similarly to the P50, the MMN abnormality is not restricted to medicated chronic schizophrenia, but has also been found in unmedicated schizophrenia patients and in recent-onset schizophrenia. Unlike the P50, the MMN deficit does not appear to be ameliorated with atypical antipsychotics.

The P300 component

The P300 (or 'P3b') component is an endogenous component of the ERP that is elicited by events that call for a revision or updating of the representation of individuals' environment in working memory (Donchin 1981; Donchin and Coles 1988). This large positive wave with a centro-parietal topography is most typically studied in the 'oddball' paradigm, in which it is elicited by rare target stimuli that are interspersed among frequent non-target standards. It is important to note the distinction between the MMN and the P300: while both components are sensitive to stimulus deviance, the MMN reflects an automatic comparison of the current stimulus with the traces of previous stimuli in echoic memory, while the P300 reflects a higher-level, post-perceptual analysis that is based on the relevance of the stimulus to the task at hand. As such, the amplitude of the P300 reflects demands on central attentional resources (Wickens *et al.* 1983), and the latency of the component is correlated with the duration of stimulus evaluation but not response selection processes (McCarthy and Donchin 1981). Since its first demonstration by Sutton *et al.* (1965), the P300 has been researched extensively in both normal and clinical populations, and has been of special interest to investigators studying cognitive dysfunction in schizophrenia.

In an oddball task, rare stimuli elicit other late ERP components besides the P300 (Spencer *et al.* 2001). The Novelty P3 (or 'P3a') component (Courchesne *et al.* 1975; Squires *et al.* 1975) is a frontally maximal positive wave that is elicited by rare events, and its amplitude is largest when these events distract from task performance (Katayama and Polich 1998; Comerchero and Polich 1998). While the latency of the Novelty P3 depends upon stimulus attributes, its peak latency is often prior to that of the P300. The classical Slow Wave has a longer latency than the P300, and is characterized by a frontal negativity and a posterior positivity that may, in fact, be separate components (Spencer *et al.* 2001).

Ever since the original report of Roth and Cannon (1972) of reduced P300 amplitude over midline electrode sites in schizophrenia patients, numerous studies have used the P300 paradigm to assess different aspects of schizophrenia pathology (for reviews see McCarley *et al.* 1991, 1993; Ford *et al.* 1992, 1999). In the quest for a biological marker of schizophrenia, in which all the components discussed so far have been considered, P300 has been examined in chronic schizophrenic men and women, relatives of schizophrenia patients, first-episode patients, and individuals with schizotypal personality disorder. The specific questions often investigated included the extent to which the P300 is a trait or state marker, additionally addressed via pharmacological studies, and the extent to which P300 provides evidence for schizophrenia being a neurodevelopmental or neurodegenerative disease. Finally, relationships between P300 and clinical symptomatology, and between P300 and brain structure, were examined in order to better understand both the functional role of processes indexed by P300 in producing clinical symptoms, and a role of possible structural abnormalities in producing reduced P300 in schizophrenia.

Trait effects

Reduced P300 amplitudes have been found in patients with clinical improvement (Blackwood *et al.* 1987; Hirayasu and Ogura 1996; Coburn *et al.* 1998; Turetsky *et al.* 1998), in remitted patients (Rao *et al.* 1995), first-episode patients (Hirayasu *et al.*

1998b; Salisbury *et al.* 1998; Brown *et al.* 2002; Demiralp *et al.* 2002), and unaffected relatives of schizophrenia, which, for many investigators, suggest that the P300 may be a marker of genetic vulnerability for schizophrenia (Blackwood *et al.* 1991; Roxborough *et al.* 1993; Frangou *et al.* 1997; Turetsky *et al.* 2000; Mathalon *et al.* 2001).

A theme closely related to the issue of reduced P300 as an enduring trait marker, is the relationship between P300 and brain structures. Reduced volume of superior temporal gyrus (STG), one of the putative generators of P300 (Halgren *et al.* 1998), has been found in schizophrenia, especially in the left hemisphere, both in chronic schizophrenia (McCarley *et al.* 1993) and in first-episode patients (see below). As a parallel finding, greater reduction of the P300 amplitude over the left relative to the right hemisphere has been reported in a number of studies (Morstyn *et al.* 1983; Faux *et al.* 1993; Salisbury *et al.* 1998). In a meta-analysis of the P300 laterality effect for studies conducted between 1966 and 1999, Jeon and Polich (2001) found a significant effect of the left-sided reduction of the P300 amplitude, especially at the TCP1 electrode. In a direct test of the relationship between P300 amplitude and brain volume, a positive correlation was found between P300 amplitude and the grey matter of the left posterior STG in chronic schizophrenia patients (McCarley *et al.* 1993). Furthermore, a similar relationship between posterior STG volumes and the left temporal (T3) scalp recorded P300 (McCarley *et al.* 2002) was found in first-episode patients, highlighting a role of this structure in the early etiology of schizophrenia.

This left-side reduction in P300 was not found in a group of patients with manic psychosis, suggesting a possible specificity to schizophrenia (McCarley *et al.* 2002). Salisbury *et al.* (1999) compared chronic schizophrenia and bipolar patients with psychotic features. The results indicated that in spite of P300 reductions in both groups, subtle topographical differences distinguished the groups: a greater P300 reduction was observed at temporal sites in schizophrenic than bipolar patients, while a greater P300 reduction was observed at frontal sites in the bipolar compared to the schizophrenia group. In addition, the schizophrenia group lacked the left > right asymmetry present in both the bipolar and normal control groups. Also, Wagner *et al.* (1997), using a single-trial analysis approach, differentiated between schizophrenia and depression patients, even though traditional, average-based ERP analyses did not.

Yet another perspective and line of evidence for the P300 as a trait marker, is a series of P300 studies in first-episode schizophrenia and unaffected relatives of schizophrenia patients, and individuals with schizophrenia spectrum disorders such as schizotypy. The argument is that if an abnormal P300 is found in these groups, then the abnormality indexed by P300 may be a genotypic marker, and not the result of medication or chronicity status. Data in support of P300 abnormalities, both in the early stages of the disease and in the unaffected relatives of schizophrenia patients, have been obtained in several recent studies. Salisbury *et al.* (1998, 2002) found that P300 amplitude was reduced in first-episode patients relative to both normal controls and affective disorder patients (Fig. 10.3). Brown *et al.* (2002) analyzed both ERPs elicited by targets and non-targets in chronic and first-episode patients, and found reduced P300s in the first-episode group.

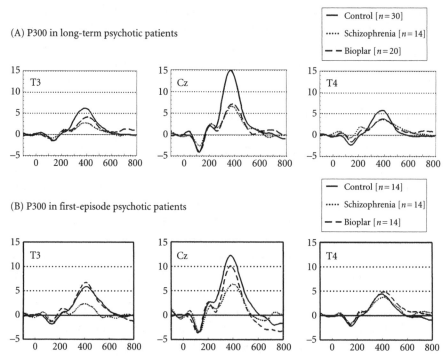

Fig. 10.3 P300 in chronic schizophrenia patients and first-episode psychotic patients (after Salisbury *et al.* 1998, 1999).

Demiralp *et al.* (2002) reported P300 amplitude reductions in first-episode patients at frontal sites rather than the temporo-parietally distributed P300 reduction reported in the Salisbury *et al.* (1998) study. Demiralp and co-workers speculated that some of the differences between the two studies may be due to medication status (in their study the patients were unmedicated), and task performance. P300 abnormalities in unaffected siblings of schizophrenia patients were also investigated as an endophenotypic marker of risk for schizophrenia (Turetsky *et al.* 2000). Chronic schizophrenia patients were found to have three reduced subcomponents of the P300: frontal, right parietal and left temporal (for right-handed subjects), relative to normal controls. At the same time, the patients did not differ significantly from their unaffected siblings. The siblings, in turn, differed from normal control subjects in the amplitude of the P3a, which the authors proposed to be a marker of genetic vulnerability for schizophrenia, and related to abnormal attentional networks. Finally, reduced P300 amplitude has been reported in schizotypal individuals (Salisbury *et al.* 1996; Trestman *et al.* 1996; Niznikiewicz *et al.* 2000).

State effects

There is also strong evidence that P300 amplitude can fluctuate with and 'track' clinical symptoms, and can thus be thought of as a valid clinical state marker (Duncan *et al.*

1987; McCarley *et al.* 1991; Pfefferbaum *et al.* 1989; Shenton *et al.* 1989; Egan *et al.* 1994). More recently, researchers have turned to longitudinal designs, and to less chronic and/or severely ill populations to better understand the role of P300 as a state-marker. In a longitudinal study of P300 amplitude changes and relations to clinical measures, Turetsky *et al.* (1998) used scalp current density to measure the P300. The results pointed to both the trait-like and state-like aspects of P300 abnormality, in that the patients showed a reduced P300 amplitude at the start of the study, and no evidence of change in P300 in spite of clinical improvements, underlying trait-like characteristics of P300 dysfunction. At the same time, however, the amplitude of the P3a was negatively correlated with auditory hallucinations, and a left temporal subcomponent was correlated with changes in the Brief Psychiatric Rating Scale (BPRS). There was also a distinction between the P3a and P300 in recent-onset schizophrenia patients, where the P3a correlated with attentional measures, and increased disorganization at intake was related to reduced P300.

The evidence for P300 as a marker of severity of the disease has been often obtained from correlations with clinical ratings (Blackwood *et al.* 1987; Pfefferbaum *et al.* 1989; Ford *et al.* 1999). In a retrospective, longitudinal study, Mathalon *et al.* (2000) examined both P3a and P300 in the auditory modality, as well as P300 in the visual modality. The ERP sessions were repeated 2–7 times per individual subject, and included both medicated and unmedicated periods for schizophrenia patients. The results supported both the finding of enduring P300 reduction even when the patients were least symptomatic, suggesting a trait-like quality to P300 abnormalities, as well as correlations between P300 amplitudes and BPRS ratings, suggesting that P300 amplitude can be a useful state marker.

The relationship between thought disorder and P300 amplitude has been more recently examined by applying factor-analytic techniques to Positive and Negative Syndrome Scale (PANSS) items (Higashima *et al.*, 1998). This approach resulted in generating five factors, including thought disorder, negative, hostile/excitable, delusional, and depressive factors. Only the thought disorder factor was correlated with P300 amplitude at parieto-temporal locations.

Age effects

In comparing early as opposed to late onset schizophrenia, Olichney *et al.* (1998) found a reduction of P300 in early onset patients, as previously reported in literature, but a normal range P300 amplitude in the late-onset patient group. The authors suggested that these results may indicate two different groups of schizophrenia patients, differentially impacted by a pathological process leading to overt signs of schizophrenia.

Along with indications that the neurocognitive deficits observed in schizophrenia and indexed by P300 appear in at-risk populations, first- or recent-onset schizophrenia, as discussed above, which suggest a neurodevelopmental aspect of the disease, researchers have also found a possible neurodegenerative aspect of the P300 in schizophrenia (O'Donnell *et al.* 1995; Mathalon *et al.* 2000). O'Donnell and co-workers examined changes in P300 latency across time, and found that the slope of P300 prolongation was steeper in schizophrenia patients relative to normal controls. Similar conclusions were reached by Mathalon *et al.* (2000). In that study, the P300 amplitude was smaller in patients with an early age of illness onset-results similar to those obtained by Olichney *et al.* (1998).

Summary

As one of the more thoroughly researched components in schizophrenia, the P300, in distinction from the P50 and MMN components, indexes central information processing mechanisms that are influenced by attention. Over the years, P300 paradigms have identified both trait and state features of such a dysfunction. The research to date suggests that the P300 is sensitive to abnormalities brought about by both a clinical state and by enduring changes in cognition independent of current clinical presentation. The abnormalities in the cognitive processes indexed by P300 seem to be related to abnormal anatomical substrates.

The N400 component

The N400 is a negative component peaking around 400 ms after the presentation of the stimulus. Identified for the first time by Kutas and Hillyard (1980), it has been reported in numerous studies using stimuli that carry semantic meaning, such as words, pictures, sentences, and paragraphs (Neville *et al.* 1986; Friedman 1990; Holcomb and Neville 1990; Brown and Hagoort 1993; Holcomb 1993; Deacon *et al.* 1999; Federmeier and Kutas 1999; Van Berkum *et al.* 1999; Van Petten *et al.* 1999). In the broadest sense, the N400 seems to be sensitive to the ease with which a word's semantic properties can be accessed (Kutas and Hillyard 1989; Holcomb 1993) and/or the ease with which it can be fitted into the available context. As such, it is a useful tool in probing different aspects of semantic processing. The N400 amplitude is larger (more negative) if words/pictures are preceded by little context, or when they do not fit the context, and, conversely, it is smaller (less negative) when the word easily fits into the context. For example, the N400 elicited by each word in a sentence diminishes as more context is provided for each consecutive word (Van Petten and Kutas 1990). On the other hand if, for example, the final word violates the context, as in *John drank the coffee with sugar and socks,* the N400 elicited by 'socks' is larger than the N400 elicited by the other words. In word-pair paradigms, the N400 elicited by the second word is smaller if the two words are related, as in *doctor–nurse*, than when the two words are unrelated, e.g. *paint–flower* (e.g. Kutas and Hillyard 1984).

Theoretical background

Given the well-documented abnormalities in the use of language in schizophrenia (Maher 1972; Chapman *et al.* 1976; Manschreck *et al.* 1988; Kwapil *et al.* 1990; Docherty *et al.* 1996; Aloia *et al.* 1998), the N400 has been used to generate evidence in a debate on what theoretical model would adequately describe the nature of language difficulties in schizophrenia. The two prevailing models that specify how language difficulties may arise in schizophrenia, posit dysfunction at opposite stages of semantic processing: (1) overactivation in semantic networks (early processing) (Spitzer 1993), and (2) inefficient use of context (late stages of processing) (Barch *et al.* 1996).

According to the first model, the characteristic loosening of associations and aberrant speech may stem from overactivation in semantic networks, where an excessively broad activation of meanings may lead to speech lacking a focus and haphazardly connected. The other model holds that language dysfunction in schizophrenia results from an inability to utilize context efficiently, such that, in the absence of effective contextual constraints, schizophrenic speech becomes disorganized, derailed, and driven by local rather than global associations.

In psycholinguistic research, processes within semantic networks are often probed with priming paradigms, where pairs of words are presented together and the subject's task is a lexical decision. It has been demonstrated repeatedly that if the first (priming) word is related to the second (primed) word, the subject is able to make a faster judgment as to whether the second word is a real word or not, than in cases where the two words are not related. Furthermore, the temporal distance, or stimulus–onset asynchrony (SOA), between the prime and target is of crucial theoretical importance: short SOAs, under about 500 ms, are believed to tap into early automatic processes of activation within semantic networks, while long SOAs (over 500 ms) are believed to tap into controlled processes such as semantic matching or context utilization (Neely 1991).

Thus, assuming the functional characteristics of N400 as described above, one would expect that if schizophrenia is associated with overactivation within semantic networks, then smaller N400s would be expected in schizophrenia patients relative to normal controls at short SOAs. On the other hand, if schizophrenia is associated with difficulties with context utilization, then larger N400s would be expected in schizophrenia patients relative to normal controls for long SOAs and in paradigms that use sentences or paragraphs as stimuli.

Empirical observations

Most studies to date have focused on late processes of context utilization. Using a long SOA word-pair paradigm, Grillon *et al.* (1991) and Koyama *et al.* (1991) reported reduced N400 difference waveforms in schizophrenic patients. However, the use of the difference waveform in these studies makes it somewhat difficult to interpret the results. The N400 difference waveform often used in studies of normal population indicates the priming effect, or the extent to which the N400 elicited by unrelated/unprimed targets is larger relative to related/primed targets. While this process works well in normal controls, using N400 values for related targets as a baseline is problematic in schizophrenia, as these values themselves may be abnormal (see Niznikiewicz *et al.* 1997). In fact, examination of waveforms in these early studies suggests that the N400 elicited by related items was larger for schizophrenia patients relative to normal subjects, suggesting the poor use of context.

This reduced N400 effect related to differences between patients and healthy individuals in processing related items was also noted by Bobes *et al.* (1996), who used a picture semantic matching task, and Koyama *et al.* (1994), who used a word recognition task, and Matsuoka *et al.* (1999), who used a semantic categorization task. The failure to attenuate N400 amplitude to related words was also reported by Condray *et al.* (1999), who used a lexical decision task with word pairs that varied in semantic relationship and expectancy, which led the authors to suggest that the semantic processes of schizophrenics are characterized by a pattern of indiscriminate activation within semantic networks.

Reduced N400 effects, i.e. diminished differences between N400 to congruent versus incongruent items, were also reported by Mitchell *et al.* (1991), in a study of active and passive attention using sentence frames as primes, and was interpreted in terms of the maintenance of active semantic memory and its ongoing integration with context. Similar conclusions were drawn by Andrews *et al.* (1993). Schizophrenic deficits in maintaining context in working memory and using it to constrain available choices have been documented in a number of studies using sentences as stimuli (Adams *et al.* 1993; Andrews *et al.* 1993; Nestor *et al.* 1997; Olichney *et al.* 1997; Niznikiewicz *et al.* 1997; Ohta *et al.* 1999). Similar conclusions of contextual maintenance problems in schizophrenia were reached by Salisbury *et al.* (2000) in a study that used short sentences containing ambiguous nouns (homographs; e.g. panel, toast) that ended with disambiguating adjectives or verb phrases for either dominant or subordinate noun meanings. Unlike controls, patients showed large N400 to both types of meanings (Fig. 10.4). In a follow-up study that explored the effects of activating the dominant meaning of a noun on processing of information in a subsequent subordinate clause (Sitnikova *et al.* 2002), schizophrenia patients were found to have deficits in the efficient suppression of context-inappropriate meanings of homographs. An indication of

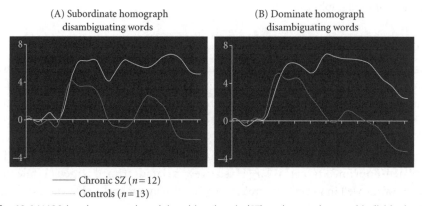

(A) Subordinate homograph disambiguating words

(B) Dominate homograph disambiguating words

——— Chronic SZ (*n* = 12)
········· Controls (*n* = 13)

Fig. 10.4 N400 in a homograph task in schizophrenic (SZ) and normal control individuals. See Plate 11(b) of the plate section at the centre of this book.

reduced influence of context was also provided by the Strandburg *et al.* (1997) study of the processing of idiomatic phrases by schizophrenic and healthy individuals.

Evidence for inefficient use of context was also found in schizotypy individuals (Niznikiewicz *et al.* 1999; Kimble *et al.* 2000), suggesting that inefficient processing of information found with earlier ERP components among both schizophrenia and schizophrenia spectrum individuals also exists for language processes.

Very few published ERP studies have focused expressly on the early processes of semantic activation. Mathalon *et al.* (2002), using a picture–word paradigm with short SOAs, found evidence of reduced N400s to target words in schizophrenia patients relative to controls. Also, Niznikiewicz *et al.* (2002) showed reduced N400 to related words in a short SOA word-pair paradigm in schizotypal individuals relative to normal controls (Fig. 10.5). Both of these studies suggest that the early processes of activation within semantic networks may be faster acting and/or reach more semantic nodes than in healthy individuals.

Taken together, the growing evidence for the abnormal processes of context utilization, and emerging evidence for abnormal processes of overactivation in the early stages of semantic processing, suggest a particularly profound impairment in the

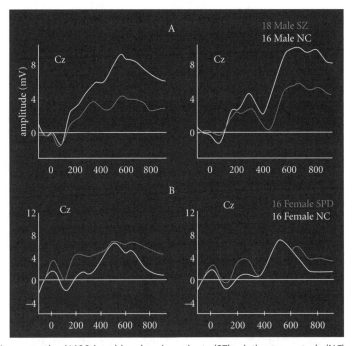

Fig. 10.5 More negative N400 in schizophrenic patients (SZ) relative to controls (NC) recorded to final words in sentences at long stimulus–onset asynchronies (SOA) (A); less negative N400 amplitude in schizotypal personality disorder (SPD) relative to normal control individuals at short SOA (B). (After Niznikiewicz *et al.* 1999, 2002.)

processing of language. According to this evidence, the excessive number of semantic meanings activated early may coincide with inefficient mechanisms in using context to suppress words with inappropriate meanings, resulting in speech that is characterized by derailment, tangentiality, loose association, and the lack of a coherent theme.

Gamma-band synchrony

The study of abnormalities in gamma-band synchrony is a new frontier in schizophrenia research. Research in this area has been stimulated by the findings that the brain can code information not just by the firing rate of neurons (rate coding), but by the relationships between neurons' firing patterns (temporal coding). The idea that temporal correlations between neuronal firing patterns could serve as a means of representation was originally proposed by Milner (1974) and von der Malsburg and Schneider (1986), and the first experimental evidence was reported by Eckhorn et al. (1988) and Gray et al. (1989). In their classic study, Gray and co-workers recorded from cells in the primary visual cortex of anesthetized cats. Light bars were passed across the cells' receptive fields, which did not overlap. When the bars moved together in the same direction, suggesting the appearance of a single coherent object, the cells' firing patterns became closely synchronized, with a nearly 0 ms lag between spikes. When the bars did not move together, no such correlated firing was seen. The cells' firing rates did not differ between the stimulus conditions, only the degree of synchrony between their firing patterns. These data suggested that temporally correlated or synchronous neuronal firing might serve as a mechanism whereby individual stimulus features could be bound together into coherent representations of complex objects. An important corollary finding was that neural synchrony was often accompanied by high-frequency oscillations in local field potentials (LFPs), which are generated by synchronous activity in local populations of neurons (Eckhorn et al. 1988; Gray and Singer 1989). These oscillations were found in the 'gamma' band (30–100 Hz), often near the frequency of 40 Hz.

A number of studies have replicated and extended the findings of these initial reports. In brief, evidence for neural synchrony in spike trains and LFP oscillations in the gamma band have been observed in awake and responding cats and primates (Kreiter and Singer 1992), between cells in separate visual areas (Engel et al. 1991), and between visual, somatosensory, association, and motor areas (Bressler et al. 1993; Roelfsema et al. 1997). Furthermore, evidence suggests that gamma-band neural synchrony is involved not just in perceptual feature-binding, but in conscious perception (Engel et al. 1999), working memory (Pesaran et al. 2002), selective attention (Steinmetz et al. 2000; Fries et al. 2001), and motor control (Riehle et al. 1997; Jackson et al. 2003). Current views propose that neural synchrony is a general mechanism for dynamically linking together cells coding related pieces of information into assemblies. Synchrony can thus act as a gating mechanism whereby only active cells that fire synchronously can influence cells at subsequent stages of processing (Singer 1999; Salinas and Sejnowski 2001).

Investigations into the neural mechanisms underlying synchrony have demonstrated that interactions between inhibitory interneurons are critical for generating synchrony among local networks of neurons (reviewed by McBain and Fisahn 2001). These inhibitory interactions involve both GABAergic synapses and gap junctions. Oscillations among inhibitory interneurons are driven and modulated by excitatory input from pyramidal cells (Traub *et al.* 1996) involving NMDA receptors (Grunze *et al.* 1996). Synchrony between neurons in distant cortical columns may be mediated in part by reciprocal cortico-thalamic projections (Steriade and Amzica 1996), as well as by intrinsic neuronal firing frequencies in the gamma band. Synchronized oscillations in the cortex are also dependent upon reticular system activation (Herculano-Houzel *et al.* 1999).

The importance of neural synchrony in feature-binding and cell assembly formation in general suggests that abnormal neural synchrony could be involved in aspects of schizophrenia, such as loose associations, reality distortions, or attention deficits. Early accounts of schizophrenia characterized it as a failure of the integration of thought and personality (Bleuler 1911/1950). A possible link between neural synchrony and schizophrenia has been suggested by post-mortem studies of the brains of persons with schizophrenia. These studies have found abnormalities in the morphology and distribution of certain types of neurons in schizophrenia, particularly inhibitory interneurons (Selemon and Goldman-Rakic 1999; Benes 2000; Lewis 2000; Whittington *et al.* 2000). In addition, studies have shown that excitatory neurotransmission via NMDA receptors is abnormal in schizophrenia (Javitt and Zukin 1991; Tsai and Coyle 2002), so schizophrenic abnormalities in pyramidal cells (Lewis and Gonzalez-Burgos 2000) could impair the NMDA-mediated glutamate projections from pyramidal cells to interneurons. Hence, schizophrenia may involve abnormalities in neural circuitry, which might be manifested by impaired neural synchrony in the gamma band.

Methods

The evidence for neural synchrony reviewed above consists mainly of single-unit and LFP studies in animals. These techniques are, in general, not possible to use with human subjects, so how might neural synchrony be studied in humans? The scalp-recorded EEG (and also the MEG) detect the spatial and temporal summation of post-synaptic potentials from thousands of pyramidal cells beneath the sensors. Since synchrony can be measured in LFP recordings, it is possible that synchrony across a large number of neurons can be detected with non-invasive measures at macroscopic levels. In fact, a number of EEG and MEG studies have indeed provided evidence of neural synchrony in humans (reviewed in Tallon-Baudry and Bertrand 1999; Varela *et al.* 2001). Evidence for gamma-band neural synchrony has been reported in perception (Tallon-Baudry *et al.* 1996; Rodriguez *et al.* 1999), attention (Müller *et al.* 2000; Herrmann and Mecklinger 2001), working memory (Tallon-Baudry *et al.* 1998), language (Pulvermüller 1996), and classical conditioning (Miltner *et al.* 1999), and long-term memory (Fell *et al.* 2001).

Neural synchrony in the EEG and MEG is measured using time-frequency methods, typically wavelet analysis or short-time windowed Fast Fourier Transforms (FFTs). These methods are used to decompose a time series into time–frequency maps that represent changes in spectral parameters during the epoch. The spectral parameters that are measured at each time point and frequency are the *power* (or amplitude), indicating the amount of energy in the signal, and the *phase* of the signal. Using these methods, two general types of oscillatory activity have been described (Pantev 1995):

1 *Evoked* oscillations are time-locked to stimulus onset and hence detectable in the average ERP. Early stimulus-evoked oscillations have been reported in the visual, auditory, and somatosensory modalities (Pantev 1995). One technique for examining evoked oscillations uses steady-state stimulation (e.g. click trains in the auditory modality, or flickering in the visual modality) to drive the relevant neural circuits (Galambos *et al.* 1981).

2 *Induced* oscillations are jittered in latency with respect to stimulus onset and tend to be washed out in the average ERP.

The power of evoked oscillations may be studied by spectral analysis of the average ERP signal; while measuring the power of induced oscillations requires averaging over single trials. Recently there has been interest in using phase measures to study evoked oscillations. The distribution of phases across single trials can be measured by computing the circular variance (Tallon-Baudry *et al.* 1996), which reflects the degree to which a set of signals match in phase, or are phase-locked. With steady-state oscillations, phase-locking can also be computed between peaks in the average evoked response and stimulus onset times (Kwon *et al.* 1999).

Neural synchrony can also be measured between sensor positions, providing measures of functional connectivity in the human brain. Power coherence computes the correlation in power between two signals, while phase coherence computes the phase-locking between two signals using the circular variance measure (Lachaux *et al.* 1999; Rodriguez *et al.* 1999; Varela *et al.* 2001). Phase coherence, in particular, may be expected to reveal the kinds of zero time-lag neural synchrony phenomena that have been detected with invasive recordings in animals.

Studies of schizophrenia

Research into gamma-band neural synchrony in schizophrenia is in the pioneering stage. Studies have found evidence for schizophrenia abnormalities in both evoked and induced gamma-band responses, using power and phase-locking measures, in a variety of tasks. Our review will start with studies of sensory evoked responses and then move into the cognitive domain.

The first study investigating sensory evoked gamma-band responses in schizophrenia was reported by Clementz *et al.* (1997*a*), who examined the early auditory evoked 40 Hz response. This response overlaps in time and scalp topography with the P50, and has been hypothesized to be related to this component (Pantev *et al.* 1993). Clementz and co-workers used the paired-click paradigm commonly used to measure P50 suppression effects in schizophrenia. They found that the auditory 40 Hz response showed abnormal suppression in schizophrenia patients, as with the P50 response. Clementz *et al.* obtained a better discrimination between patient and control groups with suppression of the 40 Hz response than with the P50, suggesting that paired-click suppression of the evoked gamma-band oscillation was more closely related to schizophrenic deficits than P50 suppression.

Kwon *et al.* (1999) studied steady-state auditory evoked responses in schizophrenia. Click trains were delivered to subjects at stimulation rates of 20, 30, and 40 Hz (Fig. 10.6). In the healthy control subjects, 40 Hz stimulation elicited the largest responses, as expected. The schizophrenia patients' responses were reduced in power compared to controls, only for 40 Hz stimulation. (Interestingly, the patients' 20 Hz subharmonic during 40 Hz stimulation was non-significantly larger than that of the controls.) Kwon and co-workers also analyzed the phase-locking of the 40 Hz steady-state response to the click train. In healthy controls, the steady-state response began to synchronize with the clicks after a few cycles, with the phase delay decreasing until the end of the click train, after which it rebounded to an intermediate value. The patients' responses were slower to phase-lock with the click trains. and the phase lag never reached the same minimum as controls. The authors suggested that their findings could be due to the

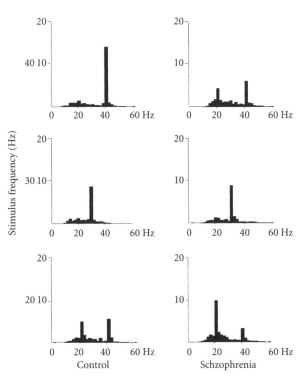

Fig. 10.6 Mean power (μV^2) spectra for EEG recorded to clicks at the three stimulus rates: 40 Hz, 30 Hz, and 20 Hz. The schizophrenic patients showed decreased power at 40 Hz stimulation relative to normal control subjects, with no group differences observed for the other two frequencies of stimulation. (After Kwon *et al.* 1999.)

dysfunction of recurrent inhibition in neural circuits in auditory cortex, consistent with neuroanatomical findings from post-mortem studies.

Examining narrow-band (37–41 Hz) gamma activity in an auditory oddball task, Haig *et al.* (2000) found that the amplitude of a response elicited by rare target stimuli in the latency range of the P300 was decreased at left hemisphere sites and increased at right hemisphere sites, compared to controls. The decrease of the response to targets in the patients was proportional to the number of schizophrenia symptoms, as measured by the PANSS general category. A later response elicited by frequent standard stimuli was also reduced. In follow-up analyses of the same data set, in which a factor analysis was performed on the PANSS ratings of the patients, Gordon *et al.* (2001) reported that the amplitude of the target response was positively correlated with the reality distortion symptom factor and the amplitude of the standard response was negatively correlated with the disorganization factor.

Gamma-band neural synchrony has been classically linked to feature-binding processes, both in animal (Gray *et al.* 1989) and human studies (Tallon-Baudry *et al.* 1996). Spencer *et al.* (2003) investigated gamma-band feature-binding mechanisms in schizophrenia, using a task in which subjects discriminated between squares formed by illusory contours (square condition) and a perceptual control condition (no-square). In an analysis of phase-locking responses, they found abnormalities in the early visual evoked gamma-band response in schizophrenia patients compared to healthy controls. For the controls, the occipital portion of the early visual gamma-band response elicited greater phase-locking for the illusory square than the no-square stimuli in the 40 Hz range. The size of this difference was correlated with the controls' difference in reaction time between the conditions, suggesting that the occipital phase-locking response reflected an early feature-binding mechanism in visual cortex. However, for the schizophrenia patients, neither the square nor the no-square condition elicited any phase-locking responses, suggesting dysfunction of early visual feature-binding processes. While the fronto-central portion of the early visual gamma-band response was present in the patients, it was abnormal in topography, latency, and frequency. The frequency of the response to no-square stimuli was negatively correlated with symptoms on the PANSS, particularly delusions, conceptual disorganization, and poor attention.

Spencer *et al.* (2003) also examined functional connectivity in this data set by analyzing gamma-band phase coherence between electrode sites. They found that schizophrenia patients' responses to the illusory square stimuli were characterized by decreases in phase coherence between the cerebral hemispheres at posterior electrodes in the 40 Hz range. In contrast, the controls' responses to the illusory square stimuli involved increases in coherence between anterior and posterior sites. These results suggested that functional interactions between distant brain areas are abnormal in schizophrenia, and that the 40 Hz frequency range of the EEG might be particularly important in normal cognition.

Kissler *et al.* (2000) used MEG to examine cognitive gamma-band activity in schizophrenia. In their study, spontaneous MEG was recorded from schizophrenia patients and healthy controls during a resting condition and while the subjects performed a complex mental arithmetic task that engaged working memory processes. The mental arithmetic task was internally driven, without the presentation of stimuli or the production of responses. For the controls, task performance was associated with increases in gamma-band power over anterior regions of the left hemisphere, while this effect was absent for the patients in the 30–45 Hz band, and showed a reverse laterality in the 45–71 Hz band, being larger during task performance than resting at right hemisphere sites. For the patients, gamma-band power in the 60–71 Hz range was reduced in both conditions compared to controls across a wide range of sensors. The findings of Kissler and co-workers are consistent with reports of structural and functional impairments of the left hemisphere and working memory dysfunction in schizophrenia.

Finally, a case study reported by Baldeweg *et al.* (1998) is of note. These authors recorded the EEG from a patient while he experienced somatic hallucinations, which were associated with periods of high-amplitude gamma-band waves with a mean frequency close to 40 Hz. The topography of the gamma waves could be accounted for by dipoles located in somatosensory and association areas, the functions of which were consistent with the nature of the patient's hallucinations.

Summary

Studies of neural synchrony in the gamma band of the EEG are beginning to provide new insights into schizophrenia. Schizophrenic abnormalities in gamma-band power and phase-locking are often found in the 40 Hz range, where studies of animals and healthy humans have often reported effects (Gray and Singer 1989; Herrmann and Mecklinger 2001). The sensitivity of gamma-band synchrony to the integrity of neural circuits makes this approach a promising tool in research into the neural substrates of schizophrenia and other neuropsychiatric disorders.

Future studies should attempt to relate gamma-band synchrony to specific information processing deficits in schizophrenia, by using tasks that directly tap schizophrenic impairments, such as working memory or semantic priming. To date, researchers have not reported any correlations between medication dosage and gamma-band effects, but it will be interesting to see if any such correlations emerge, given the hypothesized relationship between gamma-band synchrony and neural circuitry in schizophrenia. It is also important for researchers to examine a broad range of the frequency spectrum rather than just a narrow range around 40 Hz—otherwise, interesting phenomena could go undetected.

Concluding remarks

Over the years, the contributions of electrophysiological studies to our understanding of schizophrenia have been quite substantial. Hundreds of ERP studies of information processing in schizophrenia have provided strong evidence that it is a disease with biological correlates, by demonstrating how different aspects of cognition are associated with statistical differences between patients and healthy controls in the electrochemical processes that accompany these aspects of cognition.

Methodological advances

The development and use of each of the paradigms discussed in this review should be regarded as an advance in and of itself, as each of these methodologies allowed a more detailed understanding of cognition at different levels of processing, ranging from pre-attentive processes of stimulus filtering and orienting to the post-perceptual, cognitive processes of language processing. In addition, progress has been seen not only in recording from more dense electrode arrays (Potts *et al.* 1998; Kasai *et al.* 2002*a*), but also in reporting data taking into account multiple electrode sites. Different techniques to identify brain sources of scalp-recorded potentials have been implemented for both MMN (Pekkonen *et al.* 2002*b*; Youn *et al.* 2002) and P300 components (Frodl-Bauch 1999; Turetsky *et al.* 2000). In addition, there are reports using single trial analysis to measure more accurately ERP components, such as the P50 (Zouridakis *et al.* 1997; Patterson *et al.* 2000) and the P300 (Ford *et al.* 1994; Wagner *et al.* 1997, 2000).

Analytic techniques described above for gamma processes constitute a welcome addition to the traditional average ERP-based techniques of describing neural events. ERP designs are also being implemented in fMRI paradigms, to the extent that this is practical.

General summary

Electrophysiological approaches to the study of cognition in schizophrenia have seen substantial progress in identifying areas of abnormal function. Across the several domains discussed in this review, patients with schizophrenia have evinced impaired inhibitory processes in the sensory processing of auditory information, as demonstrated by the P50 and MMN components; working memory and attentional processes, as demonstrated by the P300; abnormal language processes, as demonstrated by the N400; as well as abnormal integrity of neural circuits, as demonstrated by measures of gamma-band neural synchrony. The studies reviewed shed more light on which aspects of information processing are abnormal in schizophrenia, but also on what might be the neurochemical and structural abnormalities associated with abnormalities. Furthermore, studies are beginning to provide data on the genetic bases of schizophrenia and schizophrenic abnormalities in information processing. What is emerging is an appreciation of how regional neural networks interact with each other, and how these interactions are influenced by neurochemical actions to produce neural events that become cognitive operations, and how abnormalities at any of these levels can result in disturbed cognition.

What is still an open question is the extent to which schizophrenia may be regarded as a disease of specific brain regions interconnected with each other, or a disease affecting neural function at a level low enough to affect most aspects of information processing. One can expect that the recent trend of combining electrophysiological techniques with neurochemical and genetic approaches within the context of explicit models of schizophrenia dysfunction, and in conjunction with the use of more sophisticated methods of data analysis, will further extend our understanding of schizophrenia.

Acknowledgements

This research was supported in part by the National Institute of Mental Health MH R01 63360 (MAN), by a Veterans Administration Merit Award (MAN-Co-PI), NARSAD Young Investigator Award and NIMH F23 MH 13022 (K.M.S.), RO1 NIMH MH 58704 (D.F.S.), and RO1 MH 40799 (R.W.M.). The authors also wish to acknowledge Lisa Lucia, Sarah Rabbitt, and Meredith Klump for their assistance in manuscript preparation.

References

Adams, J., Faux, S. F., Nestor, P. G., Shenton, M., Marcy, B., Smith, S., *et al.* (1993). ERP abnormalities during semantic processing in schizophrenia. *Schizophrenia Research,* **10** (3), 247–57.

Adler, L. E., Pachtman, E., Franks, R. D., Pecevich, M., Waldo, M. C., and Freedman, R. (1982). Neurophysiological evidence for a deficit in inhibitor mechanisms involved in sensory gating in schizophrenia. *Biological Psychiatry,* **17**, 639–54.

Adler, L. E., Gerhardt, G. A., Franks, R., Baker, N., Nagamoto, H., Drebing, C., *et al.* (1990). Sensory physiology and catecholamines in schizophrenia and mania. *Psychiatry Research,* **31**, 297–309.

Adler, L. E., Nagamoto, H. *et al.* (1991). *Impaired auditory sensory gating in patients with 20 years of combat post-traumatic stress disorder and depression.* American Psychiatric Association, New Orleans.

Adler, L. E., Hoffer, L. J., Griffith, J., Waldo, M. C., and Freedman, R. (1992). Normalization by nicotine of deficient auditory sensory gating in the relatives of schizophrenics. *Biological Psychiatry,* **32**, 607–16.

Adler, L. E., Olincy, A., Waldo, M., Harris, J. G., Griffith, J., Stevens, K. *et al.* (1998). Schizophrenia, sensory gating, and nicotinic receptors. *Schizophrenia Bulletin,* **24** (2), 189–202.

Adler, L. E., Freedman, R., Ross, R. G., Olincy, A., and Waldo, M. C. (1999). Elementary phenotypes in the neurobiological and genetic study of schizophrenia. *Biological Psychiatry,* **46**, 8–18.

Alain, C., Hargrave, R., and Woods, D. L. (1998). Processing of auditory stimuli during visual attention in patients with schizophrenia. *Biological Psychiatry,* **44**, 1151–9.

Alho, K., Houtilainen, M. *et al.* (1995). Are memory traces for simple and complex sounds located in different regions of auditory cortex? Recent MEG studies. *Electroencephalography and Clinical Neurophysiology—Supplement,* **44**, 197–203.

Aloia, M. S., Gourovitch, M. L., Gourovitch, M. L., Missar, D., Pickar, D., and Weinberger, D. R. (1998). Cognitive substrates of thought disorder, II: Specifying a candidate cognitive mechanism. *American Journal of Psychiatry,* **155**, 1667–84.

Andrews, S., Shelley, A. M., Ward, P. B., Fox, A., Catts, S. V., and McConaghy, N. (1993). Event-related potential indices of semantic processing in schizophrenia. *Biological Psychiatry,* **34** (7), 443–58.

Baker, N., Adler, L. E., Franks, R. D., Waldo, M., Berry, S., Nagamoto, H., *et al.* (1987). Neurophysiological assessment of sensory gating in psychiatric inpatients: comparison between schizophrenia and other diagnoses. *Biological Psychiatry, 22,* 603–17.

Baldeweg, T., Spence, S., Hirsch, S. R., and Gruzelier, J. (1998). Gamma-band electroencephalographic oscillations in a patient with somatic hallucinations. *Lancet, 352,* 620–1.

Baldeweg, T., Richardson, A., Watkins, S., Foale, C., and Gruzelier, J. (1999). Impaired auditory frequency discrimination in dyslexia detected with mismatch evoked potentials. *Annals of Neurology, 45,* 495–503.

Barch, D. M., Cohen, J. D., Servan-Schreiber, D., Steingard, S., Cohen, J. D., Steinhauer, S. S. *et al.* (1996). Semantic priming in schizophrenia: an examination of spreading activation using word pronunciation and multiple SOAs. *Journal of Abnormal Psychology, 105,* 592–601.

Benes, F. M. (2000). Emerging principles of altered neural circuitry in schizophrenia. *Brain Research Reviews, 31,* 251–69.

Blackwood, D., Whalley, L., Christie, J. E., Blackburn, I. M., St Clair, D. M., and McInnes, A. (1987). Changes in auditory P3 event-related potential in schizophrenia and depression. *British Journal of Psychiatry, 150,* 154–60.

Blackwood, D. H. R., St. Clair, D. M., Muir, W. J., and Duffy, J. C. (1991). Auditory-P300 and eye tracking dysfunction in schizophrenic pedigrees. *Archives of General Psychiatry, 48,* 899–909.

Bleuler, E. (1950/1911). *Dementia praecox or the group of schizophrenias.* International University Press, New York.

Bobes, M. A., Lei, Z. X., Ibanez, S., Yi, H., and Valdes-Sosa, M. (1996). Semantic matching of pictures in schizophrenia: a cross-cultural ERP study. *Biological Psychiatry, 40* (3), 189–202.

Boutros, N. N., Belger, A., Campbell, D., D'Souza, C., and Krystal, J. (1999). Comparison of four components of sensory gating in schizophrenia and normal subjects: a preliminary report. *Psychiatry Research, 88,* 119–30.

Bressler, S. L., Coppola, R., and Nakamura, R. (1993). Episodic multiregional cortical coherence at multiple frequencies during visual task performance. *Nature, 366,* 153–6.

Broadbent, D. E. (1971). *Decision and stress.* Academic Press, London, England.

Brown, C. M. and Hagoort, P. (1993). The processing nature of the N400: Evidence from masked primes. *Journal of Cognitive Neurosciences, 5* (1), 34–44.

Brown, K. J., Gonsalvez, C. J., Harris, A. W., Williams, L. M., and Gordon, E. (2002). Target and non-target ERP disturbances in first episode vs. chronic schizophrenia. *Clinical Neurophysiology, 113,* 1754–63.

Cadenhead, K. S. and Braff, D. L. (2002). Endophenotyping schizotypy: a prelude to genetic studies within the schizophrenia spectrum. *Schizophrenia Research, 54,* 47–57.

Cadenhead, K. S., Light, G. A., Geyer, M. A., McDowell, J. E., and Braff, D. L. (2002). Neurobiological measures of schizotypal personality disorder: defining an inhibitory endophenotype. *American Journal of Psychiatry, 159,* 869–71.

Cardenas, V. A., Gill, P., and Fein, G. (1997). Human P50 suppression is not affected by variations in wakeful alertness. *Biological Psychiatry, 41,* 891–901.

Catts, S. V., Shelley, A. M. *et al.* (1994). Brain potential evidence for an echoic memory deficit in schizophrenia. *American Journal of Psychiatry, 152,* 213–19.

Catts, S. V., Shelley, A. M., Ward, P. B., Liebert, B., McConaghy, N., Andrews, S. (1995). Brain potential evidence for an auditory sensory memory deficit in schizophrenia. *American Journal of Psychiatry, 152,* 213–19.

Chapman, L. J., Chapman, J. P. *et al.* (1976). Schizophrenic inability to disattend from strong aspects of meaning. *Journal of Abnormal Psychology, 85,* 35–40.

Clementz, B. A., Blumenfeld, L. D., and Cobb, S. (1997*a*). The gamma band response may account for poor P50 suppression in schizophrenia. *Neuroreport*, **8**, 3889–93.

Clementz, B. A., Geyer, M. A., and Braff, D. L. (1997*b*). Poor P50 suppression among schizophrenia and normal comparison subjects: a methodological analysis. *Biological Psychiatry*, **41**, 1035–44.

Clementz, B. A., Geyer, M. A., and Braff, D. L. (1998). Multiple site evaluation of P50 suppression among schizophrenia and normal comparison subjects. *Schizophrenia Research*, **30**, 71–80.

Coburn, K. L., Shillcutt, S. D., Tucker, K. A., Estes, K. M., Brin, F. B., Merai, P. (1998). P300 delay and attenuation in schizophrenia: Reversal by neuroleptic medicine. *Biological Psychiatry*, **44**, 466–74.

Comerchero, M. D. and Polich, J. (1998). P3a, perceptual distinctiveness, and stimulus modality. *Cognitive Brain Research*, **7**, 41–8.

Condray, R., Steinhauer, S. E., Cohen, J. D., van Kammen, D. P., and Kasparek, A. (1999). Modulation of language processing in schizophrenia effects of context and haloperidol on the event-related potential. *Biological Psychiatry*, **45**, 1336–55.

Courchesne, E., Hillyard, S. A., and Galambos, R. (1975). Stimulus novelty, task relevance and the visual evoked potential in man. *Electroencephalography and Clinical Neurophysiology*, **39** (2), 131–43.

Cowan, N. (1984). On short and long auditory stores. *Psychological Bulletin*, **96**, 341–70.

Cowan, N. (1988). Evolving concepts of memory storage, selective attention and their mutual constraints within the human information-processing system. *Psychological Bulletin*, **104**, 163–91.

Cowan, N., Winkler, I., Teder, W., and Naatanen, R. (1993). Memory prerequisites of the mismatch negativity in the auditory event-related potential. *Journal of Experimental Psychology: Learning, Memory, and Cognition*, **19**, 909–21.

Croft, R. J., Lee, A., Bertolot, J., and Gruzelier, J. H. (2001). Associations on P50 suppression and desensitization with perceptual and cognitive features of 'unreality' in schizotypy. *Biological Psychiatry*, **50**, 441–6.

Csëpe, V., Pantev, C., Hoke, M., Hampson, S., and Ross, B. (1992). Evoked magnetic responses of the human auditory cortex to minor pitch changes: localization of the mismatch field. *Electroencephalography and Clinical Neurophysiology*, **84**, 538–48.

Cullum, C. M., Harris, J. G., Waldo, M. C., Smernoff, E., Madison, A., Nagamoto, H. T. *et al.* (1993). Neurophysiological and neuropsychological evidence for attentional dysfunction in schizophrenia. *Schizophrenia Research*, **10**, 131–41.

Davis, H., Mast, T., Yoshie, N., and Zerlin, S. (1966). The slow response of the human cortex to auditory stimuli: Recovery process. *Electroencephalography and Clinical Neurophysiology*, **21**, 105–13.

Deacon, D., Uhm, T.-J., Ritter, W., Hewitt, S., and Dynowska, A. (1999). The lifetime of automatic semantic priming effects may exceed two seconds. *Cognitive Brain Research*, **7**, 465–72.

Demiralp, T., Üçok, A., Devrim, M., Isoglu-Alkac, U., Tecer, A., and Polich, J. (2002). N2 and P3 components of event-related potential in first-episode schizophrenic patients: scalp topography, medication, and latency effects. *Psychiatry Research*, **111**, 167–79.

Docherty, N. M., Hawkins, K. A., Hoffman, R. E., Quinlan, D. M., Rakfeldt, J., and Sledge, W. H. (1996). Working memory, attention, and communication disturbances in schizophrenia. *Journal of Abnormal Psychology*, **105** (2), 212–19.

Donchin, E. (1981). Presidential address, 1980. Surprise! . . . Surprise? *Psychophysiology*, **18** (5), 493–513.

Donchin, E. and Coles, M. G. H. (1988). Is the P300 component a manifestation of context updating? *Brain Behavior and Science*, **11**, 357–74.

Duncan, C. C., Morihisa, J. M., Fawcett, R. W., and Kirch, D. G. (1987). P300 in schizophrenia: State or trait marker? *Psychopharmacological Bulletin*, **23**, 497–501.

Eckhorn, R., Bauer, R., Jordan, W., Brosch, M., Kruse, W., Munk, M. *et al.* (1988). Coherent oscillations: a mechanism of feature linking in the visual cortex? Multiple electrode and correlation analyses in the cat. *Biological Cybernetics,* **60**, 121–30.

Egan, M.-F., Duncan, C. C., Suddath, R. L., Kirch, D. G., Mirsky, A. F., and Wyatt, R. J. (1994). Event-related abnormalities correlate with structural brain alterations and clinical features in patients with chronic schizophrenia. *Schizophrenia Research,* **11**, 259–71.

Engel, A. K., Kreiter, A. K., Konig, P., and Singer, W. (1991). Synchronization of oscillatory neuronal responses between striate and extrastriate visual cortical areas of the cat. *Proceedings of the National Academy of Sciences USA,* **88**, 6048–52.

Engel, A. K., Fries, P., Konig, P., Brecht, M., and Singer, W. (1999). Temporal binding, binocular rivalry, and consciousness. *Consciousness and Cognition,* **8**, 128–51.

Erwin, R. J. and Rao, S. M. (2000). Convergence of functional magnetic resonance imaging and event-related potential methodologies. *Brain and Cognition,* **42**, 53–5.

Erwin, R. J., Turetsky, B. I., Moberg, P., Gur, R. C., and Gur, R. E. (1998). P50 abnormalities in schizophrenia: relationship to clinical and neuropsychological indices of attention. *Schizophrenia Research,* **33**, 157–67.

Faux, S. F., McCarley, R. W., Nestor, P. G., Shenton, M.E., Pollak, S. D., and Penhune, V. (1993). P300 topographic asymmetries are present in enmedicated schizophrenics. *Electroencephalography and Clinical Neurophysiology,* **88**, 32–41.

Federmeier, K. D. and Kutas, M. (1999). A rose by any other name: Long-term structure and sentence processing. *Journal of Memory and Language,* **41**, 469–95.

Fein, G., Biggins, C., and MacKay, S. (1996). Cocaine abusers have reduced auditory P50 amplitude and suppression compared to both normal controls and alcoholics. *Biological Psychiatry,* **39**, 955–65.

Fell, J., Klaver, P., Lehnertz, K., Grunwald, T., Schaller, C., and Elger, C.E. (2001). Human memory formation is accompanied by rhinal–hippocampal coupling and decoupling. *Nature Neuroscience,* **4**, 1259–64.

Ford, J. M. (1999). Schizophrenia: The broken p300 and beyond. *Psychophysiology,* **36**, 667–82.

Ford, J. M., Pfefferbaum, A. and Roth, W. T. (1992). P3 and schizophrenia. *Annals of the New York Academy of Sciences,* **658**, 146–62.

Ford, J. M., White, P. M., Csernansky, J. G., Faustman, W. O., Roth, W. T., and Pfefferbaum, A. (1994). ERP's in schizophrenia: Effects of antipsychotic medication. *Biological Psychiatry,* **36**, 153–70.

Ford, J. M., Mathalon, D. H., Marsh, L., Faustman, W. O., Harris, D., Hoff, A. L. (1999). P300 amplitude is related to clinical state in severely and moderately ill schizophrenics. *Biological Psychiatry,* **46**, 94–101.

Frangou, S., Sharma, T. , Alarcon, G., Sigmudsson, T., Takei, N., and Binnie, C. *et al.* (1997). The Maudsley family study. II. Endogenous event-related potentials in familial schizophrenia. *Schizophrenia Research,* **23**, 45–53.

Franks, R., Adler, L. E., Waldo, M. C., Alpert, J., and Freedman, R. (1983). Neurophysiological studies of sensory gating in mania: Comparison with schizophrenia. *Biological Psychiatry,* **18**, 989–1005.

Freedman, R., Adler, L. E. *et al.* (1982). Neurophysiology of sensory inhibition in psychosis. *American Psychiatric Association,* **54**.

Freedman, R., Adler, L. E., Waldo, M. C., Pachtman, E., and Franks, R. D. (1983). Neurophysicological evidence for a defect in inhibitory pathways in schizophrenia: comparison of medicated and drug-free patients. *Biological Psychiatry,* **18** (5), 537–51.

Freedman, R., Waldo, M., Bickford-Wimer, P., and Nagamoto, H. (1991). Elementary neuronal dysfunctions in schizophrenia. *Schizophrenia Research,* **4**, 233–43.

Freedman, R., Adler, L. E., Bickford, P., Byerley, W., Coon, H., Cullum, C. M. *et al.* (1994). Schizophrenia and nicotinic receptors. *Harvard Review of Psychiatry,* **2**, 179–92.

Freedman, R., Adler, L. E., Myles-Worsley, M., Nagamoto, H. T., Miller, C., Kisley. M. (1996). Inhibitory gating of an evoked response to repeated auditory stimuli in schizophrenic and normal subjects: human recordings, computer stimulation, and an animal model. *Archives of General Psychiatry*, **53** (12), 1114–21.

Freedman, R., Coon, H., Myles-Worsley, M., Orr-Urtreger, A., Olincy, A., Davis, A. (1997). Linkage of a neurophysiological deficit in schizophrenia to a chromosome 15 locus. *Proceedings of the National Academy of Science*, **94**, 587–92.

Freedman, R., Adler, L. E., Nagamoto, H. T., and Waldo, M. C. (1998). Selection of digital filtering parameters and P50 amplitude. *Biological Psychiatry*, **43**, 921–2.

Freedman, R., Leonard, S., Gault, J. M., Hopkins, J., Cloninger, C. R., Kaufmann, C. A. (2001). Linkage disequilibrium for schizophrenia at the chromosome 15q13–14 locus of the alpha7-nicotinic acetylcholine receptor subunit gene (CHRNA7). *American Journal of Medical Genetics*, **105**, 20–2.

Friedman, D. (1990). Cognitive event-related potential components during continuous recognition memory for pictures. *Psychophysiology*, **27**, 136–48.

Fries, P., Reynolds, J. H., Rorie, A. E., and Desimone, R. (2001). Modulation of oscillatory neuronal synchronization by selective visual attention. *Science*, **291**, 1560–3.

Frodl-Bauch, T., Kathmann, N., Moller, H. J., and Hegerl, U. (1997). Dipole localization and test retest reliability of frequency and duration mismatch negativity generator processes. *Brain Topography*, **10**, 3–8.

Frodl-Bauch, T., Gallinat, J., Meisenzahl, E.M., Moller, H.J., and Hegerl, U. (1999). P300 Subcomponents reflect different aspects of psychophathology in schizophrenia. *Biological Psychiatry*, **45**, 116–26.

Galambos, R., Makeig, S., and Talmachoff, P.J. (1981). A 40-Hz auditory potential recorded from the human scalp. *Proceedings of the National Academy of Sciences USA*, **78**, 2643–7.

Giard, M. H., Perrin, F., Pernier, J., and Bouchet, P. (1990). Brain generators implicated in the processing of auditory stimulus deviance: a topographic event-related potential study. *Psychophysiology*, **27**, 627–40.

Giard, M. H., Lavikainen, J., Reinikainen, K., Perrin, F., Bertrand, O., Pernier, J. (1995). Separate representation of stimulus frequency, intensity, and duration in auditory sensory memory: an event-related potential and dipole-model analysis. *Journal of Cognitive Neuroscience*, **7**, 133–43.

Gillette, G. M., Skinner, R. D., Rasco, L.M., Fielstein, E.M., Davis, D.H., Pawelak, J.E. (1997). Combat veterans with posttraumatic stress disorder exhibit decreased habituation of the P1 midlatency auditory evoked potential. *Life Science*, **61** (14), 1421–34.

Goff, D. C., Henderson, D. C., and Amico, E. (1992). Cigarette smoking in schizophrenia: Relationship to psychopathology and medication side effects. *American Journal of Psychiatry*, **149**, 1189–94.

Gordon, E., Williams, L. M., Haig, A.R., Wright, J. and Meares, R.A. (2001). Symptom profile and 'gamma' processing in schizophrenia. *Cognitive Neuropsychiatry*, **6**, 7–19.

Gray, C. M. and Singer, W. (1989). Stimulus-specific neuronal oscillations in orientation columns of cat visual cortex. *Proceedings of the National Academy of Sciences USA*, **86**, 1698–1702.

Gray, C. M., König, P., Engel, A.K., and Singer, W. (1989). Oscillatory responses in cat visual cortex exhibit inter-columnar synchronization which reflects global stimulus properties. *Nature*, **338**, 334–7.

Griffith, J. M., Waldo, M., Adler, L. E., and Freedman, R. (1993). Normalization of auditory sensory gating in schizophrenic patients after a brief period for sleep. *Psychiatry Research*, **49**, 29–39.

Griffith, J., Hoffer, L. D., Adler, L.E., Zerbe, G.O., and Freedman, R. (1995). Effects of sound intensity on a midlatency evoked response to repeated auditory stimuli in schizophrenic and normal subjects. *Psychophysiology*, **32**, 460–6.

Griffith, J. M., O'Neill, J. E., Petty, F., Garver, D., Young, D., and Freedman, R. (1998). Nicotinic receptor desensitization and sensory gating deficits in schizophrenia. *Biological Psychiatry,* **44**, 98–106.

Grillon, C., Ameli, R., and Glazer, W.M. (1991). N400 and semantic categorization in schizophrenia. *Biological Psychiatry,* **29**, 467–80.

Grunze, H. C., Rainnie, D. G., Hasselmo, M.E., Barkai, E., Hearn, E.F., McCarley, R.W. *et al.* (1996). NMDA-dependent modulation of CA1 local circuit inhibition. *Journal of Neuroscience,* **16**, 2034–43.

Haig, A. R., Gordon, E., De Pascalis, V., Meares, R.A., Bahramali, H., and Harris, A. (2000). Gamma activity in schizophrenia: evidence of impaired network binding? *Clinical Neurophysiology,* **111**, 1461–8.

Halgren, E., Marinkovic, K., and Chauvel, P. (1998). Generators of the late cognitive potentials in auditory and visual oddball tasks. *Electroencephalography and clinical neuropshysiology,* **106**, 156–64.

Hari, R., Hämäläinen, M., Ilmoniemi, R., Kaukoranta, E., Reinikainen, K., Salminen, J., *et al.* (1984). Responses of the primary auditory cortex to pitch changes in a sequence of tone pips: neuromagnetic recordings in man. *Neuroscience Letters,* **50**, 127–32.

Hasselmo, M. E., Schnell, E., and Barkai, E. (1995). Dynamics of learning and recall at excitatory recurrent synapes and cholinergic modulation in rat hippocampal region CA3. *Journal of Neuroscience,* **15**, 5249–62.

Herculano-Houzel, S., Munk, M. H., Neuenschwander, S., and Singer, W. (1999). Precisely synchronized oscillatory firing patterns require electroencephalographic activation. *Journal of Neuroscience,* **19**, 3992–4010.

Herrmann, C. S. and Mecklinger, A. (2001). Gamma activity in human EEG is related to high-speed memory comparisons during object selective attention. *Visual Cognition,* **8**, 593–608.

Higashima, M., Urata, K., Kawasaki, Y., Maeda, Y., Sakai, N., Mizukoshi, C., (1998). P300 and the thought disorder factor extracted by factor-analytic procedures in schizophrenia. *Biological Psychiatry,* **44** (2), 115–20.

Hirayasu, Y. and Ogura, C. (1996). Event-related potential (ERP) abnormalities in schizophrenia: Effects of subtype, clinical course, neuroleptic medication and clinical symptoms. In *Recent advances in event-related brain potential research,* (ed. C. Ogura, Y. Koga, and M. Shimokochi), pp. 922–9. Elsevier, Amsterdam.

Hirayasu, Y., Potts, G. F., O'Donnell, B.F., Kwon, J.S., Arakaki, H., Akdag, S.J. *et al.* (1998*a*). Auditory mismatch negativity in schizophrenia: topographic evaluation with a high-density recording montage. *American Journal of Psychiatry,* **155**, 1281–4.

Hirayasu, Y., Asato, N., Ohta, H., Hokama, H., Arakaki, H., and Ogura, C. (1998*b*). Abnormalities of auditory event-related potentials in schizophrenia prior to treatment. *Biological Psychiatry,* **43**, 244–53.

Holcomb, P. J. (1993). Semantic priming and stimulus degradation: Implications for the role of N400 in language processing. *Psychophysiology,* **30**, 47–61.

Holcomb, P. J. and Neville, H. (1990). Auditory and semantic priming in lexical decisions: a comparison using event-related brain potentials. *Language and Cognitive Processes,* **5**, 281–312.

Jackson, A., Gee, V. J., Baker, S.N., and Lemon, R.N. (2003). Synchrony between neurons with similar muscle fields in monkey motor cortex. *Neuron,* **38**, 115–25.

Javitt, D. C. and Zukin, S. R. (1991). Recent advances in the phencyclidine model of schizophrenia. *American Journal of Psychiatry,* **48**, 1301–8.

Javitt, D. C., Doneshka, P., Zylberman, I., Ritter, W,, and Vaughan, H.G. Jr. (1993). Impairment of early cortical processing in schizophrenia: an event-related potential replication study. *Biological Psychiatry,* **33**, 513–19.

Javitt, D. C., Doneshka, P., Grochowski, S., and Ritter, W. (1995). Impaired mismatch negativity generation reflects widespread dysfunction of working memory in schizophrenia. *Archives of General Psychiatry*, **52** (7), 550–8.

Javitt, D. C., Grochowski, S., Shelley, A.M., and Ritter, W. (1998). Impaired mismatch negativity (MMN) generation in schizophrenia as a function of stimulus deviance, probability, and inter-stimulus/interdeviant interval. *Electroencephalography and Clinical Neurophysiology*, **108**, 143–53.

Javitt, D. C., Shelley, A.-M., and Ritter W. (2000). Associated deficits in mismatch negativity generation and tone matching in schizophrenia. *Clinical Neurophysiology*, **111**, 1733–7.

Jeon, Y. W. and Polich, J. (2001). P300 asymmetry in schizophrenia: A meta-analysis. *Psychiatry Research*, **104** (1), 61–74.

Jerger, K., Biggins, C., and Fein, G. (1992). P50 suppression is not affected by attentional manipulations. *Biological Psychiatry*, **31**, 365–77.

Jin, Y., Bunney, W. E. J., Sandman, C. A., Patterson, J. V., Fleming, K., Moenter, J. R. *et al.* (1998). Is P50 suppression a measure of sensory gating in schizophrenia? *Biological Psychiatry*, **43**, 873–8.

Johnson, M. R. and Adler, L. E. (1993). Transient impairment in P50 auditory sensory gating induced by a cold-pressor Test. *Biological Psychiatry*, **33**, 380–7.

Kasai, K., Okazawa, K., Nakagome, K., Hiramatsu, K., Hata, A., Fukuda, M. (1999). Mismatch negativity and N2b attenuation as an indicator for dysfunction of the preattentive and controlled processing for deviance detection in schizophrenia: a topographic event-related potential study. *Schizophrenia Research*, **35**, 141–56.

Kasai, K., Nakagome, K., Itoh, K., Koshida, I., Hata, A., Iwanami, A. (2002*a*). Impaired cortical network for preattentive detection of change in speech sounds in schizophrenia: a high-resolution event-related potential study. *American Psychiatric Association*, **159** (4), 546–53.

Kasai, K., Yamada, H., Kamio, S., Nakagome, K., Iwanami, A., Fukuda, M. (2002*b*). Do high or low doses of anxiolytics and hypnotics affect mismatch negativity in schizophrenic subjects? An EEG and MEG study. Clinical *Neurophysiology*, **113**, 141–50.

Katayama, J. and Polich, J. (1998). Stimulus context determines P3a and P3b. *Psychophysiology*, **35**, 23–33.

Kathmann, N., Wagner, M., Rendtorff, N., and Engel, R.R. (1995). Delayed peak latency of the mismatch negativity in schizophrenics and alcoholics. *Biological Psychiatry*, **37**, 754–7.

Kimble, M., Lyons, M., O'Donnell, B., Nestor, P., Niznikiewicz, M., and Toomey, R. (2000). The effect of family status and schizotypy on electrophysiological measures of attention and semantic processing. *Biological Psychiatry*, **47** (5), 402–12.

Kirino, E. and Inoue, R. (1999). The relationship of mismatch negativity to quantitative EEG and morphological findings in schizophrenia. *Journal of Psychiatric Research*, **33**, 445–6.

Kissler, J., Müller, M. M., Fehr, T., Rockstroh, B., and Elbert, T. (2000). MEG gamma band activity in schizophrenia patients and healthy subjects in a mental arithmetic task and at rest. *Clinical Neurophysiology*, **111**, 2079–87.

Koyama, S., Nageishi, Y., Shimokochi, M., Hokama, H., Miyazato, Y., and Miyatani, M. *et al.* (1991). The N400 component of event-related potentials in schizophrenic patients: A preliminary study. *Electroencephalography and clinical neurophysiology*, **78** (2), 124–32.

Koyama, S., Hokama, H., Miyatani, M., Ogura, C., Nageishi, Y., and Shimokochi, M. *et al.* (1994). ERPs in schizophrenic patients during word recognition tasks and reaction times. *Electroencephalography and clinical neurophysiology*, **92**, 546–54.

Kraepelin, E. (1899). *Psychiatrie. Ein lehrbuch fur studirende und aerzte.* Verlag von Johann Ambrosius Barth, Leipzig.

Kreiter, A. K. and Singer, W. (1992). Oscillatory neuronal responses in the visual cortex of the awake macaque monkey. *European Journal of Neuroscience*, **4**, 369–75.

Krystal, J. H., Karper, L. P., Seibyl, J.P., Freeman, G.K., Delaney, R., Bremner, J.D. *et al.* (1994). Subanesthetic effects of the non-competitive NMDA antagonist, ketamine, in humans. Psychotomimetic, perceptual, cognitive, and neuroendicrine responses. *Archives of General Psychiatry*, **51**, 199–214.

Kutas, M. and Hillyard, S. A. (1980). Reading senseless sentences: Brain potentials reflect semantic incogruity. *Science*, **207**, 203–5.

Kutas, M. and Hillyard, S. A. (1984). Brain potentials during reading reflect word expectancy and semantic association. *Nature*, **307**, 161–3.

Kutas, M. and Hillyard, S. A. (1989). An electrophysiological probe of incidental semantic association. *Journal of Cognitive Neuroscience*, **1**, 38–48.

Kwapil, T. R., Hegley, D. C., Chapman, L.J., and Chapman, J.P. (1990). Facilitation of word recognition by semantic priming in schizophrenia. *Journal of Abnormal Psychology*, **99**, 215–21.

Kwon, J. S., O'Donnell, B., Wallenstein, G.V., Greene, R.W., Hirayasu, Y., Nestor, P.G. (1999). Gamma frequency-range abnormalities to auditory stimulation in schizophrenia. *Archives of General Psychiatry*, **56**, 1001–5.

Lachaux, J.-P., Rodriguez, E., Martinerie, J., and Varela, F.J. (1999). Measuring phase synchrony in brain signals. *Human Brain Mapping*, **8**, 194–208.

Lembreghts, M. and Timsit-Berthier, M. (1993). The value of cognitive psychophysiological studies in a comprehensive approach to schizophrenia. *Acta Psychiatrica Belgica*, **93**, 322–42.

Leonard, S., Adams, C., Breese, C.R., Adler, L.E., Bickford, P., Byerley, W. (1996). Nicotinic receptor function in schizophrenia. *Schizophrenia Bulletin*, **22** (3), 431–45.

Leonard, S., Gault, J. M., Hopkins, J., Logel, J., Vianzon, R., Short, M. (2002). Association of promoter variants in the alpha7 nicotinic acetylcholine receptor subunit gene with an inhibitory deficit found in schizophrenia. *Archives of General Psychiatry*, **59** (12), 1085–96.

Lewis, D. A. (2000). GABAergic local circuit neurons and prefrontal cortical dysfunction in schizophrenia. *Brain Research Reviews*, **31**, 270–6.

Lewis, D. A. and Gonzales-Burgos, G. (2000). Intrinsic excitatory connections in the prefrontal cortex and the pathophysiology of schizophrenia. *Brain Research Bulletin*, **52**, 309–17.

Light, G. A., Malaspina, D., Geyer, M.A., Luber, B.M., Coleman, E.A., Sackeim, H.A. (1999). Amphetamine disrupts P50 suppression in normal subjects. *Biological Psychiatry*, **46**, 990–6.

Light, G., Geyer, M., Clementz, B. A., Cadenhead, K. S., and Braff, D. L. (2000). Normal P50 suppression in schizophrenia patients treated with atypical antipsychotic medications. *American Journal of Psychiatry*, **157** (5), 767–71.

Maher, B. (1972). The language of schizophrenia: a review and interpretation. *British Journal of Psychiatry*, **120**, 3–17.

Manschreck, T. C., Maher, B. A., Milavetz, J.J., Ames, D., Weisstein, C.C., and Schneyer, M.L. (1988). Semantic priming in thought disordered schizophrenic patients. *Schizophrenia Research*, **1**, 61–6.

Mathalon, D. H., Ford, J. M., and Pfefferbaum, A. (2000). Trait and state aspects of P300 amplitude reduction in schizophrenia: a retrospective longitudinal study. *Biological Psychiatry*, **47**, 434–49.

Mathalon, D. H., Sullivan, E. V, Lim, K.O., and Pfefferbaum, A. (2001). Progressive brain volume changes and the clinical course of schizophrenia in men: a longitudinal magnetic resonance imaging study. *Archives of General Psychiatry*, **58**, 148–57.

Mathalon, D. H., Faustman, W. O., and Ford, J.M. (2002). N400 and automatic semantic processing abnormalities in patients with schizophrenia. *Archives of General Psychiatry*, **59**, 641–8.

Mathiak, K., Hertrich, I., Lutzenberger, W., and Ackermann, H. (2002). Functional cerebral asymmetries of pitch processing during dichotic stimulus application: a whole-head magnetoencephalography study. *Neuropsychologia*, **6**, 585–93.

Matsuoka, H., Matsumoto, K., Yamazaki, H., Sakai, H., Miwa, S., Yoshida, S. (1999). Lack of repetition priming effect on visual event-related potentials in schizophrenia. *Biological Psychiatry,* **46** (1), 137–40.

McBain, C. J. and Fisahn, A. (2001). Interneurons unbound. *Nature Reviews Neuroscience,* **2**, 11–23.

McCarley, R. W., Faux, S. F., Shenton, M.E., Nestor, P.G., and Adams, J. (1991). Event-related potentials in schizophrenia pathophysiology. *Schizophrenia Research,* **4**, 209–31.

McCarley, R. W., Shenton, M. E., O'Donnell, B.F., Faux, S.F., Kikinis, R., Nestor, P.G. (1993). Auditory P300 abnormalities and left posterior superior temporal gyrus volume reduction in schizophrenia. *Archives of General Psychiatry,* **50**, 190–7.

McCarley, R. W., Salisbury, D. F., Hirayasu, Y., Yurgelun-Todd, D.A., Tohen, M., Zarate, C. (2002). Association between similar left posterior superior temporal gyrus volume on magnetic resonance imaging and smaller left temporal P300 amplitude in first-episode schizophrenia. *Archives of General Psychiatry,* **59**, 321–31.

McCarthy, G. and Donchin, E. (1981). A metric for thought: a comparison of P300 latency and reaction time. *Science,* **211** (4477), 77–80.

McGhie, A. and Chapman, J. S. (1961). Disorders of attention and perception in early schizophrenia. *British Journal of Medical Psychology,* **34**, 103–16.

Michie, P. T., Budd, T. W., Todd, J., Rock, D., Wichmann, H., Box, J. *et al.* (2000). Duration and frequency mismatch negativity in schizophrenia. *Clinical Neurophysiology,* **111**, 1054–65.

Michie, P. T., Innes-Brown, H., Todd, J., and Jablensky, A.V. (2002). Duration mismatch negativity in biological relatives of parents with schizophrenia spectrum disorders. *Biological Psychiatry,* **52**, 749–58.

Milner, P. M. (1974). A model for visual shape recognition. *Psychological Review,* **81**, 521–35.

Miltner, W. H., Braun, C., Arnold, M., Witte, H., and Taub, E. (1999). Coherence of gamma-band EEG activity as a basis for associative learning. *Nature,* **397**, 434–6.

Mitchell, P. F., Andrews, S., Fox, A.M., Catts, S.V., Ward, P.B., and McConaghy, N. (1991). Active and passive attention in schizophrenia: An ERP study of information processing in a lingustic task. *Biological Psychiatry,* **32**, 101–24.

Morstyn, R., Duffy, F. H., and McCarley, R.W. (1983). Altered P300 topography in schizophrenia. *Archives of General Psychiatry,* **40**, 729–34.

Müller, M. M., Gruber, T., and Keil, A. (2000). Modulation of induced gamma band activity in the human EEG by attention and visual information processing. *International Journal of Psychophysiology,* **38**, 283–99.

Murakami, T., Nakagome, K., Kamio, S., Kasai, K., Iwanami, A., Hiramatsu, K. *et al.* (2002). The effects of benzodiazepines on event-related potential indices of automatic and controlled processing in schizophrenia: a preliminary report. *Progress in Neuro-Psychopharmacology and Biological Psychiatry,* **26** (4), 651–61.

Näätänen, R. (1992). The mismatch negativity. In *Attention and brain function,* (ed. R. Näätänen), pp. 136–200. Lawrence Erlbaum Associates, Hillsdale, New Jersey.

Näätänen, R., Paavilainen, P., and Reinikainen, K. (1989). Do event-related potentials to infrequent decrements in duration of auditory stimuli demonstrate a memory trace in man? *Neuroscience Letters,* **107**, 347–52.

Nagamoto, H. T., Adler, L. E., Waldo, M. C.,Griffith, J., and Freedman, R. (1991). Gating of auditory response in schizophrenics and normal controls: effects of changing stimulation interval. *Schizophrenia Research,* **4**, 31–40.

Nagamoto, H. T., Lawrence, E. A., Hea, R. A., Griffith, J. M., McRae, K. A., and Freedman, R. (1996). Gating of Auditory P50 in Schizophrenics: Unique Effects of Clozapine. *Biological Psychiatry,* **40**, 181–8.

Nagamoto, H. T., Adler, L. E., McRae, K.A., Huettl, P., Cawthra, E., Gerhardt, G. *et al.* (1999). Auditory P50 in schizophrenics on clozapine: Improved gating parallels clinical improvement and changes in pMHPG. *Neuropsychobiology,* **39**, 10–17.

Neely, J. H. (1991). Semantic priming effects in visual word recognition: A selective review of current findings and theories. In *Basic processes in reading: Visual word recognition,* (ed. D. Besner and G. W. Humphreys), pp. 264–336. Erlbaum Associates, Hillsdale, New Jersey.

Nestor, P. G., Kimble, M. O., O'Donnell, B.F., Smith, L., Niznikiewicz, M., Shenton, M.E. (1997). Aberrant semantic activation in schizophrenia: A neurophysiological study. *American Journal of Psychiatry,* **154** (5), 640–6.

Neville, H. and Kutas, M. (1986). Event-related brain potentials during initial encoding and recognition memory of congruous and incongruous words. *Journal of Memory and Language,* **25**, 75–92.

Niznikiewicz, M. A., O'Donnell, B. F. , Nestor, P.G., Smith, L., Law, S., Karapelou, M. *et al.* (1997). ERP assesment of visual and auditory language processing in schizophrenia. *Journal of Abnormal Psychology,* **106**, 85–94.

Niznikiewicz, M. A., Voglmaier, M., Shenton, M.E., Seidman, L.J., Dickey, C.C., Rhoads, R. *et al.* (1999). Electrophysiological correlates of language processing in schizotypal personality disorder. *American Journal of Psychiatry,* **156** (7), 1052–8.

Niznikiewicz, M. A., Volgamaier, M. M., Shenton, M.E., Dickey, C.C., Seidman, L.J., The, E. *et al.* (2000). Lateralized P3 deficit in schizotypal personality disorder. *Biological Psychiatry,* **48**, 702–5.

Niznikiewicz, M., Shenton, M. E., Voglmaier, M., Nestor, P.G., Dickey, C.C., Frumin, M. *et al.* (2002). Semantic dysfunction in women with schizotypal personality disorder. *American Journal of Psychiatry,* **159** (10), 1767–74.

O'Donnell, B. F., Hokama, H., McCarley, R.W., Smith, R.S., Salisbury, D.F., Mondrow, E. *et al.* (1994). Auditory ERPs to non-target stimuli in schizophrenia: relationship to probability, task-demands, and target ERPs. *International Journal of Psychophysiology,* **17**, 219–31.

O'Donnell, B. F., Faux, S. F., McCarley, R.W., Kimble, M.O., Salisbury, D.F., Nestor, P.G. *et al.* (1995). Increased rate of P300 latency prolongation with age in schizophrenia: electrophysiological evidence for a neurodegenerative process. *Archives of General Psychiatry,* **52** (7), 544–9.

Ohta, H., Uchiyama, M., Matsushima, E., and Toru, M. (1999). An event-related potential study in schizophrenia using Japanese sentences. *Schizophrenia Research,* **40** (2), 159–70.

Olichney, J. M., Iragui, V. J., Kutas, M., Nowacki, R., and Jeste, D.V. (1997). N400 abnormalities in late-life schizophrenia and related psychoses. *Biological Psychiatry,* **42** (1), 13–23.

Olichney, J. M., Iragui, V. J., Kutas, M., Nowacki, R., Morris, S., and Jeste, D.V. (1998). Relationship between auditory P300 amplitude and age of onset of schizophrenia in older patients. *Psychiatry Research,* **79** (3), 241–54.

Olincy, A., Ross, R. G., Harris, J.G., Young, D.A., McAndrews, M.A., Cawthra, E. (2000). The P50 auditory event-evoked potential in adult attention-deficit disorder: Comparison with schizophrenia. *Biological Psychiatry,* **47**, 969–77.

Opitz, B., Mecklinger, A., Von Cramon, D.Y, and Kruggel, F. (1999). Combining electrophysiological and hemodynamic measures of the auditory oddball. *Psychophysiology,* **36**, 142–7.

Oranje, B., , Gispen-de Wied, C.C., Verbaten, M.N., and Kahn, R.S. (2002). Modulating sensory gating in healthy volunteers: the effects of ketamine and haloperidol. *Biological Psychiatry,* **52**, 887–95.

Pantev, C. (1995). Evoked and induced gamma-band avtivity of the human cortex. *Brain Topography,* **7**, 321–30.

Pantev, C., Elbert, T, Makeig, S., Hampson, S., Eulitz, C., and Hoke, M. (1993). Relationship of transient and steady-state auditory evoked fields. *Electroencephalography and Clinical Neuropshysiology,* **88**, 389–96.

Park, H.-J., Kwon, J. S., Youn, T., Pae, J.S., Kim, J.J., Kim, M.S. *et al.* (2002). Statistical parametric mapping of LORETA using high density EEG and individual MRI: application to mismatch negativities in schizophrenia. *Human Brain Mapping*, **17**, 168–78.

Patterson, J. V., Jin, Y., Gierczak, M., Hetrick, W.P., Potkin, S., Bunney, W.E. Jr. *et al.* (2000). Effects of temporal variability on P50 and the gating ratio in schizophrenia: a frequency domain adaptive filter single-trial analysis. *Archives of General Psychiatry*, **57**, (1), 57–64.

Pekkonen, E., Hirvonen, J., Ahveninen, J., Kahkonen, S., Kaakkola, S., Huttunen, J. *et al.* (2002*a*). Memory-based comparison process not attenuated by haloperidol: a combined MEG and EEG study. *Neuroreport*, **13**, (1), 177–81.

Pekkonen, E., Heikki, K., Katila, H., Ahveninen, J., Karhu, J., Huotilainen, M. *et al.* (2002*b*). Impaired temporal lobe processing of preattentive auditory discrimination in schizophrenia. *Schizophrenia Bulletin*, **28**, (3), 467–74.

Pesaran, B., Pezaris, J. S., Sahani, M., Mitra, P.P., and Andersen, R.A. (2002). Temporal structure in neuronal activity during working memory in macaque parietal cortex. *Nature Neuroscience*, **5**, 805–11.

Pfefferbaum, A., Ford, J. M., White, P.M., and Roth, W.T. (1989). P3 in schizophrenia is affected by stimulus modality, response requirements, medication status and negative symptoms. *Archives of General Psychiatry*, **46**, 1035–46.

Potts, G. F., Hirayasu, Y., O'Donnell, B.F., Shenton, M.E., and McCarley, R.W. (1998). High density recording and topographic analysis of the auditory oddball event-related potential in patients with schizophrenia. *Biological Psychiatry*, **44**, 982–9.

Pulvermüller, F. (1996). Hebb's concept of cell assemblies and the psychophysiology of word processing. *Psychophysiology*, **33**, 317–33.

Rao, K. M., Ananthnarayanan, C. V., Gangadhar, B.N., and Janakiramaiah, N. (1995). Smaller auditory P300 amplitudes in schizophrenics in remission. *Neuropsychobiology*, **32**, 171–4.

Reite, M., Teale, P., Zimmerman, J., Davis, K., Whalen, J., and Edrich, J. (1988). Source origin of a 50-msec latency auditory evoked field component in young schizophrenic men. *Biological Psychiatry*, **24**, 495–506.

Riehle, A., Grün, S., Diesmann, M., and Aertsen, A. (1997). Spike synchronization and rate modulation differentially involved in motor cortical function. *Science*, **278**, 1950–3.

Rodriguez, E., George, N., Lachaux, J.P., Martinerie, J., Renault, B., and Varela, F.J. (1999). Perception's shadow: long-distance synchronization of human brain activity. *Nature*, **397**, 430–3.

Roelfsema, P. R., Engel, A. K., Konig, P., and Singer, W. (1997). Visuomotor integration is associated with zero time-lag synchronization among cortical areas. *Nature*, **385**, 157–61.

Roth, W. T. and Cannon, E. H. (1972). Some features of the auditory evoked response in schizophrenics. *Archives of General Psychiatry*, **27**, 466–71.

Roxborough, H., Muir, W. J., Blackwood, D.H., Walker, M.T., and Blackburn, I.M. (1993). Neuropsychological and P300 abnormalities in schizophrenics and their relatives. *Psychological Medicine*, **23**, 305–14.

Salinas, E. and Sejnowski, T. J. (2001). Correlated neuronal activity and the flow of neural information. *Nature Reviews Neuroscience*, **2**, 539–50.

Salisbury, D. F., Voglmaier, M., Seidman, L.J., and McCarley, R.W. (1996). Topographic abnormalities of P3 in schizotypal personality disorder. *Biological Psychiatry*, **40**, 165–72.

Salisbury, D. F., Shenton, M. E., Sherwood, A.R., Fischer, I.A., Yurgelun-Todd, D.A., Tohen, M. *et al.* (1998). First episode schizpophrenic psychosis differs from first episode affective psychosis and controls in P300 amplitudes over left temporal lobe. *Archives of General Psychiatry*, **55**, 173–80.

Salisbury, D. F., Shenton, M. E., and McCarley, R.W. (1999). P300 topography differs in schizophrenia and manic psychosis. *Biological Psychiatry*, **45**, 99–106.

Salisbury, D. F., O'Donnell, B. F., McCarley, R.W., Nestor, P.G., and Shenton, M.E. (2000). Event-related potentials elicited during a context-free homograph task in normal versus schizophrenic subjects. *Psychophysiology*, **37**, 456–63.

Salisbury, D. F., Bonner-Jackson, A., Griggs, C.B., Bonner-Jackson, A., and McCarley, R.W. (2001a). Mismatch negativity in schizophrenia: does MMN amplitude decline with disease duration? *Biological Psychiatry*, **49** (suppl.), 85.

Salisbury, D. F., Rutherford, B., Shenton, M.E., and McCarley, R.W. (2001b). Button pressing affects P300 amplitude and scalp topography. *Clinical Neurophysiology*, **112**, 1676–84.

Salisbury, D. F., Shenton, M. E., Griggs, C.B., Bonner-Jackson, A., and McCarley, R.W. *et al.* (2002). Mismatch negativity and first-episode schizophrenia. *Archives of General Psychiatry*, **59**, 686–94.

Salisbury, D. F., Kasai K., Shenton, M. E., and McCarley, R. W. (2003). Mismatch negativity amplitude and Heschl's gyrus volume in first episode schizophrenia. *Schizophrenia Research*, **60**, S259.

Schall, U., Catts, S. V., Chaturvedi, S., Liebert, B., Redenbach, J., Karayanidis, F. *et al.* (1995). The effect of clozapine therapy on psychometric and event-related potential (ERP) measures on cognitive dysfunction in schizophrenia. *Schizophrenia Research*, **15**, 164.

Selemon, L. D. and Goldman-Rakic, P. S. (1999). The reduced neuropil hypothesis: a circuit based model of schizophrenia. *Biological Psychiatry*, **45**, 17–25.

Shelley, A.-M., Ward, P. B., Catts, S.V., Michie, P.T., Andrews, S., and McConaghy, N. (1991). Mismatch negativity: an index of a preattentive processing deficit in schizophrenia. *Biological Psychiatry*, **30**, 1059–62.

Shelley, A.-M., Silipo, G., and Javitt, D C. (1999). Diminished responsiveness of ERPs in schizophrenic subjects to changes in auditory stimulation parameters: implications for theories of cortical dysfunction. *Schizophrenia Research*, **37**, 65–79.

Shenton, M. E., Solovay, M. R., Holzman, P.S., Coleman, M., and Gale, H.J. (1989). Thought disorder in relatives of psychotic patients. *Archives of General Psychiatry*, **46**, 897–901.

Singer, W. (1999). Neuronal synchrony: a versatile code for the definition of relations? *Neuron*, **24**, 49–65, 111–25.

Sitnikova, T., Salisbury, D. F., Kuperberg, G., and Holcomb, P.I. (2002). Electrophysiological insights into language processing in schizophrenia. *Psychophysiology*, **39**, 851–60.

Spencer, K. M., Dien, J., and Donchin, E. (2001). Spatiotemporal analysis of the late ERP responses to deviant stimuli. *Psychophysiology*, **38** (2), 343–58.

Spencer, K. M., Nestor, P. G., Niznikiewicz, M. A., Salisbury, D. F., Shenton, M. E., and McCarley, R. W. (2003) Abnormal neural synchrony in schizophrenia. *Journal of Neuroscience*, **23**, 7407–11.

Spitzer, M. (1993). *The psychopathology, neuropsychology, and neurobiology of associative and working memory in schizophrenia.* Ruprecht-Karls-Universitat, Psychiatrische Klinik, Heidelberg, Germany.

Squires, N. K., Squires, K. C., and Hillyard, S.A. (1975). Two varieties of long-latency positive waves evoked by unpredictable auditory stimuli in man. *Electroencephaolography and Clinical Neurophysiology*, **38**, 387–401.

Steinmetz, P. N., Roy, A., Fitzgerald, P.J., Hsiao, S.S., Johnson, K.O., and Niebur, E. (2000). Attention modulates synchronized neuronal firing in primate somatosensory cortex. *Nature*, **404**, 187–90.

Steriade, M. and Amzica, F. (1996). Intracortical and corticothalamic coherency of fast spontaneous oscillations. *Proceedings of the National Academy of Science*, **93**, 2533–8.

Strandburg, R. J., Marsh, J. T., Brown, W.S., Asarnow, R.F., Guthrie, D., Harper, R. *et al.* (1997). Event-related potential correlates of linguistic information processing in schizophrenics. *Biological Psychiatry*, **42** (7), 596–608.

Sutton, S., Braren, M., Zubin, J., and John, E.R. (1965). Evoked potential correlates of stimulus uncertainty. *Science,* **150**, 1187–8.

Tallon-Baudry, C. and Bertrand, O. (1999). Oscillatory gamma activity in humans and its role in object representation. *Trends in Cognitive Sciences,* **3**, 151–62.

Tallon-Baudry, C., Bertrand, O., Delpuech, C., and Pernier, J. (1996). Stimulus specificity of phase-locked and non-phase-locked 40 Hz visual responses in humans. *Journal of Neuroscience,* **16**, 4240–9.

Tallon-Baudry, C., Bertrand, O., Peronnet, F., and Pernier, J. (1998). Induced gamma-band activity during the delay of a visual short-term memory task in humans. *Journal of Neuroscience,* **18**, 4244–54.

Tiitinen, H., Alho, K., Huotilainen, M., Ilmoniemi, R.J., Simola, J., and Naatanen, R. (1993). Tonotopic auditory cortex and the magnetoencephalographic (MEG) equivalent of the mismatch negativity. *Psychophysiology,* **30**, 537–40.

Traub, R. D., Whittington, M. A., Stanford, I.M., and Jefferys, J.G. (1996). A mechanism for generation of long-range synchronous fast oscillations in the cortex. *Nature,* **383**, 621–4.

Trestman, R. L., Horvath, T., Kalus, O., Peterson, A.E., Coccaro, E., Mitropoulou, V. (1996). Event-related potentials in schizotypal personality disorder. *Journal of Neuropsychiatry and Clinical Neurosciences,* **8** (1), 33–40.

Tsai, G. and Coyle, J. T. (2002). Glutamatergic mechanisms in schizophrenia. *Annual Review of Pharmacology and Toxicology,* **42**, 165–79.

Tsai, G., Passani, L. A., Slusher, B.S., Carter, R., Baer, L., Kleinman, J.E. *et al.* (1995). Abnormal excitatory neurotransmitter metabolism in schizophrenic brains. *Archives of General Psychiatry,* **52**, 829–36.

Turetsky, B., Colbath, E. A., and Gur, R.E. (1998). P300 subcomponent abnormalities in schizophrenia: I. Physiological evidence for gender and subtype specific differences in regional pathology. *Biological Psychiatry,* **43**, 84–96.

Turetsky, B. I., Cannon, T. D., and Gur, R.E. (2000). P300 subcomponent abnormalities in schizophrenia: III. Deficits in Unaffected siblings of schizophrenic probands. *Biological Psychiatry,* **47**, 380–90.

Umbricht, D., Javitt, D., Novak, G., Bates, J., Pollack, S., Lieberman, J. *et al.* (1998). Effects of clozapine on auditory event-related potentials in schizophrenia. *Biological Psychiatry,* **44**, 716–25.

Umbricht, D., Javitt, D., Novak, G., Bates, J., Pollack, S., Lieberman, J. *et al.* (1999). Effects of risperidone on auditory event-related potentials in schizophrenia. *International Journal of Neuropsychopharmacology,* **2**, 299–304.

Umbricht, D., Koller, R., Vollenweider, F.X., and Schmid, L. (2002). Mismatch negativity predicts psychotic experiences induced by NMDA receptor antagonist in healthy volunteers. *Biological Psychiatry,* **51** (5), 400–6.

Van Berkum, J., Hagoort, P., and Brown, C.M. (1999). Semantic integration in sentences and discourse: evidence from the N400. *Journal of Cognitive Neuroscience,* **11** (6), 657–71.

Van Petten, C., and Kutas, M. (1990). Interactions between sentence context and word frequency in event-related brain potentials. *Memory and Cognition,* **18**, 380–93.

Van Petten, C., Coulson, S., Rubin, S., Plante, E., and Parks, M. (1999). Time course of word identification and semantic integration in spoken language. *Journal of Experimental Psychology: Learning, Memory, and Cognition,* **25** (2), 394–417.

Varela, F. J., Lachaux, J. -P., Rodriguez, E., and Martinerie, J. (2001). The brainweb: phase synchronization and large-scale integration. *Nature Reviews Neuroscience,* **2**, 229–39.

Venables, P. (1964). Input dysfunction in schizophrenia. In *Progress in experimental personality research,* (ed. B. A. Maher), pp. 1–47. Academic Press, New York.

Vinogradov, S., Solomon, S., Ober, B. A., Biggins, C. A., Shenaut, G. K., and Fein, G. (1996). Do semantic priming effects correlate with sensory gating in schizophrenia? *Biological Psychiatry,* **39**, 821–4.

von der Malsburg, C. and Schneider, W. (1986). A neural cocktail-party processor. *Biological Cybernetics,* **54**, 29–40.

Wagner, P., Roschke, J., Fell, J., and Frank, C. (1997). Differential pathophysiological mechanisms of reduced P300 amplitude in schizophrenia and depression: a single trial analysis. *Schizophrenia Research,* **25**, 221–9.

Wagner, P., Roschke, J., Grozinger, M., and Mann, K. (2000). A replication study on P300 single trial analysis in schizophrenia: confirmation of a reduced number of 'true positive' P300 waves. *Journal of Psychiatric Research,* **34**, 255–9.

White, P. M. and Yee, C. M. (1997). Effects of attentional and stressor manipulations on the P50 gating response. *Psychophysiology,* **34**, 703–11.

Whittington, M., Faulkner, H. J., Doheny, H.C., and Traub, R.D. (2000). Neuronal fast oscillations as a target site for psychoactive drugs. *Pharmacology and Therapeutics,* **86**, 171–90.

Wible, C. G., Kubicki, M., Yoo, S.S., Kacher, D.F., Salisbury, D.F., Anderson, M.C. *et al.* (2001). A functional magnetic resonance imaging study of auditory mismatch in schizophrenia. *American Journal of Psychiatry,* **158**, 938–43.

Wickens, C., Kramer, A., Vanasse, L., and Donchin, E. (1983). Performance of concurrent tasks: a psychophysical analysis of the reciprocity of information processing resources. *Science,* **221**, 1080–2.

Woldorff, M. H., Hillyard, S. A., Gallen, C.C., Hampson, S.R., and Bloom, F.E. (1998). Magnetoencephalographic recordings demonstrate attentional modulation of mismatch-related neural activity in human auditory cortex. *Psychophysiology,* **35**, 283–92.

Yee, C. M., Nuechterlein, K. H., Morris, S.E., and White, P.M. (1998). P50 suppression in recent-onset schizophrenia: clinical correlates and risperidone effects. *Journal of Abnormal Psychology,* **107** (4), 691–8.

Youn, T., Park, H.-J., Kim, J.J., Kim, M.S., and Kwon, J.S. (2002). Altered hemispheric asymmetry and positive symptoms in schizophrenia: equivalent current dipole of auditory mismatch negativity. *Schizophrenia Research,* **59**, 253–60.

Zouridakis, G., Boutros, N. N., and Jansen, B.H.(1997). A fuzzy clustering approach to study the auditory P50 component in schizophrenia. *Psychiatry Research,* **69**, 169–81.

Chapter 11

Magnetoencephalography

Timm Rosburg and Heinrich Sauer

Introduction

Magnetoencephalography (MEG) devices permit the observation of magnetic fields stemming from electrical brain activity. MEG is, therefore, like electroencephalography (EEG), a method to record brain activity with a time resolution of milliseconds. The high temporal resolution is an important feature for the study of human brain function, as recent findings have stressed the importance of high-frequency signals in cortical information processing. Gamma-band activity (in the range of 40 Hz) is thought to play a key role in human information processing (Varela *et al.* 2001) and some sensory information seems to be processed even at much higher frequencies (~600 Hz) (Curio *et al.* 1994). Although EEG and MEG share some similarities, there are some considerable differences, which lead to slightly different applications. The differences between the methods are discussed here briefly—the reader who is interested in methodological and practical issues of MEG in more detail is referred to Hämäläinen *et al.* (1993) or Elbert (1998).

Methodological considerations

MEG is more sensitive to sources which are orientated tangentially to the head surface than for radial sources, while EEG is equally sensitive to both. Therefore, MEG is well suited for the detection of activity generated in the walls of the sulci, i.e. especially cortical activity evoked by sensory stimulation. If these components are the focus of research, MEG can be regarded as a more sensitive method than EEG, while signals from radial sources, generated on the top of the gyri, are much better detected by EEG. Furthermore, since the magnetic signal decreases with the square of the distance between the source and the sensor, MEG is primarily suited for the detection of signals generated in the neo-cortex (but for exceptions see, for example, Tesche 1996; Lütkenhöner *et al.* 2000; Tesche and Karhu 2000).

From the very beginning, MEG was used as a method for source reconstruction, i.e. on the basis of the measured neuromagnetic field the source which presumably generated the field is determined. As different source configurations can, in principle, generate the same field, the calculation can, however, only be performed with additional assumptions. In the case of a least-square algorithm, the source (or dipole) is

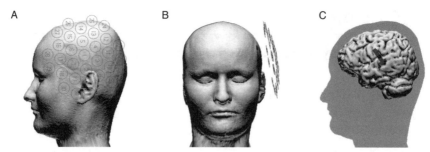

Fig. 11.1 (A) and (B) The position of the sensory array over the head for the individual whose data are shown in Fig. 11.2. Each MEG channel is indicated by a circle and a number. (C) The source of the N100 m is projected on the reconstructed surface of the brain. The midpoint of the black arrow indicates the position, and its direction the orientation of the dipole. (Modified with a different data set from Rosburg *et al.* 2002.)

calculated which produces the lowest deviance between the measured and reconstructed field. Since such a solution is not necessarily anatomically meaningful, it is necessary to validate the assumed location and number of sources by other methods, if possible by invasive recordings in animals or humans. In source reconstruction it is important to note that the electrical signal is strongly influenced by the conductivity and homogeneity of intervening tissues between the source and the electrode, as, for example, by the cranium or cerebrospinal fluid, while the neuromagnetic field is not influenced by these tissues. This makes source reconstruction with EEG a more demanding task than with MEG. Moreover, for the recording of an EEG signal a reference is needed; there are different reference solutions and the use of different references can make it difficult to compare study results. MEG, in contrast, is a reference-free method.

Another considerable difference between EEG and MEG for clinical research is the time needed for the preparation of subjects for measurement. The first MEG studies in psychiatric research were performed with 1- and 7-channel systems. In order to obtain a complete picture of the brain activity in one certain area, the stimulation procedure had to be repeated several times and the neuromagnetometer had to be placed over various scalp positions. When whole-head MEG systems were developed, it became possible to record neuromagnetic brain activity simultaneously from all parts of the scalp with a relatively high spatial resolution, requiring only a comparatively short preparation time. Latest MEG systems have up to 306 channels (e.g. Vectorview system, 4-D Neuroimaging, San Diego, California, USA). Subjects can now be prepared for MEG measurement in 5-15 minutes, which improves the compliance of (psychiatric) patients. Usually, the preparation will take longer for EEG measurements.

Applications of MEG in schizophrenia research

From the beginning, magnetoencephalographic studies of schizophrenia took advantage of the inherent possibility of calculating the sources of evoked cortical activity and focused on the investigation of functional hemispheric asymmetries. When whole-head systems became available, MEG was then used with paradigms already established in EEG research. e.g. auditory sensory gating or the quantification of brain activity in certain frequency bands. Nowadays, the broad spectrum of MEG application includes various aspects of higher cognitive processing, such as face recognition, and the investigation of drug effects.

Auditory evoked fields and hemispheric asymmetry

Schizophrenia is known to affect a wide range of cognitive functions, and one of the aims of brain imaging in schizophrenia research is to reveal the biological correlates of cognitive dysfunctions in order to deduce possible pathogenetic processes. Aberrations in the development and manifestation of hemispheric asymmetry have been regarded as one possible key to the aetiology of schizophrenia (Crow 1990). Auditory stimuli elicit a number of neuromagnetic field components (Figs 11.1 and 11.2). The N100m, as the neuromagnetic correspondent to the electrical N100, represents the most

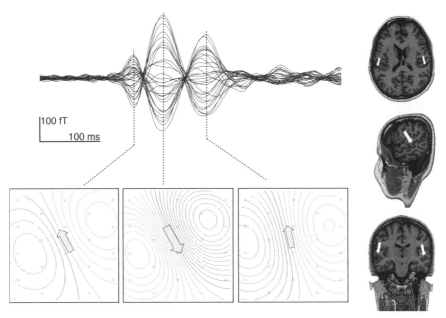

Fig. 11.2 Left top: a prototypical auditory evoked field (AEF) of a single subject with the three main deflections, P50m, N100m and P200m. The 31 MEG channels of the Philips system are plotted over each other. Left bottom: the phase reversal from P50m to N100m and N100m to P200m is also visible in the inversion of the dipole directions; the contour lines of the magnetic field are separated by 20 fT; only the central array of the neuromagnetometer with 20 channels, each indicated by little squares, is depicted. Right column: the reconstructed sources of the N100m, projected on a horizontal, sagittal and coronal MR image. The midpoint of the arrow indicates the location of the dipole, the direction of the arrow its direction. The right hemispheric dipole (right side) is located further anteriorly than the left hemispheric dipole.

reliable auditory evoked field (AEF) component and exhibits some characteristics of hemispheric asymmetry. The generators of the N100m are located bilaterally in the superior temporal gyrus, normally with right hemispheric sources anterior to left hemispheric sources (Mäkelä *et al.* 1993; Nakasato *et al.* 1995; Kanno *et al.* 1998). The hemispheric asymmetry in N100m dipole location is more evident in males than in females (Kanno *et al.* 1998) and might be related to some extent to structural asymmetry of the left and right temporal lobe, as the left temporal lobe of right-handed people is, on average, posterior to the right (Geschwind and Levitzky 1968). Another feature of the N100m is its contralateral dominance, i.e. the response to stimulation is larger on the contralateral than on the ipsilateral side (Mäkelä *et al.* 1993). The exact location of the N100m dipole depends, among other factors, on the pitch of the stimuli ('tonotopy'): the higher the stimulus pitch the more medially the source of the N100m is located (Pantev *et al.* 1988).

The study of the N100m asymmetry in schizophrenia was initiated by Martin Reite and co-workers. They reported a reduced N100m asymmetry in male patients, affecting both dipole location and orientation (Reite *et al.* 1989; Reite 1990). Although nearly all further clinical studies on the N100m revealed changes in N100m asymmetry in schizophrenic patients, the findings are not particularly consistent (see Table 11.1). Differences between schizophrenic patients and controls include: dipole orientation (Reite 1990; Hajek *et al.* 1997*a*, *b*), a reduced asymmetry in dipole location in male schizophrenics (Reite 1990; Reite *et al.* 1997; Teale *et al.* 2000), an enlarged asymmetry in dipole location in female schizophrenics (Reite *et al.* 1997), a reduced asymmetry in dipole location in both male and female schizophrenics (Rockstroh *et al.* 2001; Rojas *et al.* 2002), a reversed asymmetry in dipole location in a subgroup of patients (Tiihonen *et al.* 1998), alterations of the tonotopy (Rosburg *et al.* 2000*b*; Rojas *et al.* 2002), and the absence of contralateral dominance (Rockstroh *et al.* 1998, 2001). Alterations of the hemispheric asymmetry have also been reported in the auditory steady state response (SSR) (Teale *et al.* 2002) and the latency of the P50m (Pekkonen *et al.* 1999) in schizophrenia patients; as well as for the somatosensory evoked field component N20m in patients with schizoaffective disorder (Reite *et al.* 1999*b*).

It is rather difficult to summarize these findings on N100m lateralisation. While most findings lack confirmation, there is some replicated evidence for a reduced hemispheric asymmetry of the N100m dipole location in male patients with schizophrenia. However, there is a considerable variance in the hemispheric asymmetry of the N100m location in healthy subjects (Rosburg *et al.* 2000*b*). Furthermore, as all study samples consisted of medicated patients, a possible impact of antipsychotic medication has yet to be ruled out. In this context, a study of first-episode patients is highly desirable, as an altered hemispheric asymmetry of the auditory cortex of patients could also be related to structural changes and/or auditory hallucinations. The lack of N100m asymmetry was, however, not associated with reductions in structural location asymmetry in one study (Rojas *et al.* 1997). Acute auditory hallucinations are thought to

Table 11.1 A summary of studies on hemispheric N100m asymmetry in schizophrenia research

Study	Patient Sample	Asymmetry in N100m dipole location on average	Other study findings
Reite (1990)	6 M, 4 F	Reduced in male patients. No difference in females	Reduced asymmetry in N100m dipole orientation in male patients
Reite et al. (1997)	11 M, 9 F	Reduced in male patients. Enlarged in female patients	Smaller superior temporal gyri in male patients
Hajek et al. (1997a)	8 F	No difference	Reduced asymmetry in N100m dipole orientation in female patients
Hajek et al. (1997b)	10 M	No difference	Reduced asymmetry in N100m dipole orientation in male patients
Tiihonen et al. (1998)	13 M, 6 F	No difference	Reversed asymmetry of N100m dipole location in patients subgroup
Rockstroh et al. (1998)	7 M, 3 F	No difference	In patients contralateral dominance missing
Rosburg et al. (2000b)	16 M, 12 F	No difference	No group differences in N100m dipole orientation
Teale et al. (2000)	14 M	Reduced in male patients	Reduced asymmetry in N100m dipole location also in schizoaffective patients
Rockstroh et al. (2001)	12 M, 5 F	Reduced in patients	In patients contralateral dominance partly missing
Rojas et al. (2002)	13 M, 6 F	Reduced in patients	Less pronounced tonotopy in patients

have at least an impact on N100m latency and amplitude (Tiihonen *et al.* 1992). Future studies on the effects of varying the stimulus material (stimuli of different tone pitch, tones versus syllables) might help to elucidate possible functional shifts within the auditory cortex of schizophrenia patients (Rosburg *et al.* 2000*b*; Rockstroh *et al.* 2001; Rojas *et al.* 2002).

Sensory gating

In contrast to studies on hemispheric asymmetry, in which the location of the cortical generator represents the central feature, studies of sensory gating focus on energetic aspects. During a sensory gating study-in a paradigm which has a more than 20-year-long tradition in clinical EEG research-individuals are subjected to two auditory click stimuli, usually separated by an interval of 500 ms. Sensory gating is defined as the decrease of the cortical response from the first to the second stimulus, measured electrophysiologically as the amplitude of the positive deflection at the vertex after 50 ms (P50). Patients with schizophrenia have frequently been reported to exhibit deficient sensory gating, i.e. they show only a slight decrease of their second response (see, for example, Freedman *et al.* 1983).

Clementz and co-workers applied this paradigm in magnetoencephalographic investigations. In their first study, Clementz *et al.* (1997) combined MEG with simultaneous EEG recordings and analysed the P50 gating, as well as the suppression of the evoked gamma-band response (GBR) and N100 from the first to the second stimulus. The evoked GBR occurs 30–130 ms after onset of the acoustic stimulus and is phase-locked. Schizophrenia patients were shown to exhibit deficient sensory gating of the electrical P50, neuromagnetic evoked GBR and N100m. In contrast, the suppression of the neuromagnetic P50m, electrical GBR and N100 did not differentiate between groups. In a first follow-up study, comparing the effects of ipsi-, contra- and bilateral stimulation, only a deficient gating of the N100m in schizophrenic patients was confirmed, while differences in the gating of the neuromagnetic GBR failed to reach significance (Blumenfeld and Clementz 1999). The group differentiation for the N100m suppression were larger with binaural than with monaural stimulation. However, in a second follow-up study, using binaural stimulation, only a difference in the N100m amplitude on the first of the two stimuli between the patient and control group was detected, but no group differences in the sensory gating (Blumenfeld and Clementz 2001). Two recent combined EEG and MEG studies of sensory gating are also at variance: Moses *et al.* (2002) found group differences, but Weisbrod *et al.* (2002) did not, regardless of whether the EEG or MEG data were analysed.

In summary, the most consistent finding seems to be that the evoked GBR is unaffected in schizophrenia—see also Rosburg *et al.* (1999). The conflicting findings on sensory gating may, however, be explained by small study groups and the influences of antipsychotic medications. While deficient sensory gating in schizophrenia was thought to be independent of medication with typical antipsychotics (Freedman *et al.* 1983), some EEG studies of patients treated with 'atypical' antipsychotics have found P50 suppression in the normal range (Light *et al.* 2000) and medication with clozapine has been found to improve deficient gating (Nagamoto *et al.* 1999). A possible influence of clozapine on N100m habituation has also been shown (Rosburg *et al.* 2000*a*). The increased use of atypicals in the treatment of schizophrenia in recent years means that the proportion of patients on atypicals is relatively high in MEG studies on sensory gating, and could have decreased the likelihood of detecting deficits in this function.

Quantified MEG

Electrical and neuromagnetic brain activity can also be analysed in the frequency domain; typically divided into bands: delta (>4 Hz), theta (4–8 Hz), alpha (8–13 Hz), beta (13–25 Hz), and gamma (>25 Hz). For spontaneous brain activity and complex tasks, the average spectral power values of frequency bands are usually calculated over time. The technique was originally established in EEG research and termed quantified EEG (QEEG). QEEG studies of schizophrenia have reported, for example, an alpha slowing (Shagass 1976) and an increased theta power (Omori *et al.* 1995).

Quantified MEG (QMEG) in schizophrenia was first reported by Canive *et al.* (1996) and Sperling *et al.* (1996). Canive *et al.* (1996) found a decrease in alpha power and peak frequency during spontaneous brain activity in patients with schizophrenia compared to controls. Moreover, a large proportion of unmedicated patients showed abnormalities in delta power and slow waves, while medicated patients did not. Sperling *et al.* (1996) investigated the spontaneous activity in three schizophrenic patients during auditory hallucinations and reported an increase of fast activity (>12.5 Hz) over temporal regions compared to controls. Complementary to this finding, an increased gamma-band activity (on EEG) in the somatosensory brain areas was described in a patient with somatic hallucinations (Baldeweg *et al.* 1998). In another case report, however, auditory hallucinations were associated with increased neuromagnetic theta activity in the left superior temporal gyrus (Ishii *et al.* 2000). Canive *et al.* (1996) found a bitemporal activity in the theta range in one subject reporting auditory hallucinations during the recordings. Elevated levels of high-frequency activity might also be associated with certain types of medication, e.g. clozapine (Sperling *et al.* 1999).

In a QMEG study using a cognitive task, Kissler *et al.* (2000) observed no overall differences in gamma-band activity between schizophrenia patients and healthy controls, but topographical differences. Whereas control individuals exhibited a left frontal and fronto-temporal increase in gamma power during an arithmetic task, schizophrenia patients failed to exhibit such an effect, or had enhanced activity over the right hemisphere. This research group has also reported increases in spontaneous delta and theta activity in schizophrenia (Fehr *et al.* 2001).

Summing up, QMEG suggests that alterations of neuromagnetic activity occur in the course of schizophrenia, especially during hallucinations. Alterations of the delta and theta band, on the one hand, and gamma band on the other, do not contradict each other, as both frequency bands are assumed to be functionally connected (Lisman and Idiart 1995; Llinas *et al.* 1999). However, the effects of a number of possible confounding factors, including medication, have yet to be clarified.

Alterations of higher cortical functions

There are only a few MEG studies of higher cortical functions in schizophrenia. This may be due to the fact that higher brain functions generally involve a distributed network of cortical generators, resulting in relatively small signal-to-noise ratios. Furthermore, older MEG devices (7–37-channel systems) were only capable of covering parts of the head surface, thus making, for example, the simultaneous observation of frontal and temporal brain activity impossible.

Since whole-head MEG systems became available, this kind of study has been much easier. Most studies of higher cognitive functions in schizophrenia have focused on auditory memory and attention processes. Reite *et al.* (1996) reported a disturbed early auditory memory function in schizophrenic patients. The authors analysed the duration and intensity of alpha suppression over the left and right temporal lobes during an auditory memory task. Compared to controls, a shorter alpha suppression in schizophrenic patients became apparent over the left temporal lobe, while over the right temporal lobe patients exhibited a stronger alpha suppression than controls. Since the performance was the same in both groups, the authors speculated that a left-hemispheric dysfunction in schizophrenia patients could be compensated by a stronger right-hemispheric activation.

The mismatch negativity (MMN) represents an auditory evoked component which is related to the storage of auditory information, early discrimination, and attention processes. The MMN is elicited by infrequent, discernible deviant sounds in a sequence of repetitive auditory stimuli, even in absence of directed attention, which makes it a favourable tool for clinical investigations. Deficits in MMN generation in schizophrenic patients have been reported in both EEG (for an overview see Michie 2001) and MEG studies (Kreitschmann-Andermahr *et al.* 1999; Mathiak *et al.* 2002; Pekkonen *et al.* 2002*b*). As yet, there is hardly any evidence for hemispheric differences of the MMN deficit in schizophrenia. In their combined MEG and fMRI study, Mathiak *et al.* (2002) reported a right hemispherically pronounced MMNm (neuromagnetic MMN) response in healthy subjects for duration deviants, while schizophrenia patients had reduced and more symmetric MMNm responses. However, an alteration of hemispheric asymmetry was not apparent for the MMNm of intensity deviants and in functional magnetic resonance imaging (fMRI) data the haemodynamic response on both intensity and frequency deviants was reduced equally over both hemispheres in patients.

As shown in EEG studies, the deficit in MMN generation is observable in both medicated and unmedicated patients (Catts *et al.* 1995; Javitt *et al.* 1995), and is not affected by newer drugs such as clozapine and risperidone (Umbricht *et al.* 1998, 1999). Furthermore, the finding of a reduced MMN in schizophrenia patients is unlikely to be dependent on the dose of anxiolytic or hypnotic medication, since, according to EEG and MEG data, the MMN did not differ between patients treated with high or low doses of those medications (Kasai *et al.* 2002). In contrast, a possible involvement of the glutamatergic system in MMN generation was apparent in animal experiments (Javitt *et al.* 1996) and the effects of the *N*-methyl-D-aspartate (NMDA) antagonist ketamine in humans suggested that a dysfunction in the glutamatergic system could result in a deficient MMN (EEG: Umbricht *et al.* 2000; MEG: Kreitschmann-Andermahr *et al.* 2001), thus supporting the idea of a NMDA hypofunction in schizophrenia.

While alpha suppression and MMN are related to relatively basic information processing, higher levels of cortical processing were investigated in a recent study on the recognition of facial expressions of emotion (Streit *et al.* 2001). In schizophrenic subjects, hypoactivity was shown in a number of regions, suggesting that the deficient recognition of facial affect in patients might be referred to a dysfunctional cortical network, but sparing the visual cortex.

Taken together, studies on alpha suppression and MMN showed that there is a disruption of cortical information processing in schizophrenia at an early stage. The investigation of model psychoses induced, for example, by ketamine is a very promising tool for future schizophrenia research. In principle, the suitability of MEG for the investigation of higher cortical dysfunctions is well established.

Modulation of cortical activity by drugs

Neuroimaging techniques are useful ways of examining drug effects on cortical activity. In clinical research on medicated patients it is important to know whether observed effects can be related to the disease itself or are due to medication. The investigation of drug effects may also indicate which neurotransmitters are involved in certain brain functions, thus explaining drug effects on the behavioural level. Finally, drugs can be applied to induce a model psychosis and elucidate the pathophysiology of psychotic symptoms.

The first MEG study of drug effects was published by Sinton *et al.* in 1986. In this single-subject investigation, a decrease of the N100m and P200m amplitude was observed after the application of benzodiazepines. In later years the impact of drugs on AEF (and auditory evoked potentials) was studied mainly by Finnish research groups. Scopolamine, an antagonist at muscarinergic acetylcholine receptors, was found to reduce the MMNm amplitude in response to frequency, but not duration deviants, to increase P50m amplitude and to delay N100m latency (Pekkonen *et al.* 2001*a*). Furthermore, scopolamine was reported to increase the evoked neuromagnetic GBR in both young and elderly subjects (Ahveninen *et al.* 1999, 2002*a*), while both benzodiazepines and ethanol were reported to suppress the evoked electric GBR (Jääskeläinen *et al.* 1999, 2000). In a combined EEG/MEG study, the effects of 2 mg haloperidol were studied in healthy subjects (Ahveninen *et al.* 2000). While the neuromagnetic GBR was unaffected for both attended and unattended stimuli, haloperidol suppressed the electric GBR if tones were attended to. Additionally, the neuromagnetic MMN for frequency deviants was accelerated by haloperidol, but the electrical MMN remained unaffected (Pekkonen *et al.* 2002*a*). However, in another series, haloperidol had neither an impact on the neuromagnetic MMNm of frequency deviants (Kähkönen *et al.* 2001), nor were the amplitudes and latencies of the P50m, N100m and P200m significantly influenced by the intake of haloperidol (Kähkönen *et al.* 2001; Pekkonen *et al.* 2002*a*). Finally, tryptophan depletion may affect the MMN latency but not its amplitude (Ahveninen *et al.* 2002*b*).

In sum the results suggest that the deficient MMN generation in schizophrenia is probably not the result of insufficient dopaminergic neurotransmission, as the amplitude of the MMN is not, or at best marginally, modulated by D_2 receptor antagonism. Furthermore, although schizophrenia is associated with increased, and Parkinson's disease with decreased, dopaminergic activity, an attenuated MMN is observed in both groups of patients (Pekkonen *et al.* 1995; Kreitschmann-Andermahr *et al.* 1999). Studies on NMDA antagonists suggest a glutamatergic modulation of the MMN (Javitt *et al.* 1996; Umbricht *et al.* 2000, 2002; Kreitschmann-Andermahr *et al.* 2001). However, the impact of NMDA antagonists and other neurotransmitters has to be investigated in more detail.

MEG research in other neuropsychiatric diseases

Apart from its application in schizophrenia research, MEG has been used as a research tool in a wide range of other neuropsychiatric diseases-including bipolar disorder, stuttering, Parkinson's disease (PD), and Alzheimer's disease (AD)-albeit less extensively than in schizophrenia. Reite *et al.* (1999*a*) extended their studies on the somatosensory evoked field component N20m in patients with schizoaffective disorder (Reite *et al.* 1999*b*) to the investigation on patients with bipolar disorder with and without psychotic symptoms. Psychotic bipolar patients exhibited a reduced N20m asymmetry compared to controls, while non-psychotic bipolar subjects were similar to controls, supporting the hypothesis that a reduced cerebral asymmetry is a feature of psychotic disorders in general (Reite *et al.* 1999*a*).

Salmelin *et al.* (2000) investigated single-word reading in developmental stutterers, and revealed a reversed sequence of cortical activation within the first 400 ms after seeing the word compared to controls, with an early left motor cortex activation followed by a delayed left inferior frontal signal. Stutterers thus appeared to initiate motor programmes before preparation of the articulatory code. In PD patients, MEG was used to study deficient motor activity (Volkmann *et al.* 1996; Halliday *et al.* 2000; Salenius *et al.* 2002). However, Pekkonen *et al.* (1998) were able to show that PD also affects auditory information processing: The latencies of the ipsilateral P50m and N100m were significantly prolonged on left-ear stimulation, pointing toward a possible predominantly left-hemispheric degeneration of the auditory cortex in PD.

In AD, a similar impairment of auditory information processing was revealed (Pekkonen *et al.* 1996). The latencies of the ipsilateral P50m and N100m were significantly increased in patients compared to controls, while the latencies of the contralateral P50m and N100m were unaffected. An attenuated MMN at long but not at short interstimulus intervals (ISIs) was observed by means of EEG and interpreted as a faster decay of the sensory memory trace in AD patients (Pekkonen *et al.* 1994). In accordance with this finding, a recent MEG study by Pekkonen *et al.* (2001*b*) revealed no diminution of the MMN amplitude at short ISIs, but a delay of MMN latency over the left hemisphere ipsilaterally to the stimulated ear. The QMEG in AD patients was analysed first in a pilot study of Berendse *et al.* (2000). The authors found the absolute low-frequency magnetic power significantly and rather diffusely increased relative to controls. A similar finding was obtained by Fernandez *et al.* (2002) on calculation of dipole densities in the delta and theta bands. Slow-wave activity differed significantly between groups in temporo-parietal regions of both hemispheres. The calculation of the so-called synchronization likelihood of MEG recordings gave further evidence for alterations in the gamma-band activity in AD (Stam *et al.* 2002). In a memory task, patients with AD exhibited a lower number of activity sources over the temporal and parietal cortex between 400 and 700 ms, compared to controls, probably reflecting a deficient functioning of the phonological store in patients (Maestu *et al.* 2001).

MEG studies have therefore identified disturbances in information processing in several neuropsychiatric disorders. Comparing the findings to those obtained in schizophrenia research may increase our understanding of neuromagnetic fields in schizophrenia. For example, the finding of an increased slow-wave activity in AD resembles findings in schizophrenia and probably reflects a down-regulation of cortical activity.

Outlook

MEG offers the possibility of describing and quantifying cognitive deficits in schizophrenia with a high time resolution. Separate cognitive functions can be analysed in the time domain, making it possible to disentangle disturbances at one step of information processing from another. One has to be aware, however, that a disturbance at one stage of information processing can affect later, parallel, and even earlier stages. Moreover, the functional state of the brain as a whole influences all steps of information processing. The study of functional relations is facilitated by the increasing availability of whole-head MEG systems, providing information about simultaneous neuromagnetic activity in different brain regions and, therefore, enabling the study of hemispheric and other cortico-cortical interactions.

However, currently very little is known about how observed alterations of neuromagnetic activity in schizophrenia are related to each other; whether, for example, larger slow-wave activity in patients, possibly reflecting a down-regulated cortical activity, increases the likelihood of a decreased MMNm or deficient sensory gating. A better understanding about the relationship between altered neuromagnetic fields and the characteristics of investigated patient samples is also required. It has to be clarified, for instance, to what extent the reduced lateralization of the N100m is associated with structural deficits, psychopathologic symptoms, or a dysfunction in neurotransmitter systems.

MEG can also usefully study the core cognitive dysfunctions of schizophrenia, and evaluate the efficacy of antipsychotics in their treatment. Subject to gains in knowledge about the relation between cognitive and neurotransmitter dysfunctions, MEG could have a role as a diagnostic and therapeutic aid-by identifying patients with particular cognitive deficits, who would benefit from a certain type of pharmacological intervention.

References

Ahveninen, J., Tiitinen, H., Hirvonen, J., Pekkonen, E., Huttunen, J., Kaakola, S. *et al.* (1999). Scopolamine augments transient auditory 40-hz magnetic response in humans. *Neuroscience Letters*, **277**, 115–18.

Ahveninen, J., Kähkönen, S., Tiitinen, H., Pekkonen, E., Huttunen, J., Kaakola, S. *et al.* (2000). Suppression of transient 40-Hz auditory response by haloperidol suggests modulation of human selective attention by dopamine D(2) receptors. *Neuroscience Letters*, **292**, 29–32.

Ahveninen, J., Jääskeläinen, I. P., Kaakkola, S., Tiitinen, H., and Pekkonen, E. (2002*a*). Aging and cholinergic modulation of the transient magnetic 40-Hz auditory response. *Neuroimage*, **15**, 153–8.

Ahveninen, J., Kähkönen, S., Pennanen, S., Liesivuori, J., Ilmoniemi, R. J., and Jääskeläinen, I. P. (2002*b*. Tryptophan depletion effects on EEG and MEG responses suggest serotonergic modulation of auditory involuntary attention in humans. *Neuroimage*, **16**, 1052–61.

Baldeweg, T., Spence, S., Hirsch, S. R., and Gruzelier, J. (1998). Gamma-band electroencephalographic oscillations in a patient with somatic hallucinations. *Lancet*, **352**, 620–1.

Berendse, H. W., Verbunt, J. P., Scheltens, P., van Dijk, B. W., and Jonkman, E. J. (2000). Magnetoencephalographic analysis of cortical activity in Alzheimer's disease: a pilot study. *Clinical Neurophysiology*, **111**, 604–12.

Blumenfeld, L. D. and Clementz, B. A. (1999). Hemispheric differences on auditory evoked response suppression in schizophrenia. *Neuroreport*, **10**, 2587–91.

Blumenfeld, L. D. and Clementz, B. A. (2001). Response to the first stimulus determines reduced auditory evoked response suppression in schizophrenia: single trials analysis using MEG. *Clinical Neurophysiology*, **112**, 1650–9.

Canive, J. M., Lewine, J. D., Edgar, J. C., Davis, J. T., Torres, F., Roberts, B. *et al.* (1996). Magnetoencephalographic assessment of spontaneous brain activity in schizophrenia. *Psychopharmacological Bulletin*, **32**, 741–50.

Catts, S. V., Shelley, A. M., Ward, P. B., Liebert, B., McConaghy, N., Andrews, S. *et al.* (1995). Brain potential evidence for an auditory sensory memory deficit in schizophrenia. *American Journal of Psychiatry*, **152**, 213–19.

Clementz, B. A., Blumenfeld, L. D., and Cobb, S. (1997). The gamma band response may account for poor P50 suppression in schizophrenia. *Neuroreport*, **8**, 3889–93.

Crow, T. J. (1990). Temporal lobe asymmetries as the key to the etiology of schizophrenia. *Schizophrenia Bulletin*, **16**, 433–43.

Curio, G., Mackert, B. M., Burghoff, M., Koetitz, R., Abraham-Fuchs, K., and Harer, W. (1994). Localization of evoked neuromagnetic 600 Hz activity in the cerebral somatosensory system. *Electroencephalography and Clinical Neurophysiology*, **91**, 483–7.

Elbert, T. (1998). Neuromagnetism. In *Magnetism in medicine: a handbook*, (ed. W. Andrä and H. Nowak), pp. 190–261. Wiley-VCH, Berlin.

Fehr, T., Kissler, J., Moratti, S., Wienbruch, C., Rockstroh, B., and Elbert, T. (2001). Source distribution of neuromagnetic slow waves and MEG-delta activity in schizophrenic patients. *Biological Psychiatry*, **50**, 108–16.

Fernandez, A., Maestu, F., Amo, C., Gil, P., Fehr, T., Wienbruch, C. *et al.* (2002). Focal temporoparietal slow activity in Alzheimer's disease revealed by magnetoencephalography. *Biological Psychiatry*, **52**, 764–70.

Freedman, R., Adler, L. E., Waldo, M. C., Pachtman, E., and Franlis, R. D. (1983). Neurophysiological evidence for a defect in inhibitory pathways in schizophrenia: comparison of medicated and drug-free patients. *Biological Psychiatry*, **18**, 537–51.

Geschwind, N. and Levitsky, W. (1968). Human brain: left-right asymmetries in temporal speech region. *Science*, **161**, 186–7.

Halliday, D. M., Conway, B. A., Farmer, S. F., Shahani, U., Russell, A. J., and Rosenberg, J. R. (2000). Coherence between low-frequency activation of the motor cortex and tremor in patients with essential tremor *Lancet*, **355**, 1149–53.

Hämäläinen, M., Hari, R., Ilmoniemi, R. J., Knuutila, J., and Lounasmaa, O. V. (1993). Magnetoencephalography-theory, instrumentation, and its applications to noninvasive studies of working human brain. *Review of Modern Physics*, **65**, 414–97.

Hajek, M., Boehle, C., Huonker, R., Volz, H. P., Nowak, H., Schrott, P. R. *et al.* (1997*a*). Abnormalities of auditory evoked magnetic fields in the right hemisphere of schizophrenic females. *Schizophrenia Research*, **24**, 329–32.

Hajek, M., Huonker, R., Boehle, C., Volz, H. P., Nowak, H., and Sauer, H. (1997*b*). Abnormalities of auditory evoked magnetic fields and structural changes in the left hemisphere of male schizophrenics—a magnetoencephalographic-magnetic resonance imaging study. *Biological Psychiatry*, **42**, 609–16.

Ishii, R., Shinosaki, K., Ikejiri, Y, Ukai, S., Yamashita, K., Iwase, M. *et al.* (2000). Theta rhythm increases in left superior temporal cortex during auditory hallucinations in schizophrenia: a case report. *Neuroreport*, **11**, 3283–7.

Jääskeläinen, I. P., Hirvonen, J., Saher, M. *et al.* (1999). Benzodiazepine temazepam suppresses the transient auditory 40-Hz response amplitude in humans. *Neuroscience Letters*, **268**, 105–7.

Jääskeläinen, I. P., Hirvonen, J., Saher, M. *et al.* (2000). Dose-dependent suppression by ethanol of transient auditory 40-Hz response. *Psychopharmacology*, **148**, 132–5.

Javitt, D. C., Doneshka, P., Grochowski, S., and Ritter, W. (1995). Impaired mismatch negativity generation reflects widespread dysfunction of working memory in schizophrenia. *Archives of General Psychiatry*, **52**, 550–8.

Javitt, D. C., Steinschneider, M., Schroeder, C. E., and Arezzo, J. C. (1996). Role of cortical N-methyl-D-aspartate receptors in auditory sensory memory and mismatch negativity generation: implications for schizophrenia. *Proceedings of the National Academy of Sciences USA*, **93**, 11962–7.

Kähkönen, S., Ahveninen, J., Jääskeläinen, I. P., Kaakola, S., Naatanen, R., Huttunen, J. *et al.* (2001). Effects of haloperidol on selective attention: a combined whole-head MEG and high-resolution EEG study. *Neuropsychopharmacology*, **25**, 498–504.

Kanno, A., Nakasato, N., Hatanaka, K. Ohtomo, S., Suzuki, K., Fujiwara, S. *et al.* (1998). Interhemispheric asymmetry exists in female in the N100m source position of the auditory evoked magnetic fields. *No To Shinkei,* 50, 367–71.

Kasai, K., Yamada, H., Kamio, S., Nakagome, K., Iwanami, A., Fukuda, M. *et al.* (2002). Do high or low doses of anxiolytics and hypnotics affect mismatch negativity in schizophrenic subjects? An EEG and MEG study. *Clinical Neurophysiology,* 113, 141–50.

Kissler, J., Müller, M. M., Fehr, T., Rockstroh, B., and Elbert, T. (2000). MEG gamma band activity in schizophrenia patients and healthy subjects in a mental arithmetic task and at rest. *Clinical Neurophysiology,* 111, 2079–87.

Kreitschmann-Andermahr, I., Rosburg, T., Meier, T., Volz, H. P., Nowak, H., and Sauer, H. (1999). Impaired sensory processing in male patients with schizophrenia: a magnetoencephalographic study of auditory mismatch detection. *Schizophrenia Research,* 35, 121–9.

Kreitschmann-Andermahr, I., Rosburg, T., Demme, U., Gaser, E., Nowak, H., and Sauer, H. (2001). Effect of ketamine on the neuromagnetic mismatch field in healthy humans. *Cognitive Brain Research,* 12, 109–16.

Light, G. A., Geyer, M. A., Clementz, B. A., Cadenhead, K. S., and Braff, D. L. (2000). Normal P50 suppression in schizophrenia patients treated with atypical antipsychotic medications. *American Journal of Psychiatry,* 157, 767–71.

Lisman, J. E., and Idiart, M. A. (1995). Storage of 7 ± 2 short-term memories in oscillatory subcycles. *Science,* 267, 1512–15.

Llinas, R. R., Ribary, U., Jeanmonod, D., Kronberg, E., and Mitra, P. P. (1999). Thalamocortical dysrhythmia: A neurological and neuropsychiatric syndrome characterized by magnetoencephalography. *Proceedings of the National Academy of Sciences USA,* 96, 15222–7.

Lütkenhöner, B., Lammertmann, C., Ross, B., and Pantev, C. (2000). Brain stem auditory evoked fields in response to clicks. *Neuroreport,* 11, 913–18.

Maestu, F., Fernandez, A., Simos, P. G., Gil-Gregorio, P., Amo, C., Rodriguez, R. *et al.* (2001). Spatio-temporal patterns of brain magnetic activity during a memory task in Alzheimer's disease. *Neuroreport,* 12, 3917–22.

Mäkelä, J. P., Ahonen, A., Hämäläinen, M. *et al.* (1993). Functional differences between auditory cortices of the two hemispheres revealed by whole-head neuromagnetic recordings. *Human Brain Mapping,* 1, 48–56.

Mathiak, K., Kircher, T. T. J., Rapp, A. *et al.* (2002). Mismatch response in schizophrenia: comparative fMRI and whole-head MEG study. In *Proceedings BIOMAG 2002, 13th International Conference on Biomagnetism,* (ed. H. Nowak, J. Haueisen, F. Gießler, and R. Huonker), pp. 202–4. VDE Verlag, Berlin.

Michie, P. T. (2001). What has MMN revealed about the auditory system in schizophrenia? *International Journal of Psychophysiology,* 42, 177–94.

Moses, S. N., Thoma, R. J., Hanlon, F. M. *et al.* (2002). Impaired left hemisphere M50 gating in patients with schizophrenia. In *Proceedings BIOMAG 2002, 13th International Conference on Biomagnetism,* (ed. H. Nowak, J. Haueisen, F. Gießler, and R. Huonker), p. 207. VDE Verlag, Berlin.

Nagamoto, H. T., Adler, L. E., McRae, K. A. Huettl, P., Cawthra, E., Gerhardt, G. *et al.* (1999). Auditory P50 in schizophrenics on clozapine: improved gating parallels clinical improvement and changes in plasma 3-methoxy-4-hydroxyphenylglycol. *Neuropsychobiology,* 39, 10–17.

Nakasato, N., Fujita, S., Seki, K., Kawamura, T., Matani, A., Tamura, I. *et al.* (1995). Functional localization of bilateral auditory cortices using an MRI-linked whole head magnetoencephalography (MEG) system. *Electroencephalography and Clinical Neurophysiology,* 94, 183–90.

Omori, M., Koshino, Y., Murata, T., Murata, I., Nishio, M., Sakamoto, K. *et al.* (1995). Quantitative EEG in never-treated schizophrenic patients. *Biological Psychiatry*, **38**, 305–9.

Pantev, C., Hoke, M., Lehnertz, K., Lütkenhöner, B., Anogianakis, G., and Wittkowski, W. (1988). Tonotopic organization of the human auditory cortex revealed by transient auditory evoked magnetic fields. *Electroencephalography and Clinical Neurophysiology*, **69**, 160–70.

Pekkonen, E., Jousmäki, V., Kononen, M., Reinikainen, K., and Partanen, J. (1994). Auditory sensory memory impairment in Alzheimer's disease: an event-related potential study. *Neuroreport*, **5**, 2537–40.

Pekkonen, E., Jousmäki, V., Reinikainen, K., and Partanen, J. (1995). Automatic auditory discrimination is impaired in Parkinson's disease. *Electroencephalography and Clinical Neurophysiology*, **95**, 47–52.

Pekkonen, E., Huotilainen, M., Virtanen, J., Näätänen, R., Ilmoniemi, R. J., and Erkinjuntti, T. (1996). Alzheimer's disease affects parallel processing between the auditory cortices. *Neuroreport*, **7**, 1365–8.

Pekkonen, E., Ahveninen, J., Virtanen, J., and Teravainen, H. (1998). Parkinson's disease selectively impairs preattentive auditory processing: an MEG study. *Neuroreport*, **14**, 2949–52.

Pekkonen, E., Huotilainen, M., Katila, H., Karhu, J., Näätänen, R., and Tiihonen, J. (1999). Altered parallel auditory processing in schizophrenia patients. *Schizophrenia Bulletin*, **25**, 601–7.

Pekkonen, E., Hirvonen, J., Jääskeläinen, I. P., Kaakkola, S., and Huttunen, J. (2001*a*). Auditory sensory memory and the cholinergic system: implications for Alzheimer's disease. *Neuroimage*, **14**, 376–82.

Pekkonen, E., Jääskeläinen, L. P., Erkinjuntti, T., Hietanen, M., Huotilainen, M., Ilmoniemi, R. J. *et al.* (2001*b*). Preserved stimulus deviance detection in Alzheimer's disease. *Neuroreport*, **12**, 1649–52.

Pekkonen, E., Hirvonen, J., Ahveninen, J. *et al.* (2002*a*). Memory-based comparison process not attenuated by haloperidol: a combined MEG and EEG study. *Neuroreport*, **13**, 177–81.

Pekkonen, E., Katila, H., Ahveninen, J., Karhu, J., Huotilainen, M., and Tiihonen, J. (2002*b*). Impaired temporal lobe processing of preattentive auditory discrimination in schizophrenia. *Schizophrenia Bulletin*, **28**, 467–74.

Reite, M. (1990). Magnetoencephalography in the study of mental illness. *Advances in Neurology*, **54**, 207–22.

Reite, M., Teale, P., Goldstein, L., Whalen, J., and Linnville, S. (1989). Late auditory magnetic sources may differ in the left hemisphere of schizophrenic patients. A preliminary report. *Archives of General Psychiatry*, **46**, 565–72.

Reite, M., Teale, P., Sheeder, J., Rojas, D. C., and Schneider, E. E. (1996). Magnetoencephalographic evidence of abnormal early auditory memory function in schizophrenia. *Biological Psychiatry*, **40**, 299–301.

Reite, M., Sheeder, J., Teale, P., Adams, M., Richardson, D., Simon, J. *et al.* (1997). Magnetic source imaging evidence of sex differences in cerebral lateralization in schizophrenia. *Archives of General Psychiatry*, **54**, 433–40.

Reite, M., Teale, P., Rojas, D. C., Arciniegas, D., and Sheeder, J. (1999*a*). Bipolar disorder: anomalous brain asymmetry associated with psychosis. *American Journal of Psychiatry*, **156**, 1159–63.

Reite, M., Teale, P., Rojas, D. C., Sheeder, J., and Arciniegas, D. (1999*b*). Schizoaffective disorder: evidence for reversed cerebral asymmetry. *Biological Psychiatry*, **46**, 133–6.

Rockstroh, B., Clementz, B. A., Pantev, C., Blumenfeld, L. D., Sterr, A., and Elbert, T. (1998). Failure of dominant left hemispheric activation to right-ear stimulation in schizophrenia. *Neuroreport*, **9**, 3819–22.

Rockstroh, B., Kissler, J., Mohr, B., Eulitz, C., Lommen, U., Wienbruch, C. *et al.* (2001). Altered hemispheric asymmetry of auditory magnetic fields to tones and syllables in schizophrenia. *Biological Psychiatry*, **49**, 694–703.

Rojas, D. C., Teale, P., Sheeder, J., Simon, J., and Reite, M. (1997). Sex-specific expression of Heschl's gyrus functional and structural abnormalities in paranoid schizophrenia. *American Journal of Psychiatry*, **154**, 1655–62.

Rojas, D. C., Bawn, S. D., Carlson, J. P., Arciniegas, D. B., Teale, P. D., and Reite, M. L. (2002). Alterations in tonotopy and auditory cerebral asymmetry in schizophrenia. *Biological Psychiatry*, **52**, 32–9.

Rosburg, T., Ugur, T., Haueisen, J., Kreitschmann-Andermahr, I., and Sauer, H. (1999). Enlarged gamma band response of neuromagnetic auditory evoked fields in a visually impaired subject. *Neuroreport*, **10**, 3791–5.

Rosburg, T., Kreitschmann-Andermahr, I., Nowak, H., and Sauer, H. (2000*a*). Habituation of the auditory evoked field component N100m in male patients with schizophrenia. *Journal of Psychiatric Research*, **34**, 245–54.

Rosburg, T., Kreitschmann-Andermahr, I., Ugur, T., Nestmann, H., Nowak, H., and Sauer, H. (2000*b*). Tonotopy of the auditory-evoked field component N100m in patients with schizophrenia. *Journal of Psychophysiology*, **14**, 131–41.

Rosburg, T., Haueisen, J., and Sauer, H. (2002). Habituation of the auditory evoked field component N100m and its dependence on stimulus duration. *Clinical Neurophysiology*, **113**, 421–8.

Salenius, S., Avikainen, S., Kaakkola, S., Hari, R., and Brown, P. (2002). Defective cortical drive to muscle in Parkinson's disease and its improvement with levodopa. *Brain*, **125**, 491–500.

Salmelin, R., Schnitzler, A., Schmitz, F., and Freund, H. J. (2000). Single word reading in developmental stutterers and fluent speakers. *Brain*, **123**, 1184–202.

Shagass, C. (1976). An electrophysiological view of schizophrenia. *Biological Psychiatry*, **11**, 3–30.

Sinton, C. M., McCullough, J. R., Ilmoniemi, R. J., and Etienne, P. E. (1986). Modulation of auditory evoked magnetic fields by benzodiazepines. *Neuropsychobiology*, **16**, 215–18.

Sperling, W., Möller, M., Kober, H., Vieth, J., and Barocka, A. (1996). Spontaneous slow and fast MEG activity in schizophrenics with auditory hallucinations. *Neurology, Psychiatry and Brain Research*, **4**, 225–30.

Sperling, W., Vieth, J., Martus, M., Demling, J., and Barocka, A. (1999). Spontaneous slow and fast MEG activity in male schizophrenics treated with clozapine. *Psychopharmacology*, **142**, 375–82.

Stam, C. J., van Cappellen van Walsum, A. M., Pijnenburg, Y. A., Berendse, H. W., de Munck, J. C., Scheltens, P. *et al.* (2002). Generalized synchronization of MEG recordings in Alzheimer's Disease: evidence for involvement of the gamma band. *Journal of Clinical Neurophysiology*, **19**, 562–74.

Streit, M., Ioannides, A., Sinnemann, T., Wolwer, W., Dammers, J., Zilles, K. *et al.* (2001). Disturbed facial affect recognition in patients with schizophrenia associated with hypoactivity in distributed brain regions: a magnetoencephalographic study. *American Journal of Psychiatry*, **158**, 1429–36.

Teale, P., Reite, M., Rojas, D. C., Sheeder, J., and Arciniegas, D. (2000). Fine structure of the auditory M100 in schizophrenia and schizoaffective disorder. *Biological Psychiatry*, **48**, 1109–12.

Teale, P., Reite, M., Carlson, J., and Rojas, D. (2002). Schizophrenics patients demonstrate reduced laterality of the A/P source location for generators of the auditory steady state response. In *Proceedings BIOMAG 2002, 13th International Conference on Biomagnetism*, (ed. H. Nowak, J. Haueisen, F. Gießler, and R. Huonker), pp. 209. VDE Verlag, Berlin.

Tesche, C. D. (1996). MEG imaging of neuronal population dynamics in the human thalamus. *Electroencephalography and Clinical Neurophysiology Supplement*, **47**, 81–90.

Tesche, C. D. and Karhu, J. (2000). Theta oscillations index human hippocampal activation during a working memory task. *Proceedings of the National Academy of Sciences USA*, **97**, 919–24.

Tiihonen, J., Hari, R., Naukkarinen, H., Rimon, R., Jousmaki, V., and Kajola, M. (1992). Modified activity of the human auditory cortex during auditory hallucinations. *American Journal of Psychiatry*, **149**, 255–7.

Tiihonen, J., Katila, H., Pekkonen, E., Jaakskelainen, I. P., Huotilainen, M., Aronen, H. J. *et al.* (1998). Reversal of cerebral asymmetry in schizophrenia measured with magnetoencephalography. *Schizophrenia Research*, **30**, 209–19.

Umbricht, D., Javitt, D., Novak, G., Bates, J., Pollach, S., Lieterman, J. *et al.* (1998). Effects of clozapine on auditory event-related potentials in schizophrenia. *Biological Psychiatry*, **44**, 716–25.

Umbricht, D., Javitt, D., Novak, G., Bates, J., Pollach, S., Lieberman, J. *et al.* (1999). Effects of risperidone on auditory event-related potentials in schizophrenia. *International Journal of Neuropsychopharmcology*, **2**, 299–304.

Umbricht, D., Schmid, L., Koller, R., Vollenweider, F. X., Hell, D., and Javitt, D. C. (2000). Ketamine-induced deficits in auditory and visual context-dependent processing in healthy volunteers: implications for models of cognitive deficits in schizophrenia. *Archives of General Psychiatry*, **57**, 1139–47.

Umbricht, D., Koller, R., Vollenweider, F. X., and Schmid, L. (2002). Mismatch negativity predicts psychotic experiences induced by NMDA receptor antagonist in healthy volunteers. *Biological Psychiatry*, **51**, 400–6.

Varela, F., Lachaux, J. P., Rodriguez, E., and Martinerie, J. (2001). The brainweb: phase synchronization and large-scale integration. *Nature Reviews Neuroscience*, **2**, 229–39.

Volkmann, J., Joliot, M., Mogilner, A., Ioannides, A. A., Lado, F., Fazzini, E. *et al.* (1996). Central motor loop oscillations in parkinsonian resting tremor revealed by magnetoencephalography. *Neurology*, **46**, 1359–70.

Weisbrod, M., Roehrig, M., Schroeder, J., Scherg, M., and Rupp, A. (2002). Sensory gating in schizophrenic patients. In *Proceedings BIOMAG 2002, 13th International Conference on Biomagnetism*, (ed. H. Nowak, J. Haueisen, F. Gießler, and R. Huonker), p. 201. VDE Verlag, Berlin.

Chapter 12

Spatial analysis of ERP and EEG data

Werner K. Strik and Thomas Koenig

Novel approaches to electroencephalography (EEG)

The extended scalp potential differences that are measured by electroencephalography (EEG), magnetoencephalography (MEG), and event related potentials (ERPs) result directly from the coherent firing of large, predominantly cortical, neural populations. Theoretically, EEG and ERPs, therefore, offer views on brain functions that no other non-invasive technique can provide; these include different modes of oscillation (frequency analysis), transient functional coupling of brain regions (event related synchronization and desynchronization), or temporal sequencing of brain events in the sub-second time domain (microstates). Each of these views might be relevant for the understanding of brain functions during schizophrenia. However, the exploitation of these advantages has suffered seriously from a series of methodological problems that limited the interpretability and scientific impact of EEG and ERP research. The main source of these problems has probably been a misconception about the basic entity upon which to base the analysis: EEG and ERPs are usually viewed as sets of waves representing the time-varying potential at the recording electrodes. The analysis of these wave shapes has then often assumed that the activity at the analysed electrode corresponds more or less to the activity of the brain areas underlying the recording electrode. This lacks a sound physical foundation and introduces the various problems of wave-shape analysis in EEG: the results depend on the recording reference, increasing the number of electrodes produces an increasing amount of increasingly redundant results, the identification of components depends on location and ends up being arbitrary, and volume conduction is not taken into account in the analysis.

Overcoming these problems requires a different approach. In terms of physics, each active neuron in the brain can be considered as a single dipolar electric source. Any dipolar source in the brain produces an electric field on the scalp with a positive and a negative pole equal in size, and extending over the entire head, except for a zero line with no spatial extent (Fig. 12.1). This holds also for the sum of all neuronal activity (i.e. the momentary brain electric state), where the fields that are produced by all active neurons sum up to form a single scalp electric field. Given this tight relation between intra-cerebral sources of brain electric activity and the topography of the scalp electric field, and given a focus of interest that lies initially on the global state of the entire

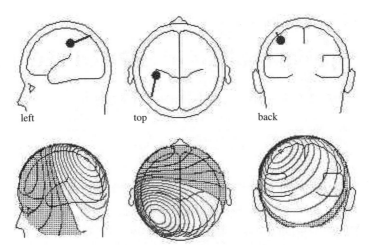

Fig. 12.1 Brian electric field topography generated by a single model dipole source. The upper row shows the three-dimensional location of the dipole. The lower row shows the field generated by that dipole shown with equipotential field lines (shaded [blue] = negative, clear [red] = positive). Note that although a point-like source model has been used, the fields obtained extend over the entire scalp. Picture generated using the Dipole Simulator by Patrick Berg. See Plate 12(a) of the plate section at the centre of this book.

brain, we will thus consider the brain electric field topography as the basic entity of analysis and centre this chapter on the different possibilities for analysing and interpreting brain electric field topographies in spontaneous EEG and in ERPs.

Quantitative topography of evoked brain electrical fields

One of the most studied paradigms in electroencephalographic schizophrenia research is the auditory P300. This is an event-related potential which appears after the recognition of an attended auditory stimulus embedded in a series of irrelevant sounds. It is an expression of the neuronal mass activiation related to the conscious experience of detecting and attributing a meaning to a sensory event.

It has been known since the 1970s that the P300 is reduced in amplitude in schizophrenia. Although this finding was consistently replicated, it lacked both a meaningful interpretation and diagnostic specificity and validity. Many other psychiatric disorders—including depression, dementia, and alcoholism—have reduced amplitudes, and there is a large overlap even between schizophrenics and normals. However, when the P300 topography was considered, a relative amplitude reduction in left temporal regions in schizophrenics compared to normals was observed (Morstyn *et al.* 1983), which was not only specific to schizophrenia, but was also compatible with theories about hemispheric imbalance (Gruzelier *et al.* 1999). Unfortunately, the hemispheric asymmetry of the P300 component was inconsistent across studies and patient populations.

Only when using simple descriptors of the configuration of the brain electric field, such as centres of gravity, and when combining this novel approach with a detailed

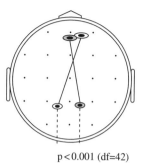

p<0.001 (df=42)

Fig. 12.2 Position of the centres of gravity of the positive (circle) and negative (rectangle) map areas for controls (white areas) and schizophrenic patients (grey areas). The size of the ellipses denotes the standard errors.

psychopathology and subgrouping of the schizophrenic patient groups, was it possible to confine pathologically asymmetric P300 fields to a subgroup of chronic and subchronic schizophrenic patients (Fig. 12.2) (Strik *et al.* 1994 *a*). Further studies showed that the finding is related to verbal memory and, therefore, to language functions (Heidrich and Strik 1997). This is consistent with the specialization of left hemispheric regions for language and with the evidence that the P300 asymmetry is most consistently found in studies which applied silent counting instead of a motor response to the target stimulus as attention control; because silent counting activates language-related functions. Functional MRI (fMRI) studies have shown that target detection during a classical P300 paradigm activated the left superior temporal gyrus bilaterally, with a predominance of the left side (Linden *et al.* 1999). Interestingly, the primary auditory cortex in that region has also been demonstrated to be activated during auditory hallucinations in schizophrenia (Dierks *et al.* 1999). Although it is not yet possible to link these findings on a pathophysiological level, the convergence of evidence of a functional deficit in left temporal regions in a subgroup of chronic and subchronic schizophrenics invites future research to focus: (1) on this specific brain region; and (2) on a restricted, more homogeneous patient population within schizophrenia.

The specificity of left temporal functional deficits for a subgroup of schizophrenics has been further clarified with more recent studies which defined the P300 alterations in other psychotic disorders. In particular, the group of schizophrenia-like acute remitting psychoses (acute polymorphous psychosis in ICD-10; in Europe traditionally known as cycloid psychosis, bouffées delirante, or acute reactive psychosis; cf. brief reactive psychosis in DSM-IV) was found to have normal topography, but increased P300 amplitudes. This was interpreted as an expression of a general state of cerebral hyperexcitation (hyperarousal) clearly distinct from the regional functional deficit found in schizophrenia (Strik *et al.* 1996). Mania may also have distinct P300 features. Since this is a hyperactive state and there are some similarities in the emotional state of mania and cycloid psychosis, one might expect similar findings of hyperarousal. Instead, the P300 amplitudes were found to be normal, but a reduced P300 activity was observed over frontal regions (Fig. 12.3) (Strik *et al.* 1998*b*). This finding was

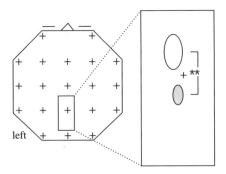

Fig. 12.3 Position of the centres of gravity of the positive map areas for controls (white area) and manic patients (grey area). Again, the size of the ellipses denotes the standard error.

interpreted as a sign of frontal disinhibition and was later supported by a PET study which demonstrated orbito-frontal hypoactivity in mania (Blumberg *et al.* 1999). The contrary finding of frontal hyperactivity in depression with three-dimensional brain electrical source imaging (LORETA; Pizzagalli *et al.* 2002) is consistent with this interpretation and supports the hypothesis of state-dependent changes of right frontal lobe functions in affective disorders.

Brain electrical microstates

In terms of firing rate, the temporal performance of neurons is much worse than that of a computer processor. They have, however, an enormous number of connections with other neurons. This and other evidence suggest that cerebral information processing is encoded in widely distributed spatio-temporal activation patterns. Modern neurophysiological and functional imaging studies have shown that mental operations activate distant brain regions simultaneously, including modality-specific areas. Similar patterns were found during the expectation of sensory input and were interpreted as active templates to structure perception (Freeman *et al.* 1983). It has been further suggested that the subjective experience of consciousness might be identical with the sequence of electrochemical cortical activation patterns during complex information processing and that changes of the mind states are reflected by changes of the brain electrical activation patterns. Electroencephalography allows measuring these activation patterns at the scalp with a time resolution compatible with the speed of change of neural activity, although the limited spatial resolution inherently reduces the number of distinguishable brain states (Lehmann 1990).

In order to reduce data and extract a comprehensive time-domain description of spontaneously occurring brain functional states from the ongoing stream of EEG data, one can establish rules that define, moment by moment, whether some brain field topographies are considered to belong to the same type. Applying such rules has consistently shown that brain field topographies come in packages (microstates) that remain quasi-stable for a brief period of time before quickly changing into another topography (Fig. 12.4). During awake resting, those microstates have an average

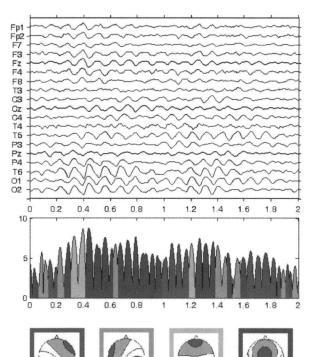

Fig. 12.4 Example of a 2-second multichannel EEG segment (upper part) parsed into spatially defined microstates. The middle section of the figure shows the momentary field strength (Global Field Power, vertical), colour-scale coded with the microstate class identified as function of time (horizontal axis): The microstate topographies with their colour-scale code are shown in the lower part, they were constructed from a large normative population (Koenig *et al.* 2002). See Plate 12(b) of the plate section at the centre of this book.

duration of around 100 ms, ranging from 50 to 1400 (Strik and Lehmann 1993). This is consistent with the time needed for single steps of cognitive operations, as is known from evoked potential and neuropsychological studies. To support the link between brain microstate topography and short-lasting cognitive states, a correlation between the microstate topography and subjective contents of consciousness was demonstrated (Lehmann *et al.* 1998). Furthermore, there are significant changes in microstate characteristics during child development that coincide with cognitive stages postulated by developmental psychologists (Koenig *et al.* 2002).

The first study of microstates in schizophrenia was performed in a group of residual schizophrenic patients. The average topography of the microstates differed significantly from controls, showing a more right posterior–left anterior pattern. This indicates differences in the hemispheric balance and is consistent with the findings in evoked potential studies showing a right posterior deviation from normals (Strik *et al.* 1994*b*). A more recent study on antipsychotic-naive schizophrenic patients was performed with a classification algorithm in order to allow statistics about the reappearance of topographically similar microstates over time. The microstates were assigned to four individual microstate classes. One microstate class differed significantly in topography and duration from controls. This microstate was shorter and the duration correlated inversely with the severity of paranoid symptoms. No group differences were found in the other microstates. The results were interpreted as an intermittent occurrence of deviant brain microstates resulting in inadequate processing strategies and context information (Koenig *et al.* 1999). Interestingly, the state that was reduced in the patients was also found to be reduced in healthy teenagers aged 16–18 years, which coincides with the typical age of onset of the prodromal phase of schizophrenia (Koenig *et al.* 2002).

What can microstate analysis contribute to the understanding of schizophrenia? First, brain information processing is always an interaction between incoming information and the momentary brain state. This state might include dimensions such as emotion, arousal, past experience, neuroendocrinological variables or drug effects. Investigating brain states before the arrival of information may thus target the seed point of aberrant processing of information that is observed during schizophrenia and account for the broad range of paradigms where behavioural and ERP abnormalities have been described in patients with schizophrenia. Secondly, parsing EEG into sub-second microstates may be a way to account for the nature of the observed psychopathology that is intermittent and spontaneously occurring.

Estimation of spatial complexity in time and frequency domain

Without further assumptions about the location and distribution of active sources in the brain, the high time resolution of EEG data can be used to distinguish brain states where the neural activity appears to be well coordinated in time from periods where several brain processes appear to operate independently. This question has become an issue in schizophrenia research as the hypothesis of a functional disconnection of brain regions has been suggested to be a core problem during schizophrenia (Andreasen 1997). In the time domain, a method called Omega complexity has been introduced to estimate the minimal number of independent processes observed during an EEG analysis period (Wackermann 1999) that is based on the entropy of the spectrum of the eigenvalues of the spatial principal components. The omega complexity has indeed been found to be increased over anterior regions of the brain in acute, neuroleptic-naïve schizophrenics (Saito *et al.* 1998), which has been interpreted as loosened cooperativity of in these regions.

An alternate approach has been chosen by Koenig *et al.* (2001), who used frequency-transformed EEG data to establish, frequency by frequency, how much of the multi-channel EEG data can be explained by a common phase; this measure was called GFS (global field synchronization). Applying global field synchronization to two datasets of neuroleptic-naïve schizophrenics from independent laboratories, a significant decrease of common phase was found, but limited to the theta frequency band. Since EEG theta activity has previously been shown to be positively correlated with frontal-lobe working memory functions, it was speculated that the finding reflected a loss of mutual interdependence of working memory functions in patients with acute schizophrenia (Koenig *et al.* 2001).

The appeal of both omega complexity and GFS is that although they are based on the EEG topography, they are spatially global and provide information on the system level, which means that the origins of changes in complexity and synchronization do not need to be the same within and across subjects. When considering the heterogeneity of schizophrenic psychology, this level of description might well be appropriate.

Brain electrical source localization

The physics that defines the brain electric field generated by any combination of electric sources in the brain (the so-called forward problem) is now well established. It is also known how the potentials propagate through the surrounding tissues (cerebrospinal fluid, skull, skin), and realistic head volume conductor models are available. However, the localization of the electric sources in the brain from a given brain electric field (the so-called inverse problem) is difficult, as the brain electric and magnetic measurements do not contain enough information about the generators. This means that mathematically, there is more than one solution for the localization of the sources of a given field, and additional assumptions are required to obtain a unique solution. The typical assumptions concern the solution space, the spatial distribution of the solution, the time course of the regional activation, and the number and/or symmetry of neuronal generators.

In the past decade, methodological developments have investigated systematically, and refined, the different possibilities to localize EEG sources, ranging from models with a few point sources to various distributed solutions. When focal activity is being investigated (i.e. activity in primary sensory or motor regions or epileptic seizures), models with a few point-like sources have yielded physiologically plausible and valuable results. When more widespread activity is under investigation, a method called low-resolution electromagnetic tomography (LORETA) has gained particular interest, and several methodological and clinical papers have been published using this method in the past few years. The special appeal of LORETA consists in the localization of the generators in the three-dimensional head space and in the minimal amount of pre-assumptions about the sources. The space constraints restrict the solution to the head space, and in a recent version to the grey matter of the Talairach brain space. Neighbouring neurons are assumed to be simultaneously active and therefore, a mathematically smooth (i.e. spatially continuous) solution is the physiologically most realistic. The three-dimensional resolution accepts, furthermore, the methodologically intrinsic low spatial resolution, resulting in a 'blurred' localization of the generators (Fig. 12.5). The resolution can be estimated at around 10–15 mm. A comparison with other localization methods based on simulated data has shown that LORETA gives valid and meaningful solutions (Pascual-Marqui *et al.*, 1994).

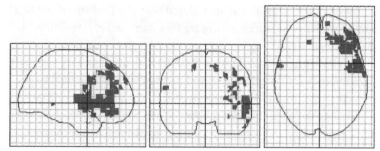

Fig. 12.5 Sample of a LORETA solution in Talairach space, obtained from a single subject performing a Continuous Performance Task (CPT). The figure shows areas where the estimated electric activity evoked by the NoGo condition (requiring a response inhibition) exceeds the activity of the Go condition (requiring the execution of a previously prepared action). The areas shown as activated are identified by voxelwise t-tests ($P < 0.01$) computed over all stimulus presentations (single-sweep analysis). Brain seen from right side, behind, and above

LORETA and other source models are today used as well-founded hypotheses of the loci of different brain functions. For this purpose, statistical parametric maps, i.e. the loci of the statistical differences between two conditions of brain activity, or between two defined groups of subjects or patients, are calculated. The results can then be used to get broad hints about the brain regions involved in particular brain functions or pathologies. Furthermore, they are extremely useful for a triangulation with other functional imaging techniques to mutually complete the data with maximal information about time course and location of the observed phenomena. Similar interpretations must, however, consider the inherent limitations due to the above-mentioned inverse problem and should be validated by experiments that prove the identity of the events found in matching locations and conditions in the measurements with different techniques. In any case, a convergence of findings can be very helpful for the development of hypotheses for further experiments.

The validity of the LORETA solutions has been shown in several studies. Although there are some known limitations, such as a probable underestimation of deep sources and a regression to the mean in some circumstances, the method is valid and useful in combination with morphological and metabolical imaging. In particular, there have been studies that showed the consistency of the localization with the current knowledge from fMRI and PET, and at the same time were able to add important information about the time course of the brain phenomenon. In epilepsy, for example, it was possible to demonstrate that the LORETA solution was consistent with event related activation, i.e. the epileptic discharge, on fMRI; and, in addition, reveal the temporal sequence of the regional excitatory neuronal activity in the subsecond range (Lantz *et al.* 1997). A further validation was done with measurements during the Continuous Performance Test, a cognitive paradigm which activates inhibitory (NoGo) brain functions. The LORETA solution was consistent with the activation patterns described in fMRI and PET studies. In addition, however, due to its high temporal resolution, it also disentangled the inhibitory (NoGo) from the executive (Go) component that rapidly alternate during the test. LORETA, in fact, localized the brain activity specifically associated with behavioural inhibition to the right medial frontal lobe and to the time range of a few hundred milliseconds after the relevant stimulus (Strik *et al.* 1998a).

The LORETA method has only been applied in a few schizophrenia studies to date. Pascual-Marqui *et al.* (1999) investigated nine acute and antipsychotic-naive schizophrenic patients during their first psychotic episode. The control group consisted of 36 healthy subjects. Schizophrenics showed a pattern of bilateral frontal inhibitory (delta frequency range) and right parietal excitatory (beta) activity along with a left central and left temporal deficit of normal resting (alpha) activity. The authors emphasized the capacity of the method to combine the functional information of the ongoing EEG that is contained in the different frequency bands with the localization of the sources in three-dimensional brain space. Mulert *et al.* (2001) investigated 18 drug-free patients and 25 controls with an auditory choice reaction task. The LORETA solution was calculated for the N1 component of the evoked potentials. An early N1 component was localized in the auditory cortex in both the schizophrenic and the control group, while a later component at 120–130 ms was related to an activation of the anterior cingulate gyrus. Only the latter differed between the groups and was decreased in the schizophrenics. The LORETA sources of the late component of the P300 have also been shown to relate to a reduced activity in the left hemisphere, including the left temporal lobe, in a group of schizophrenics compared to controls (Winterer *et al.* 2001). This is consistent with the findings and interpretations of earlier P300 studies (Heidrich and Strik 1997). In a recent evoked potential study based on an auditory discrimination paradigm (the mismatch negativity, MMN), Park *et al.* (2002) combined the LORETA solution with the individual morphological data of 14 schizophrenics and 14 matched controls. The EEGs were recorded with 128 electrodes. The brain electrical sources of the MMN were localized in frontal, parietal, and superior temporal areas, with a clear left hemispheric predominance in controls. Schizophrenics showed significantly reduced activity in the left superior temporal lobe and in the left inferior parietal lobe compared to controls. This supports the important role of the left auditory cortex in schizophrenia.

Combined use of electrophysiology and other functional imaging methods

EEG has unrivalled capability in temporal resolution, depicting different modes of electrical neuronal mass activity in real time, but is limited in spatial resolution. This suggests great potential in combining it with modern functional imaging methods that disclose reliable localizations of brain activity, but lack temporal resolution. At the current level of technical development, the most appealing combination is with functional MRI, which allows disentangling brain events in the sub-second range and, therefore, the application of rapid cognitive activation paradigms and studies of brain connectivity. The method is, on the other hand, limited by not directly reflecting the neuronal discharges, but the more inert local metabolic reactions (overshoot of oxygenated blood supply) to the neuronal activity.

A rather uncomplicated approach to the combined investigation with fMRI or other methods, such as PET or SPECT, and EEG is the separate measurement of the same paradigm in repeated sessions. This is suited to mutually validate time and space information from the different methods when the experimental conditions can be repeated. An example is the behavioural inhibition (NoGo) part of the Continuous Performance Test (CPT). With fMRI, a right medial frontal region was shown to be active during the entire CPT, and ERP source localization showed that the corresponding brain electrical activation appeared at 300–400 ms, but only after the NoGo stimulus and not after the trigger releasing the behavioural response (Go). This combined evidence supports the view that the right medial frontal region is involved in behavioural inhibition (Strik *et al.* 1998*a*). A further example is face perception, where a specialized area can be identified reliably and specifically in the fusiform gyrus with fMRI; event-related potentials together with source localization have demonstrated that the related brain electrical discharges occur as early as 150-200 ms after the visual presentation of the face and with a consistent brain electrical potential (Herrmann *et al.* 2002).

In schizophrenia research, this strategy has been applied to the investigation of hallucinations. An fMRI study had previously shown that, during schizophrenic hallucinations, the primary auditory cortex co-activates pathologically with Broca's area in the left frontal lobe (Dierks *et al.* 1999); the latter activation is typical of internal speech or verbal thoughts and tends to inhibit the primary auditory cortex in normals (Frith and Dolan 1997). This result raised the question whether the brain electrical activity of the auditory cortex, which is assumed to be reflected by the N100 component of acoustic ERPs, is influenced by the presence of hallucinations. Preliminary data suggest that the N100 response to external stimuli is attenuated in the same individual during auditory hallucinations compared to hallucination–free moments (Hubl *et al.* 2003). This indicates that the described metabolic hyperactivity of Heschl's gyrus reflects increased intrinsic processing and not excessive sensitivity to stimuli from the outer world.

A technically much more demanding approach is the co-registration of EEG during fMRI acquisition. The problems arise because of strong magnetic fields inside the MR scanner that severely restrict the use of metallic objects for electrical measurements and sensory stimulation and cause important artefacts in the EEG recording. However, EEG recording systems, including electrodes, cables, and amplifiers, are now available that can acquire reliable EEG from within the MR magnet. The MR scanning artefacts in the EEG records, on the other hand, can be handled by empirically optimized mathematical algorithms.

The complexity of co-registration is counterbalanced by the possibility to correlate simultaneously two aspects of the same brain physiological phenomenon, i.e. the electrical discharge and the local metabolic response. This is interesting from several aspects. Not all brain regions that are metabolically active produce a visible EEG; especially not subcortical structures. However, the very same structures have been postulated to act as pacemakers for the rhythmical electric oscillations that are so predominant in EEG but are not visible on fMRI. Combined EEG and fMRI may thus give important new insights into how interactions between cortical and subcortical regions are organized (Goldman *et al.* 2002). Furthermore, EEG data can be interpreted as they are, whereas resting fMRI data are difficult to interpret. Resting fMRI therefore needs some state markers to become interpretable, and since EEG is a very sensitive brain-state marker, the combination is ideal. Only a few co-registered fMRI/EEG studies which are relevant to psychiatry, and in particular to schizophrenia, have been published until now. However, recent results on multistable perception of illusionary motion (Müller *et al.* 2002) show that this novel strategy is able to contribute substantially to the understanding of the brain regions and physiological mechanisms involved in perceptual distortions controlled by attention, determined by top-down processing, and guided by experience-based expectations.

Outlook and future perspectives

The existing EEG and ERP findings have been criticized as just describing formal differences in brain electrical parameters without meaningful interpretations in terms of brain localization or physiology. The recent topographical P300 findings, based on diagnostic or psychopathological subgrouping, described above are, therefore, an important step towards a comprehensive view of the brain dysfunctions in functional psychosis at a global system physiological level. This novel strategy searches for evidence by triangulation of convergent results from different methodologies, and for mutual validation.

The demonstration of different electrophysiological patterns in different psychotic subgroups, as well as functionally and spatially interpretable results, allows them to be related to the results obtained using fMRI and PET. Beyond the simple statement that different electrophysiological brain activation patterns must be generated by different brain functional states, the results from combined modern techniques can inform the generation of new, testable, pathophysiological hypotheses. Such multi-modal imaging could, for example, address questions such as: 'What is the precise role of the left auditory cortex in auditory hallucinations?' and 'Is arousal combined with hypofrontality the key feature of manic disinhibition?' Future studies which cleverly utilize and combine the available methods with their specific time-, space-, and metabolic resolutions will make a substantial contribution to schizophrenia research in the forthcoming decade.

From the methodological perspective, these developments are equally challenging. Although there have been many improvements in EEG/ERP source localization, and there has been a considerable improvement in the time resolution of fMRI measurements, brain electrical data will never give a complete picture of all active brain regions (not all neural activity generates a scalp field) and fMRI is relatively insensitive to the frequency of neural oscillations. Current views of higher-level brain information processing emphasize the importance of the transient functional binding of localized brain regions through different modes of coherent neural oscillations in order to form short-lasting, widespread functional units. Any adequate study of such processes can thus neither rely on one method alone, be it EEG, MEG or fMRI, but needs to consider the functional interrelations between the methods. Great efforts are being made to allow the simultaneous recording of EEG and ERPs and fMRI data, and the first results are being published (Müller *et al.* 2002). Once such data can be gathered in a more routine fashion, it will be possible to study the normal and abnormal formation of transient neuro-functional units in the brain with high resolution in time, space, and frequency, and to establish their relation to normal and dysfunctional human cognition and behaviour.

References

Andreasen, N. C. (1997). Linking mind and brain in the study of mental illnesses: a project for a scientific psychopathology. *Science*, **275**, 1586–93.

Blumberg, H. P., Stern, E., Ricketts, S., Martinez, D., de Asis, J., White, T. *et al.* (1999). Rostral and orbital prefrontal cortex dysfunction in the manic state of bipolar disorder. *American Journal of Psychiatry*, **156**, 1986–8.

Dierks, T., Linden, D. E., Jandl, M., Formisano, E., Goebel, R., Lanfermann, H. *et al.* (1999). Activation of Heschl's gyrus during auditory hallucinations. *Neuron*, **22**, 615–21.

Freeman, R. D., Sclar, G., and Ohzawa, I. (1983). An electrophysiological comparison of convergent and divergent strabismus in the cat: visual evoked potentials. *Journal of Neurophysiology*, **49**, 227–37.

Frith, C. and Dolan, R. J. (1997). Brain mechanisms associated with top-down processes in perception. *Philosophical Transactions of the Royal Society of London. Series B: Biological Sciences*, **352**, 1221–30.

Goldman, R. I., Stern, J. M., Engel, J., Jr, and Cohen, M. S. (2002). Simultaneous EEG and fMRI of the alpha rhythm. *Neuroreport*, **13**, 2487–92.

Gruzelier, J., Wilson, L., and Richardson, A. (1999). Cognitive asymmetry patterns in schizophrenia: retest reliability and modification with recovery. *International Journal of Psychophysiology*, **34**, 323–31.

Heidrich, A. and Strik, W. K. (1997). Auditory P300 topography and neuropsychological test performance: evidence for left hemispheric dysfunction in schizophrenia. *Biological Psychiatry*, **41**, 327–35.

Herrmann, M. J., Aranda, D., Ellgring, H., Mueller, T. J., Strik, W. K., Heidrich, A. *et al.* (2002). Face-specific event-related potential in humans is independent from facial expression. *International Journal of Psychophysiology*, **45**, 241–4.

Hubl, D., Koenig, T., Federspiel, A., and Dierks, T. (2003). Left temporal dysfunction during auditory hallucinations investigated with auditory evoked potentials (AEP). *Brain Topography*, **15**, 267.

Koenig, T., Lehmann, D., Merlo, M. C. G., Kochi, K., Hell, D., and Koukkou, M. (1999). A deviant EEG brain microstate in acute, neuroleptic-naive schizophrenics at rest. *European Archives of Psychiatry and Clinical Neuroscience*, **249**, 205–11.

Koenig, T., Lehmann, D., Saito, N., Kuginuki, T., Kinoshita, T., and Koukkou, M. (2001). Decreased functional connectivity of EEG theta-frequency activity in first-episode, neuroleptic-naive patients with schizophrenia: preliminary results. *Schizophrenia Research*, **50**, 55–60.

Koenig, T., Prichep, L., Lehmann, D., Sosa, P. V., Braeker, E., Kleinlogel, H. *et al.* (2002). Millisecond by millisecond, year by year: normative EEG microstates and developmental stages. *Neuroimage*, **16**, 41–8.

Lantz, G., Michel, C. M., Pascual-Marqui, R. D., Spinelli, L., Seeck, M., Seri, S. *et al.* (1997). Extracranial localization of intracranial interictal epileptiform activity using LORETA (low resolution electromagnetic tomography). *Electroencephalography and Clinical Neurophysiology*, **102**, 414–22.

Lehmann, D. (1990). Brain electric microstates and cognition: the atoms of thought. In *Machinery of the Mind* (ed. E.R. John), pp. 209–24. Birkhäuser, Boston.

Lehmann, D., Strik, W. K., Henggeler, B., Koenig, T., and Koukkou, M. (1998). Brain electric microstates and momentary conscious mind states as building blocks of spontaneous thinking: I. Visual imagery and abstract thoughts. *International Journal of Psychophysiology*, **29**, 1–11.

Linden, D. E., Prvulovic, D., Formisano, E., Vollinger, M., Zanella, F. E., Goebel, R. *et al.* (1999). The functional neuroanatomy of target detection: an fMRI study of visual and auditory oddball tasks. *Cerebral Cortex*, **9**, 815–23.

Morstyn, R., Duffy, F. H., and McCarley, R. W. (1983). Altered P300 topography in schizophrenia. *Archives of General Psychiatry*, **40**, 729–34.

Mulert, C., Gallinat, J., Pascual-Marqui, R., Dorn, H., Frick, K., Schlattmann, P. *et al.* (2001). Reduced event-related current density in the anterior cingulate cortex in schizophrenia. *Neuroimage*, **13**, 589–600.

Müller, T. J., Federspiel, A., Lövblad, K., Lehmann, C., Dierks, D., and Strik, W. K. (2002). Distributed brain activity during multistable events as obtained by simultaneous EEG and fMRI. *European Archives of Psychiatry and Clinical Neuroscience*, Suppl. **1**, 14.

Park, H. J., Kwon, J. S., Youn, T., Pae, J. S., Kim, J. J., Kim, M. S. *et al.* (2002). Statistical parametric mapping of LORETA using high density EEG and individual MRI: application to mismatch negativities in schizophrenia. *Human Brain Mapping*, **17**, 168–78.

Pascual-Marqui, R. D., Michel, C. M., and Lehmann, D. (1994). Low resolution electromagnetic tomography: a new method for localizing electrical activity in the brain. *International Journal of Psychophysiology*, **18**, 49–65.

Pascual-Marqui, R. D., Lehmann, D., Koenig, T., Kochi, K., Merlo, M. C., Hell, D. *et al.* (1999). Low resolution brain electromagnetic tomography (LORETA) functional imaging in acute, neuroleptic-naive, first-episode, productive schizophrenia. *Psychiatry Research*, **90**, 169–79.

Pizzagalli, D. A., Nitschke, J. B., Oakes, T. R., Hendrick, A. M., Horras, K. A., Larson, C. L. *et al.* (2002). Brain electrical tomography in depression: the importance of symptom severity, anxiety, and melancholic features. *Biological Psychiatry*, **52**, 73–85.

Saito, N., Kuginuki, T., Yagyu, T., Kinoshita, T., Koenig, T., Pascual-Marqui, R. D. *et al.* (1998). Global, regional, and local measures of complexity of multichannel electroencephalography in acute, neuroleptic-naive, first-break schizophrenics. *Biological Psychiatry*, **43**, 794–802.

Strik, W. K. and Lehmann, D. (1993). Data-determined window size and space-oriented segmentation of spontaneous EEG map series. *Electroencephalography and Clinical Neurophysiology*, **87**, 169–74.

Strik, W. K., Dierks, T., Franzek, E., Stober, G., and Maurer, K. (1994*a*). P300 asymmetries in schizophrenia revisited with reference-independent methods. *Psychiatry Research*, **55**, 153–66.

Strik, W. K., Dierks, T., Franzek, E., Stober, G., and Maurer, K. (1994*b*). P300 asymmetries in schizophrenia revisited with reference-independent methods. *Psychiatry Research*, **55**, 153–66.

Strik, W. K., Dierks, T., Kulke, H., Maurer, K., and Fallgatter, A. (1996). The predictive value of P300-amplitudes in the course of schizophrenic disorders. *Journal of Neural Transmission*, **103**, 1351–9.

Strik, W. K., Fallgatter, A. J., Brandeis, D., and Pascual-Marqui, R. D. (1998*a*). Three-dimensional tomography of event-related potentials during response inhibition: evidence for phasic frontal lobe activation. *Electroencephalography and Clinical Neurophysiology*, **108**, 406–13.

Strik, W. K., Ruchsow, M., Abele, S., Fallgatter, A. J., and Mueller, T. J. (1998*b*). Distinct neurophysiological mechanisms for manic and cycloid psychoses: evidence from a P300 study on manic patients. *Acta Psychiatrica Scandinavica*, **98**, 459–66.

Wackermann, J. (1999). Towards a quantitative characterisation of functional states of the brain: from the non-linear methodology to the global linear description. *International Journal of Psychophysiology*, **34**, 65–80.

Winterer, G., Mulert, C., Mientus, S., Gallinat, J., Schlattmann, P., Dorn, H. *et al.* (2001). P300 and LORETA: comparison of normal subjects and schizophrenic patients. *Brain Topography*, **13**, 299–313.

Chapter 13

Towards an integrated imaging of schizophrenia

Stephen M. Lawrie, Eve C. Johnstone,
and Daniel R Weinberger

Introduction

The preceding chapters in this book demonstrate both the great advances in technology applied to brain imaging and knowledge of schizophrenia gained from these techniques over the past 25 years or so. In this chapter, we aim to synthesize the findings from these studies, in the light of other improvements in our understanding of schizophrenia and related neuropsychiatric conditions—particularly those deriving from genetics, epidemiology, and cognitive neuropsychology. We consider the conceptual and methodological problems of the field, and indicate where we think definite progress is likely in the foreseeable future (e.g. scanning both special and representative populations, multi-modal imaging, employing complementary approaches to study disconnectivity, and using neuroimaging databases).

It is hoped that these technologies will illuminate the precise pathophysiological mechanisms by which the aetiological factors produce the clinical picture of schizophrenia-rather than, for example, schizophrenia spectrum or affective disorders. This effort inevitably relies upon overarching conceptualizations of what schizophrenia is (e.g. as defined in DSM-IV) and how findings should be interpreted (e.g. in a neurodevelopmental model); both of which are likely to be refined by such research. Almost all informed observers agree that schizophrenia is multifactorial but highly genetic, polygenic in almost all cases, and that various neurodevelopmental disruptions are evident in childhood and adolescence (Marenco and Weinberger 2000). It is very difficult to obtain other reliable information until after illness onset, such that widely accepted roles for stress and illicit drugs as precipitants in the predisposed remain at least scientifically controversial (Cannon and Jones 1996; Murray *et al.* 2002). At diagnosis, patients have pronounced psychotic symptoms, cognitive deficits, and social dysfunctions, some of which are ameliorated by dopamine blockade. In the context of using neuroimaging to elucidate mechanisms of brain dysfunction in schizophrenia, genes have been identified that are likely to be valid causative factors. In contrast to all the very substantial neuroimaging findings, genes transcend phenomenology and represent, by definition, mechanisms of disease. Thus, they are likely to transform any future applications of neuroimaging to the study of schizophrenia. We will attempt to address this as well.

The earlier chapters in this book make it clear that, despite notable heterogeneity, groups of patients with schizophrenia have demonstrable abnormalities on structural and functional imaging. The gross neuropathology of schizophrenia includes a slight global reduction in brain tissue and a general increase in cerebrospinal-fluid-containing volumes—observable on pneumoencephalography and CT (Chapter 1), sMRI (Chapters 2, 3, and 6) and at post-mortem (Harrison 1999). sMRI studies suggest that volume reductions are most marked in grey matter, especially in parts of the temporal lobe; but, while the cellular basis appears to be small neurons and reduced neuropil, it is unclear that the structural changes observed with neuroimaging directly reflect this. Convincing reductions in *N*-acetyl-aspartate (NAA) on MRS (Chapter 4), and demonstrations of altered white matter integrity on DTI (Chapter 5), also require neuropathological explanations. With functional imaging, matters are yet more complex—not least because of the possibility that structural deficits may underlie them. While it is clear that patients with schizophrenia have a variety of information processing deficits that are not simply iatrogenic (Chapters 10–12), these are related to clinical status and performance effects in as yet unclear ways (Chapter 9). Dopaminergic dysfunction remains the most robust neurochemical explanation of the disorder (Chapters 7 and 8) but it may only be indirectly involved.

These uncertainties can guide the formulation of critical questions which can be addressed by brain imaging in schizophrenia. The key issues include:

◆ When are structural and functional changes first evident, and which genetic and environmental factors interact to cause these?

◆ Are the structural changes reconcilable with the post-mortem tissue histopathology, or are they reflecting different processes?

◆ Can psychosocial stress, substance abuse, and other brain insults precipitate further structural and functional abnormalities?

◆ In which particular sub-regions/nuclei are changes most pronounced?

◆ Do the structural changes reflect an actual loss of parenchymal volume or physiological compensations for altered activity?

◆ Is the neuropathology primarily one of disordered neuroplasticity or neurotoxicity?

◆ Is dopaminergic dysfunction primary or secondary?

◆ Do functional abnormalities have structural causes or effects?

◆ Which general and/or specific information-processing deficits cause the functional imaging abnormalities in schizophrenia?

◆ Do imaging findings relate to clinical features of the disorder? and perhaps most importantly,

◆ Are there useful clinical parameters that can emerge from imaging data?

Imaging risk factors and their interactions

There is little doubt that schizophrenia is primarily a genetic disorder—with a heritability in the region of 80% (Cannon *et al.* 1998; Cardno and Gottesman 2000; McGuffin *et al.* 2002). This is an obvious starting point for risk factor imaging, which has focused, until very recently, on studies of unaffected relatives. While familial effects are apparent, particularly in terms of reduced medial temporal volumes on sMRI (see Chapter 2), and abnormal prefrontal activity on fMRI (Callicott *et al.* 2003; Whalley *et al.* 2004), this approach can only allude to familial effects and much more specific data is required. On the other hand, a similar pattern of deficits in healthy siblings as in ill subjects strongly implicates the pattern as a phenotypic expression of genetic risk rather than an epiphenomenon.

Genomics

A potent known genetic risk factor for a schizophrenia-like illness is the DiGeorge or velo-cardio-facial syndrome (VCFS), which may increase the risk of schizophrenia 20-fold (Goodman 2003), although VCFS is phenotypically promiscuous and is associated with other psychiatric phenotypes as well. It is attributable in the vast majority of cases to a 22q11 deletion, of about 30 genes. VCFS is associated with sMRI abnormalities which resemble to some degree those found in schizophrenia (Reiss *et al.* 2000), but these may be as non-specific as the protean phenotypic manifestations of the syndrome.

Recent work has identified a number of genes that may increase susceptibility to schizophrenia, some of which have been greeted with enthusiasm from commentators due to their statistical robustness and neurobiological plausibility. Most persuasively, two novel genes with impressive functional significance have been described (Cloninger 2002; Harrison and Owen 2003):

◆ neuroregulin 1 (NRG1)-NRG1 has roles in neuronal migration, *N*-methyl-*D*-asparate (NMDA) receptor regulation, and synaptic plasticity;

◆ G72 and D-amino acid oxidase (DAAO) genes-G72 is primate-specific, interacts with DAAO and metabolizes D-serine, which modulates NMDA receptors.

Both of these genes were identified by association analysis targeting areas highlighted in linkage analyses, and probably reduce glutamate neurotransmission with a secondary disinhibition of limbo-cortical activity. The best replicated results are for NRG1, while the strongest effect may come from the interaction of G72 and DAAO. It should be noted, however, that a functional variation in the DNA sequence of these genes has yet to be identified, and the G72 DAAO interaction has yet to be demonstrated *in vivo*.

Two additional likely genes for schizophrenia do possess functional variants and could be expected to impact directly on the imaging findings in schizophrenia:

◆ D_2 receptor (DRD$_2$) gene—in which the Cys311 variant is associated with less inhibition of cyclic AMP (cAMP) synthesis (Glatt *et al.* 2003; Jönsson *et al.* 2003);

◆ catechol-*O*-methyl-transferase (COMT) enzyme gene—in which a Val158/108Met polymorphism influences enzyme activity.

D_2 receptor function is very likely to be disturbed in schizophrenia (see Chapters 7 and 8). A small number of ligand studies have examined the effects of other DRD$_2$ polymorphisms in controls, but with inconsistent results (Martinez *et al.* 2001). The time is therefore ripe for studies of the association between the DRD$_2$ Ser311Cys gene and D_2 ligand binding, and perhaps of its effects on dopaminergic function in pharmacological fMRI experiments, to examine the impact of the polymorphism on *in vivo* function in health and disease; although the allele frequency of only 3% means large numbers of potential participants will need to be screened first.

Ideally, genetic associations should be reliably replicated several times, and have demonstrable effects *in vitro* and *in vivo*, before examinations of their possible effects with imaging in patients. COMT is a good example of this. COMT is one of the genes implicated in VCFS, has impressive supporting biological evidence, including imaging studies in healthy controls and schizophrenics, and appears to be especially important in regulating prefrontal dopamine signalling. Egan *et al.* (2001*a*) confirmed the original observation that the Val allele was preferentially transmitted to schizophrenic offspring in families, and demonstrated a dose effect of COMT genotype expression and performance on the Wisconsin Cart Sorting Test. Several other groups have also observed effects of COMT on frontal cortex function. In the study by Egan *et al.*, COMT allelic expression was further related to brain physiology during a working memory task, in that the Met allele load predicted a stronger response in prefrontal cortex. This was subsequently confirmed in an independent sample by Mattay *et al.* (2003). The Val allele is also associated with increased tyrosine hydroxylase gene expression in striatal projections in postmortem normal human brain tissue (Akil *et al.* 2003). These findings suggest that the COMT Val allele may raise the liability to schizophrenia by disturbing striatal presynaptic dopamine and prefrontal function (see Chapter 7).

The research priorities in combined gene-imaging studies therefore include studies: to replicate and extend the COMT results on fMRI, examining D_2 ligand binding in people with the DRD$_2$ Ser311Cys polymorphism, and to conduct pilot sMRI (and perhaps MRS) studies in those with NRG1 polymorphisms. Other genes that may not increase the risk for schizophrenia may still have important modifiying effects on imaging-based manifestations of the disease (e.g. Hariri *et al.* 2002*b*; Egan *et al.* 2003). Financial and practical considerations inevitably mean that multiple genes, imaging modalities, and measures will be examined—with the ability to assess additive or multiplicative genetic effects, but the downside of more data dredging analyses and false leads. The number of observations now available from genetic microarray and image voxel-based analyses means that many false-positive findings will emerge unless imaging researchers exercise caution before embarking on such exciting work. Almost any gene–scan association could meet the rather vague biological plausibility criterion for causation. For example, some of the best evidence for genetic effects on brain structure and function in schizophrenia is for the prefrontal cortex (see Chapters 2 and 7), but the number of genes expressed in these areas and/or with relevant developmental effects (over a 30-year period!) includes the lion's share of the entire human genome.

These studies will also have to wrestle with genetic and phenotypic heterogeneity; and many potential gene–environment correlations and interactions (additive or multiplicative). Remarkable variations in the phenotypes associated with, for example, VCFS and Fragile X demonstrate that overlapping gene family effects, and the various gene–gene (epistatic), stochastic, and developmental influences on transcription control, render the relations between genes and pathology complex (Rutter 2002). Some gene expression abnormalities in schizophrenia are likely to be secondary, possibly compensatory, effects, unrelated to the disease *per se*. There may be age- or sex-specific effects that need to be controlled for or examined in suitably large cohorts. Identifying protective or resilience genetic factors, including those that protect against environmental hazards, may be most important of all for the development of novel therapeutic approaches. It is none the less likely that combined gene–imaging studies will, in time, clarify how particular susceptibility genes relate to specific aspects of the pathophysiology of schizophrenia.

Other risk factors

In comparison with family history, the evidence for other risk factors is not strong and the putative effects are themselves relatively weak (Cannon and Jones 1996; Murray *et al.* 2002). Apart from obstetric complications (OCs), their associations with imaging findings have been little studied (Lawrie 2004). Further, these 'risk factors' could be on the causal pathway between genes and psychosis, fixed-trait markers (e.g. schizoid behaviour), epiphenomenal indicators of an increased risk of several neurodevelopmental disorders (e.g. developmental delay), or early disease manifestations. How they might interrelate is almost completely unknown. These uncertainties demand more research rather than less. Indeed, the strength of the evidence, the increased risk conferred, and the integrative work thus far for some specific OCs is comparable to that for particular genes. Individual OCs can be usefully considered as complications of pregnancy (e.g. bleeding), fetal growth (e.g. low birth weight), and delivery (e.g. emergency section), and some of them have summary odds ratios of about 2–4 (Cannon *et al.* 2002) and replicated sMRI associations. In patients with schizophrenia, and their relatives, pregnancy complications and low birth weight have been related to ventriculomegaly and 'atrophy' on CT and sMRI (see Chapters 1 and 2), while hypoxia during delivery appears to reduce hippocampal volumes. Both relationships are likely to reflect gene–environment interaction, rather than correlation, but multiple genes and disease processes may be involved. Certainly, low birth weight and hypoxia are interrelated, and linked to similar structural abnormalities of the brain, as observed in schizophrenia; and yet they are more likely to lead on to generalized cognitive and motor deficits, specific developmental disorders, and attention deficit hyperactivity disorder (ADHD), than psychosis.

Establishing the role and imaging correlates of precipitants in a disorder with as long a gestation as schizophrenia is difficult. The role of 'stress' has been much better established in anxiety and affective disorders than in schizophrenia. However, our own prospective high-risk study has suggested that major stressors can trigger psychosis (Miller *et al.* 2001), at least in the genetically predisposed, and the convincing evidence that life events can precipitate psychotic relapses (Butzlaff and Hooley 1998) is unlikely to reflect an entirely secondary phenomenon. The regular use of illicit drugs, and cannabis in particular, are more clearly linked to the onset of psychotic symptoms and schizophrenia (Miller *et al.* 2001; Semple *et al.* 2004), than to anxiety or depression. Stress and cannabis may, however, act in very similar ways across disorders, at least at a gross regional level. The acute effects of cannabis and other psychotomimetics on fronto-limbic activity in healthy controls (Hariri *et al.* 2002*a*) are noticeably similar to those induced by cognitive and pharmacological challenge studies in anxiety states, mood disorders, and schizophrenia (see Chapters 7 and 8; Phillips *et al.* 2003; Steele and Lawrie 2004). Dopamine and other monoaminergic pathways mediate these effects and are implicated in the processes of behavioural sensitization and reduced neuroplasticity that may maintain psychotic disorders (see, for example, Moore *et al.* 1999). Of course, there are likely to be critical differences in such disruptions between schizophrenia and the affective disorders, but establishing them will probably require direct comparison of disease-specific effects and a move away from simply examining one system in one disorder.

Phenotype definition

The development of reliable, operationalized diagnoses was one of the major achievements in psychiatry during the twentieth century. These have undoubtedly facilitated the acquisition of the knowledge we now have about the psychoses, but recurrent replication failures and the heterogeneity evident in the biological associations of schizophrenia have led to calls for alternative non-diagnosis-based approaches. For example, common symptom factors might relate to distinguishable disease processes, which combine in various ways in different disorders—but the results are also inconsistent (see Chapter 2). The amount of variance explained in these models is generally low and might be improved by including, for example, developmental and social data. More progress has been made in mapping individual psychotic symptoms (see Chapters 2, 7, and 9) but these are arguably too unstable, unreliably elicited, and non-specific (some being found even in healthy adolescents), to reliably index the biology of schizophrenia. The clinical distinction between depressed mood and flat affect, or between flight of ideas and loosening of associations, is not straightforward and subject to observer bias. These considerations have led to an increasing interest in inherited risk factors or endophenotypes.

Endophenotypes

The concept of endophenotypes, borrowed from psychiatric genetics, is increasingly used in the design and interpretation of neurobiological studies of schizophrenia and their relatives. In addition to furthering genetic analysis, they may clarify classification and diagnosis and foster the development of animal models. An endophenotype can be usefully defined as a variable that is heritable (preferably demonstrated by association with a candidate gene or gene region, but at least inferred from relative risk for the disorder in relatives), and associated with the disease. Gottesman and Gould (2003) recently proposed the following criteria:

- The endophenotype is associated with illness in the population.
- The endophenotype is heritable.
- The endophenotype is state-independent (manifests in an individual whether or not illness is active).
- Within families, endophenotype and illness co-segregate.
- The endophenotype found in affected family members is found in non-affected family members at a higher rate than in the general population.

There is certainly cause for optimism that this approach may bring new insights. Functional imaging measures are probably more accurate assays of genetic effects on information processing than are behavioural tests (Hariri *et al.* 2002*a,b*; Egan *et al.* 2003). The same may also be true of structural imaging, in as much as both CT and sMRI studies have reported stronger statistical relationships between regional brain volumes and genetic markers than between anatomy and disease status (Shihabuddin *et al.* 1996; Wassink *et al.* 2003). Endophenotypes may, in turn, be more accurately measured than clinical features, and may have fewer determinants. They will certainly be more practical and powerful measures in most familial studies of genetic and imaging effects due to the numbers required. There is also no shortage of candidate markers. A host of information-processing abnormalities have been suggested as endophenotypic markers, but await demonstrable genetic underpinnings (see Chapter 10). Several functional and structural imaging parameters have been proposed more recently, particularly in prefrontal (Egan *et al.* 2001*a*) and medial temporal lobes (Lawrie *et al.* 2003). In the Edinburgh High Risk Study (EHRS), we have also found that the extent of the reduction in thalamus volume is related to the degree of genetic risk (Lawrie *et al.* 2001) and that those with the smallest thalami are most likely to become ill (Johnstone *et al.*, 2004). The same may be true of thalamic dysfunction on fMRI (Whalley *et al.* 2004) and as ascertained with various tests of 'sensory gating'.

However, there are some limitations of this approach. Clearly, it is the difference between affected and unaffected relatives (ill versus well) that is of central interest, rather than the common extended phenotypic markers, although the difference between well relatives and well-matched, not at increased risk controls is of equal importance. Additional genetic and other factors are presumably required to explain why there are more people with imaging and neuropsychological markers of risk than will develop schizophrenia or any related disorder (Faraone *et al.* 1995; Johnstone *et al.*, 2004). The polygenic and multifactorial aetiology of schizophrenia suggests that there are multiple pathophysiological routes to schizophrenia—some of which may be characterizable as schizophrenia-specific endophenotypes, but could equally be associated with more than one disease. Varying combinations of endophenotypes and environmental factors may lead, for example, to overlapping abnormalities in brain structure and function in schizophrenia spectrum and affective disorders, and of disrupted neurodevelopment in autistic spectrum disorders and schizophrenia. Groups of people at these fuzzy boundaries may share some key biological abnormalities but not others. Endophenotypes may also be shared between less obviously similar disorders; for example, working memory impairment and dopaminergic dysfunction have been proposed as endophenotypes for both schizophrenia and ADHD (Castellanos and Tannock 2002).

These concerns make the term 'intermediate phenotype', as one between genotype and clinical phenotype, preferable to endophenotype. It simply brings the observable phenotype closer to the basic genetic mechanism of dysfunction (Weinberger *et al.* 2001). Establishing which genes account for variation in these traits, and how they interact with each other and other background factors to modify the emergent clinical phenotype, is a complicated but tractable approach to the otherwise mysterious genetic and phenotypic heterogeneity in schizophrenia. Such studies will at least allow more precise scientific study of these possibilities and offer the prospect of more refined tests of diagnostic specificity.

Disease specificity

None of the identified biological associations of schizophrenia can be said to be specific: in some respects the aetiopathogenesis is similar to that of affective disorder, but more severe. Yet this resemblance is unlikely to simply reflect the existence of a 'unitary psychosis'—given the differences in typical symptoms, course, and treatment responses, and clear demonstration that there is segregation of genes (Cannon *et al.* 1998; Cardno and Gottesman 2000). By focusing on hospital-and clinic-based samples, rather than representative populations, we may have reduced specificity by indexing common developmental risk factors and diagnostic co-morbidities in more severe cases. These biases may have been compounded by arbitrarily excluding people with related disorders such as, for example, delusional disorder, reactive psychoses, and even mental retardation. On the other hand, there may only be a narrow range of ways in which brains 'fail', making it very difficult to distinguish disorders by the time they present clinically. It is even possible that small hippocampi are risk markers for a wide range of conditions, including severe anxiety (Gilbertson *et al.* 2002). This gives rise to the discomforting thought that imaging may have a limited ability to delineate fundamental mechanisms.

At present, before genetic factors are better elucidated, the best bet for distinguishing schizophrenia and affective disorder (from indirect comparisons of replicated findings in the disorders) is that the amygdala may be large and 'hyperfunctional' in active affective disorder, but small and hypofunctional as a trait abnormality in schizophrenia (Phillips *et al.* 2003). There are also direct demonstrations of differences between these disorders in 'hypofrontality', mismatch negativity, and the P300 (see Chapters 9 and 10), and promising candidates in the sMRI differences between childhood psychoses and ADHD (Chapter 3) and the dopamine receptor response to amphetamine in schizophrenia and depression (Chapter 8). However, these intriguing findings have yet to be replicated with sufficient frequency to be confident that they represent qualitative rather than quantitative effects.

Imaging overlapping disruptions in neuronal networks across different disorders may therefore index overlapping phenotypes but in different combinations, or establish different underpinnings of these dysfunctions that are not evident at the behavioural level. Improvements in imaging technology and knowledge of basic neuroscience may be sufficient to give greater differentiation, but the critical differences between disorders may be in more subtle disintegrations of brain structure and function, in terms of anatomical, functional, and effective disconnectivities, rather than the gross regional abnormalities mainly examined to date (see below). Given the obvious clinical differences between some conditions mentioned here, it is difficult to envisage how there could not be differences at the neuronal and possibly even sub-regional level.

A detailed neuroanatomy of schizophrenia

Although non-specific and of unclear cause, it is none the less no longer questionable that groups of patients with schizophrenia have abnormal brain structure (see Chapter 2). Now that this has been shown with a variety of post-mortem, hand-tracing, and automated approaches, artefactual explanations are unlikely. A sceptic might argue that the abnormalities represent the effects of co-morbid alcohol or drug use, or antipsychotic medication, are epiphenomena of ill-defined disease processes, and/or markers of more severe illness in the male patients who are typically studied. It may be said against such arguments that many studies exclude the substance-dependent, alcoholics do not exhibit the temporal lobe abnormalities that characterize schizophrenia (Mathalon *et al.* 2003), and cannabis is not apparently associated with structural change. Similarly, the most disturbed patients are not suitable for imaging studies, and there are no consistent sex or severity effects. Further, relatives and high-risk studies demonstrate that at least some of the changes are not direct consequences of the illness or its effects. A large, population-based study of the effects of drugs, sex and severity on sMRI measures in schizophrenia would bolster these arguments, but there are higher priorities.

Clarifying disease processes and clinical associations

Refining our knowledge of the anatomy of schizophrenia is an inevitable corollary of improving scanner resolution, more precise region of interest (ROI) tracing protocols, and the increasing use of automated techniques. These will facilitate the study of the determinants and time course of normal and abnormal neurodevelopment. In schizophrenia research, these studies would best focus on medial temporal and prefrontal structures, such as specific amygdala and thalamic nuclei, and frontal and (para)hippocampal subfields. Notwithstanding the arguments that psychotic symptoms may be influenced by many factors, and are probably attributable to distributed network pathologies that are better assessed with other techniques, there is enough evidence that prefrontal cortex volume and chemical composition relate to negative symptoms (Chapters 2 and 4), and anterior/posterior superior temporal gyrus volumes are correlated with hallucinations/thought disorder, respectively (Chapter 2), to suggest that refined studies are worthwhile. Indeed, progress could simply be made by more careful measurement and analysis of clinical associations in larger numbers of patients, or by employing multivariate statistical approaches applied to functional imaging data sets (Nestor *et al.* 2002). Symptom severity may, however, be more closely associated with the regional differences between patients and controls, than with a variably reduced raw volume.

Establishing whether there are changes in brain structure around the onset of psychosis, when they occur, and what their causes and clinical associations might be, is arguably the greatest priority for sMRI and related techniques. The impressive evidence that relatives and subjects at high risk have reduced volumes of the medial temporal lobes and probably also have some ventriculomegaly (Chapter 2; Lawrie 2003) that fall short of the changes usually found in patients themselves, suggests that at least some of these changes predate frank psychosis and associated behaviours. Greater abnormality may predict psychosis, but there may also be further structural reductions as the illness develops, particularly in the frontal and temporal lobes (Lawrie *et al.* 2002; Pantelis *et al.* 2003). What could and should be done with existing data is to relate changes to key clinical developments in pre- and peri-morbid symptoms and cognitive dysfunction.

Increasing automation

Automated techniques are inherently more suitable for identifying the subtle disturbances which may underlie complex phenomena. Ever improving software for brain extraction, image registration, and tissue-type segmentation (see Chapter 6) will improve resolution in automated studies. Specific techniques such as (sub)cortical flattening to improve registration and shape analysis offer much in this regard. Shape analysis has the potential to localize abnormalities in the ventricles, may better discriminate patients and controls than volumetry in, for example, the hippocampus (Wang *et al.* 2001), and can highlight potential areas of disconnectivity based upon that localization. Refinements of voxel-based morphometry (VBM), comparing translation vectors or tensors, in deformation- and tensor-based morphometry (DBM and TBM), should further improve sensitivity. DBM has already been applied to study differences in brain size and shape in schizophrenia, with promising results (Volz et al. 2000).

However, there are several limitations to these approaches, perhaps particularly as applied to developmental rather than degenerative disorders. The typical stages of co-registration, segmentation, and smoothing each introduce noise which could explain the less than perfect agreement with ROI (Wright et al. 1999; Job et al. 2003). All stereotaxic comparison methods are vulnerable to global effects confounding local differences; so voxel-level effects need to be adjusted for the dependency of warping fields on brain scale (Chapter 6). On the other hand, volume differences may not be identified by VBM methods, unless structures are near perfectly aligned using high-dimensional registration (Bookstein 2001). DBM preserves regional volumes and should theoretically provide even greater agreement with ROI studies, but may be sensitive to confounding neurodevelopmental deviations in brain and skull size and shape—such as, for example, increasing evidence that schizophrenia may be associated with relatively wide but shorter skulls (Moorhead et al. 2004). The effective resolution and ability to conduct clinical studies are all limited by the 4–12 mm smoothing necessary to combine images and analyse them in accordance with Gaussian random field theory. Perhaps most fundamental, given the typical study size, is the fact that automated analyses do not lend themselves to meta-analysis, and data sharing will be required (see below). None the less, the array of automated techniques available, and their relative speed of use, makes them the analysis mode of choice—the precise method to be determined by the study question and the data available. For example, high-dimensional registration may be best for detecting differential changes over time in two or more groups (see TBM in Chapter 6), but there are many factors (such as intensity non-uniformity, different contrasts in the repeated scans, etc.) that could make the 'pure' VBM approach better under some circumstances. Ideally, however, all such studies should be validated using ROI methods as the 'gold standard'.

However, the fundamental question remains, what do such changes reflect at a neuronal level? The sMRI studies finding progressive changes post-onset tend to do so while symptoms are generally improving in first-episode schizophrenia, or are static in chronic cases; with little or no evidence of neuronal stress on post-mortem (PM) (Weinberger and McClure 2002). It is possible that antipsychotic medication alterations in neuroplasticity are responsible. Alternatively, one could speculate that the medication reduces symptoms while simultaneously correcting state-related factors—such as changes in perfusion and blood volume, and level of glucocorticoid hormones—that might cause reversible increases in brain volumes against a background of, presumably genetically mediated, trait reductions. The problem is that it is impossible to examine these possibilities in vivo at a cellular level, and the necessary improvements in imaging resolution are at present only an aspiration. Further, the difficulties in obtaining large representative PM samples are insurmountable, at least in the UK. Until we get one or the other, we are forced to skirt the critical anatomical questions.

What do structural imaging indices measure?

Post-mortem studies suggest that the microscopic neuroanatomy of schizophrenia is primarily a reduction in neuropil volume and an accompanying increase in neuronal density (Harrison 1999). sMRI studies generally use T_1-weighted sequences that differentiate grey and white matter to identify case-control differences in regional tissue volume or density. Arbitrary voxel intensity values are arbitrarily classified as representing grey or white matter. None the less, when a labour-intensive ROI study compares volumes, it is probably doing just that, as it is usually the summed volume of tissue (and fluid) within structures that are traced, and the interpretation is straightforward. There are sufficient inconsistencies between the PM and ROI sMRI literature to arouse some concern, e.g. for the amygdala and hippocampus, but these might be attributable to generally lower power in smaller PM studies, which a meta-analysis could address. While a T_1 scan will not register microscopic structure, a sMRI study of PM brains in patients and controls might significantly add to our understanding of the relationship between neuropil and regional volumes (after Chance *et al.* 2003).

In contrast to ROI studies, automated VBM-like methods use the voxel intensity values to register brains in common space, delineate tissue boundaries, and then compare the likelihoods that tissue concentrations differ at particular voxels. Partial volume effects mean that a single voxel can be occupied by more than one tissue type. When a VBM study compares local volumes, e.g. from a grey matter (GM) distribution, the voxel intensities represent the likelihood of GM at that point in averaged stereotactic space, given the transformation from native space and any control for potential confounds applied. Although ROI and VBM have been cross-validated and provide similar results in schizophrenia studies (e.g. Job *et al.* 2003), VBM studies typically find few areas of increased GM density, as would be expected in the basal ganglia.

If schizophrenia has effects on T_1 or T_2 values, this would confound all structural imaging assessments of the disease. Both might impact on volume measures, and large T_2 differences could artefactually reduce signals on MRS (Chapter 4) or DTI (Chapter 5) in patients. Fortunately, there does not appear to be such an effect, although the possibility has only rarely been addressed. Proton MRS has repeatedly found reduced NAA in the temporal lobes, which used to be interpreted as evidence both of atrophy in dementia and of reduced 'integrity' in schizophrenia, but is now more consistently regarded as indicative of energy metabolism dysfunction (Moretti *et al.* 2003). Similarly, the findings on DTI and MTI (Chapter 5) can be loosely interpreted as evidence of reduced white matter 'integrity', but more usefully as indices of disrupted axonal structure with functional implications.

Bridging the structure–function divide

The MR and neuropathological literatures support a relative functional deficiency of widespread neuronal circuits associated with reduced neuropil in schizophrenia (Weinberger 1999). However, they do not establish whether the structural changes reflect an actual loss of parenchymal volume (i.e. neuropil and/or somal), or physiological compensations (e.g. dendritic, vascular, osmotic, etc.) to altered activity. Combinations of various types of imaging offer the best current approaches to these uncertainties.

MRS and DTI may provide as yet ambiguous information, but they are particularly suitable for multi-modal studies. Indeed, as a structural scan is typically acquired for co-registration purposes, this potential has already been exploited. Typical T_1-weighted structural scans have better resolution than the T_2-weighted images for MRS/DTI, but it is at least reassuring to know that a number of studies have shown that the 'functional' changes indexed by MRS/DTI are not simply attributable to grey and/or white matter volume decrements (see Chapters 4 and 5). However, there is an almost complete lack of studies in schizophrenia which have used available sMRI data to interrogate SPECT, PET, and fMRI findings. Initial combined MRS–PET studies have already provided important insights into the influences of prefrontal cortex on the activity in working memory and dopaminergic systems, and demonstrate that MRS and PET measure dissociable disruptions of energy utilization (see Chapter 4). The combination of fMRI and DTI is likely to be helpful in determining the biological basis of distributed activity in the normal brain, and the derangement of these networks in disease states. MEG may have particular advantages, with a tighter link to synaptic activity and lesser variability than fMRI, for combined assessments of cortical connectivity.

The most obvious and thus far applied form of multi-modal imaging is the use of fMRI and various electrophysiological techniques to provide complementary spatial and temporal resolution in functional imaging. The blood oxygenation level dependent (BOLD) signal does not reflect neural activation directly, but is coupled with an increase in the postsynaptic field potential (Kim 2003)—as are the EEG and MEG (Chapter 10). The neurovascular coupling is, however, variably delayed across brain regions, making it difficult to reveal precise temporal sequences. Even sophisticated analysis using more of the signal (Bellgowan et al. 2003), or data-driven approaches rather than predefined models of the haemodynamic response function (HRF) (Formisano and Goebel 2003), or 'magnetic-source MRI' (Xiong et al. 2003), with appropriate tasks, are limited to a temporal resolution of about 100 ms at best. Event related potentials (ERPs) and EEG data give fine temporal resolution of neural activity from sources capable of generating far-field potentials, but have poor spatial resolution. The combination of ERPs and fMRI improves localization of neural generators as well as enhancing temporal resolution of BOLD activation foci. This approach has already located the source of alterations in electrophysiological indices in schizophrenia to specific parts of the (left) superior temporal gyrus (Chapters 10–12).

As opposed to event-related studies, where the exact onset of an external stimulus needs to be known, continuous EEG/fMRI permits correlating spontaneous intrinsic fluctuations of (electrical) brain micro-states with changes in the BOLD signal, without the need for a baseline or explicit task condition, and with better resolution than with EEG/PET (see Chapter 12). Ongoing cortical activity modulates stimulus-evoked activity, and is correlated with behaviour; and could therefore represent the brain's 'internal context', and influence memory, perception, and behaviour (Kenet *et al.* 2003).

Multi-modal imaging comes with attendant but tractable difficulties in data collection, co-registration, computation, and storage. Even the sophisticated use of these techniques, or of novel methods which have, or promise, improved resolution (e.g. perfusion fMRI, near infra-red spectroscopy) will, however, not in themselves answer the fundamental question of whether structural or functional deficits. This will require prospective studies, and preferably of subjects pre- and post-onset; as follow-up studies in patients when ill and then well may simply index compensatory and medication effects. Ultimately, however, this crucial question may require an intermediate level of analysis—a bridge between physiological and psychological functions.

Cognitive neuropsychology and functional imaging

There is no doubt that patients with schizophrenia, as a group, exhibit deficits on a variety of information-processing and neuropsychological tasks, especially in IQ, executive function, and memory (see, for example, Heinrichs and Zakzanis 1998). However, there remain fundamental difficulties demonstrating deficits over and above reductions in general intelligence, the sedative and motor effects of antipsychotics (and dysmnesic effects of anticholinergics), the amotivation that characterizes some patients, and the distracting effects of acute psychotic symptoms in others, and the effects of co-morbid substance abuse. Simple task difficulty differences can also confound differential deficits on specific tasks. None the less, it is clear that at least some patients have focal deficits in the context of essentially intact IQ (Weickert *et al.* 2000). The effects of various drugs also appear to be less severe than those of the disorder, and there is quite good evidence that antipsychotics improve cognitive function in acute psychosis (e.g. verbal fluency, Heinrichs and Zakzanis 1998). There are also a number of robust studies showing that specific deficits remain after controlling for the psychometric properties of tasks—at least for some memory tests. Certainly, there are good data that the healthy sibs (Egan *et al.* 2001*b*) and children of patients (Byrne *et al.* 2003) have a similar pattern of deficits to patients, without any of the attendant problems associated with schizophrenia.

What underlies task failure?

It is equally clear from electrophysiological studies (Chapter 10) and examinations of simple sensori-motor and more complex function with fMRI (Chapter 9) that schizophrenia is associated with basic information processing problems, but more marked impairment of higher cortical functions (see also Callicott 2003). However, these studies still have to wrestle with longstanding difficulties in establishing the neural explanations for poor patient performance. The best replicated functional imaging abnormality in schizophrenia remains 'hypofrontality' (Chapters 7 and 9), but the extent to which this reflects a fundamental neuronal deficit, a failure to complete the task used, and even a lack of motivation to do so, is unclear. What is known, however, is that tasks can be delivered, for example at a steady rate, in such a way as to allow patients to do them and produce a tendency to 'hyperfrontality'. This suggests that the neural paresis is relative and can be compensated for, at least up to a certain level of difficulty, beyond which performance falls off, i.e. that the load–response curve is shifted to the left (Manoach 2003). Such additional neuronal recruitment for a given performance is compatible with fMRI studies in relatives (Callicott *et al.* 2003) and subjects at high risk (Whalley *et al.* 2004), and is likely to apply to other regional activations and tasks. However, it is also possible that underactivation can accompany normal performance, e.g. amygdala activation on facial emotion processing (Gur *et al.* 2002), which might index a similar neuronal inefficiency that might only have behavioural effects on more demanding tasks. In short, even these sophisticated SPECT, PET, and blocked fMRI studies still do not clarify what goes wrong when patients perform poorly.

A region that is not significantly activated in comparison to controls, especially in the small studies so typical of schizophrenia research, is not necessarily inactive or even less active—it may just reflect a relatively lesser activation from a more active 'resting' state, or a more dissipated or maldistributed activation, for example. Similarly, 'hotter' regions during task performance are not necessarily involved in performing that task, particularly in subtraction analyses comparing activity with rest, where, for example, less of a decrease in one area appears as a relative increase (Gusnard and Raichle 2001). Correlational analyses between task performance and neuronal activity are required to clarify these ambiguities, but assume a linear demand-response relationship. This relationship can be specified more precisely if event-related designs are incorporated into studies which use enough stimuli (and subjects) to conduct *post hoc* error exclusion and/or right versus wrong comparison analyses within (see, for example, Jessen *et al.* 2003) or between subjects matched for performance. We also need to design tasks that fractionate cognitive processes in, for example, working memory and cognitive control (e.g. Dreher and Berman 2002; Dehaene *et al.* 2003), so that how one or more deficits interact to produce impaired performance in patients can be better understood. These would benefit from including a range of load-response examinations within and between tasks, bearing in mind that there are many ways that the brain can complete a task, both in terms of neuronal organization and top-down strategic effects. Alternative approaches, such as factorial designs, can also map such interactions (Honey *et al.* 2002). Such design refinements would go some way to correcting the current over-reliance on demonstrating underactivations in patients and using this to impute a deficit in this region of the brain. One has to remember, however, that cognitive processes are not dissociated in everyday life and are prone to confounding by task design (McIntosh *et al.* 2001).

Technical refinements in image acquisition and analysis might also help. For example, Bayesian analysis gives likelihoods of activation rather than the probability of (not) being activated. Using the novel approach of combined blocked and event-related designs to separate sustained and task-specific effects could tease out motivational and attentional deficits from specific cognitive dysfunctions (Visscher *et al.* 2003). Improved temporal resolution could be used to distinguish discrete information processing stages from general task effects (Bellgowan *et al.* 2003). However, technology is not *the* solution—improved spatial resolution, for example, might simply highlight an increased variability in functional segregation. Fundamentally, we need to determine the conditions under which function, especially of the pre-frontal lobe, is impaired or preserved. This will require identifying the important contextual effects on function—in terms of activity in other regions, structural constraints, and top-down and bottom-up influences (McIntosh *et al.* 2001). Greater attention might also be paid to the rather neglected properties of the 'resting brain' in schizophrenia, perhaps particularly at the point it moves to action—for example, in changes of fronto-parietal coherence underlying the alpha rhythm (see below) and the EEG during 'spontaneously' occurring symptoms (Chapter 12).

An alternative approach is to side-step the complex issues in evaluating patient-control differences by examining the neuro-cognitive associations of particular symptoms in patients with and without them. The underlying model is that dissociable cognitive disturbances reflect distinct disease processes and mediate particular symptoms. This approach has been conspicuously successful in elucidating the cognitive (source memory, self–other distinction) and neural bases of certain types of auditory hallucination (see Chapters 7 and 9), but the model struggles to accommodate evidence for persistent cognitive deficits despite successfully treated acute symptoms. There are also notable inconsistencies in studies that have attempted to localize other symptoms or the disease processes implicit in factorial dimensions.

A disorder of social cognition?

Schizophrenia is characterized not just by such psychotic symptoms but also, and perhaps more fundamentally, by social dysfunction. The cognitive tests used most frequently to date were usually devised to assess the effects of gross brain lesions in hospital-based studies rather than the more subtle, integrated use of cognition in everyday life. While they demonstrate that schizophrenia has an 'organic' basis, they show little consistent relation to indices of everyday function-with the possible exception of some memory and executive deficits (Green *et al.* 2000). This has led to recent interest in the emotional and subjective aspects of mnemonic function, and the contextual influences on information processing, in schizophrenia, both of which appear to be abnormal—although their relation to clinical factors is still unclear (Hall *et al.*

2004). More promising, perhaps, are studies of 'theory of mind' abilities, and especially the refined and novel measures of social cognition now available. It may be, for example, that the irreconcilable heterogeneity between older studies of facial emotion processing, which found generalized versus specific deficits (Mandal *et al.* 1998), can be attributed to global trait deficits and additional state-specific effects (Hall *et al.* 2004). These tasks still need further refinement, both for imaging and behavioural studies, to capture ecologically valid aspects of real-life tasks, where the social stimulus is accompanied by specific inter-subjective questions (such as 'What is this person thinking?') rather than the less informative aspects of how the presentation of stimuli influence response. It is arguably these specific factors that underpin social disability.

The single best demonstration (but as yet unreplicated) of the importance of this inter-subjectivity comes from the Swedish conscript study where a semi-structured 'officer interview' to assess suitability for officer training was the best predictor of subsequent schizophrenia (Fearon and Murray 2002). This is redolent of the rather unreliable 'praecox feeling' that used to be favoured in clinical practice and could obviously have been influenced by appearance, early signs of psychosis, etc., but also attests to the importance of another virtually unstudied area in psychosis research—language. The notorious replication failures of much early work and the shear complexity of linguistics are probable reasons for this, but the imaging community is going to have to face up to these (see Chapter 10 for some early examples). After all, we elicit most symptoms and many disabilities by communicating with patients, and most of our research tasks include at least some linguistic components. Regardless, the increasingly appreciated, impressive explanatory power and localizing abilities of social tasks (Phillips *et al.* 2003)—and the simple need for more studies of emotion, facial, and stress processing in schizophrenia—makes it likely that such studies are going to be a real growth area in functional imaging. This being said, we also must acknowledge the caveat that phenomenology in schizophrenia, whether in terms of descriptive psychopathology by earlier generations of researchers or in neuroimaging now, has never been limited in the directions it could pursue. Whether social cognition studies will turn out to be another such adventure into emergent phenomena rather than primary pathology, is a reasonable concern.

Cognitive psychopharmacology

The ligand-binding and pharmacological stimulation studies reviewed in Chapters 7 and 8 make it clear that dopaminergic dysfunction is at least indirectly involved in schizophrenia, and that overactivity is associated in particular with positive symptoms; while MRS studies (Chapter 4) provide strong evidence for the role of the prefrontal cortex in mediating negative symptoms and in regulating dopamine release in the basal ganglia. Indeed, these imaging studies are now the most convincing support for this long-serving neurochemical model of schizophrenia. Further support arises from evidence that psychotomimetics, such as amphetamine and cannabis, stimulate dopamine release, activate fronto-limbic regions, and can precipitate symptoms and psychosis in the predisposed (Hariri *et al.* 2002*a,b*; Phillips *et al.*, 2003; Steele and Lawrie 2004). None the less, it remains unclear how schizophrenia can apparently be associated with both a hypo- and hyper-dopaminergia, and similarly mixed disruptions of the NMDA receptor systems; how some dopamine agonists (e.g. methylphenidate) do not appear to cause psychosis and yet NMDA receptor antagonists (e.g. ketamine, phencyclidine) commonly can. However, it is already possible to propose a common conceptual framework, from recent advances in imaging and other studies, bridging the dopamine and NMDA hypotheses of schizophrenia. For example, NMDA receptor hypofunction is implicated in deficient homeostatic control of dopaminergic cell activity and excess dopamine release under stressful conditions (Frankle *et al.* 2003).

Dopamine interactions with other neurotransmitter systems are clearly important, although the much lauded (and far from convincing) cognitive and other benefits of 'atypical' antipsychotics are less likely to reflect 'novel' dopamine: serotonin receptor binding profiles than dose and anticholinergic medication effects. The critical interactions are at least as likely to be with other monoaminergic, GABA and NMDA systems (see Chapters 4, 7, and 8). Indeed, there is already good evidence from electrophysiological studies of the importance of NMDA in mediating the mismatch negativity signal, and modulating cholinergic and dopaminergic influences on higher-level attentional tasks (Chapters 10 and 11). Because these play an integral role in basic information processing, they are also likely to impact on the efficacy of higher functions. Pharmacological fMRI and the MRS techniques that are able to measure GABA, glutamate, etc. are at an early stage of development, but of great potential interest, and could provide complementary information to PET ligand studies. It is already established that changes in ligand binding can be induced by cognitive tasks (e.g. Koepp *et al.* 1998), and that dopamine-mediated changes in activation and performance can be observed with PET and fMRI (e.g. Dolan *et al.* 1995; Honey *et al.* 2003). There are, of course, substantial methodological hurdles in co-registering and comparing the results from images of metabolite concentrations, neurotransmitter transport, binding potential and release, and activation maps. However, studying these interactions is likely to be necessary to provide a coherent cognitive psychopharmacology, i.e. an understanding of how neurotransmitter systems may interact, mediate, and moderate cognitive processes in health and disease. The greatest challenge may actually prove to be in providing the conceptual framework to integrate these findings with the effects of certain genes, various stressors, and other risk factors—as well as those of antipsychotic medication—and their interactions, on these systems. An important start in this endeavour, is the demonstration that individuals with the Met/Met COMT genotype are at increased risk of reduced working memory processing efficiency by amphetamine, whereas Val/Val people showed improvements (Mattay *et al.* 2003). The final challenge will be to integrate all these data with information about the functioning of distributed neuronal networks.

Disconnectivity

If one thing is clear from more than 20 years of concerted functional imaging in patients with schizophrenia, it is that the disorder is not simply a regional disease of, for example, the prefrontal lobe. Rather, as suggested when Bleuler first coined the term, schizophrenia is increasingly regarded as a disorder of co-ordinated brain function and probably structure—a disconnection disorder. This is a very appealing notion, with the potential to integrate what is known about schizophrenia from clinical, imaging, and other perspectives, and has the merit of providing specific testable hypotheses (Friston 2002). However, the concept has been reified and embraced without a clear sense of what it really represents. The brain does not function as a confederation of independent processing nodes, so, in fact, any brain disease could be viewed as a disconnectivity disorder. Nevertheless, reasonable questions have been raised about whether the symptoms and deficits of schizophrenia reflect specific abnormalities of how information is shared between cortical regions, i.e. the process of distributed parallel processing. Another possibility is whether the pathology of schizophrenia itself is in the wiring of connections, i.e. large white matter tracts. These are very different variations on the disconnectivity theme.

Part of the current appeal is simply attributable to the fact that we have only recently had the opportunity to examine connectivity *in vivo*. There are many different types of connectivity, and even more ways of measuring them, which bear little demonstrable relation to each other. For example, DTI tractography, EEG/MEG coherence, PET between subjects' variance maps, and fMRI time series analysis across tasks (with or without modelled tasks effects) index fundamentally different types of neural interactions (Horwitz 2003; Lee *et al.* 2003). Macro- and microscopic structural (anatomical) connectivity need not map on to functional connectivity, and there may only be a relatively slight degree of dependence, and that possibly only due to indirect connections, for example (Koch *et al.* 2002). In diseases, such as schizophrenia, connectivity could be disrupted between or within hemispheres, and short- or long-range. Although we tend to think of it as a reduction in connectivity, it is quite possible that other increases could co-exist. Any such disconnectivity is, of course, potentially attributable to all the usual confounders and to compensatory changes. A neurocognitive abnormality with associated functional disconnectivity, for example, could reflect an anatomical disruption, a generalized or localized functional energy failure, a primary disorganization of neural activity, or medication effects; while even normal performance and disconnectivity might simply index secondary cognitive or neuropharmacological reorganization to achieve a given task (Glabus *et al.* 2003). Most fundamentally, in the context of functional imaging studies, it is difficult to distinguish (differential) co-activation of a network involved in a task (Lowe *et al.* 2002), possible up- and downstream effects of defects in local circuit processing, and true 'disconnectivity'. None the less, there is an array of increasingly sophisticated approaches to these problems, and some persuasive evidence from several sources for a variety of disconnectivities in schizophrenia.

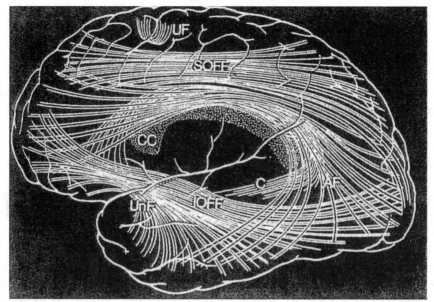

Fig. 13.1 Drawing of association and commissural white matter tracts. UF, U fibres; CC, corpus callosum; SOFF, superior occipitofrontal fasiculus; IOFF, inferior occipitofrontal fasiculus; AF, arcuate fasiculus; UnF, uncinate fasiculus; C, cingulum. (Reprinted with permission from Filley 1995.)

Structural disconnectivity

Macroscopic 'anatomical disconnectivity' in schizophrenia has been suggested by findings of abnormal regional inter-correlations of volume, structural asymmetry, abnormalities of gyrification and DTI, sMRI, and PM studies of white matter tracts. Regional inter-correlational abnormalities are, however, very inconsistent, both in terms of the regions implicated and whether correlations are increased or decreased. The evidence for cerebral asymmetry is much more convincing, at least for language-related areas in the temporal lobe (Sommer *et al.* 2001), but has no clear interpretation. It could simply reflect a general neurodevelopmental disruption, or even a reduced specialization of the schizophrenic brain. Studies of gyral complexity and the 'gyrification index' (the ratio of outer to inner cortical surface area) are of more immediate interest as they may directly measure non-genetic, mainly intra-uterine influences on brain morphology. Although inconsistent, it is possible to synthesize them as indicative of a generally reduced connectivity with increases in specific parts of the prefrontal and perhaps temporal lobes (Harris *et al.* 2004).

By far the most consistent and convincing evidence for a macroscopic anatomical disconnectivity comes from the DTI studies described in Chapter 5. While the parts of the corpus callosum and the association tracts implicated are those that connect the frontal and the temporal lobes (see Fig. 13.1), they do not necessarily indicate anything more than disorganized axonal fibre trajectories and may simply be reduced in volume or may be artefactually affected by shape (e.g. bowing) effects (Chapter 2). Despite this, and an increasing body of microscopic evidence that schizophrenia involves molecular changes in oligodendrocytes (Davis *et al.* 2003), all the foregoing are ambiguous as to which, if any, developmental processes—myelination, synatic pruning, dendritic arborization—are implicated, and say nothing about the specific nature of any synaptic dysfunction. The post-mortem literature does, however, include repeated findings of reduced neuropil (dendritic density) and synaptophysin expression (and other markers of synaptic activity), which at least strongly suggest that schizophrenia is a disorder of neuronal plasticity (Harrison 1999).

Functional and effective disconnectivity

Functional connectivity simply refers to evidence of neuronal activity in distinct (anatomical) regions which is related statistically—usually as a correlation or co-variance. Reduced functional connectivity of this type has been repeatedly demonstrated with EEG, PET, and fMRI in schizophrenia, but usually in the context of impaired task performance in medicated patients. Although many EEG 'coherence' studies have consistently found reductions in cross-correlated activity, which didn't appear to simply reflect task failure and/or medication effects, and was in some cases related to positive symptoms, there has been little precise replication. This may relate to the inherent limitations of such an approach to analysis, which will probably be replaced by measures of non-linear interdependence and phase synchronization (Breakspear *et al.* 2003). Refined techniques, such as examining gamma-band synchrony (Chapter 10), utilizing the reduced variability of MEG (Chapter 11), and interrogating the entire frequency range in 'global field synchronization' analyses (Chapter 12), also show promise. Gamma-band oscillations and dynamic ERPs are of particular interest as they are increasingly thought to reflect transiently coupled neuronal assemblies underlying, for example, the formation of memories.

Support for functional disconnectivity in schizophrenia is most frequent and consistent from PET and fMRI studies. There are replicated findings of reduced fronto-frontal, -temporal and -parietal connectivity (Meyer-Lindenberg *et al.* 2001; Lawrie *et al.* 2002; Kim *et al.* 2003), and suggestions that these patterns are not simply attributable to task performance or medication (Meyer-Lindenberg *et al.* 2001) and may be associated with auditory hallucinations (Lawrie *et al.* 2002). However, the methods used to extract this information amount to correlations between activations in disparate brain regions, such that reductions could reflect, at least in part, some combination of increased variance in patients (see Welchew *et al.* 2002), regional differences in the HRF, and localized dysfunction. There is therefore a move to use data-driven methods, such as principal or independent components analysis, and to 'de-convolve' the HRF from the neural activation patterns using, for example, a Bayesian approach to fit the data (Gitelman *et al.* 2003). Distinguishing functional disintegration from dissegregation might, however, also require event-related studies across various levels of task difficulty (cf. Manoach 2003).

Establishing effective disconnectivity in schizophrenia is, in principle, a more interesting objective, as it can clarify which region in a disrupted network is driving the dysfunction, but the methods are still in their infancy. The established methods for estimating effective connectivity from neurophysiological time series include structural equation modelling (also know as path analysis) and models based on multivariate autoregressive processes. Differences in latency between regions cannot be used to infer the dynamics of (effective) connectivity in fMRI because there are region-specific differences in the coupling of neuronal activity to BOLD response that obscure any differences due to neuronal latency—although it can be useful in EEG/MEG. Structural equation modelling is the only approach applied to patients with schizophrenia thus far. The two studies used PET/fMRI, different tasks, data driven/hypothetical approaches to node selection, and only had one region in common. None the less, both studies implicated dorsolateral prefrontal cortex, made it clear that effective disconnectivity in schizophrenia was not global, and provide results that are in keeping with current theoretical approaches and with findings of functional disconnectivity (Jennings *et al.* 1998; Schlosser *et al.* 2003). However, path analysis has several limitations: it assumes that interactions are linear, does not actually provide a time-series model, and is unreliable if the overall model fits the data poorly or subject groups unevenly. Multivariate autoregression models and their spectral equivalents, such as coherence analysis, are also restricted to linear interactions, and assume the system is driven by stochastic (unknown) inputs. Friston *et al.* (2003) have recently described the novel approach of 'dynamic causal modeling', which was designed to assess changes in connectivity induced by experimental design factors in a hypothesis-led fashion, by perturbing the system and measuring the response. This is a critical departure from conventional approaches to causal modelling in neuroimaging, and brings the analysis of effective connectivity much closer to the conventional analysis of region-specific effects, and indeed to computational modelling of neurobiology.

Neuroinformatics

Progress in neuroimaging research has been dependent upon advances in information technology, both in image acquisition and analysis, but has not yet taken advantage of developments in neuroinformatics. The amount of data generated by techniques such as structural, and particularly functional, imaging demands novel approaches to storage, and provides largely untapped opportunities for analysing all of the available information. A central theme in neuroinformatics is the application of computational tools to archive, integrate, and share neuroscience data, thus enabling these to be examined in greater detail than with traditional approaches. These kinds of tools were crucial to the success of the Human Genome Project and, adapted to deal with neural data, have the potential to advance dramatically our understanding of the brain in health and disease. This is also true of another central theme in neuroinformatics—the development of explanatory computational models of processes in the nervous system, and computational tools to create, manage, simulate, and analyse the properties of these models.

Computational models

Computational models of biological nervous systems and the mechanisms underlying their operation have to reflect their complexity and sophistication, while remaining comprehensible and manageable enough to allow neuroscientists to engage in the modelling process (Goddard *et al.* 2002). They are mathematical descriptions of selected dynamic processes, either as theoretical simulations or data-driven, usually from a cognitive connectionist perspective. Models have been devised at the single cell, ensemble, and systems levels to investigate successfully the integrative properties of neurons, how they behave collectively, and regional interconnectivity. They contributed to elucidating the dendritic basis of ERP and MEG signals, but their potential to elucidate various aspects of the neural basis of other functional imaging signals, and to take connectivity analyses from correlations towards couplings, remains largely untapped (Horwitz and Sporns 1994).

At worst, these models are little more than abstractions, with no clear relation to neural events; but at their most impressive, they can generate novel predictions that have been tested and confirmed (O'Reilly and Norman 2002). In schizophrenia, notable models of delusions, hallucinations, priming, emotion recognition, semantic, and working memory have been proposed, which have at least prompted researchers to make their assumptions about such phenomena explicit, and allowed them to think about these phenomena in terms of neuromodulation and plasticity. Such models also permit empirical testing of the effects of particular 'lesions' introduced into the system, as an alternative to the obvious inadequacies of animal models. Probably the best example is the pioneering work of Hoffman and colleagues, which finds that auditory hallucinations may be related to the extent of cortical pruning during adolescence (e.g. McGlashan and Hoffman 2000). This work awaits a suitable technique for *in vivo* assessment of synaptic density, but imaging applications for other computational models have already been found. Perhaps the most impressive body of work is that of Cohen *et al.* (1996). They described a model of dopamine-modulated prefrontal function in schizophrenia which led to a new theory that the 'internal representation of context' could explain several aspects of patients' cognitive disturbances, which in turn led to novel behavioural and fMRI studies that have supported this view and have received some external replication. Neural networks have already shown promise in distinguishing the functional connectivity patterns of patients and controls (Josin and Liddle 2001), and are an important preliminary to effective connectivity analyses (e.g. Schlosser *et al.* 2003). Trained pattern recognition systems have been used to (semi)automatically measure regional brain volumes (compatible with ROI data) and could be applied to automating these and complementary measures of, for example, gyral complexity in large data sets.

Information management

The relatively discrete nature of quantitative neuroimaging data makes it ideal for developing systems designed to facilitate data archiving, analysis, and sharing (Shepherd *et al.* 1998). The databases are designed to accommodate the highly diverse data researchers obtain, reflecting the complexity of biological nervous systems and their outputs. Traditionally, each main data type (e.g. clinical, cognitive, imaging) is stored and analysed separately, and once the essential details are published, it (and associated descriptive data, e.g. experimental protocols) is forgotten and often irretrievable. Neuroinformatics approaches to data storage, organization, and mining of the vast amount of imaging and other data in schizophrenia studies, would facilitate integrative analyses and meta-analyses (e.g. Steele and Lawrie 2004) and could serve as a template for collaborative storage and analyses of multi-centre data in the future. Such large group analyses would be able to detect subtle differences between psychotic disorders. They may even be essential for studies of relatively rare but potentially very important gene effects, e.g. of the DRD_2 Ser311Cys gene polymorphism on D_2 ligand binding or dopaminergic function in pharmacological fMRI.

There are, of course, important technical issues to deal with in combining scans obtained on different machines. The quality of MRI images is determined by a host of factors affecting signal strength, image contrast, and signal to noise ratio, which together with image processing and storage parameters contribute to the final signal intensity as viewed or analysed. Inevitable signal intensity differences and coil inhomogeneities between identical scanners set up in the same way, let alone different machines, can be corrected for in automated analyses by, for example, optimized normalization or using (data driven) template-free segmentation approaches. Spatial distortions are likely to be a greater problem, especially if regionally variable, but it may also be possible to deal with these. If, for example, representative subpopulations of interest were scanned on both scanners, and controls had greater than expected subregional changes, it would be possible to use phantom scans on both machines to identify the extent of these and either control or mask for them.

There are also political or sociological issues about data sharing, in terms of access and ownership (Toga 2002). One solution is to simply store descriptive details of particular studies, and to allow access to original data subject to the original investigators' approval, but this obviously would limit one of the main advantages of the venture. An alternative is to establish both the data acquisition and sharing arrangements from the outset of new collaborative ventures. Several imaging centres in the USA have already embarked on such a project, utilizing the Brain Informatics Research Network, and are establishing the factors that influence image variation with a view to developing a standardized approach to imaging patients with schizophrenia in 10 centres. These issues will have to be addressed if the potential of multi-centre studies to increase sample sizes and generate robust results is to be realized.

Clinical utility

All the foregoing is as nothing unless it ultimately succeeds in improving the diagnosis and management of schizophrenia. This is not the place to rehearse hyperbolic discussion of the clinical potential of imaging necessary for grant applications, but rather to specify where success can really be envisaged, based on existing work. This is, at first thought, a daunting task. The oft-cited clinical and biological heterogeneity of the disorder has made replication in group studies of patients difficult, let alone single cases. On the other hand, one has to remember that all that is required is to improve on current practice in predicting and differentiating disorders, and their therapeutic response or prognosis.

Improving diagnostic practice

The clinical utility of any type of structural or functional imaging in psychiatry is at present limited to excluding neurological disorders in patients with atypical symptoms and signs. Routine neuroradiology of even first-episode psychosis cannot be justified, due to the very low yield of clinically significant findings that alter management (Lawrie *et al.* 1997). Viewing sMRI scans of hippocampal volumes, for example, is also unlikely to be of much assistance—although Suddath *et al.* (1990) found this could differentiate affected and unaffected monozygotic twins in almost all cases, such a reference group is impractical in everyday practice.

The approaches that are likely to be helpful are automated analyses of especially sMRI and fMRI data, in which individual subjects can be compared with appropriate norms (see, for example, Salmond *et al.* 2003). Early diagnoses of Alzheimer's disease can now be made as accurately with assessments of hippocampal volume, or temporo-parietal perfusion, as they can be clinically (Frisoni *et al.* 2003). Technological improvements and combining imaging and biological indices might well surpass clinical prediction in the near future. In the EHRS, small amygdalo-hippocampal and thalamus volumes are predictive of schizophrenia up to 5 or so years in advance, but not with anything like the predictive power required to justify exposure to antipsychotics in young healthy people (Johnstone *et al.*, 2004). On VBM the greater difference is in changes over time in hippocampal volume (Job *et al.* 2004), but changes are more prey to measurement error than single scan predictors unless registration is optimized (see Chapter 6). Both sMRI and fMRI might have a role in the differential diagnosis of first-episode psychosis, at least between schizophrenia and depression, although acutely psychotic patients are particularly difficult to scan. However, the additional complication with fMRI is that many, if not all, tasks will require some standardization in the scanner according to the individual's load–response profile on the task in question. Single-subject fMRI studies over time will also have to deal with the lower reliability of the technique in individuals than within and across groups.

Improving treatment

Several studies have examined the associations of treatment response or outcome in schizophrenia (see, for example, Lawrie *et al.* 1995), but almost all have been cross-sectional. The small number of PET and SPECT studies of therapeutic response prediction are inconsistent (Chapters 7 and 8) and there is, to date, only one prospective sMRI study of outcome predictors. However, a few EEG studies have suggested that early alpha activity changes on exposure to antipsychotics can predict later response (Galderisi and Mucci 2002). Several imaging indices have also been shown to change in association with effective treatment, which may provide measures of predictive value. Ligand-binding studies have already provided clinically useful information on the optimal (average) dosages of several drugs and the basis of 'atypicality' (Seeman and Tallerico 1999).

More speculatively, it is at least conceivable that natural history studies might inform the development of novel treatments. For example, studying premorbid compensatory processes in those at risk, identifying developmental 're-mediators' in those with intermediate phenotypes who do not get ill, better characterization of social cognition deficits in patients, and imaging auditory hallucinations as they become pseudo-hallucinations may all provide the basis for novel interventions. It is, however, difficult to escape the conclusion that the best use of imaging for developing new treatments would be to increase knowledge of pathophysiology, that might then be applied in more accurate animal models.

Concluding remarks

The immense cost and effort expended on structural and functional imaging in schizophrenia over the past 25 years or so has established that there are biological or 'organic' associations of the disorder and of certain risk factors for it. The greatest limitation of this endeavour has been in the tendency to conduct essentially small replication studies, which have all too often resulted in replication failures, rather than coherent hypothesis building and testing. Many of the apparent volumetric inconsistencies turn out, on systematic reviews and meta-analyses of the literature, to be more indicative of limited study power than true heterogeneity; but almost all of the structural imaging abnormalities appear to be non-specific, possibly because they represent final common pathways in disrupted brains. While functional imaging is likely to index clinical features more closely, there may be substantial limitations to the progress that can be made from studying phenomenology, and the complexities of such studies make them less amenable to data pooling and synthesis. There is clearly a major problem when both relative decreases and increases in functional activations are interpreted as indicating neuronal inefficiency. It is, however, possible to synthesize this very variable and, to a considerable degree, inconsistent functional imaging literature as indicating that patients with schizophrenia process environmental information—whether cognitive, sensory, or emotional—differently from healthy controls, and that their (un)conscious strategies for organizing and engaging the necessary neuronal circuitry are anomalous. This might be epiphenomenal, but is more likely to represent a more fundamental synaptic abnormality manifest at the neurofunctional level. In a nutshell, functional imaging tells us how patients are using their brains during the procedure, the challenge is to provide useful accounts of how they are using them—in particular, how disruptions at a systems level relate to key risk factors, core features of the illness and performance on everyday tasks.

Imaging researchers interested in schizophrenia need to re-think their approach. The single greatest research opportunity is that afforded by advances in the knowledge of the molecular genetics of schizophrenia. Genes are the most mechanistic insight we have about biological causation, and are probably the strongest and most specific risk factors for psychosis. The most profitable focus of future imaging work will therefore probably be on elucidating the effects of specific genes and refining phenotypic descriptions for particular disorders. This effort requires standardized definitions of disease phenotypes and intermediate biological measures associated with risk, well-defined populations in unbiased samples which are large enough to detect small effects, and the concurrent use of both genetic and environmental risk measures (Burke 2003). The recent demonstrations that the short allele of the serotonin transporter gene polymorphism is associated with amygdala activity on viewing fearful faces (Hariri *et al.* 2002*b*), and with depression in response to stressful events (Caspi *et al.* 2003), is a good example of the integrative research that could be conducted profitably in schizophrenia.

However, there is one crucial additional need—to distinguish primary and secondary changes in gene expression, brain structure, and function. Establishing such precise disease mechanisms can arguably only be achieved in large prospective studies of people as they move from being at risk to prodromal to ill. This is, in any case, a *sine qua non* if any of the imaging work in schizophrenia is to be clinically useful for prediction and prevention. It will also help to define the nature of the maturational events that interact with developmental vulnerability, and to clarify the influences on synaptic transmission and plasticity around this critical period. The difficulties in assembling and retaining such cohorts are, however, likely to demand data sharing, multi-centre studies, and possibly even international collaboration. Several American centres have already established a benchmark for this approach. Researchers in Europe and the rest of world may have some advantages in being able to scan more epidemiologically representative populations, but will need to join such networks or create their own to avoid being left behind doing small 'pilot' studies.

Ultimately, the greatest challenges are in integration: between levels of explanation; between neurons, regions, and systems; and between imaging modes and centres; and, most importantly, between large studies and the single-case approach that is required if any of this is to have clinical impact.

References

Akil, M., Kolachana, B. S., Rothmond, D. A., Hyde, T. M., Weinberger, D. R., and Kleinman, J. E. (2003). Catechol-O-methyltransferase genotype and dopamine regulation in the human brain. *Journal of Neuroscience,* **23,** 2008–13.

Bellgowan, P. S., Saad, Z. S., and Bandettini, P. A. (2003). Understanding neural system dynamics through task modulation and measurement of functional MRI amplitude, latency, and width. *Proceedings of the National Academy of Sciences USA,* **100,** 1415–19.

Bookstein, F. L. (2001). 'Voxel-based morphometry' should not be used with imperfectly registered images. *Neuroimage,* **14,** 1454–62.

Breakspear, M., Terry, J. R., Friston, K. J., Harris, A. W., Williams, L. M., Brown, K. *et al.* (2003). A disturbance of nonlinear interdependence in scalp EEG of subjects with first episode schizophrenia. *Neuroimage,* **20,** 466–78.

Burke, W. (2003). Genomics as a probe for disease biology. *New England Journal of Medicine,* **349,** 969–74.

Butzlaff, R. L. and Hooley, J. M. (1998). Expressed emotion and psychiatric relapse: a meta-analysis. *Archives of General Psychiatry,* **55,** 547–52.

Byrne, M., Clafferty, B. A., Cosway, R., Grant, L., Hodges, A., Whalley, H. C. *et al.* (2003). Neuropsychology, genetic liability and the development of psychotic symptoms in those at high risk of schizophrenia. *Journal of Abnormal Psychology* **112,** 38–48

Callicott, J. H. (2003). An expanded role for functional neuroimaging in schizophrenia. *Current Opinion in Neurobiology,* **13,** 256–60.

Callicott, J. H., Egan, M. F., Mattay, V. S., Bertolino, A., Bone, A. D., Verchinshi, B. *et al.* (2003). Abnormal fMRI response of the dorsolateral prefrontal cortex in cognitively intact siblings of patients with schizophrenia. *American Journal of Psychiatry,* **160,** 709–19.

Cannon, M. and Jones, P. (1996). Schizophrenia. *Journal of Neurology, Neurosurgery and Psychiatry,* **61,** 604–13.

Cannon, M., Jones, P. B., and Murray, R. M. (2002). Obstetric complications and schizophrenia: Historical and meta-analytic review. *American Journal of Psychiatry,* **159,** 1080–92.

Cannon, T. D., Kaprio, J., Lönnqvist, J., Huttunen, M., and Koskenvvo, M. (1998). The genetic epidemiology of schizophrenia in a Finnish twin cohort. *Archives of General Psychiatry,* **55,** 67–74.

Cardno, A. G., and Gottesman, I. I. (2000). Twin studies of schizophrenia: from bow-and-arrow concordances to star wars Mx and functional genomics. *American Journal of Medical Genetics,* **97,** 12–17.

Castellanos, F. X. and Tannock, R. (2002). Neuroscience of attention-deficit/hyperactivity disorder: the search for endophenotypes. *Nature Review Neuroscience,* **3,** 617–28.

Chance, S. A., Esiri, M. M., and Crow, T. J. (2003). Ventricular enlargement in schizophrenia: a primary change in the temporal lobe? *Schizophrenia Research,* **62,** 123–31.

Cloninger, C. R. (2002). The discovery of susceptibility genes for mental disorders. *Proceedings of the National Academy of Sciences USA,* **99,** 13365–7.

Cohen, J. D., Braver, T. S., and O'Reilly, R. C. (1996). A computational approach to prefrontal cortex, cognitive control and schizophrenia: recent developments and current challenges. *Philosophical Transactions of the Royal Society of London,* **351,** 1515–27.

Davis, K. L., Stewart, D. G., Friedman, J. I., Buchsbaum, M., Harvey, P. D., Hof, P. R. *et al.* (2003). White matter changes in schizophrenia: evidence for myelin-related dysfunction. *Archives of General Psychiatry,* **60,** 443–56.

Dehaene, S., Artiges, E., Naccache, L., Martelli, C., Viard, A., Schurhoff, F. *et al.* (2003). Conscious and subliminal conflicts in normal subjects and patients with schizophrenia: the role of the anterior cingulate. *Proceedings of the National Academy of Sciences USA,* **100,** 13722–7.

Dolan, R. J., Fletcher, P., Frith, C. D., Friston. K. J., Frackowiak, K. S., and Grasby, P. M. (1995). Dopaminergic modulation of impaired cognitive activation in the anterior cingulate cortex in schizophrenia. *Nature*, **378**, 180–2.

Dreher, J. C. and Berman, K. F. (2002). Fractionating the neural substrate of cognitive control processes. *Proceedings of the National Academy of Sciences USA*, **99**, 14595–600.

Egan, M. F., Goldberg, T. E., Kolachana, B. S., Callicott. J. H., Mazzanti. C. M., Straub, R. E. *et al.* (2001*a*). Effect of COMT Val108/158 Met genotype on frontal lobe function and risk for schizophrenia. *Proceedings of the National Academy of Sciences USA*, **98**, 6917–22.

Egan, M. F., Hyde, T. M., Bonomo, J. B. Mattay, V. S., Bigelour, L. B., Goldberg, T. E. *et al.* (2001*b*). Relative risk of neurological signs in siblings of patients with schizophrenia. *American Journal of Psychiatry*, **158**, 1827–34.

Egan, M. F., Kojima, M., Callicott, J. H. Goldberg, T. E., Kolachana, B. S., Bertolino, A. *et al.* (2003). The BDNF val66met polymorphism affects activity-dependent secretion of BDNF and human memory and hippocampal function. *Cell*, **112**, 257–69.

Fallgatter, A. J. and Strik, W. K. (2000). Reduced frontal functional asymmetry in schizophrenia during a cued continuous performance test assessed with near-infrared spectroscopy. *Schizophrenia Bulletin*, **26**, 913–19.

Faraone, S. V., Kremen, W. S., Lyons, M. J., Repple, J. R., Seidman, L. J., Tsuang, M. T. *et al.* (1995). Diagnostic accuracy and linkage analysis: how useful are schizophrenia spectrum phenotypes? *American Journal of Psychiatry*, **152**, 1286–90.

Fearon, P. and Murray, R. (2002). Intellectual function and schizophrenia. *British Journal of Psychiatry*, **181**, 276–7.

Filley, C. M. (2001). *The behavioural neurology of white matter.* Oxford University Press, Oxford.

Formisano, E. and Goebel, R. (2003). Tracking cognitive processes with functional MRI mental chronometry. *Current Opinion in Neurobiology*, **13**, 174–81.

Frankle, W. G., Lerma, J., and Laruelle, M. (2003). The synaptic hypothesis of schizophrenia. *Neuron*, **39**, 205–16.

Frisoni, G. B., Scheltens, P., Galluzzi, S., Nobili, F. M., Fox, N. C., Robert, P. H. *et al.* (2003). Neuroimaging tools to rate regional atrophy, subcortical cerebrovascular disease, and regional cerebral blood flow and metabolism: consensus paper of the EADC. *Journal of Neurology, Neurosurgery and Psychiatry*, **74**, 1371–81.

Friston, K. J. (2002) Dysfunctional connectivity in schizophrenia. *World Psychiatry*, **1** (2), 66–71.

Friston, K. J., Harrison, L., and Penny, W. (2003). Dynamic causal modelling. *Neuroimage*, **19**, 1273–302.

Galderisi, S. and Mucci, A. (2002). Psychophysiology in psychiatry: new perspectives in the study of mental disorders. *World Psychiatry*, **1** (3), 166–8.

Gilbertson, M. W., Shenton, M. E., Ciszewski, A. Kasai, K., Lasko, N. B., Orr, S. P. *et al.* (2002). Smaller hippocampal volume predicts pathologic vulnerability to psychological trauma. *Nature Neuroscience*, **5**, 1242–7.

Gitelman, D. R., Penny, W. D., Ashburner, J. and Friston, K. J. (2003). Modeling regional and psychophysiologic interactions in fMRI: the importance of hemodynamic deconvolution. *Neuroimage*, **19**, 200–7.

Glabus, M. F., Horwitz, B., Holt, J. L. Kohn, P. D., Gerton, B. K., Callicott, J. H. *et al.* (2003). Interindividual differences in functional interactions among prefrontal, parietal and parahippocampal regions during working memory. *Cerebral Cortex*, **13**, 1352–61.

Glatt, S. J., Faraone, S. V., and Tsuang, M. T. (2003). Meta-analysis identifies an association between the dopamine D2 receptor gene and schizophrenia. *Molecular Psychiatry*, **8**, 911–15.

Goddard, N., Hucka, M., Howell, F., Cornelis, H., Shankar, K., and Beeman, D. (2002). Towards NeuroML: Model description methods for collaborative modelling in neuroscience. *Philosophical Transactions of the Royal Society of London*, **356**, 1209–28.

Goodman, F. R. (2003). Congenital abnormalities of body patterning: embryology revisited. *Lancet*, **362**, 651–62.

Gottesman, I. I. and Gould, T. D. (2003). The endophenotype concept in psychiatry: etymology and strategic intentions. *American Journal of Psychiatry*, **160**, 636–45.

Green, M. F., Kern, R. S., Braff, D. L., and Mintz, J. (2000). Neurocognitive deficits and functional outcome in schizophrenia: are we measuring the 'right stuff'? *Schizophrenia Bulletin*, **26**, 119–36.

Gur, R. E., McGrath, C., Chan, R. M., Schroeder, L., Turner, T., Turetsky, B. I. *et al.* (2002). An fMRI study of facial emotion processing in patients with schizophrenia. *American Journal of Psychiatry*, **159**, 1992–9.

Gusnard, D. A. and Raichle, M. E. (2001). Searching for a baseline: functional imaging and the resting human brain. *Nature Review Neuroscience*, **2**, 685–94.

Hall, J., Harris, J. M., Sprengelmeyer, R., Sprengelmeyer, A., Young, A. W., Santos, I. M. *et al.* (2004). Social cognition and face processing in schizophrenia. *British Journal of Psychiatry*, **185**, 169–70.

Hariri, A. R., Mattay, V. S., Tessitore, A., Fera, F., Smith, W. G., and Weinberger, D. R. (2002a). Dextroamphetamine modulates the response of the human amygdala. *Neuropsychopharmacology*, **27**, 1036–40.

Hariri, A. R., Mattay, V. S., Tessitore, A., Kolachana, B., Fera, F., Goldman, D. *et al.* (2002b). Serotonin transporter genetic variation and the response of the human amygdala. *Science*, **297**, 400–3.

Harris, J. M., Yates, S., Miller, P., Best, J. J., Johnstone, E. C., and Lawrie, S. M. (2004). Gyrification in first-episode schizophrenia: A morphometric study. *Biological Psychiatry*, **55**, 141–7.

Harrison, P. J. (1999). The neuropathology of schizophrenia. A critical review of the data and their interpretation. *Brain*, **122**, 593–624.

Harrison, P. J. and Owen, M. J. (2003). Genes for schizophrenia? Recent findings and their pathophysiological implications. *Lancet*, **361**, 417–19.

Heinrichs, R. W. and Zakzanis, K. K. (1998). Neurocognitive deficit in schizophrenia: a quantitative review of the evidence. *Neuropsychology*, **12**, 426–45.

Honey, G. D., Fletcher, P. C., and Bullmore, E. T. (2002). Functional brain mapping of psychopathology. *Journal of Neurology, Neurosurgery and Psychiatry*, **72**, 432–9.

Honey, G. D., Suckling, J., Zelaya, F., Long, C., Routledge, C., Jackson, S. *et al.* (2003). Dopaminergic drug effects on physiological connectivity in a human cortico-striato-thalamic system. *Brain*, **126**, 1767–81.

Horwitz, B. (2003). The elusive concept of brain connectivity. *Neuroimage*, **19**, 466–70.

Horwitz, B. and Sporns, O. (1994). Neural modeling and functional neuroimaging. *Human Brain Mapping*, **1**, 269–83.

Jennings, J. M., McIntosh, A. R., Kapur, S. Zipursky, R. B., and Houle, S. (1998). Functional network differences in schizophrenia: a rCBF study of semantic processing. *Neuroreport*, **9**, 1697–700.

Jessen, F., Scheef, L., Germeshausen, L. Tawo, Y., Kockler, M., Kuhn, K. U. *et al.* (2003). Reduced hippocampal activation during encoding and recognition of words in schizophrenia patients. *American Journal of Psychiatry*, **160**, 1305–12.

Job, D. E., Whalley, H. C., McConnell, S. Glabus, M., Johnstone, E. C., and Lawrie, S. M. (2003). Voxel based morphometry of grey matter densities in subjects at high risk of schizophrenia. *Schizophrenia Research*, **64**, 1–13

Job, D. E., Whalley, H. C., Johnstone, E. C., Lawrie, S. M. (in press). Grey matter changes over time in high risk subjects developing Schizophrenia. *Neuroimage* (in Press).

Johnstone, E. C., Byrne, M., Miller, P., Ebmeier, K. P., Owens, D. C. G., and Lawrie, S. M. (2004). Predicting schizophrenia: results from the Edinburgh High Risk Study. *British Journal of Psychiatry,* in press.

Jönsson, E. G., Sillen, A., Vares, M. Ekholm, B., Terenius, L., and Sedvell, G. C. (2003). Dopamine D2 receptor gene Ser311Cys variant and schizophrenia: association study and meta-analysis. *American Journal of Medical Genetics,* **119B**, 28–34.

Josin, G. M. and Liddle, P. F. (2001). Neural network analysis of the pattern of functional connectivity between cerebral areas in schizophrenia. *Biological Cybernetics,* **84**, 117–22.

Kenet, T., Bibitchkov, D., Tsodyks, M. Grinvald, A., and Arieli, A. (2003). Spontaneously emerging cortical representations of visual attributes. *Nature,* **425**, 954–6.

Kim, J. J., Kwon, J. S., Park, H. J., Young, T., Kangdo, H., Kim, M. S. *et al.* (2003). Functional disconnection between the prefrontal and parietal cortices during working memory processing in schizophrenia: a[^{15}(O)]H2O PET study. *American Journal of Psychiatry,* **160**, 919–23.

Kim, S.-G. (2003). Progress in understanding functional imaging signals. *Proceedings of the National Academy of Sciences USA,* **100**, 3550–2.

Koch, M. A., Norris, D. G., and Hund-Georgiadis, M. (2002). An investigation of functional and anatomical connectivity using magnetic resonance imaging. *Neuroimage,* **16**, 241–50.

Koepp, M. J., Gunn, R. N., Lawrence, A. D. Cunningham, V. J., Daghes, A., Jones, T. *et al.* (1998). Evidence for striatal dopamine release during a video game. *Nature,* **393**, 266–8.

Lawrie, S.M. (2004). Premorbid structural abnormalities in schizophrenia. In: *Neurodevelopment and schizophrenia,* (ed. M. Keshavan, J. Kennedy, and R. Murray). Cambridge University Press, Cambridge (in press).

Lawrie, S. M., Ingle, G. T., Santosh, C. G. Rogers, A. C., Rimmimgton, J. E., Naidu, K. P. *et al.* (1995). Magnetic resonance imaging and single photon emission tomography in treatment-responsive and treatment-resistant schizophrenia. *British Journal of Psychiatry,* **167**, 202–10.

Lawrie, S. M., Abukmeil, S. S., Chiswick, A. Egan, V., Santhosh, C. G., and Best, J. J. (1997). Qualitative cerebral morphology in schizophrenia: a magnetic resonance imaging study and systematic literature review. *Schizophrenia Research,* **25**, 155–66.

Lawrie, S. M., Whalley, H. C., Abukmeil, S. S. Kestelman, J. N., Donnelly, L., Miller, P. *et al.* (2001). Brain structure, genetic liability and psychotic symptoms in subjects at high risk of developing schizophrenia. *Biological Psychiatry,* **49**, 811–23.

Lawrie, S. M., Buechel, C., Whalley, H. C. Frith, C. D., Friston, K. J., and Johnstone, E. C. (2002). Reduced frontotemporal functional connectivity in schizophrenia associated with auditory hallucinations. *Biological Psychiatry,* **51**, 1008–11.

Lawrie, S. M., Whalley, H. C., Job, D. E., and Johnstone, E. C. (2003). Structural and functional abnormalities of the amygdala in schizophrenia. *Annals of the New York Academy of Sciences,* **985**, 445–60.

Lee, L., Harrison, L. M., and Mechelli, A. (2003). A report of the functional connectivity workshop, Dusseldorf 2002. *Neuroimage,* **19**, 457–65.

Lowe, M. J., Dzemidzic, M., Lurito, J. T. Matthews, V. P., and Phillips, M. D. (2000). Correlations in low-frequency BOLD fluctuations reflect cortico-cortical connections. *Neuroimage,* **12**, 582–7.

Mandal, M. K., Pandey, R., and Prasad, A. B. (1998). Facial expressions of emotions and schizophrenia: a review. *Schizophrenia Bulletin,* **24**, 399–412.

Manoach, D. S. (2003). Prefrontal cortex dysfunction during working memory performance in schizophrenia: reconciling discrepant findings. *Schizophrenia Research,* **60**, 285–98.

Marenco, S. and Weinberger, D. R. (2000). The neurodevelopmental hypothesis of schizophrenia: following a trail of evidence from cradle to grave. *Developmental Psychopathology*, **12**, 501–27.

Martinez, D., Broft, A., and Laruelle, M. (2001). Imaging neurochemical endophenotypes: promises and pitfalls. *Pharmacogenomics*, **2**, 223–37.

Mathalon, D. H., Pfefferbaum, A., Lim, K. O. Rosenbloom, M. J., and Sullivan, E. V. (2003). Compounded brain volume deficits in schizophrenia–alcoholism comorbidity. *Archives of General Psychiatry*, **60**, 245–52.

Mattay, V. S., Goldberg, T. E., Fera, F., Hariri, A. R., Tessitore, A., Egan, M. F., *et al.* (2003). Catechol O-methyltransferase val158 met genotype and individual variation in the brain response to amphetamine. *Proceedings of the National Academy of Sciences USA*, **100**, 6186-91.

McGlashan, T. H. and Hoffman, R. E. (2000). Schizophrenia as a disorder of developmentally reduced synaptic connectivity. *Archives of General Psychiatry*, **57**, 637–48.

McGuffin, P., Owens, M. J. and Gottesman, I. I. (2002). *Psychiatric genetics and genomics*. Oxford University Press, New York.

McIntosh, A. R., Fitzpatrick, S. M., and Friston, K. J. (2001). On the marriage of cognition and neuroscience. *Neuroimage*, **14**, 1231–7.

Meyer-Lindenberg, A., Poline, J. B., Kohn, P. D., Holt, J. L., Egan, M. F., Weinberger, D. R. *et al.* (2001). Evidence for abnormal cortical functional connectivity during working memory in schizophrenia. *American Journal of Psychiatry*, **158**, 1809–17.

Miller, P., Lawrie, S. M., Hodges, A., Clafferty, R., Cosway, K., and Johnstone, E. C. (2001). Genetic liability, illicit drug use, life stress and psychotic symptoms: preliminary findings from the Edinburgh study of people at high risk for schizophrenia. *Social Psychiatry and Psychiatric Epidemiology*, **36**, 338–42.

Moore, H., West, A. R., and Grace, A. A. (1999). The regulation of forebrain dopamine transmission: relevance to the pathophysiology and psychopathology of schizophrenia. *Biological Psychiatry*, **46**, 40–55.

Moorhead, T. W. J., Job, D. E., Whalley, H. C., Sanderson, T. L., Johnstone, E. C., and Lawrie, S. M. (2004). Voxel-based morphometry of comorbid schizophrenia and learning disability. *Neuroimage*, **22**, 188–202.

Moretti, A., Gorini, A., and Villa, R. F. (2003). Affective disorders, antidepressant drugs and brain metabolism. *Molecular Psychiatry*, **8**, 773–85.

Murray, R. M., Jones, P. B., Susser, E., Van Os, J., and Cannon, M. *et al.* (2002). *The epidemiology of schizophrenia*. Cambridge University Press, Cambridge.

Nestor, P. G., O'Donnell, B. F., McCarley, R. W., Niznikiewicz, M., Barnard, J., Jen Shen, Z. *et al.* (2002). A new statistical method for testing hypotheses of neuropsychological/MRI relationships in schizophrenia: partial least squares analysis. *Schizophrenia Research*, **53**, 57–66.

O'Reilly, R. C. and Norman, K. A. (2002). Hippocampal and neocortical contributions to memory: advances in the complementary learning systems framework. *Trends in Cognitive Sciences*, **6**, 505–10.

Pantelis, C., Velakoulis, D., McGorry, P. D., Wood, S. J., Suckling, J., Phillips, L.J., *et al.* (2003). Neuroanatomical abnormalities before and after onset of psychosis: a cross-sectional and longitudinal MRI comparison. *Lancet* **361**, 281-8.

Phillips, M. L., Drevets, W. C., Rauch, S. L., and Lane, R. (2003). Neurobiology of emotion perception II: Implications for major psychiatric disorders. *Biological Psychiatry*, **54**, 515–28.

Reiss, A. L., Eliez, S., Schmitt, J. E., Patwardhan, A., and Haberecht, M. (2000). Brain imaging in neurogenetic conditions: Realizing the potential of behavioral neurogenetics research. *Mental Retardation and Developmental Disabilities Research Reviews*, **6**, 186–97.

Rutter, M. (2002). The interplay of nature, nurture, and developmental influences: the challenge ahead for mental health. *Archives of General Psychiatry,* **59**, 996–1000.

Salmond, C. H., de Haan, M., Friston, K. J., Gadian, D. G., and Vargha-Khadem, F. (2003). Investigating individual differences in brain abnormalities in autism. *Philosophical Transactions of the Royal Society of London Biological Sciences,* **358**, 405–13.

Schlosser, R., Gesierich, T., Kaufmann, B., Vucurevic, G., Hunsche, S., Gawehn, J. *et al.* (2003). Altered effective connectivity during working memory performance in schizophrenia: a study with fMRI and structural equation modeling. *Neuroimage,* **19**, 751–63.

Seeman, P. and Tallerico, T. (1999). Rapid release of antipsychotic drugs from dopamine D2 receptors: an explanation for low receptor occupancy and early clinical relapse upon withdrawal of clozapine or quetiapine. *American Journal of Psychiatry,* **156**, 876–84.

Semple, D. M. and Lawrie, S. M. (2004). Structural and functional brain imaging studies of the effects of cannabis: a systematic review. *Biological Psychiatry,* submitted.

Semple, D. M., McIntosh, A. M., and Lawrie, S. M. (2004) Cannabis as a risk factor for psychosis: systematic review. *Journal of Psychopharmacology,* in press.

Shepherd, G. M., Mirsky, J. S., Healy, M. D., Singer, M. S., Shoufos, E., Hines, M. S. *et al.* (1998). The Human Brain Project: neuroinformatics tools for integrating, searching and modeling multidisciplinary neuroscience data. *Trends in Neurosciences,* **21**, 460–8.

Shihabuddin, L., Silverman, J. M., Buchsbaum, M. S., Seiver, L. J., Luu, C., Germans, M. K. *et al.* (1996). Ventricular enlargement associated with linkage marker for schizophrenia-related disorders in one pedigree. *Molecular Psychiatry,* **1**, 215–22.

Sommer, I., Aleman, A., Ramsey, N., Kahn, R., and Bouma, A. (2001). Handedness, language lateralisation and anatomical asymmetry in schizophrenia: meta-analysis. *British Journal of Psychiatry,* **178**, 344–51.

Steele, J. D. and Lawrie, S. M. (2004). Segregation of cognitive and emotional function in the prefrontal cortex: A stereotactic meta-analysis. *Neuroimage,* **21**, 868–75.

Suddath, R. L., Christison, G. W., Torrey, E. F., Casanova, M F., Weinberger, D. R. (1990). Anatomical abnormalities in the brains of monozygotic twins discordant for schizophrenia. *New England Journal of Medicine,* **322**, 789–94.

Toga, A. W. (2002). Neuroimage databases: the good, the bad and the ugly. *Nature Review Neuroscience,* **3**, 302–9.

Visscher, K. M., Miezin, F. M., Kelly, J. E., Buckner, R. I., Donaldson, D. I., McAvoy, M. P. (2003). Mixed blocked/event-related designs separate transient and sustained activity in fMRI. *Neuroimage,* **19**, 1694–708.

Volz, H., Gaser, C., and Sauer, H. (2000). Supporting evidence for the model of cognitive dysmetria in schizophrenia—a structural magnetic resonance imaging study using deformation-based morphometry. *Schizophrenia Research,* **46**, 45–56.

Wang, L., Joshi, S.C., Miller, M. I., and Csernansky, J. G. (2001) Statistical analysis of hippocampal asymmetry in schizophrenia. *Neuroimage* **14**, 531–45.

Wassink, T. H., Nopoulos, P., Pietila, J., Crowe, R. R., and Andreasson, N. C. (2003). NOTCH4 and the frontal lobe in schizophrenia. *American Journal of Medical Genetics,* **118B**, 1–7.

Weickert, T. W., Goldberg, T. E., Gold, J. M., Bigelow, L. B., Egan, M. F., and Weinberger, D. R. (2000). Cognitive impairments in patients with schizophrenia displaying preserved and compromised intellect. *Archives of General Psychiatry,* **57**, 907–13.

Weinberger, D. R. (1987). Implications of normal brain development for the pathogenesis of schizophrenia. *Archives of General Psychiatry,* **44**, 660–9.

Weinberger, D. R. (1999) Cell biology of the hippocampal formation in schizophrenia. *Biological Psychiatry* **45**, 395–402.

Weinberger, D. R. and McClure, R. K. (2002). Neurotoxicity, neuroplasticity, and magnetic resonance imaging morphometry: what is happening in the schizophrenic brain? *Archives of General Psychiatry, 59,* 553–8.

Weinberger, D. R., Egan, M. F., Bertolino, A., Callicott, J. H., Mattay, V. S., Lipska, B. K. *et al.* (2001). Prefrontal neurons and the genetics of schizophrenia. *Biological Psychiatry* 50, 825-44.

Welchew, D. E., Honey, G. D., Sharma, T., Robbins, T. W., and Bullmore, E. T. (2002). Multidimensional scaling of integrated neurocognitive function and schizophrenia as a disconnexion disorder. *Neuroimage, 17,* 1227–39.

Whalley, H. C., Simonotto, E., Flett, S., Marshall, I., Ebmeier, K. P., Owens, D. G. *et al.* (2004). fMRI correlates of state and trait effects in subjects at genetically enhanced risk of schizophrenia. *Brain, 127,* 478–90.

Wright, I. C., Ellison, Z. R., Sharma, T., Friston, K. J., Murray, R. M., and McGuire, P. K. (1999) Mapping of grey matter changes in schizophrenia. *Schizophrenia Research* 35, 1-14.

Xiong, J., Fox, P. T., and Gao, J. H. (2003). Directly mapping magnetic field effects of neuronal activity by magnetic resonance imaging. *Human Brain Mapping, 20,* 41–9.

Index

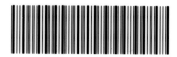
DATE DUE

MAR 31 2010			
MAR 31 2010			

GAYLORD   PRINTED IN U.S.A.